CPT 1996 **on Magnetic Tape** speeds up the whole coding procedure for mainframe users. It's licensed by the AMA and available in two formats—a short description tape and a full procedure tape.

The *CPT 1996* Short Description Tape has a database file constructed in 80-byte line records. Each record contains one abbreviated procedure description and a 5-digit CPT procedure code. Nine-track magnetic, 28-character line, fixed block record format.

Make coding faster and easier on the mainframe.

Field specifications:
CPT procedure number: Positic
Procedure data: Positions 6-33
Blanks: Positions 34-80

Upper case only

1600 BPI, EBCDIC	Order #: OP060496UM
6250 BPI, EBCDIC	Order #: OP060596UM
1600 BPI, ASCII	Order #: OP061096UM
6250 BPI, ASCII	Order #: OP061196UM

License fee: $385

The *CPT 1996* Full Procedure Tape is designed for more complex activities. It contains the complete procedural text of CPT, along with the 5-digit CPT procedure codes. Nine-track magnetic, 80-character line, fixed block record format. For longer descriptions, the CPT code is repeated and the sequence number is increased by one (01, 02, 03, etc).

Field Specifications:
CPT procedure number: Positions 1-5
Sequence numbers: Positions 6-7
Special procedure codes: Position 8*
Procedure data: Positions 9-80

Upper and lower case

1600 BPI, EBCDIC	Order #: OP060196UM
6250 BPI, EBCDIC	Order #: OP060396UM
1600 BPI, ASCII	Order #: OP060796UM
6250 BPI, ASCII	Order #: OP060996UM

Upper case only

1600 BPI, EBCDIC	Order #: OP060096UM
6250 BPI, EBCDIC	Order #: OP060296UM
1600 BPI, ASCII	Order #: OP060696UM
6250 BPI, ASCII	Order #: OP060896UM

License fee: $550

* Does not include pre- and post-operative care. See introduction of *CPT 1996.*

Note: Magnetic tapes are not returnable. Please check with your computer systems professional to ensure compatibility with your system.

To order now, call toll free
800-621-8335
for all your coding needs.

MasterCard, VISA, American Express, and Optima accepted.
State sales taxes and shipping/handling charges apply.

American Medical Association
Physicians dedicated to the health of America

To help make your coding easier, *CPT Assistant* is written and produced by the same AMA coding experts who compile the CPT.

Each issue delivers helpful articles, like guides to specialty coding, case studies which detail code selection rationale, and advice on how to avoid coding mistakes. There are also news updates, special features, charts, and graphs.

Get the inside view of coding with CPT Assistant.

Plus, each year's final issue gives you a review of changes and additions to the next volume of CPT.

Let the *CPT Assistant* provide you with valuable insights on real, everyday coding situations and guide you with information from an insider's view that you can't get anywhere else.

Order #: NR000124UM
AMA member price: $85/one year; $153/two years
Nonmenber price: $135/one year; $243/two years

To order now, call toll free
800-621-8335
for all your coding needs.
MasterCard, VISA, American Express, and Optima accepted.
State sales taxes and shipping/handling charges apply.

American Medical Association
Physicians dedicated to the health of America

The AMA has the most complete selection of *Health Insurance Claim Forms* around. They are top quality, government approved, laser-printer compatible, come with or without bar codes, and are all at affordable prices. From mini packs and convenience packs for small-volume users, to special forms for large-volume users, we have the forms you need.

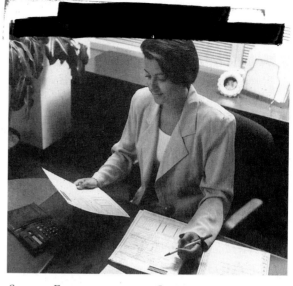

"When our office expanded, the AMA had all the claim forms we needed, in the quantities we needed."

Snap-out Form
2-part NCR, Kodak bar code

Mini Pack: 50 sheets
Order #: OP051394UM
AMA member price: $7.95
Nonmember price: $9.95

Convenience Pack: 250 sheets
Order #: OP051294UM
AMA member price: $24.95
Nonmember price: $29.95

Carton: 1000 sheets
Order #: OP050292UM
AMA member price: $49.95/carton
Nonmember price: $59.95/carton

Single Form
1-page, Kodak bar code, laser-printer compatible. Single sheet, not padded.

Mini Pack: 50 sheets
Order #: OP051194UM
AMA member price: $5.95
Nonmember price: $6.95

Convenience Pack: 250 sheets
Order #: OP050692UM
AMA member price: $17.95
Nonmember price: $21.95

Carton: 1000 sheets
Order #: OP050192UM
AMA member price: $34.95/carton
Nonmember price: $43.95/carton

Continuous Form
2-part NCR with pinfeeds for computer printers, 1000 carton

With Bar Code
Order #: OP050392UM
AMA member price: $55.95/carton
Nonmember price: $67.95/carton

Without Bar Code
Order #: OP050592UM
AMA member price: $55.95/carton
Nonmember price: $67.95/carton

To order now, call toll free
800-621-8335
for all your coding needs.

MasterCard, VISA, American Express, and Optima accepted.
State sales taxes and shipping/handling charges apply.

American Medical Association
Physicians dedicated to the health of America

Now you can save time and use your personal computer to help eliminate manual coding errors.

Licensed by the AMA, *CPT 1996* on disk contains all codes in short description data files on both 5 1/4" and 3 1/2" disks for your convenience. Also included are a copy of *CPT 1996*, a printed copy of the disk contents, and a disk license. Required IBM PC, XT, AT, or compatible MS or PC DOS memory sufficient to use 250K and selected program software. Not returnable.

1996 CPT On Disk
Order #: OP052496UM
AMA member license fee: $140
Nonmember license fee: $175

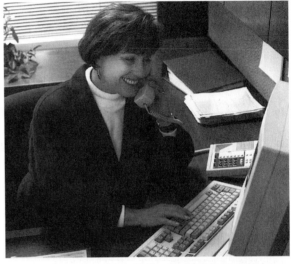

"Data entry is much faster with the CPT and ICD-9-CM on disk, so I'll be home for dinner."

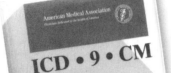

A complete data file of all 1996 ICD-9-CM codes and descriptions found in printed versions of Volumes 1 and 2. Disks for both standard size computer drives—5 1/4" double density and 3 1/2" high density floppy disks—are included. Use with any software program that allows import of an ASCII file. Requires a hard drive with 1.4 megabytes of free space and 640K RAM. Not returnable.

Note: Both products contain a data file only, not a program or automated coder. You can use the data file with any software that allows import of an ASCII file. Check with your data processing professional to ensure compatibility.

ICD-9-CM On Disk
Order #: OP050896UM
AMA member license fee: $140
Nonmember license fee: $175

To order now, call toll free
800-621-8335
for all your coding needs.

MasterCard, VISA, American Express, and Optima accepted. State sales taxes and shipping/handling charges apply.

American Medical Association
Physicians dedicated to the health of America

CPT 1996 Evaluation Form

Your satisfaction is important to the American Medical Association. We are continually trying to improve the *CPT* book to help you code more accurately and efficiently. Please give us your reactions to this book and your thoughts about how to make it better.

After completing this evaluation form, follow the mailing instructions on the back side.

1. How long have you been coding medical procedures? (Check the appropriate response.)
   - ☐ Less than one year
   - ☐ 1 to 2 years
   - ☐ 3 to 4 years
   - ☐ 5 to 6 years
   - ☐ More than 6 years

2. What other coding products do you use in your job beside *CPT*? (Check all that apply.)
   - ☐ *ICD-9*
   - ☐ *HCPCS*
   - ☐ *Medicare RBRVS*
   - ☐ *CPT Assistant*
   - ☐ Other (Please specify) _____

3. Please indicate the company from which you purchased this *CPT* book. (Check the appropriate response.)
   - ☐ American Medical Association
   - ☐ St. Anthony's
   - ☐ Medicode
   - ☐ PMIC
   - ☐ Other (Please specify) _____

4. Please indicate below the characteristics that best describe this book.
   Type of Book
   - ☐ Standard *CPT* Book
   - ☐ Professional Edition

   Style of Book
   - ☐ Soft cover
   - ☐ Hardcover
   - ☐ Spiral bound
   - ☐ Notebook binder

5. Overall, how would you rate this *CPT* book?
   - ☐ Excellent
   - ☐ Good
   - ☐ Fair
   - ☐ Poor

6. Please indicate the extent to which this *CPT* book met or did not meet you expectations.
   - ☐ Exceeded expectations
   - ☐ Met expectations
   - ☐ Did not meet expectations

7. What is there about this book that you **like?** (Please be specific as possible.)

   _____
   _____
   _____
   _____

8. What is there about this book that you **dislike?** (Please be specific as possible.)

   _____
   _____
   _____
   _____

9. Please indicate any ideas you may have for products or services that would assist you in coding. (Please be specific as possible.)

   _____
   _____
   _____
   _____

10. What is your primary employment setting?
    - ☐ Office-based medical practice
    - ☐ Billing/Consulting service
    - ☐ Hospital
    - ☐ Insurance company
    - ☐ Outpatient clinic
    - ☐ Other (Please specify) _____

11. Please complete the following questions for classification purposes.

    Name _____

    Title _____

    Company Name _____

    Address _____

    _____

Mailing Instructions

Thank you for responding to this evaluation form. We appreciate
your comments and reactions. To return this form to the AMA, remove
it from your *CPT* book, fold and seal it with a small piece of tape.
Do not use staples. Then mail it directly to the AMA. This is postage-
paid business reply mail and no stamp is necessary.

American Medical Association

Physicians dedicated to the health of America

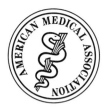

Physicians'
Current
Procedural
Terminology

cpt '96

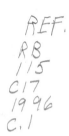

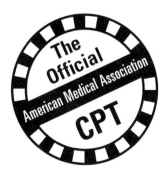

Celeste G. Kirschner, MHSA
Leann M. Frankel, BS
Joyce A. Jackson
Caryn A. Jacobson, ART, CCS
Grace M. Kotowicz, RN, BS
Gina Leoni, RRA
Mary R. O'Heron, RRA
Karen E. O'Hara, BS
Dan Reyes, BA
Desiree Rozell, MPA
Dianne M. Willard, RRA, MBA
Shelley L. Yacorella, BA
Rejina L. Young
Jill Zanutto, BS

Acknowledgements

The publication of *CPT 1996* represents a product of the combined efforts of many individuals and organizations. The editors accordingly express their gratitude to the many national medical specialty societies, state medical associations, health insurance organizations and agencies, and to the many individual physicians who devoted their energies and expertise to the preparation of this revision. Thanks are due to Jean A. Harris, Health Care Financing Administration, Claudia Bonnell, Blue Cross and Blue Shield Association, Thomas Musco, Health Insurance Association of America, Donna Pickett, American Hospital Association, and to Sue Prophet, RRA, American Health Information Management Association, for their invaluable assistance in enhancing *CPT*. Finally, the editors are grateful to Barry S. Eisenberg, Director, Division of Payment Programs, for his helpful invaluable assistance.

Foreword

Physicians' Current Procedural Terminology, Fourth Edition (*CPT*) is a listing of descriptive terms and identifying codes for reporting medical services and procedures performed by physicians. The purpose of the terminology is to provide a uniform language that will accurately describe medical, surgical, and diagnostic services, and will thereby provide an effective means for reliable nationwide communication among physicians, patients, and third parties. *CPT 1996* is the most recent revision of a work that first appeared in 1966.

CPT descriptive terms and identifying codes currently serve a wide variety of important functions in the field of medical nomenclature. This system of terminology is the most widely accepted nomenclature for the reporting of physician procedures and services under government and private health insurance programs. *CPT* is also useful for administrative management purposes such as claims processing and for the development of guidelines for medical care review. The uniform language is likewise applicable to medical education and research by providing a useful basis for local, regional, and national utilization comparisons.

The changes that appear in this revision have been prepared by the CPT Editorial Panel with the assistance of physicians representing all specialties of medicine, and with important contributions from many third party payors and governmental agencies.

The American Medical Association trusts that this revision will continue the usefulness of its predecessors in identifying, describing, and coding medical, surgical, and diagnostic services performed by practicing physicians.

James S. Todd, MD
Executive Vice President

October 1, 1995

Arnold M. Rosen, MD
American Society for Gastrointestinal Endoscopy

Richard A. Roski, MD
American Association of Neurological Surgeons

Jacob M. Rowe, MD
American Society of Hematology

Andrew C. Ruoff III, MD
The Society of Medical Consultants to the Armed Forces

Peter L. Sawchuk, MD
American College of Emergency Physicians

Chester W. Schmidt, Jr., MD
American Psychiatric Association

Jon D. Shanser, MD
American College of Radiology

Willis W. Stogsdill, MD
American Society of Anesthesiologists, Inc.

Dennis L. Stone, MD
American Medical Directors Association

Douglas L. Stringer, MD
Congress of Neurological Surgeons

Steven J. Stryker, MD
American Society of Colon & Rectal Surgeons

Roger F. Suchyta, MD
American Academy of Pediatrics

Sheldon B. Taubman, MD
College of American Pathologists

Elizabeth A. Tindall, MD
American College of Rheumatology

David G. Tinkelman, MD
American College of Allergy, Asthma, and Immunology

Susan K. Turney, MD
American Group Practice Association

F. Stephen Vogel, MD
United States & Canadian Academy of Pathology

Theodore A. Watson, MD
American Academy of Otolaryngic Allergy

Jonathan B. Weisbuch, MD
American Association of Public Health Physicians

AMA CPT Health Care Professionals Advisory Committee (HCPAC)

Tracy R. Gordy, MD, Co-Chairman
AMA CPT Editorial Panel

Robert D. Sowell, D.P.M. Co-Chairman
American Podiatric Medical Association

Helene Fearon, P.T.
American Physical Therapy Association

Carol H. Gwin, O.T.R./L.
American Occupational Therapy Association

Vivian H. Jackson, M.S.W.
National Association of Social Workers

Jerilynn S. Kaibel, DC
American Chiropractic Association

John Lahr, O.D.
American Optometric Association

Janet P. McCarty C.C.C.-S.L.P.
American Speech-Language Hearing Association

Ron L. Nelson, P.A.-C.
American Academy of Physician Assistants

Antonio Puente, Ph.D.
American Psychological Association

Ann M. Thrailkill, R.N.
American Nurses Association

Arnold Widen, MD
AMA CPT Editorial Panel

Douglas L. Wood, MD
AMA CPT Editorial Panel

Contents

Contents

Introduction

Physicians' Current Procedural Terminology, Fourth Edition (*CPT*) is a systematic listing and coding of procedures and services performed by physicians. Each procedure or service is identified with a five digit code. The use of CPT codes simplifies the reporting of services. With this coding and recording system, the procedure or service rendered by the physician is accurately identified.

Inclusion of a descriptor and its associated specific five-digit identifying code number in *CPT* is generally based upon the procedure being consistent with contemporary medical practice and being performed by many physicians in clinical practice in multiple locations. Inclusion in *CPT* does not represent endorsement by the American Medical Association of any particular diagnostic or therapeutic procedure. Inclusion or exclusion of a procedure does not imply any health insurance coverage or reimbursement policy.

The main body of the material is listed in six sections. Within each section are subsections with anatomic, procedural, condition, or descriptor subheadings. The procedures and services with their identifying codes are presented in numeric order with one exception—the entire **Evaluation and Management** section (99201-99499) has been placed at the beginning of the listed procedures. These items are used by most physicians in reporting a significant portion of their services. The **Medicine** (procedures) section now follows **Pathology**.

Section Numbers and Their Sequences

Evaluation and Management ..99201 to 99499

Anesthesiology ....00100 to 01999, 99100 to 99140

Surgery......................10040 to 69979

Radiology (Including Nuclear Medicine and Diagnostic Ultrasound) ...70010 to 79999

Pathology and Laboratory ....80002 to 89399

Medicine (except Anesthesiology) .....90701 to 99199

The first and last code numbers and the subsection name of the items appear at the top of each page (eg, "11100—11420 Surgery/Integumentary System"). The continuous pagination of *CPT* is found on the lower, outer margin of each page along with the section name.

Instructions for Use of CPT

A physician using CPT terminology and coding selects the name of the procedure or service that most accurately identifies the service performed. In surgery, it may be an operation; in medicine, a diagnostic or therapeutic procedure; in radiology, a radiograph. The physician then may list other additional procedures performed or pertinent special services. When necessary, he lists any modifying or extenuating circumstance. Any service or procedure should be adequately documented in the medical record.

It is important to recognize that the listing of a service or procedure and its code number in a specific section of this book does not restrict its use to a specific specialty group. Any procedure or service in any section of this book may be used to designate the services rendered by any qualified physician.

Format of the Terminology

CPT procedure terminology has been developed as stand-alone descriptions of medical procedures. However, some of the procedures in *CPT* are not printed in their entirety but refer back to a common portion of the procedure listed in a preceding entry. This is evident when an entry is followed by one or more indentations. This is done in an effort to conserve space.

Example

25100 Arthrotomy, wrist joint; for biopsy

25105   for synovectomy

Note that the common part of code 25100 (that part before the semicolon) should be considered part of code 25105. Therefore the full procedure represented by code 25105 should read:

25105 Arthrotomy, wrist joint; for synovectomy

Requests to Update CPT

The effectiveness of *Physicians' Current Procedural Terminology* is dependent upon constant updating to reflect changes in medical practice. This can only be accomplished through the interest and timely suggestions of practicing physicians, medical specialty societies, state medical associations, and other organizations and agencies. Accordingly, the American Medical Association welcomes correspondence, inquiries, and suggestions concerning old and new procedures, as well as other matters such as codes and indices.

For suggestions concerning the introduction of new procedures, or the coding, deleting, or revising of procedures contained in *CPT 1996*, correspondence should be directed to:

Department of Coding and Nomenclature
American Medical Association
515 North State Street
Chicago, Illinois 60610

All proposed additions to, or modifications of, *CPT 1996* will be by decision of the CPT Editorial Panel after consultation with appropriate medical specialty societies.

Guidelines

Specific "Guidelines" are presented at the beginning of each of the six sections. These Guidelines define items that are necessary to appropriately interpret and report the procedures and services contained in that section. For example, in the **Medicine** section, specific instructions are provided for handling unlisted services or procedures, special reports, and supplies and materials provided by the physician. Guidelines also provide explanations regarding terms that apply only to a particular section. For instance, **Surgery** guidelines provide an explanation of the use of the star, while in **Radiology,** the unique term, "radiological supervision and interpretation" is defined.

Starred Procedures

The star "*" is used to identify certain surgical procedures. A description of this reporting mechanism will be found in the **Surgery Guidelines.**

Modifiers

A modifier provides the means by which the reporting physician can indicate that a service or procedure that has been performed has been altered by some specific circumstance but not changed in its definition or code. The judicious application of modifiers obviates the necessity for separate procedure listings that may describe the modifying circumstance. Modifiers may be used to indicate to the recipient of a report that:

- A service or procedure has both a professional and technical component.
- A service or procedure was performed by more than one physician and/or in more than one location.
- A service or procedure has been increased or reduced.
- Only part of a service was performed.
- An adjunctive service was performed.
- A bilateral procedure was performed.
- A service or procedure was provided more than once.
- Unusual events occurred.

Example

A physician providing diagnostic or therapeutic radiology services, ultrasound or nuclear medicine services in a hospital would use either modifier '-26' or 09926 to report the professional component.

73090-26 = Professional component only for an x-ray of the forearm

or

73090 AND 09926 = Professional component only for an x-ray of the forearm

Example

Two surgeons, usually with different skills, may be required to manage a specific surgical problem. The modifier '-62' or the alternative modifier five digit code 09962 would be applicable. Modifier '-62' would be appropriate only when both surgeons are reporting the same code number and descriptor. For instance, a neurological surgeon and an otolaryngologist are working as co-surgeons in performing transsphenoidal excision of a pituitary neoplasm.

61548-62 = Hypophysectomy or excision of pitiutary tumor, transnasal or transseptal approach, nonstereotactic + two surgeons modifier

or

61548 AND 09962 = Hypophysectomy or excision of pitiutary tumor, transnasal or transseptal approach, nonstereotactic + two surgeons modifier

AND the second surgeon would report:

61548-62 = Hypophysectomy or excision of

pitiutary tumor, transnasal or transseptal approach, nonstereotactic + two surgeons modifier

or

61548 AND 09962 = Hypophysectomy or excision of pitiutary tumor, transnasal or transseptal approach, nonstereotactic + two surgeons modifier

A listing of modifiers pertinent to **Evaluation and Management, Anesthesia, Surgery, Radiology, Pathology,** and **Medicine** are located in the Guidelines of each section. A complete listing of modifiers is found in Appendix A.

Unlisted Procedure or Service

It is recognized that there may be services or procedures performed by physicians that are not found in *CPT*. Therefore, a number of specific code numbers have been designated for reporting unlisted procedures. When an unlisted procedure number is used, the service or procedure should be described. Each of these unlisted procedural code numbers (with the appropriate accompanying topical entry) relates to a specific section of the book and is presented in the Guidelines of that section.

Special Report

A service that is rarely provided, unusual, variable, or new may require a special report in determining medical appropriateness of the service. Pertinent information should include an adequate definition or description of the nature, extent, and need for the procedure; and the time, effort, and equipment necessary to provide the service. Additional items which may be included are:

Complexity of symptoms, final diagnosis, pertinent physical findings, diagnostic and therapeutic procedures, concurrent problems, and follow-up care.

Code Changes

A summary listing of additions, deletions and revisions applicable to *CPT 1996* is found in Appendix B. New procedure numbers added to *CPT* are identified throughout the text with the symbol "●" placed before the code number. In instances where a code revision has resulted in a substantially altered procedure descriptor, the symbol "▲" is placed before the code number.

Short Procedure Tape Revision

Appendix C has been included for those users who have purchased a *CPT 1995* short procedure description tape or floppy disk or have a tape/disk current through *CPT 1995*. The listing includes changes and/or corrections necessary to update the *CPT 1996* data file. For additional information regarding the availability of *CPT* magnetic computer tapes and floppy disks, see below.

Alphabetical Reference Index

A new, expanded alphabetical index is found in the back of the book. It includes listings by procedure and anatomic site. Procedures and services commonly known by their eponyms or other designations are also included.

Magnetic Computer Tapes and Floppy Disk

CPT 1996 procedure codes and descriptors are also available on magnetic computer tapes in the three formats listed below.

*CPT **Full Procedure Tape*** contains the complete procedural text of the *CPT* manual. The procedures in this tape are constructed of 80-byte line records. In cases where the procedural narrative exceeds the 80-byte line limit, the header record is followed by several trailing line records. The start of each procedure is indicated by a change in "procedure number" or the presence of 01, 02 etc. in the sequence fields.

*CPT **Short Description Tape*** also contains the complete listing of procedural codes found in the *CPT* manual; however, each has an abbreviated narrative written in non-technical or layman's terms. Each code and description is limited to 28 characters or less on a single line.

Technical Description of Tapes

Both *CPT* computer tapes are identical technically, each having the following line specifications:

record format . . . . .fixed

logical record length . . . . .80 bytes

block size. . . . . .80 bytes

label . . . . .no label

tracks 9

tape density. . . . . .1600 or 6250 BPI

content . . . . .EBCDIC or ASCII

*CPT **Floppy Disk*** is identical in content to the short description tape. That is, each code and description is limited to 28 characters or less on a single line.

Technical Description of Disk

- Standard PC format with a maximum length of 36 characters per record

- Content: ASCII

- PC requirements: IBM PC, XT, AT or compatible

- 3½″ double side/double density (720K) disk OR 5¼″ double side/double density (360K) disk

Using Compatible Software

Please bear in mind that the disks and tapes contain *only* a *CPT* data file. They are *not* programs or other operations software. We have deliberately not included programs with this data file, as each user has different needs.

Evaluation and Management (E/M) Services Guidelines

In addition to the information presented in the **Introduction,** several other items unique to this section are defined or identified here.

Classification of Evaluation and Management (E/M) Services

The E/M section is divided into broad categories such as office visits, hospital visits, and consultations. Most of the categories are further divided into two or more subcategories of E/M services. For example, there are two subcategories of office visits (new patient and established patient) and there are two subcategories of hospital visits (initial and subsequent). The subcategories of E/M services are further classified into levels of E/M services that are identified by specific codes. This classification is important because the nature of physician work varies by type of service, place of service, and the patient's status.

The basic format of the levels of E/M services is the same for most categories. First, a unique code number is listed. Second, the place and/or type of service is specified, eg, office consultation. Third, the content of the service is defined, eg, comprehensive history and comprehensive examination. (See "Levels of E/M Services," page 2, for details on the content of E/M services.) Fourth, the nature of the presenting problem(s) usually associated with a given level is described. Fifth, the time typically required to provide the service is specified. (A detailed discussion of time is provided on pages 3-4.)

Definitions of Commonly Used Terms

Certain key words and phrases are used throughout the E/M section. The following definitions are intended to reduce the potential for differing interpretations and to increase the consistency of reporting by physicians in differing specialties.

New and Established Patient

A new patient is one who has not received any professional services from the physician or another physician of the same specialty who belongs to the same group practice, within the past three years.

An established patient is one who has received professional services from the physician or another physician of the same specialty who belongs to the same group practice, within the past three years.

In the instance where a physician is on call for or covering for another physician, the patient's encounter will be classified as it would have been by the physician who is not available.

No distinction is made between new and established patients in the emergency department. E/M services in the emergency department category may be reported for any new or established patient who presents for treatment in the emergency department.

Chief Complaint

A concise statement describing the symptom, problem, condition, diagnosis or other factor that is the reason for the encounter, usually stated in the patient's words.

Concurrent Care

Concurrent care is the provision of similar services, eg, hospital visits, to the same patient by more than one physician on the same day. When concurrent care is provided, no special reporting is required. Modifier '-75' has been deleted.

Counseling

Counseling is a discussion with a patient and/or family concerning one or more of the following areas:

- diagnostic results, impressions, and/or recommended diagnostic studies;
- prognosis;
- risks and benefits of management (treatment) options;
- instructions for management (treatment) and/or follow-up;
- importance of compliance with chosen management (treatment) options;
- risk factor reduction; and
- patient and family education.

(For psychotherapy, see 90841-90857)

Family History

A review of medical events in the patient's family that includes significant information about:

- the health status or cause of death of parents, siblings, and children;
- specific diseases related to problems identified in the Chief Complaint or History of the Present Illness, and/or System Review;
- diseases of family members which may be hereditary or place the patient at risk.

History of Present Illness

A chronological description of the development of the patient's present illness from the first sign and/or symptom to the present. This includes a description of location, quality, severity, timing, context, modifying factors and associated signs and symptoms significantly related to the presenting problem(s).

Levels of E/M Services

Within each category or subcategory of E/M service, there are three to five levels of E/M services available for reporting purposes. Levels of E/M services are *not* interchangeable among the different categories or subcategories of service. For example, the first level of E/M services in the subcategory of office visit, new patient, does not have the same definition as the first level of E/M services in the subcategory of office visit, established patient.

The levels of E/M services include examinations, evaluations, treatments, conferences with or con-

cerning patients, preventive pediatric and adult health supervision, and similar medical services, such as the determination of the need and/or location for appropriate care. Medical screening includes the history, examination, and medical decision-making required to determine the need and/or location for approriate care and treatment of the patient (eg, office and other outpatient setting, emergency department, nursing facility, etc.). The levels of E/M services encompass the wide variations in skill, effort, time, responsibility and medical knowledge required for the prevention or diagnosis and treatment of illness or injury and the promotion of optimal health. Each level of E/M services may be used by all physicians.

The descriptors for the levels of E/M services recognize seven components, six of which are used in defining the levels of E/M services. These components are:

- history;
- examination;
- medical decision making;
- counseling;
- coordination of care;
- nature of presenting problem; and
- time.

The first three of these components (history, examination and medical decision making) are considered the **key** components in selecting a level of E/M services. (See "Determine the Extent of History Obtained", page 7.)

The next three components (counseling, coordination of care, and the nature of the presenting problem) are considered **contributory** factors in the majority of encounters. Although the first two of these contributory factors are important E/M services, it is not required that these services be provided at every patient encounter.

Coordination of care with other providers or agencies without a patient encounter on that day is reported using the case management codes.

The final component, time, is discussed in detail (see pages 3-4).

The actual performance of diagnostic tests/studies for which specific CPT codes are available is *not* included in the levels of E/M services. Physician performance of diagnostic tests/studies for which specific CPT codes are available should be reported separately, *in addition* to the appropriate E/M code.

Nature of Presenting Problem

A presenting problem is a disease, condition, illness, injury, symptom, sign, finding, complaint, or other reason for encounter, with or without a diagnosis being established at the time of the encounter. The E/M codes recognize five types of presenting problems that are defined as follows:

Minimal: A problem that may not require the presence of the physician, but service is provided under the physician's supervision.

Self-limited or minor: A problem that runs a definite and prescribed course, is transient in nature, and is not likely to permanently alter health status OR has a good prognosis with management/compliance.

Low severity: A problem where the risk of morbidity without treatment is low; there is little to no risk of mortality without treatment; full recovery without functional impairment is expected.

Moderate severity: A problem where the risk of morbidity without treatment is moderate; there is moderate risk of mortality without treatment; uncertain prognosis OR increased probability of prolonged functional impairment.

High severity: A problem where the risk of morbidity without treatment is high to extreme; there is a moderate to high risk of mortality without treatment OR high probability of severe, prolonged functional impairment.

Past History

A review of the patient's past experiences with illnesses, injuries, and treatments that includes significant information about:

- prior major illnesses and injuries;
- prior operations;
- prior hospitalizations;
- current medications;
- allergies (eg, drug, food);
- age appropriate immunization status;
- age appropriate feeding/dietary status.

Social History

An age appropriate review of past and current activities that includes significant information about:

- marital status and/or living arrangements;
- current employment;
- occupational history;
- use of drugs, alcohol, and tobacco;
- level of education;
- sexual history;
- other relevant social factors.

System Review (Review of Systems)

An inventory of body systems obtained through a series of questions seeking to identify signs and/or symptoms which the patient may be experiencing or has experienced. For the purposes of CPT the following elements of a system review have been identified:

- Constitutional symptoms (fever, weight loss, etc.)
- Eyes
- Ears, Nose, Mouth, Throat
- Cardiovascular
- Respiratory
- Gastrointestinal
- Genitourinary
- Musculoskeletal
- Integumentary (skin and/or breast)
- Neurological
- Psychiatric
- Endocrine
- Hematologic/Lymphatic
- Allergic/Immunologic

The review of systems helps define the problem, clarify the differential diagnoses, identify needed testing, or serves as baseline data on other systems that might be affected by any possible management options.

Time

The inclusion of time in the definitions of levels of E/M services has been implicit in prior editions of *CPT*. The inclusion of time as an explicit factor beginning in *CPT 1992* is done to assist physicians in selecting the most appropriate level of E/M services. It should be recognized that the specific times expressed in the visit code descriptors are averages, and therefore represent a range of times which may be higher or lower depending on actual clinical circumstances.

Time is *not* a descriptive component for the emergency department levels of E/M services because emergency department services are typically provided on a variable intensity basis, often involving multiple encounters with several patients over an extended period of time. Therefore, it is often difficult for physicians to provide accurate estimates of the time spent face-to-face with the patient.

Studies to establish levels of E/M services employed surveys of practicing physicians to obtain data on the amount of time and work associated with typical E/M services. Since "work" is not easily quantifiable, the codes must rely on other objective, verifiable measures that correlate with physicians' estimates of their "work". It has been demonstrated that physicians' estimations of **intra-service time** (as explained below), both within and across specialties, is a variable that is predictive of the "work" of E/M services. This same research has shown there is a strong relationship between intra-service time and total time for E/M services. Intra-service time, rather than total time, was chosen for inclusion with the codes because of its relative ease of measurement and because of its direct correlation with measurements of the total amount of time and work associated with typical E/M services.

Intra-service times are defined as **face-to-face** time for office and other outpatient visits and as **unit/ floor** time for hospital and other inpatient visits. This distinction is necessary because most of the work of typical office visits takes place during the face-to-face time with the patient, while most of the work of typical hospital visits takes place during the time spent on the patient's floor or unit.

Face-to-face time (office and other outpatient visits and office consultations): For coding purposes, face-to-face time for these services is defined as only that time that the physician spends face-to-face with the patient and/or family. This includes the time in which the physician performs such tasks as obtaining a history, performing an examination, and counseling the patient.

Physicians also spend time doing work before or after the face-to-face time with the patient, performing such tasks as reviewing records and tests, arranging for further services, and communicating further with other professionals and the patient through written reports and telephone contact.

This *non* face-to-face time for office services—also called pre- and post-encounter time—is not included in the time component described in the E/M codes. However, the pre- and post-face-to-face work associated with an encounter was included in calculating the total work of typical services in physician surveys.

Thus, the face-to-face time associated with the services described by any E/M code is a valid proxy for the total work done before, during, and after the visit.

Unit/floor time (bospital observation services, inpatient hospital care, initial and follow-up bospital consultations, nursing facility): For reporting purposes, intra-service time for these services is defined as unit/floor time, which includes the time that the physician is present on the patient's hospital unit and at the bedside rendering services for that patient. This includes the time in which the physician establishes and/or reviews the patient's chart, examines the patient, writes notes and communicates with other professionals and the patient's family.

In the hospital, pre- and post-time includes time spent off the patient's floor performing such tasks as reviewing pathology and radiology findings in another part of the hospital.

This pre- and post-visit time is not included in the time component described in these codes. However, the pre- and post-work performed during the time spent off the floor or unit was included in calculating the total work of typical services in physician surveys.

Thus, the unit/floor time associated with the services described by any code is a valid proxy for the total work done before, during, and after the visit.

Unlisted Service

An E/M service may be provided that is not listed in this section of *CPT*. When reporting such a service, the appropriate "Unlisted" code may be used to indicate the service, identifying it by "Special Report", as discussed in the following paragraph. The "Unlisted Services" and accompanying codes for the E/M section are as follows:

99429 Unlisted preventive medicine service

99499 Unlisted evaluation and management service

Special Report

An unlisted service or one that is unusual, variable, or new may require a special report demonstrating the medical appropriateness of the service. Pertinent information should include an adequate definition or description of the nature, extent, and need for the procedure; and the time, effort and equipment necessary to provide the service. Additional items which may be included are complexity of symptoms, final diagnosis, pertinent physical findings, diagnostic and therapeutic procedures, concurrent problems, and follow-up care.

Clinical Examples

Clinical examples of the codes for E/M services are provided to assist physicians in understanding the meaning of the descriptors and selecting the correct code. Each example was developed by physicians in the specialties shown.

The same problem, when seen by physicians in different specialties, may involve different amounts of work. Therefore, the appropriate level of encounter should be reported using the descriptors rather than the examples.

The examples have been tested for validity and approved by the CPT Editorial Panel. Physicians were given the examples and asked to assign a code or assess the amount of time and work involved. Only those examples that were rated consistently have been included.

Modifiers

Listed services may be modified under certain circumstances. When applicable, the modifying circumstance against general guidelines should be identified by the addition of the appropriate modifier code, which may be reported in either of two ways. The modifier may be reported by a two digit number placed after the usual procedure number, from which it is separated by a hyphen. Or, the modifier may be reported by a separate five digit code that is used in addition to the procedure code. Modifiers available in E/M are as follows:

-21 Prolonged Evaluation and Management Services: When the face-to-face or floor/unit service(s) provided is prolonged or otherwise greater than that usually required for the highest level of E/M service within a given category, it may be identified by adding modifier '-21' to the E/M code number or by use of the separate five digit modifier code 09921. A report may also be appropriate.

-24 Unrelated Evaluation and Management Service by the Same Physician During a Postoperative Period: The physician may need to indicate that an evaluation and management service was performed during a postoperative period for a reason(s) unrelated to the original procedure. This circumstance may be reported by adding the modifier '-24' to the appropriate level of E/M service, or the separate five digit modifier 09924 may be used.

-25 Significant, Separately Identifiable Evaluation and Management Service by the Same Physician on the Same Day of a Procedure or Other Service: The physician may need to indicate that on the day a procedure or service identified by a CPT code was performed, the patient's condition required a significant, separately identifiable E/M service above and beyond the other service provided or beyond the usual preoperative and postoperative care associated with the procedure that was performed. This circumstance may be reported by adding the modifier '-25' to the appropriate level of E/M service, or the separate five digit modifier 09925 may be used. **Note:** This modifier is not used to report an E/M service that resulted in a decision to perform surgery. See modifier '-57'.

-32 Mandated Services: Services related to *mandated* consultation and/or related services (eg, PRO, 3rd party payor) may be identified by adding the modifier '-32' to the basic procedure or the service may be reported by use of the five digit modifier 09932.

-52 Reduced Services: Under certain circumstances a service or procedure is partially reduced or eliminated at the physician's election. Under these circumstances the service provided can be identified by its usual procedure number and the addition of the modifier '-52,' signifying that the service is reduced. This provides a means of reporting reduced services without disturbing the identification of the basic service. Modifier code 09952 may be used as an alternative to modifier '-52.'

-57 Decision for Surgery. An evaluation and management service that resulted in the initial decision to perform the surgery, may be identified by adding the modifier '-57' to the appropriate level of E/M service, or the separate five digit modifier 09957 may be used.

Instructions for Selecting a Level of E/M Service

Identify the Category and Subcategory of Service

The categories and subcategories of codes available for reporting E/M services are shown in Table 1 below.

Review the Reporting Instructions for the Selected Category or Subcategory

Most of the categories and many of the subcategories of service have special guidelines or instructions unique to that category or subcategory. Where these are indicated, eg, "Inpatient Hospital Care", special instructions will be presented preceding the levels of E/M services.

Review the Level of E/M Service Descriptors and Examples in the Selected Category or Subcategory

The descriptors for the levels of E/M services recognize seven components, six of which are used in defining the levels of E/M services. These components are:

- history;
- examination;
- medical decision making;
- counseling;
- coordination of care;
- nature of presenting problem; and
- time.

The first three of these components (ie, history, examination, and medical decision making) should be considered the **key** components in selecting the level of E/M services. An exception to this rule is in the case of visits which consist predominantly of counseling or coordination of care (See numbered paragraph 3, page 8.)

The nature of the presenting problem and time are provided in some levels to assist the physician in determining the appropriate level of E/M service.

Table 1

Categories and Subcategories of Service

Category/Subcategory	Code Numbers	Category/Subcategory	Code Numbers
Office or Other Outpatient Services		Domiciliary, Rest Home or	
New Patient	99201-99205	Custodial Care Services	
Established Patient	99211-99215	New Patient	99321-99323
Hospital Observation Discharge Services	99217	Established Patient	99331-99333
Hospital Observation Services	99218-99220	Home Services	
Hospital Inpatient Services		New Patient	99341-99343
Initial Hospital Care	99221-99223	Established Patient	99351-99353
Subsequent Hospital Care	99231-99233	Prolonged Services	
Hospital Discharge Services	99238	With Direct Patient Contact	99354-99357
Consultations		Without Direct Patient Contact	99358-99359
Office Consultations	99241-99245	Standby Services	99360
Initial Inpatient Consultations	99251-99255	Case Management Services	
Follow-up Inpatient Consultations	99261-99263	Team Conferences	99361-99362
Confirmatory Consultations	99271-99275	Telephone Calls	99371-99373
Emergency Department Services	99281-99288	Care Plan Oversight Services	99375-99376
Critical Care Services	99291-99292	Preventive Medicine Services	
Neonatal Intensive Care	99295-99297	New Patient	99381-99387
Nursing Facility Services		Established Patient	99391-99397
Comprehensive Nursing Facility		Individual Counseling	99401-99404
Assessments	99301-99303	Group Counseling	99411-99412
Subsequent Nursing Facility Care	99311-99313	Other	99420-99429
		Newborn Care	99431-99440
		Special E/M Services	99450-99456
		Other E/M Services	99499

Determine the Extent of History Obtained

The extent of the history is dependent upon clinical judgement and on the nature of the presenting problems(s). The levels of E/M services recognize four types of history that are defined as follows:

Problem focused: chief complaint; brief history of present illness or problem.

Expanded problem focused: chief complaint; brief history of present illness; problem pertinent system review.

Detailed: chief complaint; extended history of present illness; problem pertinent system review extended to include a review of a limited number of additional systems; **pertinent** past, family, and/or social history *directly related to the patient's problems.*

Comprehensive: chief complaint; extended history of present illness; review of systems which is directly related to the problem(s) identified in the history of the present illness plus a review of all additional body systems; **complete** past, family and social history.

The comprehensive history obtained as part of the preventive medicine evaulation and management service is not problem-oriented and does not involve a chief complaint or present illness. It does, however, include a comprehensive system review and comprehensive or interval past, family and social history as well as a comprehensive assessment/history of pertinent risk factors.

Determine the Extent of Examination Performed

The extent of the examination performed is dependent on clinical judgement and on the nature of the presenting problem(s). The levels of E/M services recognize four types of examination that are defined as follows:

Problem focused: a limited examination of the affected body area or organ system.

Expanded problem focused: a limited examination of the affected body area or organ system and other symptomatic or related organ system(s).

Detailed: an extended examination of the affected body area(s) and other symptomatic or related organ system(s).

Comprehensive: a general multi-system examination or a complete examination of a single organ system. **Note:** The comprehensive examination performed as part of the preventive medicine evaulation and management service is multi-system, but its extent is based on age and risk factors identified.

For the purposes of these CPT definitions, the following body areas are recognized:

- Head, including the face
- Neck
- Chest, including breasts and axilla
- Abdomen
- Genitalia, groin, buttocks
- Back
- Each extremity

For the purposes of these CPT definitions, the following organ systems are recognized:

- Eyes
- Ears, Nose, Mouth and Throat
- Cardiovascular
- Respiratory
- Gastrointestinal
- Genitourinary
- Musculoskeletal
- Skin
- Neurologic
- Psychiatric
- Hematologic/Lymphatic/Immunologic

Determine the Complexity of Medical Decision Making

Medical decision making refers to the complexity of establishing a diagnosis and/or selecting a management option as measured by:

- the number of possible diagnoses and/or the number of management options that must be considered;
- the amount and/or complexity of medical records, diagnostic tests, and/or other information that must be obtained, reviewed and analyzed; and
- the risk of significant complications, morbidity and/or mortality, as well as comorbidities, associated with the patient's presenting problems(s), the diagnostic procedure(s) and/or the possible management options.

Four types of medical decision making are recognized: straightforward; low complexity; moderate complexity; and, high complexity. To qualify for a given type of decision making, two of the three elements in Table 2 below must be met or exceeded.

Comorbidities/underlying diseases, in and of themselves, are not considered in selecting a level of E/M services *unless* their presence significantly increases the complexity of the medical decision making.

Select the Appropriate Level of E/M Services Based on the Following

1. For the following categories/subcategories, **all of the key components,** ie, history, examination, and medical decision making, must meet or exceed the stated requirements to qualify for a particular level of E/M service: office, new patient; hospital observation services; initial hospital care; office consultations; initial inpatient consultations; confirmatory consultations; emergency department services; comprehensive nursing facility assessments; domiciliary care, new patient; and home, new patient.

2. For the following categories/subcategories, **two of the three key components** (ie, history, examination, and medical decision making) must meet or exceed the stated requirements to qualify for a particular level of E/M services: office, established patient; subsequent hospital care; follow-up inpatient consultations; subsequent nursing facility care; domiciliary care, established patient; and home, established patient.

3. In the case where counseling and/or coordination of care dominates (more than 50%) of the physician/patient and/or family encounter (face-to-face time in the office or other outpatient setting or floor/unit time in the hospital or nursing facility), then **time** is considered the key or controlling factor to qualify for a particular level of E/M services. The extent of counseling and/or coordination of care must be documented in the medical record.

Table 2
Complexity of Medical Decision Making

Number of Diagnoses or Management Options	Amount and/or Complexity of Data to be Reviewed	Risk of Complications and/or Morbidity or Mortality	Type of Decision Making
minimal	minimal or none	minimal	**straightforward**
limited	limited	low	**low complexity**
multiple	moderate	moderate	**moderate complexity**
extensive	extensive	high	**high complexity**

Evaluation and Management

Office or Other Outpatient Services

The following codes are used to report evaluation and management services provided in the physician's office or in an outpatient or other ambulatory facility. A patient is considered an outpatient until inpatient admission to a health care facility occurs.

To report services provided to a patient who is admitted to a hospital or nursing facility in the course of an encounter in the office or other ambulatory facility, see the notes for initial hospital inpatient care (page 15) or comprehensive nursing facility assessments (page 30).

For services provided by physicians in the Emergency Department, see 99281-99285.

For observation care, see 99217-99220.

For definitions of key components, see **Evaluation and Management Services Guidelines.**

New Patient

99201   **Office or other outpatient visit** for the evaluation and management of a new patient, which requires these three key components:

- **a problem focused history;**
- **a problem focused examination; and**
- **straightforward medical decision making.**

Counseling and/or coordination of care with other providers or agencies are provided consistent with the nature of the problem(s) and the patient's and/or family's needs.

Usually, the presenting problems are self limited or minor. Physicians typically spend 10 minutes face-to-face with the patient and/or family.

Examples

Initial office visit with 65-year-old male for reassurance about an isolated seborrheic keratosis on the upper back. (Dermatology/Plastic Surgery)

Initial office visit with an out-of-town visitor who needs a prescription refilled because she forgot her hay fever medication. (Allergy & Immunology/Internal Medicine)

Initial office visit with 9-month-old female with diaper rash. (Pediatrics)

Initial office visit with 10-year-old male with severe rash and itching for the past 24 hours, positive history for contact with poison oak 48 hours prior to the visit. (Family Medicine)

Initial office visit to advise for or against the removal of wisdom teeth, 18-year-old male referred by an orthodontist. (Oral & Maxillofacial Surgery)

Initial office visit with 5-year-old female to remove sutures from simple wound, placed by another physician. (Plastic Surgery)

Initial office visit for a 22-year-old male with a small area of sunburn requiring first aid. (Dermatology/Family Medicine/Internal Medicine)

Initial office visit for the evaluation and management of a contusion of a finger. (Orthopaedic Surgery)

99202   **Office or other outpatient visit** for the evaluation and management of a new patient, which requires these three key components:

- **an expanded problem focused history;**
- **an expanded problem focused examination; and**
- **straightforward medical decision making.**

Counseling and/or coordination of care with other providers or agencies are provided consistent with the nature of the problem(s) and the patient's and/or family's needs.

Usually, the presenting problem(s) are of low to moderate severity. Physicians typically spend 20 minutes face-to-face with the patient and/or family.

Examples

Initial office visit, 16-year-old male with severe cystic acne, new patient. (Dermatology)

Initial office evaluation for gradual hearing loss, 58-year-old male, history and physical examination, with interpretation of complete audiogram, air bone, etc. (Otolaryngology)

Initial evaluation and management of recurrent urinary infection in female. (Internal Medicine)

Initial office visit with 10-year-old girl with history of chronic otitis media and a draining ear. (Pediatrics)

Initial office visit for a 10-year-old female with acute maxillary sinusitis. (Family Medicine)

Initial office visit for a patient with recurring episodes of herpes simplex who has developed a clustering of vesicles on the upper lip. (Internal Medicine)

Initial office visit for a 25-year-old patient with single season allergic rhinitis. (Allergy & Immunology)

Initial office visit to plan transient dialysis for a 56-year-old stable dialysis patient who has accompanying records. (Nephrology)

99203 **Office or other outpatient visit** for the evaluation and management of a new patient, which requires these three key components:

- **a detailed history;**
- **a detailed examination; and**
- **medical decision making of low complexity.**

Counseling and/or coordination of care with other providers or agencies are provided consistent with the nature of the problem(s) and the patient's and/or family's needs.

Usually, the presenting problem(s) are of moderate severity. Physicians typically spend 30 minutes face-to-face with the patient and/or family.

Examples

Initial office visit for initial evaluation of a 48-year-old man with recurrent low back pain radiating to the leg. (General Surgery)

Initial office visit for evaluation, diagnosis and management of painless gross hematuria in new patient, without cystoscopy. (Internal Medicine)

Initial office visit with couple for counseling concerning voluntary vasectomy for sterility. Spent 30 minutes discussing procedure, risks and benefits, and answering questions. (Urology)

Initial office visit of 49-year-old male with nasal obstruction. Detailed exam with topical anesthesia. (Plastic Surgery)

Initial office visit for evaluation of 13-year-old female with progressive scoliosis. (Physical Medicine & Rehabilitation)

Initial office visit for 21-year-old female desiring counseling and evaluation of initiation of contraception. (Family Practice/Internal Medicine/Obstetrics & Gynecology)

Initial office visit for 49-year-old male presenting with painless blood per rectum associated with bowel movement. (Colon & Rectal Surgery)

Initial office visit for 19-year-old football player with 3 day old acute knee injury; now with swelling and pain. (Orthopaedic Surgery)

99204 **Office or other outpatient visit** for the evaluation and management of a new patient, which requires these three key components:

- **a comprehensive history;**
- **a comprehensive examination; and**
- **medical decision making of moderate complexity.**

Counseling and/or coordination of care with other providers or agencies are provided consistent with the nature of the problem(s) and the patient's and/or family's needs.

Usually, the presenting problem(s) are of moderate to high severity. Physicians typically spend 45 minutes face-to-face with the patient and/or family.

Examples

Initial office visit for initial evaluation of a 63-year-old male with chest pain on exertion. (Cardiology/Internal Medicine)

Initial office visit for evaluation of a 70-year-old patient with recent onset of episodic confusion. (Internal Medicine)

Initial office visit for 7-year-old female with juvenile diabetes mellitus, new to area, past history of hospitalization times three. (Pediatrics)

Initial office visit of a 50-year-old female with progressive solid food dysphagia. (Gastroenterology)

Initial office visit for 34-year-old patient with primary infertility, including counseling. (Obstetrics & Gynecology)

Initial office visit for evaluation of 70-year-old female with polyarthralgia. (Rheumatology)

Initial office visit for a patient with papulosquamous eruption involving 60% of the cutaneous surface with joint pain. Combinations of topical and systemic treatments discussed. (Dermatology)

99205 **Office or other outpatient visit** for the evaluation and management of a new patient, which requires these three key components:

- **a comprehensive history;**
- **a comprehensive examination; and**
- **medical decision making of high complexity.**

Counseling and/or coordination of care with other providers or agencies are provided consistent with the nature of the problem(s) and the patient's and/or family's needs.

Usually, the presenting problem(s) are of moderate to high severity. Physicians typically spend 60 minutes face-to-face with the patient and/or family.

Examples

Initial office evaluation of a 65-year-old female with exertional chest pain, intermittent claudication, syncope and a murmur of aortic stenosis. (Cardiology)

Initial office visit for a 73-year-old male with an unexplained 20 lb. weight loss. (Hematology/Oncology)

Initial office evaluation, patient with systemic lupus erythematosus, fever, seizures and profound thrombocytopenia. (Allergy & Immunology/Internal Medicine/Rheumatology)

Initial office evaluation and management of patient with systemic vasculitis and compromised circulation to the limbs. (Rheumatology)

Initial office visit for a 24-year-old homosexual male who has a fever, a cough, and shortness of breath. (Infectious Disease)

Initial outpatient evaluation of a 69-year-old male with severe chronic obstructive pulmonary disease, congestive heart failure, and hypertension. (Family Medicine)

Initial office visit for a 17-year-old female, who is having school problems and has told a friend she is considering suicide. The patient and her family are consulted in regards to treatment options. (Psychiatry)

Initial office visit for a female with severe hirsutism, amenorrhea, weight loss and a desire to have children. (Endocrinology/Obstetrics & Gynecology)

Initial office visit for a 42-year-old male on hypertensive medication, newly arrived to the area, with diastolic blood pressure of 110, history of recurrent renal calculi, episodic headaches, intermittent chest pain and orthopnea. (Internal Medicine)

Established Patient

99211   Office or other outpatient visit for the evaluation and management of an established patient, that may not require the presence of a physician.

Usually, the presenting problem(s) are minimal. Typically, 5 minutes are spent performing or supervising these services.

Examples

Outpatient visit with 19-year-old male, established patient, for supervised drug screen. (Addiction Medicine)

Office visit with 12-year-old male, established patient, for cursory check of hematoma one day after venipuncture. (Internal Medicine)

Office visit with 31-year-old female, established patient, for return to work certificate. (Anesthesiology)

Office visit for a 42-year-old established patient to read tuberculin test results. (Allergy & Immunology)

Office visit for 14-year-old established patient to re-dress an abrasion. (Orthopaedic Surgery)

Office visit for a 45-year-old female, established patient, for a blood pressure check. (Obstetrics & Gynecology)

Office visit for a 23-year-old established patient for instruction in use of peak flow meter. (Allergy & Immunology)

Office visit for prescription refill for a 35-year-old female, established patient, with schizophrenia who is stable but has run out of neuroleptic and is scheduled to be seen in a week. (Psychiatry)

99212   Office or other outpatient visit for the evaluation and management of an established patient, which requires at least two of these three key components:

- **a problem focused history;**
- **a problem focused examination;**
- **straightforward medical decision making.**

Counseling and/or coordination of care with other providers or agencies are provided consistent with the nature of the problem(s) and the patient's and/or family's needs.

Usually, the presenting problem(s) are self limited or minor. Physicians typically spend 10 minutes face-to-face with the patient and/or family.

Examples

Office visit, established patient, 6-year-old child with sore throat and headache. (Family Medicine/Pediatrics)

Office evaluation for possible purulent bacterial conjunctivitis with 1-2 day history of redness and discharge, 16-year-old female, established patient. (Pediatrics/Internal Medicine/Family Medicine)

Office visit with 65-year-old female, established patient, returns for 3 week follow-up for resolving severe ankle sprain. (Orthopaedic Surgery)

Office visit, sore throat, fever and fatigue in 19-year-old college student, established patient. (Internal Medicine)

Office visit with 33-year-old female, established patient, recently started on treatment for hemorrhoidal complaints, for re-evaluation. (Colon & Rectal Surgery)

Office visit with 36-year-old male, established patient, for follow-up on effectiveness of medicine management of oral candidiasis. (Oral & Maxillofacial Surgery)

Office visit for 27-year-old female, established patient, with complaints of vaginal itching. (Obstetrics & Gynecology)

Office visit for a 65-year-old male, established patient, with eruptions on both arms from poison oak exposure. (Allergy & Immunology/Internal Medicine)

99213 **Office or other outpatient visit** for the evaluation and management of an established patient, which requires at least two of these three key components:

- **an expanded problem focused history;**
- **an expanded problem focused examination;**
- **medical decision making of low complexity.**

Counseling and coordination of care with other providers or agencies are provided consistent with the nature of the problem(s) and the patient's and/or family's needs.

Usually, the presenting problem(s) are of low to moderate severity. Physicians typically spend 15 minutes face-to-face with the patient and/or family.

Examples

Office visit with 55-year-old male, established patient, for management of hypertension, mild fatigue, on beta blocker/thiazide regimen. (Family Medicine/Internal Medicine)

Outpatient visit with 37-year-old male, established patient, who is 3 years post total colectomy for chronic ulcerative colitis, presents for increased irritation at his stoma. (General Surgery)

Office visit for a 70-year-old diabetic hypertensive established patient with recent change in insulin requirement. (Internal Medicine/Nephrology)

Office visit with 80-year-old female established patient, for follow-up osteoporosis, status-post compression fractures. (Rheumatology)

Office visit for an established patient with stable cirrhosis of the liver. (Gastroenterology)

Routine, follow-up office evaluation at a three-month interval for a 77-year-old female, established patient, with nodular small cleaved-cell lymphoma. (Hematology/Oncology)

Quarterly follow-up office visit for a 45-year-old male established patient, with stable chronic asthma, on steroid and bronchodilator therapy. (Pulmonary Medicine)

Office visit for a 50-year-old female, established patient, with insulin-dependent diabetes mellitus and stable coronary artery disease, for monitoring. (Family Medicine/Internal Medicine)

99214 **Office or other outpatient visit** for the evaluation and management of an established patient, which requires at least two of these three key components:

- **a detailed history;**
- **a detailed examination;**
- **medical decision making of moderate complexity.**

Counseling and/or coordination of care with other providers or agencies are provided consistent with the nature of the problem(s) and the patient's and/or family's needs.

Usually, the presenting problem(s) are of moderate to high severity. Physicians typically spend 25 minutes face-to-face with the patient and/or family.

Examples

Office visit for a 68-year-old male, established patient, with stable angina, two months post myocardial infarction, who is not tolerating one of his medications. (Cardiology)

Weekly office visit for 5FU therapy for an ambulatory established patient with metastatic colon cancer and increasing shortness of breath. (Hematology/Oncology)

Follow-up office visit for a 60-year-old male, established patient, whose post-traumatic seizures have disappeared on medication, and who now raises the question of stopping the medication (Neurology)

Office evaluation on new onset RLQ pain in a 32-year-old woman, established patient. (Urology/General Surgery/Internal Medicine/Family Medicine)

Office evaluation of 28-year-old established patient with regional enteritis, diarrhea and low grade fever. (Family Medicine/Internal Medicine)

Office visit with 50-year-old female, established patient, diabetic, blood sugar controlled by diet. She now complains of frequency of urination and weight loss, blood sugar of 320 and negative ketones on dipstick. (Internal Medicine)

Follow-up office visit for a 45-year-old established patient with rheumatoid arthritis on gold, methotrexate, or immunosuppressive therapy. (Rheumatology)

Office visit with 63-year-old female, established patient, with familial polyposis, after a previous colectomy and sphincter sparing procedure, now with tenesmus, mucus, and increased stool frequency. (Colon & Rectal Surgery)

Office visit for 60-year-old male, established patient, 2 years post-removal of intracranial meningioma, now with new headaches and visual disturbance. (Neurosurgery)

Office visit for a 68-year-old female, established patient, for routine review and follow-up of non-insulin dependent diabetes, obesity, hypertension and congestive heart failure. Complains of vision difficulties and admits dietary noncompliance. Patient is counseled concerning diet and current medications adjusted. (Family Medicine)

99215 **Office or other outpatient visit** for the evaluation and management of an established patient, which requires at least two of these three key components:

- **a comprehensive history;**
- **a comprehensive examination;**
- **medical decision making of high complexity.**

Counseling and/or coordination of care with other providers or agencies are provided consistent with the nature of the problem(s) and the patient's and/or family's needs.

Usually, the presenting problem(s) are of moderate to high severity. Physicians typically spend 40 minutes face-to-face with the patient and/or family.

Examples

Office visit with 30-year-old male, established patient for 3 month history of fatigue, weight loss, intermittent fever, and presenting with diffuse adenopathy and splenomegaly. (Family Medicine)

Office visit for restaging of an established patient with new lymphadenopathy one year post-therapy for lymphoma. (Hematology/Oncology)

Office visit for evaluation of recent onset syncopal attacks in a 70-year-old woman, established patient. (Internal Medicine)

Follow-up visit, 40-year-old mother of 3, established patient, with acute rheumatoid arthritis, anatomical Stage 3, ARA function Class 3 rheumatoid arthritis, and deteriorating function. (Rheumatology)

Office evaluation and discussion of treatment options for a 68-year-old male, established patient, with a biopsy-proven rectal carcinoma. (General Surgery)

Follow-up office visit for a 65-year-old male, established patient, with a fever of recent onset while on outpatient antibiotic therapy for endocarditis. (Infectious Disease)

Office visit for a 75-year-old established patient with ALS (amyotrophic lateral sclerosis), who is no longer able to swallow. (Neurology)

Office visit for a 70-year-old female, established patient, with diabetes mellitus and hypertension, presenting with a 2 month history of increasing confusion, agitation and short-term memory loss. (Family Medicine/Internal Medicine)

Hospital Observation Services

The following codes are used to report evaluation and management services provided to patients designated/admitted as "observation status" in a hospital. It is not necessary that the patient be located in an observation area designated by the hospital. If such an area does exist in a hospital (as a separate unit in the hospital, in the emergency department, etc.), these codes are to be utilized if the patient is placed in such an area.

For definitions of key components and commonly used terms, please see **Evaluation and Management Services Guidelines.**

Typical times have not yet been established for this category of services.

Observation Care Discharge Services

Observation care discharge of a patient from "observation status" includes final examination of the patient, discussion of the hospital stay, instructions for continuing care, and preparation of discharge records.

99217 **Observation care discharge** day management (This code is to be utilized by the physician to report all services provided to a patient on discharge from "observation status" if the discharge is on other than the initial date of "observation status". To report services to a patient designated as "observation status" who is discharged on the same date, use only the codes for Initial Observation Services (99218-99220))

Initial Observation Care

New or Established Patient

The following codes are used to report the encounter(s) by the supervising physician with the patient when designated as "observation status." This refers to the initiation of observation status, supervision of the care plan for observation and performance of periodic reassessments. For observation encounters by other physicians, see Office or Other Outpatient Consultation codes (99241-99245).

To report services provided to a patient who is admitted to the hospital after receiving hospital observation care services on the same date, see the notes for initial hospital inpatient care (page 15). For a patient admitted to the hospital on a date subsequent to the date of observation status, the hospital admission would be reported with the appropriate Initial Hospital Care codes (99221-99223). Do not report observation discharge in conjunction with the hospital admission.

When "observation status" is initiated in the course of an encounter in another site of service (eg, hospital emergency department, physician's office, nursing facility) all evaluation and management services provided by the supervising physician in conjunction with initiating "observation status" are considered part of the initial observation care when performed on the same date. The observation care level of service reported by the supervising physician should include the services related to initiating "observation status" provided in the other sites of service as well as in the observation setting.

Evaluation and management services on the same date provided in sites that are related to initiating "observation status" should NOT be reported separately.

These codes may not be utilized for post-operative recovery if the procedure is considered part of the surgical "package." These codes apply to all evaluation and management services that are provided on the same date of initiating "observation status."

99218 **Initial observation care,** per day, for the evaluation and management of a patient which requires these three key components:

- **a detailed or comprehensive history;**
- **a detailed or comprehensive examination; and**
- **medical decision making that is straightforward or of low complexity.**

Counseling and/or coordination of care with other providers or agencies are provided consistent with the nature of the problem(s) and the patient's and/or family's needs.

Usually, the problem(s) requiring admission to "observation status" are of low severity.

99219 **Initial observation care,** per day, for the evaluation and management of a patient, which requires these three key components:

- **a comprehensive history;**
- **a comprehensive examination; and**
- **medical decision making of moderate complexity.**

Counseling and/or coordination of care with other providers or agencies are provided consistent with the nature of the problem(s) and the patient's and/or family's needs.

Usually, the problem(s) requiring admission to "observation status" are of moderate severity.

99220 **Initial observation care,** per day, for the evaluation and management of a patient, which requires these three key components:

- **a comprehensive history;**
- **a comprehensive examination; and**
- **medical decision making of high complexity.**

Counseling and/or coordination of care with other providers or agencies are provided consistent with the nature of the problem(s) and the patient's and/or family's needs.

Usually, the problem(s) requiring admission to "observation status" are of high severity.

Hospital Inpatient Services

The following codes are used to report evaluation and management services provided to hospital inpatients. Hospital inpatient services include those services provided to patients in a 'partial hospital' setting. These codes are to be used to report these partial hospitalization services. See also psychiatry notes in the full text of *CPT*.

For definitions of key components and commonly used terms, please see **Evaluation and Management Services Guidelines.** For Hospital Observation Services, see 99218-99220.

Initial Hospital Care

New or Established Patient

The following codes are used to report the first hospital inpatient encounter with the patient by the admitting physician. For initial inpatient encounters by physicians other than the admitting physician, see initial inpatient consultation codes (99251-99255) or subsequent hospital care codes (99231-99233) as appropriate.

When the patient is admitted to the hospital as an inpatient in the course of an encounter in another site of service (eg, hospital emergency department, observation status in a hospital, physician's office, nursing facility) all evaluation and management services provided by that physician in conjunction with that admission are considered part of the initial hospital care when performed on the same date as the admission. The inpatient care level of service reported by the admitting physician should include the services related to the admission he/she provided in the other sites of service as well as in the inpatient setting. Evaluation and management services on the same date provided in sites other than the hospital that are related to the admission should NOT be reported separately.

99221 **Initial hospital care,** per day, for the evaluation and management of a patient which requires these three key components:

- **a detailed or comprehensive history;**
- **a detailed or comprehensive examination; and**
- **medical decision making that is straightforward or of low complexity.**

Counseling and/or coordination of care with other providers or agencies are provided consistent with the nature of the problem(s) and the patient's and/or family's needs.

Usually, the problem(s) requiring admission are of low severity. Physicians typically spend 30 minutes at the bedside and on the patient's hospital floor or unit.

Examples

Hospital admission, examination, and initiation of treatment program for a 67-year-old male with uncomplicated pneumonia who requires IV antibiotic therapy. (Internal Medicine)

Hospital admission for an 18-month-old child with 10 percent dehydration. (Pediatrics)

Hospital admission for a 12-year-old with a laceration of the upper eyelid involving the lid margin and superior canaliculus, admitted prior to surgery for IV antibiotic therapy. (Ophthalmology)

Hospital admission for a 32-year-old female with severe flank pain, hematuria and presumed diagnosis of ureteral calculus as determined by Emergency Department physician. (Urology)

Initial hospital visit for a patient with several large venous stasis ulcers not responding to outpatient therapy. (Dermatology)

Initial hospital visit for 21-year-old pregnant patient (9 weeks gestation) with hyperemesis gravidarum. (Obstetrics & Gynecology)

Initial hospital visit for a 73-year-old female with acute pyelonephritis who is otherwise generally healthy. (Geriatrics)

Initial hospital visit for 62-year-old patient with cellulitis of the foot requiring bedrest and intravenous antibiotics. (Orthopaedic Surgery)

99222 **Initial hospital care,** per day, for the evaluation and management of a patient, which requires these three key components:

- **a comprehensive history;**
- **a comprehensive examination; and**
- **medical decision making of moderate complexity.**

Counseling and/or coordination of care with other providers or agencies are provided consistent with the nature of the problem(s) and the patient's and/or family's needs.

Usually, the problem(s) requiring admission are of moderate severity. Physicians typically spend 50 minutes at the bedside and on the patient's hospital floor or unit.

Examples

Hospital admission, young adult patient, failed previous therapy and now presents in acute asthmatic attack. (Family Medicine/Allergy & Immunology)

Hospital admission of a 62-year-old smoker, established patient, with bronchitis in acute respiratory distress. (Internal Medicine/Pulmonary Medicine)

Hospital admission, examination, and initiation of a treatment program for a 65-year-old female with new onset of right-sided paralysis and aphasia. (Neurology)

Hospital admission for a 50-year-old with left lower quadrant abdominal pain and increased temperature, but without septic picture. (General Surgery)

Hospital admission, examination, and initiation of treatment program for a 66-year-old chronic hemodialysis patient with fever and a new pulmonary infiltrate. (Nephrology)

Hospital admission for a 3-year-old with high temperature, limp and painful hip motion of 18 hours duration. (Orthopaedic Surgery)

Hospital admission for an 8-year-old febrile patient with chronic sinusitis and severe headache, unresponsive to oral antibiotics. (Allergy & Immunology)

Hospital admission for a 40-year-old male with submaxillary cellulitis and trismus from infected lower molar. (Oral & Maxillofacial Surgery)

99223 **Initial hospital care,** per day, for the evaluation and management of a patient, which requires these three key components:

- **a comprehensive history;**
- **a comprehensive examination; and**
- **medical decision making of high complexity.**

Counseling and/or coordination of care with other providers or agencies are provided consistent with the nature of the problem(s) and the patient's and/or family's needs.

Usually, the problem(s) requiring admission are of high severity. Physicians typically spend 70 minutes at the bedside and on the patient's hospital floor or unit.

Examples

Hospital admission, examination, and initiation of treatment program for a previously unknown 58-year-old male who presents with acute chest pain. (Cardiology)

Hospital admission, examination, and initiation of induction chemotherapy for a 42-year-old patient with newly diagnosed acute myelogenous leukemia. (Hematology/Oncology)

Hospital admission following a motor vehicle accident of a 24-year-old male with fracture dislocation of C5-6; neurologically intact. (Neurosurgery)

Hospital admission for a 78-year-old female with left lower lobe pneumonia and a history of coronary artery disease, congestive heart failure, osteoarthritis and gout. (Family Medicine)

Hospital admission, examination, and initiation of treatment program for a 65-year-old immunosuppressed male with confusion, fever, and a headache. (Infectious Disease)

Hospital admission for a 9-year-old with vomiting, dehydration, fever, tachypnea and an admitting diagnosis of diabetic ketoacidosis. (Pediatrics)

Initial hospital visit for a 65-year-old male who presents with acute myocardial infarction, oliguria, hypotension, and altered state of consciousness. (Cardiology)

Initial hospital visit for a hostile/resistant adolescent patient who is severely depressed and involved in poly-substance abuse. Patient is experiencing significant conflict in his chaotic family situation and was suspended from school following an attack on a teacher with a baseball bat. (Psychiatry)

Initial hospital visit for 89-year-old female with fulminant hepatic failure and encephalopathy. (Gastroenterology)

Initial hospital visit for a 42-year-old female with rapidly progressing scleroderma, malignant hypertension, digital infarcts, and oligourea. (Rheumatology)

Subsequent Hospital Care

All levels of subsequent hospital care include reviewing the medical record and reviewing the results of diagnostic studies and changes in the patient's status, (ie, changes in history, physical condition and response to management) since the last assessment by the physician.

99231 **Subsequent hospital care,** per day, for the evaluation and management of a patient, which requires at least two of these three key components:

- **a problem focused interval history;**
- **a problem focused examination;**
- **medical decision making that is straightforward or of low complexity.**

Counseling and/or coordination of care with other providers or agencies are provided consistent with the nature of the problem(s) and the patient's and/or family's needs.

Usually, the patient is stable, recovering or improving. Physicians typically spend 15 minutes at the bedside and on the patient's hospital floor or unit.

Examples

Subsequent hospital visit for a 50-year-old male with uncomplicated myocardial infarction who is clinically stable and without chest pain. (Family Medicine/Cardiology/Internal Medicine)

Subsequent hospital visit for a stable 72-year-old lung cancer patient undergoing a five day course of infusion chemotherapy. (Hematology/Oncology)

Subsequent hospital visit, two days post admission for a 65-year-old male with a CVA (cerebral vascular accident) and left hemiparesis, who is clinically stable. (Neurology/Physical Medicine and Rehabilitation)

Subsequent hospital visit for now stable, 33-year-old male, status post lower gastrointestinal bleeding. (General Surgery)

Subsequent visit on third day of hospitalization for a 60-year-old female recovering from an uncomplicated pneumonia. (Infectious Disease/Internal Medicine/Pulmonary Medicine)

Subsequent hospital visit for a 3-year-old patient in traction for a congenital dislocation of the hip. (Orthopaedic Surgery)

Subsequent hospital visit for a 4-year-old female, admitted for acute gastroenteritis and dehydration, requiring IV hydration; now stable. (Family Medicine/Internal Medicine)

Subsequent hospital visit for 50-year-old female with resolving uncomplicated acute pancreatitis. (Gastroenterology)

99232 **Subsequent hospital care,** per day, for the evaluation and management of a patient, which requires at least two of these three key components:

- **an expanded problem focused interval history;**
- **an expanded problem focused examination;**
- **medical decision making of moderate complexity.**

Counseling and/or coordination of care with other providers or agencies are provided consistent with the nature of the problem(s) and the patient's and/or family's needs.

Usually, the patient is responding inadequately to therapy or has developed a minor complication. Physicians typically spend 25 minutes at the bedside and on the patient's hospital floor or unit.

Examples

Subsequent hospital visit for a 54-year-old patient, post MI (myocardial infarction), who is out of the CCU (coronary care unit) but is now having frequent premature ventricular contractions on telemetry. (Cardiology/Internal Medicine)

Subsequent hospital visit for a patient with neutropenia, a fever responding to antibiotics, and continued slow gastrointestinal bleeding on platelet support. (Hematology/Oncology)

Subsequent hospital visit for a 50-year-old male admitted two days ago for sub-acute renal allograft rejection. (Nephrology)

Subsequent hospital visit for a 35-year-old drug addict, not responding to initial antibiotic therapy for pyelonephritis. (Urology)

Subsequent hospital visit of an 81-year-old male with abdominal distention, nausea, and vomiting. (General Surgery)

Subsequent hospital care for a 62-year-old female with congestive heart failure, who remains dyspneic and febrile. (Internal Medicine)

Subsequent hospital visit for a 73-year-old female with recently diagnosed lung cancer, who complains of unsteady gait. (Pulmonary Medicine)

Subsequent hospital visit for a 20-month-old male with bacterial meningitis treated 1 week with antibiotic therapy; has now developed a temperature of 101.0. (Pediatrics)

Subsequent hospital visit for 13-year-old male admitted with left lower quadrant abdominal pain and fever, not responding to therapy. (General Surgery)

Subsequent hospital visit for a 65-year-old male with hemiplegia and painful paretic shoulder. (Physical Medicine & Rehabilitation)

99233 **Subsequent hospital care,** per day, for the evaluation and management of a patient, which requires at least two of these three key components:

- **a detailed interval history;**
- **a detailed examination;**
- **medical decision making of high complexity.**

Counseling and/or coordination of care with other providers or agencies are provided consistent with the nature of the problem(s) and the patient's and/or family's needs.

Usually, the patient is unstable or has developed a significant complication or a significant new problem. Physicians typically spend 35 minutes at the bedside and on the patient's hospital floor or unit.

Examples

Subsequent hospital visit for a 60-year-old female, 4 days post uncomplicated inferior myocardial infarction who has developed severe chest pain, dyspnea, diaphoresis and nausea. (Family Medicine)

Subsequent hospital visit for a patient with AML (acute myelogenous leukemia), fever, elevated white count and uric acid undergoing induction chemotherapy. (Hematology/Oncology)

Subsequent hospital visit for a 38-year-old quadriplegic male with acute autonomic hyperreflexia, who is not responsive to initial care. (Physical Medicine & Rehabilitation)

Subsequent hospital visit for a 65-year-old female post-op resection of abdominal aortic aneurysm, with suspected ischemic bowel. (General Surgery)

Subsequent hospital visit for a 60-year-old female with persistent leukocytosis and a fever seven days after a sigmoid colon resection for carcinoma. (Infectious Disease)

Subsequent hospital visit for a chronic renal failure patient on dialysis, who develops chest pain, shortness of breath and new onset of pericardial friction rub. (Nephrology)

Subsequent hospital visit for a 65-year-old male with acute myocardial infarction who now demonstrates complete heart block and congestive heart failure. (Cardiology)

Subsequent hospital visit for a 25-year-old female with hypertension and systemic lupus erythematosus, admitted for fever and respiratory distress. On the third hospital day, the patient presented with purpuric skin lesions and acute renal failure. (Allergy & Immunology)

Subsequent hospital visit for a 55-year-old male with severe chronic obstructive pulmonary disease and bronchospasm; initially admitted for acute respiratory distress requiring ventilatory support in the ICU. The patient was stabilized, extubated and transferred to the floor, but has now developed acute fever, dyspnea, left lower lobe rhonchi and laboratory evidence of carbon dioxide retention and hypoxemia. (Family Medicine/Internal Medicine)

Subsequent hospital visit for 46-year-old female, known liver cirrhosis patient, with recent upper gastrointestinal hemorrhage from varices; now with worsening ascites and encephalopathy. (Gastroenterology)

Subsequent hospital visit for 62-year-old female admitted with acute subarachnoid hemorrhage, negative cerebral arteriogram, increased lethargy and hemiparesis with fever. (Neurosurgery)

Hospital Discharge Services

The hospital discharge day management codes are to be used to report the total duration of time spent by a physician for final hospital discharge of a patient. The codes include, as appropriate, final examination of the patient, discussion of the hospital stay, even if the time spent by the physician on that date is not continuous. Instructions for continuing care to all relevant caregivers, and preparation of discharge records, prescriptions and referral forms.

▲**99238** **Hospital discharge day management;** 30 minutes or less

●**99239**   more than 30 minutes

(These codes are to be utilized by the physician to report all services provided to a patient on the date of discharge, if other than the initial date of inpatient status. To report services to a patient who is admitted as an inpatient, and discharged on the same date, use only the codes for Initial Hospital Inpatient Services, 99221-99223. To report concurrent care services provided by a physician(s) other than the attending physician, use subsequent hospital care codes (99231-99233) on the day of discharge.)

(For Observation Care Discharge, use 99217)

(For discharge services provided to newborns admitted and discharged on the same date, see 99435)

Consultations

A consultation is a type of service provided by a physician whose opinion or advice regarding evaluation and/or management of a specific problem is requested by another physician or other appropriate source.

A physician consultant may initiate diagnostic and/or therapeutic services.

The request for a consultation from the attending physician or other appropriate source and the need for consultation must be documented in the patient's medical record. The consultant's opinion and any services that were ordered or performed must also be documented in the patient's medical record and communicated to the requesting physician or other appropriate source.

A "consultation" initiated by a patient and/or family, and not requested by a physician, is not reported using the initial consultation codes but may be reported using the codes for confirmatory consultation or office visits, as appropriate. If a confirmatory consultation is required, eg, by a third party payor, the modifier '-32' or 09932, mandated services, should also be reported.

Any specifically identifiable procedure (ie, identified with a specific CPT code) performed on or subsequent to the date of the initial consultation should be reported separately.

If subsequent to the completion of a consultation, the consultant assumes responsibility for management of a portion or all of the patient's condition(s), the follow-up consultation codes should not be used. In the hospital setting, the physician receiving the patient for partial or complete transfer of care should use the appropriate inpatient hospital consultation code for the initial encounter and then subsequent hospital care codes (not follow-up consultation codes). In the office setting, the appropriate established patient code should be used.

There are four subcategories of consultations: office, initial inpatient, follow-up inpatient, and confirmatory. See each subcategory for specific reporting instructions.

For definitions of key components and commonly used terms, please see **Evaluation and Management Services Guidelines.**

Office or Other Outpatient Consultations

New or Established Patient

The following codes are used to report consultations provided in the physician's office or in an outpatient or other ambulatory facility, including hospital observation services, home services, domiciliary, rest home, custodial care, or emergency department (See consultation definition, page 18).

Follow-up visits in the consultant's office or other outpatient facility that are initiated by the physician consultant are reported using office visit codes for established patients (99211-99215). If an additional request for an opinion or advice regarding the same or a new problem is received from the attending physician and documented in the medical record, the office consultation codes may be used again.

99241 **Office consultation** for a new or established patient, which requires these three key components:

- **a problem focused history;**
- **a problem focused examination; and**
- **straightforward medical decision making.**

Counseling and/or coordination of care with other providers or agencies are provided consistent with the nature of the problem(s) and the patient's and/or family's needs.

Usually, the presenting problem(s) are self limited or minor. Physicians typically spend 15 minutes face-to-face with the patient and/or family.

Examples

Office consultation with 25-year-old postpartum female with severe symptomatic hemorrhoids. (Colon & Rectal Surgery)

Office consultation with 58-year-old male, referred for follow-up of creatinine level and evaluation of obstructive uropathy, relieved two months ago. (Nephrology)

Office consultation for 30-year-old female tennis player with sprain or contusion of the forearm. (Orthopaedic Surgery)

Office consultation for a 45-year-old male, requested by his internist, with asymptomatic torus palatinus requiring no further treatment. (Oral & Maxillofacial Surgery)

99242 **Office consultation** for a new or established patient, which requires these three key components:

- **an expanded problem focused history;**
- **an expanded problem focused examination; and**
- **straightforward medical decision making.**

Counseling and/or coordination of care with other providers or agencies are provided consistent with the nature of the problem(s) and the patient(s) and/or family's needs.

Usually, the presenting problem(s) are of low severity. Physicians typically spend 30 minutes face-to-face with the patient and/or family.

Examples

Office consultation for management of systolic hypertension in a 70-year-old male scheduled for elective prostate resection. (Geriatrics)

Office consultation with 27-year-old female, with old amputation, for evaluation of existing above-knee prosthesis. (Physical Medicine & Rehabilitation)

Office consultation with 66-year-old female with wrist and hand pain, and finger numbness, secondary to suspected carpal tunnel syndrome. (Orthopaedic Surgery)

Office consultation for 61-year-old female, recently on antibiotic therapy, now with diarrhea and leukocytosis. (Abdominal Surgery)

Office consultation for a patient with papulosquamous eruption of elbow with pitting of nails and itchy scalp. (Dermatology)

Office consultation for a 30-year-old female with single season allergic rhinitis. (Allergy & Immunology)

99243 **Office consultation** for a new or established patient, which requires these three key components:

- **a detailed history;**
- **a detailed examination; and**
- **medical decision making of low complexity.**

Counseling and/or coordination of care with other providers or agencies are provided consistent with the nature of the problem(s) and the patient's and/or family's needs.

Usually, the presenting problem(s) are of moderate severity. Physicians typically spend 40 minutes face-to-face with the patient and/or family.

Examples

Office consultation for a 65-year-old female with persistent bronchitis. (Infectious Disease)

Office consultation for a 65-year-old man with chronic low-back pain radiating to the leg. (Neurosurgery)

Office consultation for 23-year-old female with Crohn's disease not responding to therapy. (Abdominal Surgery/ Colon & Rectal Surgery)

Office consultation for 25-year-old patient with symptomatic knee pain and swelling, with torn anterior cruciate ligament and/or torn meniscus. (Orthopaedic Surgery)

Office consultation for a 67-year-old patient with osteoporosis and mandibular atrophy with regard to reconstructive alternatives. (Oral & Maxillofacial Surgery)

Office consultation for 39-year-old patient referred at a perimenopausal age for irregular menses and menopausal symptoms. (Obstetrics & Gynecology)

99244 **Office consultation** for a new or established patient, which requires these three key components:

- **a comprehensive history;**
- **a comprehensive examination; and**
- **medical decision making of moderate complexity.**

Counseling and/or coordination of care with other providers or agencies are provided consistent with the nature of the problem(s) and the patient's and/or family's needs.

Usually, the presenting problem(s) are of moderate to high severity. Physicians typically spend 60 minutes face-to-face with the patient and/or family.

Examples

Office consultation with 38-year-old female, with inflammatory bowel disease, who now presents with right lower quadrant pain and suspected intra-abdominal abscess. (General Surgery/Colon & Rectal Surgery)

Office consultation with 72-year-old male with esophageal carcinoma, symptoms of dysphagia and reflux. (Thoracic Surgery)

Office consultation for discussion of treatment options for a 40-year-old female with a two-centimeter adenocarcinoma of the breast. (Radiation Oncology)

Office consultation for young patient referred by pediatrician because of patient's short attention span, easy distractibility and hyperactivity. (Psychiatry)

Office consultation for 66-year-old female, history of colon resection for adenocarcinoma 6 years earlier, now with severe mid-back pain; x-rays showing osteoporosis and multiple vertebral compression fractures. (Neurosurgery)

Office consultation for a patient with chronic pelvic inflammatory disease who now has left lower quadrant pain with a palpable pelvic mass. (Obstetrics & Gynecology)

Office consultation for a patient with long-standing psoriasis with acute onset of erythroderma, pustular lesions, chills and fever. Combinations of topical and systemic treatments discussed and instituted. (Dermatology)

99245 **Office consultation** for a new or established patient, which requires these three key components:

- **a comprehensive history;**
- **a comprehensive examination; and**
- **medical decision making of high complexity.**

Counseling and/or coordination of care with other providers or agencies are provided consistent with the nature of the problem(s) and the patient's and/or family's needs.

Usually, the presenting problem(s) are of moderate to high severity. Physicians typically spend 80 minutes face-to-face with the patient and/or family.

Examples

Office consultation in the emergency room for a 25-year-old male with severe, acute, closed head injury. (Neurosurgery)

Office consultation for a 23-year-old female with Stage II A Hodgkins disease with positive supraclavicular and mediastinal nodes. (Radiation Oncology)

Office consultation for a 27-year-old juvenile diabetic patient with severe diabetic retinopathy, gastric atony, nephrotic syndrome and progressive renal failure, now with a serum creatinine of 2.7, and a blood pressure of 170/114. (Nephrology)

Office consultation for independent medical evaluation of a patient with a history of complicated low back and neck problems with previous multiple failed back surgeries. (Orthopaedic Surgery)

Office consultation for adolescent referred by pediatrician for recent onset of violent and self-injurious behavior. (Psychiatry)

Office consultation for a 6-year-old male for evaluation of severe muscle and joint pain and a diffuse rash. Well until 4-6 weeks earlier when he developed arthralgia, myalgias, and a fever of 102° for 1 week. (Rheumatology)

Initial Inpatient Consultations

New or Established Patient

The following codes are used to report physician consultations provided to hospital inpatients, residents of nursing facilities, or patients in a partial hospital setting. Only one initial consultation should be reported by a consultant per admission.

99251   Initial inpatient consultation for a new or established patient, which requires these three key components:

- **a problem focused history;**
- **a problem focused examination; and**
- **straightforward medical decision making.**

Counseling and/or coordination of care with other providers or agencies are provided consistent with the nature of the problem(s) and the patient's and/or family's needs.

Usually, the presenting problem(s) are self limited or minor. Physicians typically spend 20 minutes at the bedside and on the patient's hospital floor or unit.

Examples

Initial inpatient consultation for a 30-year-old female complaining of vaginal itching, post orthopaedic surgery. (Obstetrics & Gynecology)

Initial inpatient consultation for a 36-year-old male on orthopaedic service with complaint of localized dental pain. (Oral & Maxillofacial Surgery)

99252   Initial inpatient consultation for a new or established patient, which requires these three key components:

- **an expanded problem focused history;**
- **an expanded problem focused examination; and**
- **straightforward medical decision making.**

Counseling and/or coordination of care with other providers or agencies are provided consistent with the nature of the problem(s) and the patient's and/or family's needs.

Usually, the presenting problem(s) are of low severity. Physicians typically spend 40 minutes at the bedside and on the patient's hospital floor or unit.

Examples

Initial inpatient consultation for recommendation of antibiotic prophylaxis for a patient with a synthetic heart valve who will undergo urologic surgery. (Internal Medicine)

Initial inpatient consultation for possible drug eruption in 50-year-old male. (Dermatology)

Preoperative inpatient consultation for evaluation of hypertension in a 60-year-old male who will undergo a cholecystectomy. Patient had a normal annual check-up in your office four months ago. (Internal Medicine)

Initial inpatient consultation for 66-year-old patient with wrist and hand pain and finger numbness, secondary to carpal tunnel syndrome. (Orthopaedic Surgery/Plastic Surgery)

Initial inpatient consultation for a 66-year-old male smoker referred for pain management immediately status post-biliary tract surgery done via sub-costal incision. (Anesthesiology/Pain Medicine)

Initial inpatient consultation for a 45-year-old male previously abstinent alcoholic, who relapsed and was admitted for management of gastritis. The patient readily accepts the need for further treatment. (Addiction Medicine)

99253   Initial inpatient consultation for a new or established patient, which requires these three key components:

- **a detailed history;**
- **a detailed examination; and**
- **medical decision making of low complexity.**

Counseling and/or coordination of care with other providers or agencies are provided consistent with the nature of the problem(s) and the patient's and/or family's needs.

Usually, the presenting problem(s) are of moderate severity. Physicians typically spend 55 minutes at the bedside and on the patient's hospital floor or unit.

Examples

Initial inpatient consultation for a 57-year-old male, post lower endoscopy, for evaluation of abdominal pain and fever. (General Surgery)

Initial inpatient consultation for rehabilitation of a 73-year-old female one week after surgical management of a hip fracture. (Physical Medicine & Rehabilitation)

Initial inpatient consultation for diagnosis/management of fever following abdominal surgery. (Internal Medicine)

Initial inpatient consultation for a 35-year-old female with a fever and pulmonary infiltrate following cesarean section. (Pulmonary Medicine)

Initial inpatient consultation for a 42-year-old non-diabetic patient, post-op cholecystectomy, now with an acute urinary tract infection. (Nephrology)

Initial inpatient consultation for 53-year-old female with moderate uncomplicated pancreatitis. (Gastroenterology)

Initial inpatient consultation for 45-year-old patient with chronic neck pain with radicular pain of the left arm. (Orthopaedic Surgery)

Initial inpatient consultation for 8-year-old patient with new onset of seizures who has a normal examination and previous history. (Neurology)

99254 **Initial inpatient consultation** for a new or established patient, which requires three key components:

- **a comprehensive history;**
- **a comprehensive examination; and**
- **medical decision making of moderate complexity.**

Counseling and/or coordination of care with other providers or agencies are provided consistent with the nature of the problem(s) and the patient's and/or family's needs.

Usually, the presenting problem(s) are of moderate to high severity. Physicians typically spend 80 minutes at the bedside and on the patient's hospital floor or unit.

Examples

Initial inpatient consultation for evaluation of a 63-year-old in the ICU with diabetes and chronic renal failure who develops acute respiratory distress syndrome 36 hours after a mitral valve replacement. (Anesthesiology)

Initial inpatient consultation for a 66-year-old female with enlarged supraclavicular lymph nodes, found on biopsy to be malignant. (Hematology/Oncology)

Initial inpatient consultation for a 43-year-old female for evaluation of sudden painful visual loss, optic neuritis and episodic paresthesia. (Ophthalmology)

Initial inpatient consultation for evaluation of a 71-year-old male with hyponatremia (serum sodium 114) who was admitted to the hospital with pneumonia. (Nephrology)

Initial inpatient consultation for a 72-year-old male with emergency admission for possible bowel obstruction. (Internal Medicine/General Surgery)

Initial inpatient consultation for a 35-year-old female with fever, swollen joints, and rash of 1 week duration. (Rheumatology)

99255 **Initial inpatient consultation** for a new or established patient, which requires these three key components:

- **a comprehensive history;**
- **a comprehensive examination; and**
- **medical decision making of high complexity.**

Counseling and/or coordination of care with other providers or agencies are provided consistent with the nature of the problem(s) and the patient's and/or family's needs.

Usually, the presenting problem(s) are of moderate to high severity. Physicians typically spend 110 minutes at the bedside and on the patient's hospital floor or unit.

Examples

Initial inpatient consultation in the ICU for a 70-year-old male who experienced a cardiac arrest during surgery and was resuscitated. (Cardiology)

Initial inpatient consultation for a patient with severe pancreatitis complicated by respiratory insufficiency, acute renal failure and abscess formation. (Gastroenterology)

Initial inpatient consultation for a 70-year-old cirrhotic male admitted with ascites, jaundice, encephalopathy, and massive hematemesis. (Gastroenterology)

Initial inpatient consultation in the ICU for a 51-year-old patient who is on a ventilator and has a fever two weeks after a renal transplantation. (Infectious Disease)

Initial inpatient consultation for evaluation and formulation of plan for management of multiple trauma patient with complex pelvic fracture, 35-year-old male. (General Surgery/Orthopaedic Surgery)

Initial inpatient consultation for a 50-year-old male with a history of previous myocardial infarction, now with acute pulmonary edema and hypotension. (Cardiology)

Initial inpatient consultation for 45-year-old male with recent, acute subarachnoid hemorrhage, hesitant speech, mildly confused, drowsy. High risk group for HIV+ status. (Neurosurgery)

Initial inpatient consultation for 36-year-old female referred by her internist to evaluate a patient being followed for abdominal pain and fever. The patient has developed diffuse abdominal pain, guarding, rigidity and increased fever. (Obstetrics & Gynecology)

Follow-Up Inpatient Consultations

Established Patient

Follow-up consultations are visits to complete the initial consultation OR subsequent consultative visits requested by the attending physician.

A follow-up consultation includes monitoring progress, recommending management modifications or advising on a new plan of care in response to changes in the patient's status.

If the physician consultant has initiated treatment at the initial consultation, and participates thereafter in the patient's management, the codes for subsequent hospital care should be used (99231-99233).

The following codes are used to report follow-up consultations provided to hospital inpatients or nursing facility residents only. For consultative services provided in other settings, the codes for office or other outpatient consultations should be reported (99241-99245).

99261   Follow-up inpatient consultation for an established patient, which requires at least two of these three key components:

- **a problem focused interval history;**
- **a problem focused examination;**
- **medical decision making that is straightforward or of low complexity.**

Counseling and/or coordination of care with other providers or agencies are provided consistent with nature of the problem(s) and the patient's and/or family's needs.

Usually, the patient is stable, recovering or improving. Physicians typically spend 10 minutes at the bedside and on the patient's hospital floor or unit.

Examples

Follow-up inpatient consultation with 35-year-old female with pulmonary embolism post-op cesarean section, now stable, for assessment of response to anticoagulation and recommended adjustment of heparin dose. (Pulmonary Medicine)

Follow-up inpatient consultation for a 74-year-old male whose postoperative facial paralysis after a cholecystectomy is now resolving. (Neurology)

Follow-up inpatient consultation with 67-year-old female, established patient for review of diagnostic studies ordered at time of first contact. (Internal Medicine)

Follow-up inpatient consultation for 78-year-old female nursing home resident for evaluation of medical management of pruritis ani. (General Surgery/Colon & Rectal Surgery)

Follow-up inpatient consultation for a 36-year-old female 2 days after spontaneous passage of 3mm stone. (Urology)

Follow-up inpatient consultation for a 94-year-old male nursing home resident for re-evaluation of hemorrhoids following conservative therapy. (Colon & Rectal Surgery/General Surgery/Geriatrics)

Follow-up inpatient consultation for a 50-year-old male, asymptomatic with borderline ECG abnormality, needs preoperative opinion after a thallium exercise perfusion scan. (Cardiology)

99262   Follow-up inpatient consultation for an established patient which requires at least two of these three key components:

- **an expanded problem focused interval history;**
- **an expanded problem focused examination;**
- **medical decision making of moderate complexity.**

Counseling and/or coordination of care with other providers or agencies are provided consistent with the nature of the problem(s) and the patient's and/or family's needs.

Usually, the patient is responding inadequately to therapy or has developed a minor complication. Physicians typically spend 20 minutes at the bedside and on the patient's hospital floor or unit.

Examples

Follow-up inpatient consultation with 72-year-old female, established patient with bullous pemphigoid on combined oral therapy steroids and immunosuppressive to evaluate progress of cutaneous care orders and adjustment of oral/parenteral therapy dosages. (Dermatology)

Follow-up inpatient consultation for a 71-year-old male who has developed a maculopapular skin rash while on antibiotics that you recommended for an uncomplicated pneumonia. (Infectious Disease)

Follow-up inpatient consultation with 68-year-old, incapacitated male, with spinal stenosis and failure to respond to bedrest, analgesics, and PT. (Neurosurgery)

Follow-up inpatient consultation with 51-year-old male, for evaluation and determination of the etiology of postoperative hyponatremia following TURP. (Family Medicine)

Follow-up inpatient consultation for reevaluation of a stroke patient, and development of plan for initial rehabilitation services. (Neurology)

Follow-up inpatient consultation with 45-year-old male, established patient for discussion of CT scan which demonstrates a cavernous hemangioma. (Ophthalmology)

Follow-up inpatient consultation for an asymptomatic 35-year-old Type I diabetic patient with hyperkalemic, hyperchloremia acidosis, to review lab results. (Nephrology)

Follow-up inpatient consultation for an elderly male with a perioperative myocardial infarction requiring adjustment of vasoactive medications. (Anesthesiology)

99263 **Follow-up inpatient consultation** for an established patient which requires at least two of these three key components:

- **a detailed interval history;**
- **a detailed examination;**
- **medical decision making of high complexity.**

Counseling and/or coordination of care with other providers or agencies are provided consistent with the nature of the problem(s) and the patient's and/or family's needs.

Usually, the patient is unstable or has developed a significant complication or a significant new problem. Physicians typically spend 30 minutes at the bedside and on the patient's hospital floor or unit.

Examples

Follow-up inpatient consultation with 72-year-old male established patient admitted for management of alcohol withdrawal, now confused and febrile. (Addiction Medicine)

Follow-up inpatient consultation for an HIV-positive patient with an increasing fever following ten days of antibiotic therapy for pneumocystis carinii pneumonia. (Infectious Disease)

Follow-up inpatient consultation with 58-year-old diabetic female, with bacterial endocarditis, continued fever after 2 weeks of intravenous antibiotic therapy, and new onset ventricular ectopia. (Cardiology)

Follow-up inpatient consultation for a 90-year-old female with urinary incontinence who has a complicated medical history requiring reassessment of multiple medical problems, recommendations for placement, further recommendation for management of incontinence and reevaluation of cognitive status because of competency issues. (Geriatrics/Psychiatry)

Follow-up inpatient consultation for 42-year-old male with persistent gastrointestinal bleeding, etiology undetermined, not responding to conservative therapy of transfusions. (General Surgery/Colon & Rectal Surgery)

Follow-up inpatient consultation for a 62-year-old female with steroid-dependent asthma, diabetes mellitus, thyrotoxicosis, abdominal pain and possible vasculitis. (Rheumatology)

Follow-up inpatient consultation for a 62-year-old male, status post-op acute small bowel obstruction; now with acute renal failure. (Family Medicine)

Confirmatory Consultations

New or Established Patient

The following codes are used to report the evaluation and management services provided to patients when the consulting physician is aware of the confirmatory nature of the opinion sought (eg, when a second/third opinion is requested or required on the necessity or appropriateness of a previously recommended medical treatment or surgical procedure).

Confirmatory consultations may be provided in any setting.

A physician consultant providing a confirmatory consultation is expected to provide an opinion and/or advice only. Any services subsequent to the opinion are coded at the appropriate level of office visit, established patient, or subsequent hospital care. If a confirmatory consultation is required, eg, by a third party payor, the modifier '-32' or 09932, mandated services, should also be reported.

(See also Consultation notes, page 18).

Typical times have not yet been established for this subcategory of services.

99271 **Confirmatory consultation** for a new or established patient, which requires these three key components:

- **a problem focused history;**
- **a problem focused examination; and**
- **straightforward medical decision making.**

Counseling and/or coordination of care with other providers or agencies are provided consistent with the nature of the problem(s) and the patient's and/or family's needs.

Usually, the presenting problem(s) are self limited or minor.

99272 **Confirmatory consultation** for a new or established patient, which requires these three key components:

- **an expanded problem focused history;**
- **an expanded problem focused examination; and**
- **straightforward medical decision making.**

Counseling and/or coordination of care with other providers or agencies are provided consistent with the nature of the problem(s) and the patient's and/or family's needs.

Usually, the presenting problem(s) are of low severity.

99273 **Confirmatory consultation** for a new or established patient, which requires these three key components:

- **a detailed history;**
- **a detailed examination; and**
- **medical decision making of low complexity.**

Counseling and/or coordination of care with other providers or agencies are provided consistent with the nature of the problem(s) and the patient's and/or family's needs.

Usually, the presenting problem(s) are of moderate severity.

99274 **Confirmatory consultation** for a patient, which requires these three key components:

- **a comprehensive history;**
- **a comprehensive examination; and**
- **medical decision making of moderate complexity.**

Counseling and/or coordination of care with other providers or agencies are provided consistent with the nature of the problem(s) and the patient's and/or family's needs.

Usually, the presenting problem(s) are of moderate to high severity.

99275 **Confirmatory consultation** for a patient, which requires these three key components:

- **a comprehensive history;**
- **a comprehensive examination; and**
- **medical decision making of high complexity.**

Counseling and/or coordination of care with other providers or agencies are provided consistent with the nature of the problem(s) and the patient's and/or family's needs.

Usually, the presenting problem(s) are of moderate to high severity.

Emergency Department Services

New or Established Patient

The following codes are used to report evaluation and management services provided in the emergency department. No distinction is made between new and established patients in the emergency department.

An emergency department is defined as an organized hospital-based facility for the provision of unscheduled episodic services to patients who present for immediate medical attention. The facility must be available 24 hours a day.

For critical care services provided in the Emergency Department, see Critical Care notes and 99291, 99292.

For evaluation and management services provided to a patient in an observation area of a hospital, see 99217-99220.

For definitions of key components and commonly used terms, see **Evaluation and Management Services Guidelines.**

99281 **Emergency department visit** for the evaluation and management of a patient, which requires these three key components:

- **a problem focused history;**
- **a problem focused examination; and**
- **straightforward medical decision making.**

Counseling and/or coordination of care with other providers or agencies are provided consistent with the nature of the problem(s) and the patient's and/or family's needs.

Usually, the presenting problem(s) are self limited or minor.

Examples

Emergency department visit for a patient for removal of sutures from a well-healed, uncomplicated laceration. (Emergency Medicine)

Emergency department visit for a patient for tetanus toxoid immunization. (Emergency Medicine)

Emergency department visit for a patient with several uncomplicated insect bites. (Emergency Medicine)

99282   Emergency department visit for the evaluation and management of a patient, which requires these three key components:

- **an expanded problem focused history;**
- **an expanded problem focused examination; and**
- **medical decision making of low complexity.**

Counseling and/or coordination of care with other providers or agencies are provided consistent with the nature of the problem(s) and the patient's and/or family's needs.

Usually, the presenting problem(s) are of low to moderate severity.

Examples

Emergency department visit for a 20-year-old student who presents with a painful sunburn with blister formation on the back. (Emergency Medicine)

Emergency department visit for a child presenting with impetigo localized to the face. (Emergency Medicine)

Emergency department visit for a patient with a minor traumatic injury of an extremity with localized pain, swelling, and bruising. (Emergency Medicine)

Emergency department visit for an otherwise healthy patient whose chief complaint is a red, swollen cystic lesion on his/her back. (Emergency Medicine)

Emergency department visit for a patient presenting with a rash on both legs after exposure to poison ivy. (Emergency Medicine)

Emergency department visit for a young adult patient with infected sclera and purulent discharge from both eyes without pain, visual disturbance or history of foreign body in either eye. (Emergency Medicine)

99283   Emergency department visit for the evaluation and management of a patient, which requires these three key components:

- **an expanded problem focused history;**
- **an expanded problem focused examination; and**
- **medical decision making of moderate complexity.**

Counseling and/or coordination of care with other providers or agencies are provided consistent with the nature of the problem(s) and the patient's and/or family's needs.

Usually, the presenting problem(s) are of moderate severity.

Examples

Emergency department visit for a sexually active female complaining of vaginal discharge who is afebrile and denies experiencing abdominal or back pain. (Emergency Medicine)

Emergency department visit for a well-appearing 8-year-old child who has a fever, diarrhea and abdominal cramps, is tolerating oral fluids and is not vomiting. (Emergency Medicine)

Emergency department visit for a patient with an inversion ankle injury, who is unable to bear weight on the injured foot and ankle. (Emergency Medicine)

Emergency department visit for a patient who has a complaint of acute pain associated with a suspected foreign body in the painful eye. (Emergency Medicine)

Emergency department visit for a healthy, young adult patient who sustained a blunt head injury with local swelling and bruising without subsequent confusion, loss of consciousness or memory deficit. (Emergency Medicine)

99284   Emergency department visit for the evaluation and management of a patient, which requires these three key components:

- **a detailed history;**
- **a detailed examination; and**
- **medical decision making of moderate complexity.**

Counseling and/or coordination of care with other providers or agencies are provided consistent with the nature of the problem(s) and the patient's and/or family's needs.

Usually, the presenting problem(s) are of high severity, and require urgent evaluation by the physician but do not pose an immediate significant threat to life or physiologic function.

Examples

Emergency department visit for a 4-year-old child who fell off a bike sustaining a head injury with brief loss of consciousness. (Emergency Medicine)

Emergency department visit for an elderly female who has fallen and is now complaining of pain in her right hip and is unable to walk. (Emergency Medicine)

Emergency department visit for a patient with flank pain and hematuria. (Emergency Medicine)

Emergency department visit for a female presenting with lower abdominal pain and a vaginal discharge. (Emergency Medicine)

99285 **Emergency department visit** for the evaluation and management of a patient, which requires these three key components within the constraints imposed by the urgency of the patient's clinical condition and mental status:

- **a comprehensive history;**
- **a comprehensive examination; and**
- **medical decision making of high complexity.**

Counseling and/or coordination of care with other providers or agencies are provided consistent with the nature of the problem(s) and the patient's and/or family's needs.

Usually, the presenting problem(s) are of high severity and pose an immediate significant threat to life or physiologic function.

Examples

Emergency department visit for a patient with a complicated overdose requiring aggressive management to prevent side effects from the ingested materials. (Emergency Medicine)

Emergency department visit for a patient with a new onset of rapid heart rate requiring IV drugs. (Emergency Medicine)

Emergency department visit for a patient exhibiting active, upper gastrointestinal bleeding. (Emergency Medicine)

Emergency department visit for a previously healthy young adult patient who is injured in an automobile accident and is brought to the emergency department immobilized and has symptoms compatible with intra-abdominal injuries or multiple extremity injuries. (Emergency Medicine)

Emergency department visit for a patient with an acute onset of chest pain compatible with symptoms of cardiac ischemia and/or pulmonary embolus. (Emergency Medicine)

Emergency department visit for a patient who presents with a sudden onset of "the worst headache of her life," and complains of a stiff neck, nausea, and inability to concentrate. (Emergency Medicine)

Emergency department visit for a patient with a new onset of a cerebral vascular accident. (Emergency Medicine)

Emergency department visit for acute febrile illness in an adult, associated with shortness of breath and an altered level of alertness. (Emergency Medicine)

Other Emergency Services

In physician directed emergency care, advanced life support, the physician is located in a hospital emergency or critical care department, and is in two-way voice communication with ambulance or rescue personnel outside the hospital. The physician directs the performance of necessary medical procedures, including but not limited to: telemetry of cardiac rhythm; cardiac and/or pulmonary resuscitation; endotracheal or esophageal obturator airway intubation; administration of intravenous fluids and/or administration of intramuscular, intratracheal or subcutaneous drugs; and/or electrical conversion of arrhythmia.

99288 **Physician direction of** emergency medical systems (EMS) emergency care, advanced life support

Critical Care Services

Critical care is the care of the unstable critically ill or unstable critically injured patient who requires constant physician attendance (the physician need not be constantly at bedside per se but is engaged in physician work directly related to the individual patient's care). Critical care services are provided to but not limited to, patients with central nervous system failure, circulatory failure, shock-like conditions, renal, hepatic or respiratory failure, postoperative complications, or overwhelming infection. Critical care is usually, but not always, given in a critical care area, such as the coronary care unit, intensive care unit, respiratory care unit, or the emergency care facility.

Services for a patient who is not critically ill but happens to be in a critical care unit are reported using subsequent hospital care codes (see 99231-99233) or hospital consultation codes (see 99251-99263) as appropriate.

The following services are included in reporting critical care when performed during the critical period by the physician providing critical care: the interpretation of cardiac output measurements (93561, 93562), chest x-rays (71010, 71020), blood gases, and information data stored in computers (eg, ECGs, blood pressures, hematologic data (99090)); gastric intubation (91105); temporary transcutaneous pacing (92953); ventilator management (94656, 94657, 94660, 94662);

---

and vascular access procedures (36000, 36410, 36415, 36600). Any services performed which are not listed above should be reported separately.

The critical care codes are used to report the total duration of time spent by a physician providing constant attention to an unstable critically ill or unstable critically injured patient, even if the time spent by the physician providing critical care services on that date is not continuous. Code 99291 is used to report the first hour of critical care on a given date. It should be used only once per date even if the time spent by the physician is not continuous on that date. Critical care of less than 30 minutes total duration on a given date should be reported with the appropriate E/M code. Code 99292 is used to report each additional 30 minutes beyond the first hour. It also may be used to report the final 15-30 minutes of critical care on a given date. Critical care of less than 15 minutes beyond the first hour or less than 15 minutes beyond the final 30 minutes is not reported separately.

The following examples illustrate the correct reporting of critical care services:

Total Duration of Critical Care	Codes
less than 30 minutes (less than 1/2 hour)	99232 or 99233
30-74 minutes (1/2 hr. – 1 hr. 14 min.)	99291 X 1
75-104 minutes (1 hr. 15 min. – 1 hr. 44 min.)	99291 X 1 AND 99292 X 1
105-134 minutes (1 hr. 45 min. – 2 hr. 14 min.)	99291 X 1 AND 99292 X 2
135 - 164 minutes (2 hr. 15 min. – 2 hr. 44 min.)	99291 X 1 AND 99292 X 3
165 - 194 minutes (2 hr. 45 min. – 3 hr. 14 min.)	99291 X 1 AND 99292 X 4

▲**99291** **Critical care, evaluation and management** of the unstable critically ill or unstable critically injured patient, requiring the constant attendance of the physician; first hour

99292 each additional 30 minutes

Neonatal Intensive Care

The following codes (99295-99297) are used to report services provided by a physician directing the care of a neonate or infant in a neonatal intensive care unit (NICU). They represent care starting with the date of admission to the NICU and may be reported only once per day, per patient. Once the neonate is no longer considered to be critically ill, the codes for Subsequent Hospital Care (99231-99233) should be utilized.

These neonatal intensive care codes are to be used in addition to codes 99360 and 99440 when the physician is present for the delivery and newborn resuscitation is required.

Care rendered includes management; monitoring and treatment of the patient including enteral and parenteral nutritional maintenance, metabolic and hematologic maintenance; pharmacologic control of the circulatory system; parent counseling; case management services, and personal direct supervision of the health care team in the performance of cognitive and procedural activities.

The following procedures are also included as part of the global descriptors: umbilical, central or peripheral vessel catheterization, oral or nasogastric tube placement, endotracheal intubation, lumbar puncture, suprapubic bladder aspiration, bladder catheterization, initiation and management of mechanical ventilation or continuous positive airway pressure (CPAP), surfactant administration, intravascular fluid administration, transfusion of blood components, vascular punctures, invasive or non-invasive electronic monitoring of vital signs, bedside pulmonary function testing, and/or monitoring or interpretation of blood gases or oxygen saturation. Any services performed which are not listed above should be reported separately.

For additional instructions, see parenthetical descriptions listed for 99295-99297.

▲**99295** **Initial neonatal intensive care,** per day, for the evaluation and management of a critically ill neonate or infant

This code is reserved for the date of admission for neonates who are critically ill. Critically ill neonates require cardiac and/or respiratory support (including ventilator or nasal CPAP), continuous or frequent vital sign monitoring, laboratory and blood gas interpretations, follow-up physician reevaluations, and constant observation by the health care team under direct physician supervision. Immediate preoperative evaluation and stabilization of neonates with life threatening surgical or cardiac conditions are included under this code.

▲99296 **Subsequent neonatal intensive care,** per day, for the evaluation and management of a critically ill and unstable neonate or infant

A critically ill and unstable neonate will require cardiac and/or respiratory support (including ventilator or nasal CPAP), continuous or frequent vital sign monitoring, laboratory and blood gas interpretations, follow-up physician reevaluations throughout a 24 hour period, and constant observation by the health care team under direct physician supervision. In addition, most will require frequent ventilator changes, intravenous fluid alterations, and/or early initiation of parenteral nutrition. Neonates in the immediate post-operative period or those who become critically ill and unstable during the hospital stay will commonly qualify for this level of care.

This code encompasses intensive care provided on dates subsequent to the admission date.

▲99297 **Subsequent neonatal intensive care,** per day, for the evaluation and management of a critically ill though stable neonate or infant

Critically ill though stable neonates require cardiac and/or respiratory support (including ventilator and nasal CPAP), continuous or frequent vital sign monitoring, laboratory and blood gas interpretations, follow-up physician re-evaluations throughout a 24 hour period, and constant observation by the health care team under direct physician supervision. Neonates at this level of care would be expected to require less frequent changes in respiratory, cardiovascular and fluid and electrolyte therapy as those included under code 99296.

This code encompasses intensive care provided on dates subsequent to the admission date.

Nursing Facility Services

The following codes are used to report evaluation and management services to patients in Nursing Facilities (formerly called Skilled Nursing Facilities (SNFs), Intermediate Care Facilities (ICFs) or Long Term Care Facilities (LTCFs)).

These codes should also be used to report evaluation and management services provided to a patient in a psychiatric residential treatment center (a facility or a distinct part of a facility for psychiatric care, which provides a 24 hour therapeutically planned and professionally staffed group living and learning environment). If procedures such as medical psychotherapy are provided in addition to evaluation and management services, these should be reported in addition to the evaluation and management services provided.

Nursing facilities that provide convalescent, rehabilitative, or long term care are required to conduct comprehensive, accurate, standardized, and reproducible assessments of each resident's functional capacity using a Resident Assessment Instrument (RAI). All RAIs include the Minimum Data Set (MDS), Resident Assessment Protocols (RAPs) and utilization guidelines. The MDS is the primary screening and assessment tool; the RAPs trigger the identification of potential problems and provide guidelines for follow-up assessments.

Physicians have a central role in assuring that all residents receive thorough assessments and that medical plans of care are instituted or revised to enhance or maintain the residents' physical and psychosocial functioning.

Two subcategories of nursing facility services are recognized: Comprehensive Nursing Facility Assessments and Subsequent Nursing Facility Care. Both subcategories apply to new or established patients. Comprehensive Assessments may be performed at one or more sites in the assessment process: the hospital, observation unit, office, nursing facility, domiciliary/non-nursing facility or patient's home.

For definitions of key components and commonly used terms, please see **Evaluation and Management Services Guidelines.**

Comprehensive Nursing Facility Assessments

New or Established Patient

When the patient is admitted to the nursing facility in the course of an encounter in another site of service (eg, hospital emergency department, physician's office), all evaluation and management services provided by that physician in conjunction with that admission are considered part of the initial nursing facility care when performed as part of the admission. The nursing facility care level of service reported by the admitting physician should include the services related to the admission he/she provided in the other sites of service as well as in the nursing facility setting. With the exception of hospital discharge services, evaluation and management services on the same date provided in sites other than the nursing facility that are related to the admission should NOT be reported separately. Hospital discharge services may be reported separately.

More than one comprehensive assessment may be necessary during an inpatient confinement.

99301 **Evaluation and management** of a new or established patient involving an annual nursing facility assessment which requires these three key components:

- a detailed interval history;
- a comprehensive examination; and
- medical decision making that is straightforward or of low complexity.

Counseling and/or coordination of care with other providers or agencies are provided consistent with the nature of the problem(s) and the patient's and/or family's needs.

Usually, the patient is stable, recovering or improving. The review and affirmation of the medical plan of care is required. Physicians typically spend 30 minutes at the bedside and on the patient's facility floor or unit.

99302 **Evaluation and management** of a new or established patient involving a nursing facility assessment which requires these three key components:

- a detailed interval history;
- a comprehensive examination; and
- medical decision making of moderate to high complexity.

Counseling and/or coordination of care with other providers or agencies are provided consistent with the nature of the problem(s) and the patient's and/or family's needs.

Usually, the patient has developed a significant complication or a significant new problem and has had a major permanent change in status.

The creation of a new medical plan of care is required. Physicians typically spend 40 minutes at the bedside and on the patient's facility floor or unit.

99303 **Evaluation and management** of a new or established patient involving a nursing facility assessment at the time of initial admission or readmission to the facility, which requires these three key components:

- a comprehensive history;
- a comprehensive examination; and
- medical decision making of moderate to high complexity.

Counseling and/or coordination of care with other providers or agencies are provided consistent with the nature of the problem(s) and the patient's and/or family's needs.

The creation of a medical plan of care is required. Physicians typically spend 50 minutes at the bedside and on the patient's facility floor or unit.

Subsequent Nursing Facility Care

New or Established Patient

The following codes are used to report the services provided to residents of nursing facilities who do not require a comprehensive assessment, and/or who have not had a major, permanent change of status.

All levels include reviewing the medical record, noting changes in the resident's status since the last visit, and reviewing and signing orders.

99311 **Subsequent nursing facility care,** per day, for the evaluation and management of a new or established patient, which requires at least two of these three key components:

- **a problem focused interval history;**
- **a problem focused examination;**
- **medical decision making that is straightforward or of low complexity.**

Counseling and/or coordination of care with other providers or agencies are provided consistent with the nature of the problem(s) and the patient's and/or family's needs.

Usually, the patient is stable, recovering or improving. Physicians typically spend 15 minutes at the bedside and on the patient's facility floor or unit.

99312 **Subsequent nursing facility care,** per day, for the evaluation and management of a new or established patient, which requires at least two of these three key components:

- **an expanded problem focused interval history;**
- **an expanded problem focused examination;**
- **medical decision making of moderate complexity.**

Counseling and/or coordination of care with other providers or agencies are provided consistent with the nature of the problem(s) and the patient's and/or family's needs.

Usually, the patient is responding inadequately to therapy or has developed a minor complication. Physicians typically spend 25 minutes at the bedside and on the patient's facility floor or unit.

99313 **Subsequent nursing facility care,** per day, for the evaluation and management of a new or established patient, which requires at least two of these three key components:

- **a detailed interval history;**
- **a detailed examination;**
- **medical decision making of moderate to high complexity.**

Counseling and/or coordination of care with other providers or agencies are provided consistent with the nature of the problem(s) and the patient's and/or family's needs.

Usually, the patient has developed a significant complication or a significant new problem. Physicians typically spend 35 minutes at the bedside and on the patient's facility floor or unit.

Domiciliary, Rest Home (eg, Boarding Home), or Custodial Care Services

The following codes are used to report evaluation and management services in a facility which provides room, board and other personal assistance services, generally on a long-term basis. The facility's services do not include a medical component.

For definitions of key components and commonly used terms, please see **Evaluation and Management Services Guidelines.**

Typical times have not yet been established for this category of services.

New Patient

99321 **Domiciliary or rest home visit** for the evaluation and management of a new patient which requires these three key components:

- **a problem focused history;**
- **a problem focused examination; and**
- **medical decision making that is straightforward or of low complexity.**

Counseling and/or coordination of care with other providers or agencies are provided consistent with the nature of the problem(s) and the patient's and/or family's needs.

Usually, the presenting problem(s) are of low severity.

99322 **Domiciliary or rest home visit** for the evaluation and management of a new patient, which requires these three key components:

- **an expanded problem focused history;**
- **an expanded problem focused examination; and**
- **medical decision making of moderate complexity.**

Counseling and/or coordination of care with other providers or agencies are provided consistent with the nature of the problem(s) and the patient's and/or family's needs.

Usually, the presenting problem(s) are of moderate severity.

99323 **Domiciliary or rest home visit** for the evaluation and management of a new patient, which requires these three key components:

- **a detailed history;**
- **a detailed examination; and**
- **medical decision making of high complexity.**

Counseling and/or coordination of care with other providers or agencies are provided consistent with the nature of the problem(s) and the patient's and/or family's needs.

Usually, the presenting problem(s) are of high complexity.

Established Patient

99331 **Domiciliary or rest home visit** for the evaluation and management of an established patient, which requires at least two of these three key components:

- **a problem focused interval history;**
- **a problem focused examination;**
- **medical decision making that is straightforward or of low complexity.**

Counseling and/or coordination of care with other providers or agencies are provided consistent with the nature of the problem(s) and the patient's and/or family's needs.

Usually, the patient is stable, recovering or improving.

99332 **Domiciliary or rest home visit** for the evaluation and management of an established patient, which requires at least two of these three key components:

- **an expanded problem focused interval history;**
- **an expanded problem focused examination;**
- **medical decision making of moderate complexity.**

Counseling and/or coordination of care with other providers or agencies are provided consistent with the nature of the problem(s) and the patient's and/or family's needs.

Usually, the patient is responding inadequately to therapy or has developed a minor complication.

99333 **Domiciliary or rest home visit** for the evaluation and management of an established patient, which requires at least two of these three key components:

- **a detailed interval history;**
- **a detailed examination;**
- **medical decision making of high complexity.**

Counseling and/or coordination of care with other providers or agencies are provided consistent with the nature of the problem(s) and the patient's and/or family's needs.

Usually, the patient is unstable or has developed a significant complication or a significant new problem.

Home Services

The following codes are used to report evaluation and management services provided in a private residence.

For definitions of key components and commonly used terms, please see **Evaluation and Management Services Guidelines.**

Typical times have not yet been established for this category of services.

New Patient

99341 **Home visit** for the evaluation and management of a new patient, which requires these three key components:

- **a problem focused history;**
- **a problem focused examination; and**
- **medical decision making that is straightforward or of low complexity.**

Counseling and/or coordination of care with other providers or agencies are provided consistent with the nature of the problem(s) and the patient's and/or family's needs.

Usually, the presenting problem(s) are of low severity.

99342 **Home visit** for the evaluation and management of a new patient, which requires these three key components:

- **an expanded problem focused history;**
- **an expanded problem focused examination; and**
- **medical decision making of moderate complexity.**

Counseling and/or coordination of care with other providers or agencies are provided consistent with the nature of the problem(s) and the patient's and/or family's needs.

Usually, the presenting problem(s) are of moderate severity.

99343 **Home visit** for the evaluation and management of a new patient, which requires these three key components:

- **a detailed history;**
- **a detailed examination; and**
- **medical decision making of high complexity.**

Counseling and/or coordination of care with other providers or agencies are provided consistent with the nature of the problem(s) and the patient's and/or family's needs.

Usually, the presenting problem(s) are of high severity.

Established Patient

99351 **Home visit** for the evaluation and management of an established patient, which requires at least two of these three key components:

- **a problem focused interval history;**
- **a problem focused examination;**
- **medical decision making that is straightforward or of low complexity.**

Counseling and/or coordination of care with other providers or agencies are provided consistent with the nature of the problem(s) and the patient's and/or family's needs.

Usually, the patient is stable, recovering or improving.

99352 **Home visit** for the evaluation and management of an established patient, which requires at least two of these three key components:

- **an expanded problem focused interval history;**
- **an expanded problem focused examination;**
- **medical decision making of moderate complexity.**

Counseling and/or coordination of care with other providers or agencies are provided consistent with the nature of the problem(s) and the patient's and/or family's needs.

Usually, the patient is responding inadequately to therapy or has developed a minor complication.

99353 **Home visit** for the evaluation and management of an established patient, which requires at least two of these three key components:

- **a detailed interval history;**
- **a detailed examination;**
- **medical decision making of high complexity.**

Counseling and/or coordination of care with other providers or agencies are provided consistent with the nature of the problem(s) and the patient's and/or family's needs.

Usually, the patient is unstable or has developed a significant complication or a significant new problem.

Prolonged Services

Prolonged Physician Service With Direct (Face-To-Face) Patient Contact

Codes 99354-99357 are used when a physician provides prolonged service involving direct (face-to-face) patient contact that is beyond the usual service in either the inpatient or outpatient setting. This service is reported in addition to other physician service, including evaluation and management services at any level. Appropriate codes should be selected for supplies provided or procedures performed in the care of the patient during this period.

Codes 99354-99357 are used to report the total duration of face-to-face time spent by a physician on a given date providing prolonged service, even if the time spent by the physician on that date is not continuous.

Code 99354 or 99356 is used to report the first hour of prolonged service on a given date, depending on the place of service. Either code also may be used to report a total duration of prolonged service of 30-60 minutes on a given date. Either code should be used only once per date, even if the time spent by the physician is not continuous on that date. Prolonged service of less than 30 minutes total duration on a given date is not separately reported because the work involved is included in the total work of the evaluation and management codes.

Code 99355 or 99357 is used to report each additional 30 minutes beyond the first hour, depending on the place of service. Either code may also be used to report the final 15-30 minutes of prolonged service on a given date. Prolonged service of less than 15 minutes beyond the first hour or less than 15 minutes beyond the final 30 minutes is not reported separately.

The following examples illustrate the correct reporting of prolonged physician service with direct patient contact in the office setting:

Total Duration of Prolonged Services	Code(s)
less than 30 minutes (less than 1/2 hour)	Not reported separately
30-74 minutes (1/2 hr. – 1 hr. 14 min.)	99354 X 1
75-104 minutes (1 hr. 15 min. – 1 hr. 44 min.)	99354 X 1 AND 99355 X 1
105-134 minutes (1 hr. 45 min. – 2 hr. 14 min.)	99354 X 1 AND 99355 X 2
135-164 minutes (2 hr. 15 min. – 2 hr. 44 min.)	99354 X 1 AND 99355 X 3
165-194 minutes (2 hr. 45 min. – 3 hr. 14 min.)	99354 X 1 AND 99355 X 4

99354 **Prolonged physician service** in the office or other outpatient setting requiring direct (face-to-face) patient contact beyond the usual service (eg, prolonged care and treatment of an acute asthmatic patient in an outpatient setting); first hour

99355 each additional 30 minutes

99356 **Prolonged physician service** in the inpatient setting, requiring direct (face-to-face) patient contact beyond the usual service (eg, maternal fetal monitoring for high risk delivery or other physiological monitoring, prolonged care of an acutely ill inpatient); first hour

99357 each additional 30 minutes

Prolonged Physician Service Without Direct (Face-To-Face) Patient Contact

Codes 99358 and 99359 are used when a physician provides prolonged service not involving direct (face-to-face) care that is beyond the usual service in either the inpatient or outpatient setting. This service is to be reported in addition to other physician service, including evaluation and management services at any level.

Codes 99358 and 99359 are used to report the total duration of non-face-to-face time spent by a physician on a given date providing prolonged service, even if the time spent by the physician on that date is not continuous. Code 99358 is used to report the first hour of prolonged service on a given date regardless of the place of service.

It may also be used to report a total duration of prolonged service of 30-60 minutes on a given date. It should be used only once per date even if the time spent by the physician is not continuous on that date.

Prolonged service of less than 30 minutes total duration on a given date is not separately reported.

Code 99359 is used to report each additional 30 minutes beyond the first hour regardless of the place of service. It may also be used to report the final 15-30 minutes of prolonged service on a given date.

Prolonged service of less than 15 minutes beyond the first hour or less than 15 minutes beyond the final 30 minutes is not reported separately.

99358 **Prolonged evaluation and management service** before and/or after direct (face-to-face) patient care (eg, review of extensive records and tests, communication with other professionals and/or the patient/family); first hour

99359 each additional 30 minutes

(To report telephone calls, see 99371-99373)

Physician Standby Services

Code 99360 is used to report physician standby service that is requested by another physician and that involves prolonged physician attendance without direct (face-to-face) patient contact. The physician may not be providing care or services to other patients during this period. This code is not used to report time spent proctoring another physician. It is also not used if the period of standby ends with the performance of a procedure subject to a "surgical package" by the physician who was on standby.

Code 99360 is used to report the total duration of time spent by a physician on a given date on standby. Standby service of less than 30 minutes total duration on a given date is not reported separately.

Second and subsequent periods of standby beyond the first 30 minutes may be reported only if a full 30 minutes of standby was provided for each unit of service reported.

99360 **Physician standby service,** requiring prolonged physician attendance, each 30 minutes (eg, operative standby, standby for frozen section, for cesarean/high risk delivery for newborn care, for monitoring EEG)

Case Management Services

Physician case management is a process in which a physician is responsible for direct care of a patient, and for coordinating and controlling access to or initiating and/or supervising other health care services needed by the patient.

Team Conferences

99361 **Medical conference** by a physician with interdisciplinary team of health professionals or representatives of community agencies to coordinate activities of patient care (patient not present); approximately 30 minutes

99362 approximately 60 minutes

Telephone Calls

99371 **Telephone call** by a physician to patient or for consultation or medical management or for coordinating medical management with other health care professionals (eg, nurses, therapists, social workers, nutritionists, physicians, pharmacists); simple or brief (eg, to report on tests and/or laboratory results, to clarify or alter previous instructions, to integrate new information from other health professionals into the medical treatment plan, or to adjust therapy)

99372 intermediate (eg, to provide advice to an established patient on a new problem, to initiate therapy that can be handled by telephone, to discuss test results in detail, to coordinate medical management of a new problem in an established patient, to discuss and evaluate new information and details, or to initiate new plan of care)

99373   complex or lengthy (eg, lengthy counseling session with anxious or distraught patient, detailed or prolonged discussion with family members regarding seriously ill patient, lengthy communication necessary to coordinate complex services of several different health professionals working on different aspects of the total patient care plan)

Care Plan Oversight Services

Care Plan Oversight Services are reported separately from codes for office/outpatient, hospital, home, nursing facility or domiciliary services. The complexity and approximate physician time of the care plan oversight services provided within a 30-day period determine code selection. Only one physician may report services for a given period of time, to reflect that physician's sole or predominant supervisory role with a particular patient. These codes should not be reported for supervision of patients in nursing facilities or under the care of home health agencies unless they require recurrent supervision of therapy.

The work involved in providing very low intensity or infrequent supervision services is included in the pre- and post-encounter work for home, office/outpatient and nursing facility or domiciliary visit codes.

Care plan oversight services provided which are less than 30 minutes during a 30-day period are considered part of patient evaluation and management and should not be reported separately.

99375 **Physician supervision** of patients under care of home health agencies, hospice or nursing facility patients (patient not present) requiring complex or multidisciplinary care modalities involving regular physician development and/or revision of care plans, review of subsequent reports of patient status, review of related laboratory and other studies, communication (including telephone calls) with other health care professionals involved in patient's care, integration of new information into the medical treatment plan and/or adjustment of medical therapy, within a 30-day period; 30-60 minutes

99376   greater than 60 minutes

Preventive Medicine Services

The following codes are used to report the preventive medicine evaluation and management of infants, children, adolescents and adults.

The extent and focus of the services will largely depend on the age of the patient. (If an abnormality/ies is encountered or a preexisting problem is addressed in the process of performing this preventive medicine evaluation and management service, and if the problem/abnormality is significant enough to require additional work to perform the key components of a problem-oriented E/M service, then the appropriate Office/Outpatient code 99201-99215 should also be reported. Modifier '-25' should be added to the Office/Outpatient code to indicate that a significant, separately identifiable Evaluation and Management service was provided by the same physician on the same day as the preventive medicine service. An insignificant or trivial problem/abnormality that is encountered in the process of performing the preventive medicine evaluation and management service and which does not require additional work and the performance of the key components of a problem-oriented E/M service, should not be reported.)

Codes 99381-99397 include counseling/anticipatory guidance/risk factor reduction interventions which are provided at the time of the initial or periodic, comprehensive preventive medicine examination. (Refer to codes 99401-99412 for reporting those counseling/anticipatory guidance/risk factor reduction interventions that are provided at an encounter separate from the preventive medicine examination).

Immunizations and ancillary studies involving laboratory, radiology, or other procedures are reported separately. For immunizations, see 90701-90749.

New Patient

99381 **Initial preventive medicine** evaluation and management of an individual including a comprehensive history, a comprehensive examination, counseling/anticipatory guidance/risk factor reduction interventions, and the ordering of appropriate laboratory/diagnostic procedures, new patient; infant (age under 1 year)

99382   early childhood (age 1 through 4 years)

99383   late childhood (age 5 through 11 years)

99384   adolescent (age 12 through 17 years)

99385   18-39 years

99386   40-64 years

99387   65 years and over

Established Patient

99391   **Periodic preventive medicine** reevaluation and management of an individual including a comprehensive history, comprehensive examination, counseling/anticipatory guidance/risk factor reduction interventions, and the ordering of appropriate laboratory/ diagnostic procedures, established patient; infant (age under 1 year)

99392   early childhood (age 1 through 4 years)

99393   late childhood (age 5 through 11 years)

99394   adolescent (age 12 through 17 years)

99395   18-39 years

99396   40-64 years

99397   65 years and over

Counseling and/or Risk Factor Reduction Intervention

New or Established Patient

These codes are used to report services provided to individuals at a separate encounter for the purpose of promoting health and preventing illness or injury.

Preventive medicine counseling and risk factor reduction interventions provided as a separate encounter will vary with age and should address such issues as family problems, diet and exercise, substance abuse, sexual practices, injury prevention, dental health, and diagnostic and laboratory test results available at the time of the encounter.

These codes are not to be used to report counseling and risk factor reduction interventions

provided to patients with symptoms or established illness. For counseling individual patients with symptoms or established illness, use the appropriate office, hospital or consultation or other evaluation and management codes. For counseling groups of patients with symptoms or established illness, use 99078.

Preventive Medicine, Individual Counseling

99401   **Preventive medicine counseling** and/or risk factor reduction intervention(s) provided to an individual (separate procedure); approximately 15 minutes

99402   approximately 30 minutes

99403   approximately 45 minutes

99404   approximately 60 minutes

Preventive Medicine, Group Counseling

99411   **Preventive medicine counseling** and/or risk factor reduction intervention(s) provided to individuals in a group setting (separate procedure); approximately 30 minutes

99412   approximately 60 minutes

Other Preventive Medicine Services

99420   **Administration and interpretation** of health risk assessment instrument (eg, health hazard appraisal)

99429   **Unlisted preventive** medicine service

Newborn Care

The following codes are used to report the services provided to normal or high risk newborns in several different settings. For newborn hospital discharge services provided on a date subsequent to the admission date of the newborn, use 99238. For discharge services provided to newborns admitted and discharged on the same date, see 99435.

99431 **History and examination** of the normal newborn infant, initiation of diagnostic and treatment programs and preparation of hospital records. (This code should also be used for birthing room deliveries.)

99432 **Normal newborn care** in other than hospital or birthing room setting, including physical examination of baby and conference(s) with parent(s)

99433 **Subsequent hospital care,** for the evaluation and management of a normal newborn, per day

●**99435** **History and examination** of the normal newborn infant, including the preparation of medical records (this code should only be used for newborns assessed and discharged from the hospital or birthing room on the same date)

(99438 has been deleted)

▲**99440** **Newborn resuscitation:** provision of positive pressure ventilation and/or chest compressions in the presence of acute inadequate ventilation and/or cardiac output

Special Evaluation and Management Services

The following codes are used to report evaluations performed to establish baseline information prior to life or disability insurance certificates being issued. This service is performed in the office or other setting, and applies to both new and established patients. When using these codes, no active management of the problem(s) is undertaken during the encounter.

If other evaluation and management services and/or procedures are performed on the same date, the appropriate E/M or procedure code(s) should be reported in addition to these codes.

Basic Life and/or Disability Evaluation Services

99450 **Basic life** and/or disability examination that includes:

■ **measurement of height, weight and blood pressure;**

■ **completion of a medical history following a life insurance pro forma;**

■ **collection of blood sample and/or urinalysis complying with "chain of custody" protocols; and**

■ **completion of necessary documentation/certificates.**

Work Related or Medical Disability Evaluation Services

99455 **Work related** or medical disability examination by the treating physician that includes:

■ **completion of a medical history commensurate with the patient's condition;**

■ **performance of an examination commensurate with the patient's condition;**

■ **formulation of a diagnosis, assessment of capabilities and stability, and calculation of impairment;**

■ **development of future medical treatment plan; and**

■ **completion of necessary documentation/certificates and report.**

99456 **Work related** or medical disability examination by other than the treating physician that includes:

■ **completion of a medical history commensurate with the patient's condition;**

■ **performance of an examination commensurate with the patient's condition;**

■ **formulation of a diagnosis, assessment of capabilities and stability, and calculation of impairment;**

■ **development of future medical treatment plan; and**

■ **completion of necessary documentation/certificates and report.**

Other Evaluation and Management Services

99499 **Unlisted evaluation and management** service

Notes

Notes

Anesthesia Guidelines

Services involving administration of anesthesia are reported by the use of the anesthesia five-digit procedure code (00100-01999) plus modifier codes (defined under "Anesthesia Modifiers" later in these Guidelines).

The reporting of anesthesia services is appropriate by or under the responsible supervision of a physician. These services may include but are not limited to general, regional, supplementation of local anesthesia, or other supportive services in order to afford the patient the anesthesia care deemed optimal by the anesthesiologist during any procedure. These services include the usual preoperative and postoperative visits, the anesthesia care during the procedure, the administration of fluids and/or blood and the usual monitoring services (eg, ECG, temperature, blood pressure, oximetry, capnography, and mass spectrometry). Unusual forms of monitoring (eg, intra-arterial, central venous, and Swan-Ganz) are not included.

Items used by all physicians in reporting their services are presented in the **Introduction.** Some of the commonalities are repeated here for the convenience of those physicians referring to this section on **Anesthesia.** Other definitions and items unique to anesthesia are also listed.

Time Reporting

Time for anesthesia procedures may be reported as is customary in the local area. Anesthesia time begins when the anesthesiologist begins to prepare the patient for the induction of anesthesia in the operating room or in an equivalent area and ends when the anesthesiologist is no longer in personal attendance, that is, when the patient may be safely placed under postoperative supervision.

Physician's Services

Physician's services rendered in the office, home, or hospital, consultation and other medical services are listed in the section entitled **Evaluation and Management Services** (99200 series)

found in the front of the book, beginning on page 1. "Special Services and Reporting" (99000 series) are presented in the **Medicine** section.

Materials Supplied by Physician

Supplies and materials provided by the physician (eg, sterile trays, drugs) over and above those usually included with the office visit or other services rendered may be listed separately. List drugs, tray supplies, and materials provided. Identify as 99070.

Separate or Multiple Procedures

It is appropriate to designate multiple procedures that are rendered on the same date by separate entries. This can be reported by using the multiple procedure modifier ('-51' or 09951). See "Anesthesia Modifiers" for modifier definitions.

Special Report

A service that is rarely provided, unusual, variable, or new may require a special report in determining medical appropriateness of the service. Pertinent information should include an adequate definition or description of the nature, extent, and need for the procedure; and the time, effort and equipment necessary to provide the service. Additional items which may be included are:

- complexity of symptoms;
- final diagnosis;
- pertinent physical findings;
- diagnostic and therapeutic procedures;
- concurrent problems;
- follow-up care.

Anesthesia Modifiers

All anesthesia services are reported by use of the anesthesia five-digit procedure code (00100-01999) plus the addition of a physical status modifier. The use of other optional modifiers may be appropriate.

Physical Status Modifiers

Physical Status modifiers are represented by the initial letter 'P' followed by a single digit from 1 to 6 defined below.

P1—A normal healthy patient.

P2—A patient with mild systemic disease.

P3—A patient with severe systemic disease.

P4—A patient with severe systemic disease that is a constant threat to life.

P5—A moribund patient who is not expected to survive without the operation.

P6—A declared brain-dead patient whose organs are being removed for donor purposes.

The above six levels are consistent with the American Society of Anesthesiologists (ASA) ranking of patient physical status. Physical status is included in *CPT* to distinguish between various levels of complexity of the anesthesia service provided.

Example: 00100-P1

Other Modifiers (Optional)

Under certain circumstances, medical services and procedures may need to be further modified. Other modifiers commonly used in **Anesthesia** are included below. A complete list of modifiers and their respective codes are listed in Appendix A.

-22 Unusual Procedural Services: When the service(s) provided is greater than that usually required for the listed procedure, it may be identified by adding modifier '-22' to the usual procedure number or by use of the separate five digit modifier code 09922. A report may also be appropriate.

-23 Unusual Anesthesia: Occasionally, a procedure which usually requires either no anesthesia or local anesthesia, because of unusual circumstances must be done under general anesthesia. This circumstance may be reported by adding the modifier '-23' to the procedure

code of the basic service or by use of the separate five digit modifier code 09923. **Note:** Modifier '-47', Anesthesia by Surgeon, (See Appendix A) would not be used as a modifier for the anesthesia procedures 00100-01999.

-32 Mandated Services: Services related to *mandated* consultation and/or related services (eg, PRO, 3rd party payor) may be identified by adding the modifier '-32' to the basic procedure, or the service may be reported by use of the five digit modifier 09932.

-51 Multiple Procedures: When multiple procedures are performed on the same day or at the same session, the major procedure or service may be reported as listed. The secondary additional, or lesser procedure(s) or service(s) may be identified by adding the modifier '-51' to the secondary procedure or service code(s) or by use of the separate five digit modifier code 09951. This modifier may be used to report multiple medical procedures performed at the same session, as well as a combination of medical and surgical procedures, or several surgical procedures performed at the same operative session.

Qualifying Circumstances

More than one may be selected.

Many anesthesia services are provided under particularly difficult circumstances, depending on factors such as extraordinary condition of patient, notable operative conditions, and/or unusual risk factors. This section includes a list of important qualifying circumstances that significantly impact on the character of the anesthesia service provided. These procedures would not be reported alone but would be reported as additional procedure numbers qualifying an anesthesia procedure or service.

99100 Anesthesia for patient of extreme age, under one year or over seventy

99116 Anesthesia complicated by utilization of total body hypothermia

99135   Anesthesia complicated by utilization of
controlled hypotension

99140   Anesthesia complicated by emergency
conditions (specify)

An emergency is defined as existing when delay in
treatment of the patient would lead to a significant
increase in the threat to life or body part.

Anesthesia

Head

00100 Anesthesia for procedures on integumentary system of head and/or salivary glands, including biopsy; not otherwise specified

00102 plastic repair of cleft lip

00103 blepharoplasty

00104 Anesthesia for electroconvulsive therapy

00120 Anesthesia for procedures on external, middle, and inner ear including biopsy; not otherwise specified

(00122 has been deleted. To report, use 00120)

00124 otoscopy

00126 tympanotomy

00140 Anesthesia for procedures on eye; not otherwise specified

00142 lens surgery

00144 corneal transplant

00145 vitrectomy

(00146 has been deleted. To report, use 00140)

00147 iridectomy

00148 ophthalmoscopy

00160 Anesthesia for procedures on nose and accessory sinuses; not otherwise specified

00162 radical surgery

00164 biopsy, soft tissue

00170 Anesthesia for intraoral procedures, including biopsy; not otherwise specified

00172 repair of cleft palate

00174 excision of retropharyngeal tumor

00176 radical surgery

00190 Anesthesia for procedures on facial bones; not otherwise specified

00192 radical surgery (including prognathism)

00210 Anesthesia for intracranial procedures; not otherwise specified

00212 subdural taps

00214 burr holes

(For burr holes for ventriculography, see 01902)

00215 elevation of depressed skull fracture, extradural (simple or compound)

00216 vascular procedures

00218 procedures in sitting position

00220 spinal fluid shunting procedures

00222 electrocoagulation of intracranial nerve

Neck

00300 Anesthesia for all procedures on integumentary system of neck, including subcutaneous tissue

00320 Anesthesia for all procedures on esophagus, thyroid, larynx, trachea and lymphatic system of neck; not otherwise specified

00322 needle biopsy of thyroid

(For procedures on cervical spine and cord, see 00600, 00604, 00670)

00350 Anesthesia for procedures on major vessels of neck; not otherwise specified

00352 simple ligation

(For arteriography, see 01916)

Thorax (Chest Wall and Shoulder Girdle)

00400   Anesthesia for procedures on anterior integumentary system of chest, including subcutaneous tissue; not otherwise specified

00402   reconstructive procedures on breast (eg, reduction or augmentation mammoplasty, muscle flaps)

00404   radical or modified radical procedures on breast

00406   radical or modified radical procedures on breast with internal mammary node dissection

00410   electrical conversion of arrhythmias

00420   Anesthesia for procedures on posterior integumentary system of chest, including subcutaneous tissue

00450   Anesthesia for procedures on clavicle and scapula; not otherwise specified

00452   radical surgery

00454   biopsy of clavicle

00470   Anesthesia for partial rib resection; not otherwise specified

00472   thoracoplasty (any type)

00474   radical procedures (eg, pectus excavatum)

(00476 has been deleted. To report, use 00470)

Intrathoracic

00500   Anesthesia for all procedures on esophagus

▲**00520**   Anesthesia for closed chest procedures (including esophagoscopy, bronchoscopy, diagnostic thoracoscopy); not otherwise specified

00522   needle biopsy of pleura

00524   pneumocentesis

(00526 has been deleted. To report, use 00520)

00528   mediastinoscopy

00530   Anesthesia for transvenous pacemaker insertion

00532   Anesthesia for access to central venous circulation

00534   Anesthesia for transvenous insertion or replacement of cardioverter/defibrillator

(For transthoracic approach, use 00560)

▲**00540**   Anesthesia for thoracotomy procedures involving lungs, pleura, diaphragm, and mediastinum (including surgical thorascoscopy); not otherwise specified

00542   decortication

00544   pleurectomy

00546   pulmonary resection with thoracoplasty

00548   intrathoracic repair of trauma to trachea and bronchi

00560   Anesthesia for procedures on heart, pericardium, and great vessels of chest; without pump oxygenator

00562   with pump oxygenator

00580   Anesthesia for heart transplant or heart/lung transplant

Spine and Spinal Cord

00600   Anesthesia for procedures on cervical spine and cord; not otherwise specified

(For myelography and diskography, see radiological procedures 01906-01914)

00604   posterior cervical laminectomy in sitting position

00620   Anesthesia for procedures on thoracic spine and cord; not otherwise specified

00622   thoracolumbar sympathectomy

00630 Anesthesia for procedures in lumbar region; not otherwise specified

00632 lumbar sympathectomy

00634 chemonucleolysis

(00650 has been deleted. To report, use 00220)

00670 Anesthesia for extensive spine and spinal cord procedures (eg, Harrington rod technique)

Upper Abdomen

00700 Anesthesia for procedures on upper anterior abdominal wall; not otherwise specified

00702 percutaneous liver biopsy

00730 Anesthesia for procedures on upper posterior abdominal wall

00740 Anesthesia for upper gastrointestinal endoscopic procedures

00750 Anesthesia for hernia repairs in upper abdomen; not otherwise specified

00752 lumbar and ventral (incisional) hernias and/or wound dehiscence

00754 omphalocele

00756 transabdominal repair of diaphragmatic hernia

00770 Anesthesia for all procedures on major abdominal blood vessels

00790 Anesthesia for intraperitoneal procedures in upper abdomen including laparoscopy; not otherwise specified

00792 partial hepatectomy (excluding liver biopsy)

00794 pancreatectomy, partial or total (eg, Whipple procedure)

00796 liver transplant (recipient)

(For harvesting of liver, use 01990)

Lower Abdomen

00800 Anesthesia for procedures on lower anterior abdominal wall; not otherwise specified

00802 panniculectomy

(00806 has been deleted. To report, see 00790, 00840)

00810 Anesthesia for intestinal endoscopic procedures

00820 Anesthesia for procedures on lower posterior abdominal wall

00830 Anesthesia for hernia repairs in lower abdomen; not otherwise specified

00832 ventral and incisional hernias

00840 Anesthesia for intraperitoneal procedures in lower abdomen including laparoscopy; not otherwise specified

00842 amniocentesis

00844 abdominoperineal resection

00846 radical hysterectomy

00848 pelvic exenteration

00850 cesarean section

00855 cesarean hysterectomy

00857 Continuous epidural analgesia, for labor and cesarean section

00860 Anesthesia for extraperitoneal procedures in lower abdomen, including urinary tract; not otherwise specified

00862 renal procedures, including upper 1/3 of ureter, or donor nephrectomy

00864 total cystectomy

●**00865** radical prostatectomy (suprapubic, retropubic)

00866 adrenalectomy

00868 renal transplant (recipient)

(For donor nephrectomy, use 00862)

(For harvesting kidney from brain-dead patient, use 01990)

00870   cystolithotomy

00872   Anesthesia for lithotripsy, extracorporeal shock wave; with water bath

00873   without water bath

00880   Anesthesia for procedures on major lower abdominal vessels; not otherwise specified

00882   inferior vena cava ligation

00884   transvenous umbrella insertion

Perineum

00900   Anesthesia for procedures on perineal integumentary system (including biopsy of male genital system); not otherwise specified

00902   anorectal procedure (including endoscopy and/or biopsy)

00904   radical perineal procedure

00906   vulvectomy

00908   perineal prostatectomy

00910   Anesthesia for transurethral procedures (including urethrocystoscopy); not otherwise specified

00912   transurethral resection of bladder tumor(s)

00914   transurethral resection of prostate

00916   post-transurethral resection bleeding

00918   with fragmentation and/or removal of ureteral calculus

00920   Anesthesia for procedures on male external genitalia; not otherwise specified

00922   seminal vesicles

00924   undescended testis, unilateral or bilateral

00926   radical orchiectomy, inguinal

00928   radical orchiectomy, abdominal

00930   orchiopexy, unilateral or bilateral

00932   complete amputation of penis

00934   radical amputation of penis with bilateral inguinal lymphadenectomy

00936   radical amputation of penis with bilateral inguinal and iliac lymphadenectomy

00938   insertion of penile prosthesis (perineal approach)

00940   Anesthesia for vaginal procedures (including biopsy of labia, vagina, cervix or endometrium); not otherwise specified

00942   colpotomy, colpectomy, colporrhaphy

00944   vaginal hysterectomy

00946   vaginal delivery

00948   cervical cerclage

00950   culdoscopy

00952   hysteroscopy

00955   Continuous epidural analgesia, for labor and vaginal delivery

Pelvis (Except Hip)

01000   Anesthesia for procedures on anterior integumentary system of pelvis (anterior to iliac crest), except external genitalia

01110   Anesthesia for procedures on posterior integumentary system of pelvis (posterior to iliac crest), except perineum

01120   Anesthesia for procedures on bony pelvis

(01122 has been deleted. To report, use 01120)

01130   Anesthesia for body cast application or revision

01140   Anesthesia for interpelviabdominal (hindquarter) amputation

01150   Anesthesia for radical procedures for tumor of pelvis, except hindquarter amputation

01160   Anesthesia for closed procedures involving symphysis pubis or sacroiliac joint

01170 Anesthesia for open procedures involving symphysis pubis or sacroiliac joint

01180 Anesthesia for obturator neurectomy; extrapelvic

01190   intrapelvic

Upper Leg (Except Knee)

01200 Anesthesia for all closed procedures involving hip joint

01202 Anesthesia for arthroscopic procedures of hip joint

01210 Anesthesia for open procedures involving hip joint; not otherwise specified

01212   hip disarticulation

01214   total hip replacement or revision

01220 Anesthesia for all closed procedures involving upper 2/3 of femur

01230 Anesthesia for open procedures involving upper 2/3 of femur; not otherwise specified

01232   amputation

01234   radical resection

01240 Anesthesia for all procedures on integumentary system of upper leg

01250 Anesthesia for all procedures on nerves, muscles, tendons, fascia, and bursae of upper leg

01260 Anesthesia for all procedures involving veins of upper leg, including exploration

01270 Anesthesia for procedures involving arteries of upper leg, including bypass graft; not otherwise specified

01272   femoral artery ligation

01274   femoral artery embolectomy

(01276 has been deleted. To report, use 00880)

Knee and Popliteal Area

01300 Anesthesia for all procedures on integumentary system of knee and/or popliteal area

01320 Anesthesia for all procedures on nerves, muscles, tendons, fascia, and bursae of knee and/or popliteal area

01340 Anesthesia for all closed procedures on lower 1/3 of femur

01360 Anesthesia for all open procedures on lower 1/3 of femur

01380 Anesthesia for all closed procedures on knee joint

01382 Anesthesia for arthroscopic procedures of knee joint

01390 Anesthesia for all closed procedures on upper ends of tibia, fibula, and/or patella

01392 Anesthesia for all open procedures on upper ends of tibia, fibula, and/or patella

01400 Anesthesia for open procedures on knee joint; not otherwise specified

01402   total knee replacement

01404   disarticulation at knee

01420 Anesthesia for all cast applications, removal, or repair involving knee joint

01430 Anesthesia for procedures on veins of knee and popliteal area; not otherwise specified

01432   arteriovenous fistula

01440 Anesthesia for procedures on arteries of knee and popliteal area; not otherwise specified

01442   popliteal thromboendarterectomy, with or without patch graft

01444   popliteal excision and graft or repair for occlusion or aneurysm

Lower Leg (Below Knee)

Includes ankle and foot.

01460 Anesthesia for all procedures on integumentary system of lower leg, ankle, and foot

01462 Anesthesia for all closed procedures on lower leg, ankle, and foot

01464 Anesthesia for arthroscopic procedures of ankle joint

01470 Anesthesia for procedures on nerves, muscles, tendons, and fascia of lower leg, ankle, and foot; not otherwise specified

01472   repair of ruptured Achilles tendon, with or without graft

01474   gastrocnemius recession (eg, Strayer procedure)

01480 Anesthesia for open procedures on bones of lower leg, ankle, and foot; not otherwise specified

01482   radical resection

01484   osteotomy or osteoplasty of tibia and/or fibula

01486   total ankle replacement

01490 Anesthesia for lower leg cast application, removal, or repair

01500 Anesthesia for procedures on arteries of lower leg, including bypass graft; not otherwise specified

01502   embolectomy, direct or with catheter

01520 Anesthesia for procedures on veins of lower leg; not otherwise specified

01522   venous thrombectomy, direct or with catheter

Shoulder and Axilla

Includes humeral head and neck, sternoclavicular joint, acromioclavicular joint, and shoulder joint.

01600 Anesthesia for all procedures on integumentary system of shoulder and axilla

01610 Anesthesia for all procedures on nerves, muscles, tendons, fascia, and bursae of shoulder and axilla

01620 Anesthesia for all closed procedures on humeral head and neck, sternoclavicular joint, acromioclavicular joint, and shoulder joint

01622 Anesthesia for arthroscopic procedures of shoulder joint

01630 Anesthesia for open procedures on humeral head and neck, sternoclavicular joint, acromioclavicular joint, and shoulder joint; not otherwise specified

01632   radical resection

01634   shoulder disarticulation

01636   interthoracoscapular (forequarter) amputation

01638   total shoulder replacement

01650 Anesthesia for procedures on arteries of shoulder and axilla; not otherwise specified

01652   axillary-brachial aneurysm

01654   bypass graft

01656   axillary-femoral bypass graft

01670 Anesthesia for all procedures on veins of shoulder and axilla

01680 Anesthesia for shoulder cast application, removal or repair; not otherwise specified

01682   shoulder spica

Upper Arm and Elbow

01700 Anesthesia for all procedures on integumentary system of upper arm and elbow

01710 Anesthesia for procedures on nerves, muscles, tendons, fascia, and bursae of upper arm and elbow; not otherwise specified

01712   tenotomy, elbow to shoulder, open

01714   tenoplasty, elbow to shoulder

01716   tenodesis, rupture of long tendon of biceps

01730   Anesthesia for all closed procedures on humerus and elbow

01732   Anesthesia for arthroscopic procedures of elbow joint

01740   Anesthesia for open procedures on humerus and elbow; not otherwise specified

01742   osteotomy of humerus

01744   repair of nonunion or malunion of humerus

01756   radical procedures

01758   excision of cyst or tumor of humerus

01760   total elbow replacement

01770   Anesthesia for procedures on arteries of upper arm and elbow; not otherwise specified

01772   embolectomy

01780   Anesthesia for procedures on veins of upper arm and elbow; not otherwise specified

01782   phleborrhaphy

01784   Anesthesia for repair of arterio-venous (A-V) fistula, congenital or acquired

Forearm, Wrist and Hand

01800   Anesthesia for all procedures on integumentary system of forearm, wrist, and hand

01810   Anesthesia for all procedures on nerves, muscles, tendons, fascia, and bursae of forearm, wrist, and hand

01820   Anesthesia for all closed procedures on radius, ulna, wrist, or hand bones

01830   Anesthesia for open procedures on radius, ulna, wrist, or hand bones; not otherwise specified

01832   total wrist replacement

01840   Anesthesia for procedures on arteries of forearm, wrist, and hand; not otherwise specified

01842   embolectomy

01844   Anesthesia for vascular shunt, or shunt revision, any type (eg, dialysis)

01850   Anesthesia for procedures on veins of forearm, wrist, and hand; not otherwise specified

01852   phleborrhaphy

01860   Anesthesia for forearm, wrist, or hand cast application, removal, or repair

Radiological Procedures

01900   Anesthesia for injection procedure for hysterosalpingography

01902   Anesthesia for burr hole(s) for ventriculography

01904   Anesthesia for injection procedure for pneumoencephalography

01906   Anesthesia for injection procedure for myelography; lumbar

01908   cervical

01910   posterior fossa

01912   Anesthesia for injection procedure for diskography; lumbar

01914   cervical

01916   Anesthesia for arteriograms, needle; carotid, or vertebral

01918   retrograde, brachial or femoral

01920   Anesthesia for cardiac catheterization including coronary arteriography and ventriculography (not to include Swan-Ganz catheter)

01921   Anesthesia for angioplasty

01922   Anesthesia for non-invasive imaging or radiation therapy

Other Procedures

01990 Physiological support for harvesting of organ(s) from brain-dead patient

01995 Regional IV administration of local anesthetic agent (upper or lower extremity)

(For intra-arterial or intravenous therapy for pain management, see 90783, 90784)

01996 Daily management of epidural or subarachnoid drug administration

01999 Unlisted anesthesia procedure(s)

Notes

Surgery Guidelines

Items used by all physicians in reporting their services are presented in the **Introduction.** Some of the commonalities are repeated here for the convenience of those physicians referring to this section on **Surgery.** Other definitions and items unique to Surgery are also listed.

Physicians' Services

Physicians' services rendered in the office, home, or hospital, consultations and other medical services are listed in the section entitled **Evaluation and Management Services** (99200 series) found in the front of the book, beginning on page 9. "Special Services and Reports" (99000 series) is presented in the **Medicine** section.

Listed Surgical Procedures

Listed surgical procedures includes the operation per se, local infiltration, metacarpal/digital block or topical anesthesia when used, and the normal, uncomplicated follow-up care. This concept is referred to as a "package" for surgical procedures. To report a postoperative follow-up visit for documentation purposes only, use 99024.

Follow-Up Care for Diagnostic Procedures

Follow-up care for diagnostic procedures (eg, endoscopy, arthroscopy, injection procedures for radiography) includes only that care related to recovery from the diagnostic procedure itself. Care of the condition for which the diagnostic procedure was performed or of other concomitant conditions is not included and may be listed separately.

Follow-Up Care for Therapeutic Surgical Procedures

Follow-up care for therapeutic surgical procedures includes only that care which is usually a part of the surgical service. Complications, exacerbations, recurrence, or the presence of other diseases or injuries requiring additional services should be reported with the identification of appropriate procedures.

Materials Supplied by Physician

Supplies and materials provided by the physician (eg, sterile trays/drugs), over and above those usually included with the office visit or other services rendered may be listed separately. List drugs, trays, supplies, and materials provided. Identify as 99070.

Multiple Procedures

It is appropriate to designate multiple procedures that are rendered on the same date by separate entries. This can be reported by using the multiple procedure modifier ('-51' or 09951). See page 55 for modifier definitions.

Separate Procedure

Some of the listed procedures are commonly carried out as an integral part of a total service, and as such do not warrant a separate identification. When, however, such a procedure is performed independently of, and is not immediately related to, other services, it may be listed as a "separate procedure." Thus, when a procedure that is ordinarily a component of a larger procedure is performed alone for a specific purpose, it may be considered to be a separate procedure.

Subsection Information

Several of the subheadings or subsections have special needs or instructions unique to that section. Where these are indicated (eg, "Maternity Care and Delivery"), special **"Notes"** will be presented preceding those procedural terminology listings, referring to that subsection specifically. If there is an "Unlisted Procedure" code number (see below) for the individual subsection, it will also be shown. Those subsections within the **Surgery** section that have **"Notes"** are as follows:

Musculoskeletal 20000-29909
Cardiovascular System 33010-37799
Laparoscopy/Peritoneoscopy/
   Hysteroscopy 56300-56399
Maternity Care and Delivery 59000-59899

Unlisted Service or Procedure

A service or procedure may be provided that is not listed in this edition of *CPT*. When reporting such a service, the appropriate "Unlisted Procedure" code may be used to indicate the service, identifying it by "Special Report" as discussed in the section below. The "Unlisted Procedures" and accompanying codes for **Surgery** are as follows:

15999   Unlisted procedure, excision pressure ulcer
17999   Unlisted procedure, skin, mucous membrane, and subcutaneous tissue
19499   Unlisted procedure, breast
20999   Unlisted procedure, musculoskeletal system, general
21299   Unlisted craniofacial and maxillofacial procedure
21499   Unlisted musculoskeletal procedure, head
21899   Unlisted procedure, neck or thorax
22899   Unlisted procedure, spine
22999   Unlisted procedure, abdomen, musculoskeletal system
23929   Unlisted procedure, shoulder
24999   Unlisted procedure, humerus or elbow
25999   Unlisted procedure, forearm or wrist
26989   Unlisted procedure, hands or fingers

27299   Unlisted procedure, pelvis or hip joint
27599   Unlisted procedure, femur or knee
27899   Unlisted procedure, leg or ankle
28899   Unlisted procedure, foot or toes
29799   Unlisted procedure, casting or strapping
29909   Unlisted procedure, arthroscopy
30999   Unlisted procedure, nose
31299   Unlisted procedure, accessory sinuses
31599   Unlisted procedure, larynx
31899   Unlisted procedure, trachea, bronchi
32999   Unlisted procedure, lungs and pleura
33999   Unlisted procedure, cardiac surgery
36299   Unlisted procedure, vascular injection
37799   Unlisted procedure, vascular surgery
38999   Unlisted procedure, hemic or lymphatic system
39499   Unlisted procedure, mediastinum
39599   Unlisted procedure, diaphragm
40799   Unlisted procedure, lips
40899   Unlisted procedure, vestibule of mouth
41599   Unlisted procedure, tongue, floor of mouth
41899   Unlisted procedure, dentoalveolar structures
42299   Unlisted procedure, palate, uvula
42699   Unlisted procedure, salivary glands or ducts
42999   Unlisted procedure, pharynx, adenoids, or tonsils
43499   Unlisted procedure, esophagus
43999   Unlisted procedure, stomach
44799   Unlisted procedure, intestine
44899   Unlisted procedure, Meckel's diverticulum and the mesentery
45999   Unlisted procedure, rectum
46999   Unlisted procedure, anus
47399   Unlisted procedure, liver
47999   Unlisted procedure, biliary tract
48999   Unlisted procedure, pancreas
49999   Unlisted procedure, abdomen, peritoneum, and omentum
53899   Unlisted procedure, urinary system
55899   Unlisted procedure, male genital system
56399   Unlisted procedure, laparoscopy, peritoneoscopy, hysteroscopy
58999   Unlisted procedure, female genital system nonobstetrical
59899   Unlisted procedure, maternity care and delivery
60699   Unlisted procedure, endocrine system
64999   Unlisted procedure, nervous system
66999   Unlisted procedure, anterior segment of eye
67299   Unlisted procedure, posterior segment
67399   Unlisted procedure, ocular muscle
67599   Unlisted procedure, orbit
67999   Unlisted procedure, eyelids
68399   Unlisted procedure, conjunctiva
68899   Unlisted procedure, lacrimal system
69399   Unlisted procedure, external ear
69799   Unlisted procedure, middle ear
69949   Unlisted procedure, inner ear
69979   Unlisted procedure, temporal bone, middle fossa approach

Special Report

A service that is rarely provided, unusual, variable, or new may require a special report in determining medical appropriateness of the service. Pertinent information should include an adequate definition or description of the nature, extent, and need for the procedure, and the time, effort, and equipment necessary to provide the service. Additional items which may be included are:

- complexity of symptoms;
- final diagnosis;
- pertinent physical findings (such as size, locations, and number of lesion(s), if appropriate);
- diagnostic and therapeutic procedures (including major and supplementary surgical procedures, if appropriate);
- concurrent problems;
- follow-up care.

Modifiers

Listed services and procedures may be modified under certain circumstances. When applicable, the modifying circumstance should be identified by the addition of the appropriate modifier code, which may be reported in either of two ways. The modifier may be reported by a two digit number placed after the usual procedure number, from which it is separated by a hyphen. Or, the modifier may be reported by a separate five digit code that is used in addition to the procedure code. If more than one modifier is used, place the "Multiple Modifiers" code '-99' immediately after the procedure code. This indicates that one or more additional modifier codes will follow. Modifiers commonly used in **Surgery** are as follows:

-20 Microsurgery: When the surgical services are performed using the techniques of microsurgery, requiring the use of an operating microscope, modifier '-20' may be added to the surgical procedure or the separate five digit modifier code 09920 may be used. Modifier '-20' is not to be used when a magnifying surgical loupe is used, whether attached to the eyeglasses or on a headband. A special report may be appropriate to document the necessity of the microsurgical approach.

-22 Unusual Procedural Services: When the service(s) provided is greater than that usually required for the listed procedure, it may be identified by adding modifier '-22' to the usual procedure number or by use of the separate five digit modifier code 09922. A report may also be appropriate.

-26 Professional Component: Certain procedures are a combination of a physician component and a technical component. When the physician component is reported separately, the service may be identified by adding the modifier '-26' to the usual procedure number or the service may be reported by use of the five digit modifier code 09926.

-32 Mandated Services: Services related to *mandated* consultation and/or related services (eg, PRO, 3rd party payor) may be identified by adding the modifier '-32' to the basic procedure or the service may be reported by use of the five digit modifier 09932.

-47 Anesthesia by Surgeon: Regional or general anesthesia provided by the surgeon may be reported by adding the modifier '-47' to the basic service or by use of the separate five digit modifier code 09947. (This does not include local anesthesia) **Note:** Modifier '-47' or 09947 would not be used as a modifier for the anesthesia procedures 00100-01999.

-50 Bilateral Procedure: Unless otherwise identified in the listings, bilateral procedures that are performed at the same operative session should be identified by the appropriate five digit code describing the first procedure. The second (bilateral) procedure is identified either by adding modifier '-50' to the procedure number or by use of the separate five digit modifier code 09950.

-51 Multiple Procedures: When multiple procedures are performed on the same day or at the same session, the major procedure or service may be reported as listed. The secondary, additional, or lesser procedure(s) or service(s) may be identified by adding the modifier '-51' to the secondary procedure or service code(s) or by use of the separate five digit modifier code 09951. This modifier may be used to report multiple medical procedures performed at the same session, as well as a combination of medical and surgical procedures, or several surgical procedures performed at the same operative session.

-52 Reduced Services: Under certain circumstances, a service or procedure is partially reduced or eliminated at the physician's election. Under these circumstances, the service provided can be identified by its usual procedure number and the addition of the modifier '-52,' signifying that the service is reduced. This provides a means of reporting reduced services without disturbing the identification of the basic service. Modifier code 09952 may be used as an alternative to modifier '-52.'

-54 Surgical Care Only: When one physician performs a surgical procedure and another provides preoperative and/or postoperative management, surgical services may be identified by adding the modifier '-54' to the usual procedure number or by use of the separate five digit modifier code 09954.

-55 Postoperative Management Only: When one physician performs the postoperative management and another physician has performed the surgical procedure, the postoperative component may be identified by adding the modifier '-55' to the usual procedure number or by use of the separate five digit modifier code 09955.

-56 Preoperative Management Only: When one physician performs the preoperative care and evaluation and another physician performs the surgical procedure, the preoperative component may be identified by adding the modifier '-56' to the usual procedure number or by use of the separate five digit modifier code 09956.

-57 Decision for Surgery: An evaluation and management service that resulted in the initial decision to perform the surgery may be identified by adding the modifier '-57' to the appropriate level of E/M service, or the separate five digit modifier 09957 may be used.

-58 Staged or Related Procedure or Service by the Same Physician During the Postoperative Period: The physician may need to indicate that the performance of a procedure or service during the postoperative period was: a) planned prospectively at the time of the original procedure (staged); b) more extensive than the original procedure; or c) for therapy following a diagnostic surgical procedure. This circumstance may be reported by adding the modifier '-58' to the staged or related procedure, or the separate five digit modifier 09958

may be used. **Note:** This modifier is not used to report the treatment of a problem that requires a return to the operating room. See modifier '-78.'

-62 Two Surgeons: Under certain circumstances, the skills of two surgeons (usually with different skills) may be required in the management of a specific surgical procedure. Under such circumstances, the separate services may be identified by adding the modifier '-62' to the procedure number used by each surgeon for reporting his services. Modifier code 09962 may be used as an alternative to modifier '-62.'

-66 Surgical Team: Under some circumstances, highly complex procedures (requiring the concomitant services of several physicians, often of different specialties, plus other highly skilled, specially trained personnel, and various types of complex equipment) are carried out under the "surgical team" concept. Such circumstances may be identified by each participating physician with the addition of the modifier '-66' to the basic procedure number used for reporting services. Modifier code 09966 may be used as an alternative to modifier '-66'.

-76 Repeat Procedure by Same Physician: The physician may need to indicate that a procedure or service was repeated subsequent to the original service. This circumstance may be reported by adding the modifier '-76' to the repeated service or the separate five digit modifier code 09976 may be used.

-77 Repeat Procedure by Another Physician: The physician may need to indicate that a basic procedure performed by another physician had to be repeated. This situation may be reported by adding modifier '-77' to the repeated service or the separate five digit modifier code 09977 may be used.

-78 Return to the Operating Room for a Related Procedure During the Postoperative Period: The physician may need to indicate that another procedure was performed during the postoperative period of the initial procedure. When this subsequent procedure is related to the first, and requires the use of the operating room, it may be reported by adding the modifier '-78' to the related procedure, or by using the separate five digit modifier 09978. (For repeat procedures on the same day, see '-76').

-79 Unrelated Procedure or Service by the Same Physician During the Postoperative Period: The physician may need to indicate that the performance of a procedure or service during the postoperative period was unrelated to the original procedure. This circumstance may be reported by using the modifier '-79' or by using the separate five digit modifier 09979. (For repeat procedures on the same day, see '-76').

-80 Assistant Surgeon: Surgical assistant services may be identified by adding the modifier '-80' to the usual procedure number(s) or by use of the separate five digit modifier code 09980.

-81 Minimum Assistant Surgeon: Minimum surgical assistant services are identified by adding the modifier '-81' to the usual procedure number or by use of the separate five digit modifier code 09981.

-82 Assistant Surgeon (when qualified resident surgeon not available): The unavailability of a qualified resident surgeon is a prerequisite for use of modifier '-82' appended to the usual procedure code number(s) or by use of the separate five digit modifier code 09982.

-90 Reference (Outside) Laboratory: When laboratory procedures are performed by a party other than the treating or reporting physician, the procedure may be identified by adding the modifier '-90' to the usual procedure number or by using the separate five digit modifier code 09990.

-99 Multiple Modifiers: Under certain circumstances, two or more modifiers may be necessary to completely delineate a service. In such situations modifier '-99' should be added to the basic procedure, and other applicable modifiers may be listed as part of the description of the service. Modifier code 09999 may be used as an alternative to modifier '-99.'

Starred (*) Procedures or Items

Certain relatively small surgical services involve a readily identifiable surgical procedure but include variable preoperative and postoperative services (eg, incision and drainage of an abscess, injection of a tendon sheath, manipulation of a joint under anesthesia, dilation of the urethra). Because of the indefinite pre- and postoperative services the usual "package" concept for surgical services (see above) cannot be applied. Such procedures are identified by a star (*) following the procedure code number.

When a star (*) follows a surgical procedure code number, the following rules apply:

1. *The service as listed includes the surgical procedure only.* Associated pre- and postoperative services are not included in the service as listed.

2. *Preoperative services are considered as one of the following:*

- When the starred (*) procedure is carried out at the time of an initial visit (new patient) and this procedure constitutes the major service at that visit, procedure number 99025 is listed in lieu of the usual initial visit as an additional service.

- When the starred (*) procedure is carried out at the time of an initial or other visit involving significant identifiable services (eg, removal of a small skin lesion at the time of a comprehensive history and physical examination), the appropriate visit is listed in addition to the starred (*) procedure and its follow-up care.

- When the starred (*) procedure is carried out at the time of a follow-up (established patient) visit and this procedure constitutes the major service at that visit, the service visit is usually not added.

- When the starred (*) procedure requires hospitalization, an appropriate hospital visit is listed in addition to the starred (*) procedure and its follow-up care.

3. *All postoperative care is added on a service-by-service basis (eg, office or hospital visit, cast change).*

4. *Complications are added on a service-by-service basis (as with all surgical procedures).*

Surgical Destruction

Surgical destruction is a part of a surgical procedure and different methods of destruction are not ordinarily listed separately unless the technique substantially alters the standard management of a problem or condition. Exceptions under special circumstances are provided for by separate code numbers.

Notes

Surgery

Skin, Subcutaneous and Accessory Structures

Incision and Drainage

(For excision, see 11400, et seq)

(10000-10020 have been deleted. To report, see 10060, 10061)

10040* Acne surgery (eg, marsupialization, opening or removal of multiple milia, comedones, cysts, pustules)

10060* Incision and drainage of abscess (eg, carbuncle, suppurative hidradenitis, cutaneous or subcutaneous abscess, cyst, furuncle, or paronychia); simple or single

10061 complicated or multiple

10080* Incision and drainage of pilonidal cyst; simple

10081 complicated

(For excision of pilonidal cyst, see 11770-11772)

(10100, 10101 have been deleted. To report, see 10060, 10061)

10120* Incision and removal of foreign body, subcutaneous tissues; simple

10121 complicated

(To report wound exploration due to penetrating trauma without laparotomy or thoracotomy, see 20100-20103, as appropriate)

10140* Incision and drainage of hematoma, seroma or fluid collection

(10141 has been deleted. To report, see 10140)

10160* Puncture aspiration of abscess, hematoma, bulla, or cyst

10180 Incision and drainage, complex, postoperative wound infection

(For secondary closure of surgical wound, see 12020, 12021, 13160)

Excision—Debridement

(For dermabrasions, see 15780-15791)

(For nail debridement, see 11700-11711)

(For burn(s), see 16000-16042)

11000* Debridement of extensive eczematous or infected skin; up to 10% of body surface

11001 each additional 10% of the body surface

11040 Debridement; skin, partial thickness

11041 skin, full thickness

11042 skin, and subcutaneous tissue

11043 skin, subcutaneous tissue, and muscle

11044 skin, subcutaneous tissue, muscle, and bone

Paring or Curettement

11050* Paring or curettement of benign hyperkeratotic skin lesion with or without chemical cauterization (such as verrucae or clavi) not extending through the stratum corneum (eg, callus or wart) with or without local anesthesia; single lesion

11051 two to four lesions

11052 more than four lesions

(11060-11062 have been deleted. To report, see 11300-11313)

Biopsy

11100 Biopsy of skin, subcutaneous tissue and/or mucous membrane (including simple closure), unless otherwise listed (separate procedure); single lesion

11101 each separate/additional lesion

(For biopsy of conjunctiva, see 68100; eyelid, see 67810)

Removal of Skin Tags

Removal by scissoring, or any sharp method or ligature strangulation including chemical or electrocauterization of wound, with or without local anesthesia.

11200* Removal of skin tags, multiple fibrocutaneous tags, any area; up to and including 15 lesions

11201 each additional ten lesions

(For electrosurgical destruction, see 17200, 17201)

Shaving of Epidermal or Dermal Lesions

Shaving is the sharp removal by transverse incision or horizontal slicing to remove epidermal and dermal lesions without a full-thickness dermal excision. This includes local anesthesia, chemical or electrocauterization of the wound. The wound does not require suture closure.

11300* Shaving of epidermal or dermal lesion, single lesion, trunk, arms or legs; lesion diameter 0.5 cm or less

11301 lesion diameter 0.6 to 1.0 cm

11302 lesion diameter 1.1 to 2.0 cm

11303 lesion diameter over 2.0 cm

11305* Shaving of epidermal or dermal lesion, single lesion, scalp, neck, hands, feet, genitalia; lesion diameter 0.5 cm or less

11306 lesion diameter 0.6 to 1.0 cm

11307 lesion diameter 1.1 to 2.0 cm

11308 lesion diameter over 2.0 cm

11310* Shaving of epidermal or dermal lesion, single lesion, face, ears, eyelids, nose, lips, mucous membrane; lesion diameter 0.5 cm or less

11311 lesion diameter 0.6 to 1.0 cm

11312 lesion diameter 1.1 to 2.0 cm

11313 lesion diameter over 2.0 cm

Excision—Benign Lesions

Excision (including simple closure) of benign lesions of skin or subcutaneous tissues (eg, cicatricial, fibrous, inflammatory, congenital, cystic lesions), including local anesthesia. See appropriate size and area below.

Excision is defined as full-thickness (through the dermis) removal of the following lesions and includes simple (non-layered) closure. The closure of defects created by incision, excision, or trauma may require intermediate (layered) closure. Layered closure involves dermal closure with separate suture closure of at least one of the deeper layers of subcutaneous and non-muscle fascial tissues. See page 62 and following for repair codes.

(For excision of lesions requiring more than simple closure, ie, requiring intermediate, complex, or reconstructive closure, see 12031-12057, 13100-13300, 14000-14300, 15000-15261, 15570-15770)

(For electrosurgical and other methods, see 17000 et seq)

11400 Excision, benign lesion, except skin tag (unless listed elsewhere), trunk, arms or legs; lesion diameter 0.5 cm or less

11401 lesion diameter 0.6 to 1.0 cm

11402 lesion diameter 1.1 to 2.0 cm

11403 lesion diameter 2.1 to 3.0 cm

11404 lesion diameter 3.1 to 4.0 cm

11406 lesion diameter over 4.0 cm

(For unusual or complicated excision, add modifier -22 or 09922)

11420 Excision, benign lesion, except skin tag (unless listed elsewhere), scalp, neck, hands, feet, genitalia; lesion diameter 0.5 cm or less

11421   lesion diameter 0.6 to 1.0 cm

11422   lesion diameter 1.1 to 2.0 cm

11423   lesion diameter 2.1 to 3.0 cm

11424   lesion diameter 3.1 to 4.0 cm

11426   lesion diameter over 4.0 cm

> (For unusual or complicated excision, add modifier -22 or 09922)

11440   Excision, other benign lesion (unless listed elsewhere), face, ears, eyelids, nose, lips, mucous membrane; lesion diameter 0.5 cm or less

11441   lesion diameter 0.6 to 1.0 cm

11442   lesion diameter 1.1 to 2.0 cm

11443   lesion diameter 2.1 to 3.0 cm

11444   lesion diameter 3.1 to 4.0 cm

11446   lesion diameter over 4.0 cm

> (For unusual or complicated excision, add modifier -22 or 09922)

> (For eyelids involving more than skin, see also 67800 et seq)

11450   Excision of skin and subcutaneous tissue for hidradenitis, axillary; with simple or intermediate repair

11451   with complex repair

11462   Excision of skin and subcutaneous tissue for hidradenitis, inguinal; with simple or intermediate repair

11463   with complex repair

11470   Excision of skin and subcutaneous tissue for hidradenitis, perianal, perineal, or umbilical; with simple or intermediate repair

11471   with complex repair

> (When skin graft or flap is used for closure, use appropriate procedure code in addition)

> (For bilateral procedure, add modifier -50 or 09950)

Excision—Malignant Lesions

Excision (including simple closure) of malignant lesion of skin or subcutaneous tissues including local anesthesia, each lesion. For removal of malignant lesions of skin by any method other than excision, as defined above, see destruction codes 17000-17999.

Excision is defined as full-thickness (through the dermis) removal of the following lesions and includes simple (non-layered) closure. The closure of defects created by incision, excision, or trauma may require intermediate (layered) closure. Layered closure involves dermal closure with separate suture closure of at least one of the deeper layers of subcutaneous and non-muscle fascial tissues.

> (For excision of lesions requiring more than simple closure, ie, requiring intermediate, complex, or reconstructive repair, see 12031-12057, 13100-13300, 14000-14300, 15000-15261, 15570-15770)

11600   Excision, malignant lesion, trunk, arms, or legs; lesion diameter 0.5 cm or less

11601   lesion diameter 0.6 to 1.0 cm

11602   lesion diameter 1.1 to 2.0 cm

11603   lesion diameter 2.1 to 3.0 cm

11604   lesion diameter 3.1 to 4.0 cm

11606   lesion diameter over 4.0 cm

11620   Excision, malignant lesion, scalp, neck, hands, feet, genitalia; lesion diameter 0.5 cm or less

11621   lesion diameter 0.6 to 1.0 cm

11622   lesion diameter 1.1 to 2.0 cm

11623   lesion diameter 2.1 to 3.0 cm

11624   lesion diameter 3.1 to 4.0 cm

11626   lesion diameter over 4.0 cm

11640   Excision, malignant lesion, face, ears, eyelids, nose, lips; lesion diameter 0.5 cm or less

11641   lesion diameter 0.6 to 1.0 cm

11642   lesion diameter 1.1 to 2.0 cm

11643   lesion diameter 2.1 to 3.0 cm

11644   lesion diameter 3.1 to 4.0 cm

11646   lesion diameter over 4.0 cm

    (For eyelids involving more than skin, see also 67800 et seq)

Nails

    (For drainage of paronychia or onychia, see 10060, 10061)

11700* Debridement of nails, manual; five or less

11701   each additional, five or less

11710* Debridement of nails, electric grinder; five or less

11711   each additional, five or less

11730* Avulsion of nail plate, partial or complete, simple; single

11731   second nail plate

11732   each additional nail plate

11740 Evacuation of subungual hematoma

11750 Excision of nail and nail matrix, partial or complete, (eg, ingrown or deformed nail) for permanent removal;

11752   with amputation of tuft of distal phalanx

    (For skin graft, if used, see 15050)

11755 Biopsy of nail unit, any method (eg, plate, bed, matrix, hyponychium, proximal and lateral nail folds) (separate procedure)

11760 Repair of nail bed

11762 Reconstruction of nail bed with graft

11765 Wedge excision of skin of nail fold (eg, for ingrown toenail)

    (For incision of pilonidal cyst, see 10080, 10081)

11770 Excision of pilonidal cyst or sinus; simple

11771   extensive

11772   complicated

Introduction

11900* Injection, intralesional; up to and including seven lesions

11901*   more than seven lesions

    (For veins, see 36470, 36471)

    (For intralesional chemotherapy administration, see 96405, 96406)

11920 Tattooing, intradermal introduction of insoluble opaque pigments to correct color defects of skin, including micropigmentation; 6.0 sq cm or less

11921   6.1 to 20.0 sq cm

11922   each additional 20.0 sq cm

11950 Subcutaneous injection of "filling" material (eg, collagen); 1 cc or less

11951   1.1 to 5.0 cc

11952   5.1 to 10.0 cc

11954   over 10.0 cc

11960 Insertion of tissue expander(s) for other than breast, including subsequent expansion

    (For breast reconstruction with tissue expander(s), see 19357)

11970 Replacement of tissue expander with permanent prosthesis

11971 Removal of tissue expander(s) without insertion of prosthesis

11975 Insertion, implantable contraceptive capsules

11976 Removal, implantable contraceptive capsules

11977 Removal with reinsertion, implantable contraceptive capsules

Repair (Closure)

Definitions

The repair of wounds may be classified as Simple, Intermediate or Complex.

Simple repair is used when the wound is superficial; eg, involving primarily epidermis or dermis, or subcutaneous tissues without significant involvement of deeper structures, and requires simple one layer closure/suturing. This includes local anesthesia and chemical or electrocauterization of wounds not closed.

Closure with adhesive strips is included in appropriate E/M service.

Intermediate repair includes the repair of wounds that, in addition to the above, require layered closure of one or more of the deeper layers of subcutaneous tissue and superficial (non-muscle) fascia, in addition to the skin (epidermal and dermal) closure. Single-layer closure of heavily contaminated wounds that have required extensive cleaning or removal of particulate matter also constitutes intermediate repair.

Complex repair includes the repair of wounds requiring more than layered closure, viz., scar revision, debridement, (eg, traumatic lacerations or avulsions), extensive undermining, stents or retention sutures. It may include creation of the defect and necessary preparation for repairs or the debridement and repair of complicated lacerations or avulsions.

Instructions for listing services at time of wound repair:

1. The repaired wound(s) should be measured and recorded in centimeters, whether curved, angular or stellate.

2. When multiple wounds are repaired, add together the lengths of those in the same classification (see above) and report as a single item.

When more than one classification of wounds is repaired, list the more complicated as the primary procedure and the less complicated as the secondary procedure, using either modifier '-51' or 09951.

3. Decontamination and/or debridement: Debridement is considered a separate procedure only when gross contamination requires prolonged cleansing, when appreciable amounts of devitalized or contaminated tissue are removed, or when debridement is carried out separately without immediate primary closure. (For extensive debridement of soft tissue and/or bone, see 11040-11044.)

4. Involvement of nerves, blood vessels and tendons: Report under appropriate system (Nervous, Cardiovascular, Musculoskeletal) for repair of these structures. The repair of these associated wounds is included in the primary procedure unless it qualifies as a complex wound, in which case either modifier '-51' or 09951 applies.

Simple ligation of vessels in an open wound is considered as part of any wound closure.

Simple "exploration" of nerves, blood vessels or tendons exposed in an open wound is also considered part of the essential treatment of the wound and is not a separate procedure unless appreciable dissection is required. If the wound requires enlargement, extension of dissection (to determine penetration), debridement, removal of foreign body(s), ligation or coagulation of minor subcutaneous and/or muscular blood vessel(s), of the subcutaneous tissue, muscle, fascia, and/or muscle, not requiring thoracotomy or laparotomy, use codes 20100-20103, as appropriate.

Repair—Simple

Sum of lengths of repairs.

12001* Simple repair of superficial wounds of scalp, neck, axillae, external genitalia, trunk and/or extremities (including hands and feet); 2.5 cm or less

12002* 2.6 cm to 7.5 cm

12004* 7.6 cm to 12.5 cm

12005 12.6 cm to 20.0 cm

12006 20.1 cm to 30.0 cm

12007 over 30.0 cm

12011* Simple repair of superficial wounds of face, ears, eyelids, nose, lips and/or mucous membranes; 2.5 cm or less

12013* 2.6 cm to 5.0 cm

12014 5.1 cm to 7.5 cm

12015 7.6 cm to 12.5 cm

12016 12.6 cm to 20.0 cm

12017 20.1 cm to 30.0 cm

12018 over 30.0 cm

12020 Treatment of superficial wound dehiscence; simple closure

12021   with packing

(For extensive or complicated secondary wound closure, see 13160)

Repair—Intermediate

Sum of lengths of repairs.

12031*   Layer closure of wounds of scalp, axillae, trunk and/or extremities (excluding hands and feet); 2.5 cm or less

12032*   2.6 cm to 7.5 cm

12034   7.6 cm to 12.5 cm

12035   12.6 cm to 20.0 cm

12036   20.1 cm to 30.0 cm

12037   over 30.0 cm

12041*   Layer closure of wounds of neck, hands, feet and/or external genitalia; 2.5 cm or less

12042   2.6 cm to 7.5 cm

12044   7.6 cm to 12.5 cm

12045   12.6 cm to 20.0 cm

12046   20.1 cm to 30.0 cm

12047   over 30.0 cm

12051*   Layer closure of wounds of face, ears, eyelids, nose, lips and/or mucous membranes; 2.5 cm or less

12052   2.6 cm to 5.0 cm

12053   5.1 cm to 7.5 cm

12054   7.6 cm to 12.5 cm

12055   12.6 cm to 20.0 cm

12056   20.1 cm to 30.0 cm

12057   over 30.0 cm

Repair—Complex

Reconstructive procedures, complicated wound closure.

Sum of lengths of repairs.

(For full thickness repair of lip or eyelid, see respective anatomical subsections)

13100   Repair, complex, trunk; 1.1 cm to 2.5 cm

(For 1.0 cm or less, see simple or intermediate repairs)

13101   2.6 cm to 7.5 cm

13120   Repair, complex, scalp, arms, and/or legs; 1.1 cm to 2.5 cm

(For 1.0 cm or less, see simple or intermediate repairs)

13121   2.6 cm to 7.5 cm

13131   Repair, complex, forehead, cheeks, chin, mouth, neck, axillae, genitalia, hands and/or feet; 1.1 cm to 2.5 cm

(For 1.0 cm or less, see simple or intermediate repairs)

13132   2.6 cm to 7.5 cm

13150   Repair, complex, eyelids, nose, ears and/or lips; 1.0 cm or less

(See also 40650-40654, 67961-67975)

13151   1.1 cm to 2.5 cm

13152   2.6 cm to 7.5 cm

13160   Secondary closure of surgical wound or dehiscence, extensive or complicated

(For packing or simple secondary wound closure, see 12020, 12021)

13300   Repair, unusual, complicated, over 7.5 cm, any area

Adjacent Tissue Transfer or Rearrangement

For full thickness repair of lip or eyelid, see respective anatomical subsections.

Excision (including lesion) and/or repair by adjacent tissue transfer or rearrangement (eg, Z-plasty, W-plasty, V-Y plasty, rotation flap, advancement flap, double pedicle flap). When applied in repairing lacerations, the procedures listed must be developed by the surgeon to accomplish the repair. They do not apply when direct closure or rearrangement of traumatic wounds incidentally result in these configurations.

Skin graft necessary to close secondary defect is considered an additional procedure.

14000   Adjacent tissue transfer or rearrangement, trunk; defect 10 sq cm or less

14001   defect 10.1 sq cm to 30.0 sq cm

14020   Adjacent tissue transfer or rearrangement, scalp, arms and/or legs; defect 10 sq cm or less

14021   defect 10.1 sq cm to 30.0 sq cm

14040   Adjacent tissue transfer or rearrangement, forehead, cheeks, chin, mouth, neck, axillae, genitalia, hands and/or feet; defect 10 sq cm or less

14041   defect 10.1 sq cm to 30.0 sq cm

14060   Adjacent tissue transfer or rearrangement, eyelids, nose, ears and/or lips; defect 10 sq cm or less

14061   defect 10.1 sq cm to 30.0 sq cm

(For eyelid, full thickness, see 67961 et seq)

14300   Adjacent tissue transfer or rearrangement, more than 30 sq cm, unusual or complicated, any area

14350   Filleted finger or toe flap, including preparation of recipient site

Free Skin Grafts

Identify by size and location of the defect (recipient area) and the type of graft; includes simple debridement of granulations or recent avulsion.

When a primary procedure such as orbitectomy, radical mastectomy, or deep tumor removal requires skin graft for definitive closure, see appropriate anatomical subsection for primary procedure and this section for skin graft.

Repair of donor site requiring skin graft or local flaps is to be added as an additional procedure.

15000   Excisional preparation or creation of recipient site by excision of essentially intact skin (including subcutaneous tissues), scar, or other lesion prior to repair with free skin graft (list as separate service in addition to skin graft)

(For appropriate skin grafts, see 15050-15261; list the free graft separately by its procedure number when the graft, immediate or delayed, is applied)

15050   Pinch graft, single or multiple, to cover small ulcer, tip of digit, or other minimal open area (except on face), up to defect size 2 cm diameter

(For tissue-cultured skin grafts, use 15100-15121. These codes include harvesting of keratinocytes. Procedures are coded by recipient site.)

15100   Split graft, trunk, scalp, arms, legs, hands, and/or feet (except multiple digits); 100 sq cm or less, or each one percent of body area of infants and children (except 15050)

15101   each additional 100 sq cm, or each one percent of body area of infants and children, or part thereof

15120   Split graft, face, eyelids, mouth, neck, ears, orbits, genitalia, and/or multiple digits; 100 sq cm or less, or each one percent of body area of infants and children (except 15050)

15121   each additional 100 sq cm, or each one percent of body area of infants and children, or part thereof

(For eyelids, see also 67961 et seq)

15200   Full thickness graft, free, including direct closure of donor site, trunk; 20 sq cm or less

15201   each additional 20 sq cm

15220   Full thickness graft, free, including direct closure of donor site, scalp, arms, and/or legs; 20 sq cm or less

15221   each additional 20 sq cm

15240 Full thickness graft, free, including direct closure of donor site, forehead, cheeks, chin, mouth, neck, axillae, genitalia, hands, and/or feet; 20 sq cm or less

(For finger tip graft, see 15050)

(For repair of syndactyly, fingers, see 26560-26562)

15241 each additional 20 sq cm

15260 Full thickness graft, free, including direct closure of donor site, nose, ears, eyelids, and/or lips; 20 sq cm or less

15261 each additional 20 sq cm

(For eyelids, see also 67961 et seq)

(Repair of donor site requiring skin graft or local flaps, to be added as additional separate procedure)

15350 Application of allograft, skin

15400 Application of xenograft, skin

(15410-15416 have been deleted. To report, use 15755)

Flaps (Skin and/or Deep Tissues)

Regions listed refer to recipient area (not donor site) when flap is being attached in transfer or to final site.

Regions listed refer to donor site when tube is formed for later or when "delay" of flap is prior to transfer.

Procedures 15570-15738 do not include extensive immobilization (eg, large plaster casts and other immobilizing devices are considered additional separate procedures).

Repair of donor site requiring skin graft or local flaps is considered an additional separate procedure.

(15500-15515 have been deleted. To report, see 15000)

(15540-15555 have been deleted. To report, see 15570-15576)

15570 Formation of direct or tubed pedicle, with or without transfer; trunk

15572 scalp, arms, or legs

15574 forehead, cheeks, chin, mouth, neck, axillae, genitalia, hands or feet

15576 eyelids, nose, ears, lips, or intraoral

15580 Cross finger flap, including free graft to donor site

(For major debridement or excisional preparation of recipient area at the time of attachment of pedicle flap, see 15570-15576)

15600 Delay of flap or sectioning of flap (division and inset); at trunk

15610 at scalp, arms, or legs

15620 at forehead, cheeks, chin, neck, axillae, genitalia, hands (except 15625), or feet

15625 section pedicle of cross finger flap

15630 at eyelids, nose, ears, or lips

15650 Transfer, intermediate, of any pedicle flap (eg, abdomen to wrist, "Walking" tube), any location

(15700-15730 have been deleted. To report, see 15570-15576)

(For eyelids, nose, ears, or lips, see also anatomical area)

(For revision, defatting or rearranging of transferred pedicle flap or skin graft, see 13100-14300)

(Procedures 15732-15738 are described by donor site of the muscle, myocutaneous, or fasciocutaneous flap)

15732 Muscle, myocutaneous, or fasciocutaneous flap; head and neck (eg, temporalis, masseter, sternocleidomastoid, levator scapulae)

15734 trunk

15736 upper extremity

15738 lower extremity

Other Flaps and Grafts

Repair of donor site requiring skin graft or local flaps should be reported as an additional procedure.

15740 Flap; island pedicle

(15745 has been deleted. To report, see 15732-15738)

15750 neurovascular pedicle

15755 Free flap (microvascular transfer)

15760 Graft; composite (eg, full thickness of external ear or nasal ala), including primary closure, donor area

15770 derma-fat-fascia

15775 Punch graft for hair transplant; 1 to 15 punch grafts

15776 more than 15 punch grafts

(For strip transplant, use 15220)

Other Procedures

15780 Dermabrasion; total face (eg, for acne scarring, fine wrinkling, rhytids, general keratosis)

15781 segmental, face

15782 regional, other than face

15783 superficial, any site, (eg, tattoo removal)

(15785 has been deleted. To report, see 15781, 15782)

15786* Abrasion; single lesion (eg, keratosis, scar)

15787 each additional four lesions or less

15788 Chemical peel, facial; epidermal

15789 dermal

(15790, 15791 have been deleted. To report, see 15788-15793)

15792 Chemical peel, nonfacial; epidermal

15793 dermal

(15800 has been deleted)

15810 Salabrasion; 20 sq cm or less

15811 over 20 sq cm

15819 Cervicoplasty

15820 Blepharoplasty, lower eyelid;

15821 with extensive herniated fat pad

15822 Blepharoplasty, upper eyelid;

15823 with excessive skin weighting down lid

(For bilateral blepharoplasty, add modifier -50 or 09950)

(See also 67916, 67917, 67923, 67924)

15824 Rhytidectomy; forehead

(For repair of brow ptosis, see 67900)

15825 neck with platysmal tightening (platysmal flap, "P-flap")

15826 glabellar frown lines

(15827 has been deleted. To report, use 15838)

15828 cheek, chin, and neck

15829 superficial musculoaponeurotic system (SMAS) flap

(For bilateral rhytidectomy, add modifier -50 or 09950)

15831 Excision, excessive skin and subcutaneous tissue (including lipectomy); abdomen (abdominoplasty)

15832 thigh

15833 leg

15834 hip

15835 buttock

15836 arm

15837 forearm or hand

15838 submental fat pad

15839 other area

(For bilateral procedure, add modifier -50 or 09950)

15840 Graft for facial nerve paralysis; free fascia graft (including obtaining fascia)

(For bilateral procedure, add modifier -50 or 09950)

15841 free muscle graft (including obtaining graft)

15842 free muscle graft by microsurgical technique

15845 regional muscle transfer

(For intravenous fluorescein examination of blood flow in graft or flap, see 15860)

(For nerve transfers, decompression, or repair, see 64830-64876, 64905, 64907, 69720, 69725, 69740, 69745, 69955)

15850 Removal of sutures under anesthesia (other than local), same surgeon

15851 Removal of sutures under anesthesia (other than local), other surgeon

15852 Dressing change (for other than burns) under anesthesia (other than local)

15860 Intravenous injection of agent (eg, fluorescein) to test blood flow in flap or graft

(15875 has been deleted. To report, see 15876-15879)

15876 Suction assisted lipectomy; head and neck

15877 trunk

15878 upper extremity

15879 lower extremity

Pressure Ulcers (Decubitus Ulcers)

15920 Excision, coccygeal pressure ulcer, with coccygectomy; with primary suture

15922 with flap closure

(15930 has been deleted. To report, use 15934)

15931 Excision, sacral pressure ulcer, with primary suture;

(15932 has been deleted)

15933 with ostectomy

15934 Excision, sacral pressure ulcer, with skin flap closure;

15935 with ostectomy

15936 Excision, sacral pressure ulcer, with muscle or myocutaneous flap closure;

15937 with ostectomy

(To identify muscle or myocutaneous flap closure, use also code number for specific flap)

15940 Excision, ischial pressure ulcer, with primary suture;

15941 with ostectomy (ischiectomy)

(15942, 15943 have been deleted. To report, use 15944-15946)

15944 Excision, ischial pressure ulcer, with skin flap closure;

15945 with ostectomy

15946 Excision, ischial pressure ulcer, with ostectomy, with muscle or myocutaneous flap closure

(To identify muscle or myocutaneous flap closure, use also code number for specific flap)

15950 Excision, trochanteric pressure ulcer, with primary suture;

15951 with ostectomy

15952 Excision, trochanteric pressure ulcer, with skin flap closure;

15953 with ostectomy

(15954 and 15955 have been deleted. To report, use appropriate debridement, closure or flap codes)

15956 Excision, trochanteric pressure ulcer, with muscle or myocutaneous flap closure;

15958 with ostectomy

(To identify muscle or myocutaneous flap closure, use also code number for specific flap)

(15960-15983 have been deleted. To report, use appropriate debridement, closure or flap codes)

15999   Unlisted procedure, excision pressure ulcer

(For free skin graft to close ulcer or donor site, see 15000 et seq)

Burns, Local Treatment

Procedures 16000-16042 refer to local treatment of burned surface only.

List percentage of body surface involved and depth of burn.

For necessary related medical services (eg, hospital visits, detention) in management of burned patients, see appropriate services in **Evaluation and Management** and **Medicine** sections.

(For skin graft, see 15100-15650)

16000   Initial treatment, first degree burn, when no more than local treatment is required

16010   Dressings and/or debridement, initial or subsequent; under anesthesia, small

16015   under anesthesia, medium or large, or with major debridement

16020*   without anesthesia, office or hospital, small

16025*   without anesthesia, medium (eg, whole face or whole extremity)

16030   without anesthesia, large (eg, more than one extremity)

16035   Escharotomy

16040   Excision burn wound, without skin grafting, employing alloplastic dressing (eg, synthetic mesh), any anatomic site; up to one percent total body surface area

16041   greater than one percent and up to nine percent total body surface area

16042   each additional nine percent total body surface area, or part thereof

(For debridement, curettement of burn wound, see 16010-16030)

Destruction

Destruction means the ablation of benign, premalignant or malignant tissues by any method, with or without curettement, including local anesthesia, and not usually requiring closure. Any method includes electrocautery, electrodesiccation, cryosurgery, laser and chemical treatment. Lesions include condylomata, papillomata, molluscum contagiosum, herpetic lesions, flat (plane, juvenile) warts, milia, or other benign, premalignant, or malignant lesions.

(For sharp removal of skin tags and fibrocutaneous lesions, see codes 11200, 11201)

(For electrosurgical destruction of skin tags, see codes 17200, 17201)

(For destruction of malignant skin lesions, see 17260-17286)

(For cryotherapy of acne, use 17340)

Destruction, Benign or Premalignant Lesions

17000*   Destruction by any method, including laser, with or without surgical curettement, all benign facial lesions or premalignant lesions in any location, or benign lesions other than cutaneous vascular proliferative lesions, including local anesthesia; one lesion

17001   second and third lesions, each

17002   over three lesions, each additional lesion

17010   complicated lesion(s)

17100*   Destruction by any method, including laser, of benign skin lesions other than cutaneous vascular proliferative lesions on any area other than the face, including local anesthesia; one lesion

17101   second lesion

17102   over two lesions, each additional lesion up to 15 lesions

17104   15 or more lesions

17105   complicated or extensive lesions

17106   Destruction of cutaneous vascular proliferative lesions (eg, laser technique); less than 10 sq cm

17107   10.0 - 50.0 sq cm

17108   over 50.0 sq cm

▲**17110*** Destruction by any method of flat warts or molluscum contagiosum, milia, up to 15 lesions

(For common or plantar warts, see 17000 or 17100 series)

(Retreatment same as office visit)

17200* Electrosurgical destruction of multiple fibrocutaneous tags; up to 15 lesions

17201 each additional ten lesions

(For excision of fibrocutaneous tags, see 11200, 11201)

17250* Chemical cauterization of granulation tissue (proud flesh, sinus or fistula)

(17250 is not to be used with removal or excision codes)

Destruction, Malignant Lesions, Any Method

17260* Destruction, malignant lesion, any method, trunk, arms or legs; lesion diameter 0.5 cm or less

17261 lesion diameter 0.6 to 1.0 cm

17262 lesion diameter 1.1 to 2.0 cm

17263 lesion diameter 2.1 to 3.0 cm

17264 lesion diameter 3.1 to 4.0 cm

17266 lesion diameter over 4.0 cm

17270* Destruction, malignant lesion, any method, scalp, neck, hands, feet, genitalia; lesion diameter 0.5 cm or less

17271 lesion diameter 0.6 to 1.0 cm

17272 lesion diameter 1.1 to 2.0 cm

17273 lesion diameter 2.1 to 3.0 cm

17274 lesion diameter 3.1 to 4.0 cm

17276 lesion diameter over 4.0 cm

17280* Destruction, malignant lesion, any method, face, ears, eyelids, nose, lips, mucous membrane; lesion diameter 0.5 cm or less

17281 lesion diameter 0.6 to 1.0 cm

17282 lesion diameter 1.1 to 2.0 cm

17283 lesion diameter 2.1 to 3.0 cm

17284 lesion diameter 3.1 to 4.0 cm

17286 lesion diameter over 4.0 cm

Mohs' Micrographic Surgery

Mohs' micrographic surgery, for the removal of complex or ill-defined skin cancer, requires a single physician to act in two integrated, but separate and distinct capacities: surgeon and pathologist. If either of these responsibilities are delegated to another physician who reports his services separately, these codes are not appropriate. If repair is performed, use separate repair, flap, or graft codes.

(17300-17302 have been deleted. To report, use 17304-17310)

(17303 has been deleted)

17304 Chemosurgery (Mohs' micrographic technique), including removal of all gross tumor, surgical excision of tissue specimens, mapping, color coding of specimens, microscopic examination of specimens by the surgeon, and complete histopathologic preparation; first stage, fresh tissue technique, up to 5 specimens

17305 second stage, fixed or fresh tissue, up to 5 specimens

17306 third stage, fixed or fresh tissue, up to 5 specimens

17307 additional stage(s), up to 5 specimens, each stage

17310 more than 5 specimens, fixed or fresh tissue, any stage

(For initiation or follow-up care of topical chemotherapy (eg, 5-FU or similar agents), see appropriate office visits)

Other Procedures

17340* Cryotherapy (CO_2 slush, liquid N_2) for acne

17360* Chemical exfoliation for acne (eg, acne paste, acid)

17380* Electrolysis epilation, each 1/2 hour

(For actinotherapy, see 96900)

17999 Unlisted procedure, skin, mucous membrane and subcutaneous tissue

Breast

Incision

19000* Puncture aspiration of cyst of breast;

19001 each additional cyst

19020 Mastotomy with exploration or drainage of abscess, deep

19030 Injection procedure only for mammary ductogram or galactogram

(For radiological supervision and interpretation, see 76086, 76088)

Excision

(All codes for bilateral procedures have been deleted. To report, add modifier -50 or 09950)

19100* Biopsy of breast; needle core (separate procedure)

(For fine needle aspiration, use 88170)

19101 incisional

19110 Nipple exploration, with or without excision of a solitary lactiferous duct or a papilloma lactiferous duct

19112 Excision of lactiferous duct fistula

19120 Excision of cyst, fibroadenoma, or other benign or malignant tumor aberrant breast tissue, duct lesion or nipple lesion (except 19140), male or female, one or more lesions

19125 Excision of breast lesion identified by preoperative placement of radiological marker; single lesion

19126 each additional lesion separately identified by a radiological marker

19140 Mastectomy for gynecomastia

19160 Mastectomy, partial;

19162 with axillary lymphadenectomy

19180 Mastectomy, simple, complete

(For immediate or delayed insertion of implant, use 19340 or 19342)

(For gynecomastia, see 19140)

19182 Mastectomy, subcutaneous

(19184-19187 have been deleted. To report, use 19182 with 19340 or 19342)

19200 Mastectomy, radical, including pectoral muscles, axillary lymph nodes

(19211-19216 have been deleted. To report, use 19200 with 19340 or 19342)

19220 Mastectomy, radical, including pectoral muscles, axillary and internal mammary lymph nodes (Urban type operation)

(19224-19229 have been deleted. To report, use 19220 with 19340 or 19342)

19240 Mastectomy, modified radical, including axillary lymph nodes, with or without pectoralis minor muscle, but excluding pectoralis major muscle

(19250-19255 have been deleted. To report, use 19240 with 19340 or 19342)

19260 Excision of chest wall tumor including ribs

19271 Excision of chest wall tumor involving ribs, with plastic reconstruction; without mediastinal lymphadenectomy

19272 with mediastinal lymphadenectomy

Introduction

19290 Preoperative placement of needle localization wire, breast;

19291 each additional lesion

(For radiological supervision and interpretation, see 76096)

▲=Revised Code   ●=New Code   ✱=Service Includes Surgical Procedure Only

Repair and/or Reconstruction

(19300-19304 have been deleted. To report, see 19316, 19318)

(19310, 19311 have been deleted. To report, use 19325)

(All codes for bilateral procedures have been deleted. To report, add modifier -50 or 09950)

19316 Mastopexy

19318 Reduction mammaplasty

19324 Mammaplasty, augmentation; without prosthetic implant

19325 with prosthetic implant

(For flap or graft, use also appropriate number)

19328 Removal of intact mammary implant

19330 Removal of mammary implant material

19340 Immediate insertion of breast prosthesis following mastopexy, mastectomy or in reconstruction

19342 Delayed insertion of breast prosthesis following mastopexy, mastectomy or in reconstruction

(For supply of implant, use 99070)

(For preparation of custom breast implant, see 19396)

19350 Nipple/areola reconstruction

19355 Correction of inverted nipples

19357 Breast reconstruction, immediate or delayed, with tissue expander, including subsequent expansion

(19360 has been deleted)

19361 Breast reconstruction with latissimus dorsi flap, with or without prosthetic implant

(19362 has been deleted. To report, see 19367-19369)

19364 Breast reconstruction with free flap

(Use also code number for specific flap)

19366 Breast reconstruction with other technique

(For microsurgical technique, add modifier -20 or 09920)

(For insertion of prosthesis, use also 19340 or 19342)

19367 Breast reconstruction with transverse rectus abdominis myocutaneous flap (TRAM), single pedicle, including closure of donor site;

19368 with microvascular anastomosis (supercharging)

19369 Breast reconstruction with transverse rectus abdominis myocutaneous flap (TRAM), double pedicle, including closure of donor site

19370 Open periprosthetic capsulotomy, breast

19371 Periprosthetic capsulectomy, breast

19380 Revision of reconstructed breast

19396 Preparation of moulage for custom breast implant

Other Procedures

19499 Unlisted procedure, breast

Musculoskeletal System

Cast and strapping procedures appear at the end of this section. The services listed below include the application and removal of the first cast or traction device only. Subsequent replacement of cast and/or traction device may require an additional listing.

Definitions

The terms "closed treatment", "open treatment", and "percutaneous skeletal fixation" have been carefully chosen to accurately reflect current orthopaedic procedural treatments.

Closed treatment specifically means that the fracture site is not surgically opened (exposed to the external environment and directly visualized). This terminology is used to describe procedures that treat fractures by three methods: 1) without manipulation 2) with manipulation 3) with or without traction.

Open treatment is used when the fracture is surgically opened (exposed to the external environment). In this instance, the fracture (bone ends) is visualized and internal fixation may be used.

Percutaneous skeletal fixation describes fracture treatment which is neither open nor closed. In this procedure, the fracture fragments are not visualized, but fixation (eg, pins) is placed across the fracture site, usually under x-ray imaging.

The type of fracture (eg, open, compound, closed) does not have any coding correlation with the type of treatment (eg, closed, open, or percutaneous) provided.

The codes for treatment of fractures and joint injuries (dislocations) are categorized by the type of manipulation (reduction) and stabilization (fixation or immobilization). These codes can apply to either open (compound) or closed fractures or joint injuries.

Skeletal traction is the application of a force (distracting or traction force) to a limb segment through a wire, pin, screw, or clamp that is attached (eg, penetrates) to bone.

Skin traction is the application of a force (longitudinal) to a limb using felt or strapping applied directly to skin only.

External fixation is the usage of skeletal pins plus an attaching mechanism/device used for tempo-rary or definitive treatment of acute or chronic bony deformity.

Codes for obtaining autogenous bone grafts, cartilage, tendon fascia lata grafts or other tissues, through separate incisions are to be used only when the graft is not already listed as part of the basic procedure.

Re-reduction of a fracture and/or dislocation performed by the primary physician may be identified by either the addition of the modifier '-76' to the usual procedure number or by use of modifier code 09976 to indicate "Repeat Procedure by Same Physician". (See Guidelines.)

Codes for external fixation are to be used only when external fixation is not already listed as part of the basic procedure.

All codes for suction irrigation have been deleted. To report, list only the primary surgical procedure performed (eg, sequestrectomy, deep incision).

Manipulation is used throughout the musculoskeletal fracture and dislocation subsections to specifically mean the attempted reduction or restoration of a fracture or joint dislocation to its normal anatomic alignment by the application of manually applied forces.

General

Incision

20000* Incision of soft tissue abscess (eg, secondary to osteomyelitis); superficial

20005 deep or complicated

(20010 has been deleted)

Wound Exploration—Trauma (eg, Penetrating Gunshot, Stab Wound)

20100-20103 relate to wound(s) resulting from penetrating trauma. These codes describe surgical exploration and enlargement of the wound, extension of dissection (to determine penetration), debridement, removal of foreign body(s), ligation or coagulation of minor subcutaneous and/or muscular blood vessel(s), of the subcutaneous tissue, muscle fascia, and/or muscle, not requiring thoracotomy or laparotomy. If a repair is done to major structure(s) or major blood vessel(s) requiring thoracotomy or laparotomy, then those specific code(s) would supersede the use of codes 20100-20103. To report Simple, Intermediate or Complex repair of wound(s) that do not require enlargement of the wound, extension of dissection, etc., as stated above, use specific Repair code(s) in the Integumentary System section.

- **20100** Exploration of penetrating wound (separate procedure); neck

- **20101** chest

- **20102** abdomen/flank/back

- **20103** extremity

Excision

(For aspiration of bone marrow, see 85095)

20200 Biopsy, muscle; superficial

20205 deep

20206* Biopsy, muscle, percutaneous needle

(For radiological supervision and interpretation, see 76360, 76942)

(For fine needle aspiration, preparation, and interpretation of smears, see 88170-88173)

(For excision of muscle tumor, deep, see specific anatomic section)

20220 Biopsy, bone, trocar, or needle; superficial (eg, ilium, sternum, spinous process, ribs)

20225 deep (vertebral body, femur)

(For bone marrow biopsy, use 85102)

20240 Biopsy, excisional; superficial (eg, ilium, sternum, spinous process, ribs, trochanter of femur)

20245 deep (eg, humerus, ischium, femur)

20250 Biopsy, vertebral body, open; thoracic

20251 lumbar or cervical

(For sequestrectomy, osteomyelitis or drainage of bone abscess, see anatomical area)

Introduction or Removal

(For injection procedure for arthrography, see anatomical area)

20500* Injection of sinus tract; therapeutic (separate procedure)

20501* diagnostic (sinogram)

(For radiological supervision and interpretation, see 76080)

20520* Removal of foreign body in muscle or tendon sheath; simple

20525 deep or complicated

20550* Injection, tendon sheath, ligament, trigger points or ganglion cyst

20600* Arthrocentesis, aspiration and/or injection; small joint, bursa or ganglion cyst (eg, fingers, toes)

20605* intermediate joint, bursa or ganglion cyst (eg, temporomandibular, acromioclavicular, wrist, elbow or ankle, olecranon bursa)

20610* major joint or bursa (eg, shoulder, hip, knee joint, subacromial bursa)

20615 Aspiration and injection for treatment of bone cyst

20650* Insertion of wire or pin with application of skeletal traction, including removal (separate procedure)

20660 Application of cranial tongs, caliper, or stereotactic frame, including removal (separate procedure)

20661 Application of halo, including removal; cranial

20662 pelvic

20663 femoral

20665* Removal of tongs or halo applied by another physician

20670* Removal of implant; superficial, (eg, buried wire, pin or rod) (separate procedure)

20680 deep (eg, buried wire, pin, screw, metal band, nail, rod or plate)

20690 Application of a uniplane (pins or wires in one plane), unilateral, external fixation system

(List 20690 in addition to code for treatment of the fracture or joint injury unless listed as part of basic procedure)

(20691 has been deleted. To report, use 20690)

20692 Application of a multiplane (pins or wires in more than one plane), unilateral, external fixation system (eg, Ilizarov, Monticelli type)

(List 20692 in addition to code for treatment of fracture or joint injury unless listed as part of basic procedure)

20693 Adjustment or revision of external fixation system requiring anesthesia (eg, new pin(s) or wire(s) and/or new ring(s) or bar(s))

20694 Removal, under anesthesia, of external fixation system

Replantation

20802 Replantation, arm (includes surgical neck of humerus through elbow joint), complete amputation

(20804 has been deleted. To report, see specific code(s) for repair of bone(s), ligament(s), tendon(s), nerve(s), or blood vessel(s) with modifier -52 Reduced Services or 09952)

20805 Replantation, forearm (includes radius and ulna to radial carpal joint), complete amputation

(20806 has been deleted. To report, see specific code(s) for repair of bone(s), ligament(s), tendon(s), nerve(s), or blood vessel(s) with modifier -52 Reduced Services or 09952)

20808 Replantation, hand (includes hand through metacarpophalangeal joints), complete amputation

(20812 has been deleted. To report, see specific code(s) for repair of bone(s), ligament(s), tendon(s), nerve(s), or blood vessel(s) with modifier -52 Reduced Services or 09952)

20816 Replantation, digit, excluding thumb (includes metacarpophalangeal joint to insertion of flexor sublimis tendon), complete amputation

(20820 has been deleted. To report, see specific code(s) for repair of bone(s), ligament(s), tendon(s), nerve(s), or blood vessel(s) with modifier -52 Reduced Services or 09952)

20822 Replantation, digit, excluding thumb (includes distal tip to sublimis tendon insertion), complete amputation

(20823 has been deleted. To report, see specific code(s) for repair of bone(s), ligament(s), tendon(s), nerve(s), or blood vessel(s) with modifier -52 Reduced Services or 09952)

20824 Replantation, thumb (includes carpometacarpal joint to MP joint), complete amputation

(20826 has been deleted. To report, see specific code(s) for repair of bone(s), ligament(s), tendon(s), nerve(s), or blood vessel(s) with modifier -52 Reduced Services or 09952)

20827 Replantation, thumb (includes distal tip to MP joint), complete amputation

(20828 has been deleted. To report, see specific code(s) for repair of bone(s), ligament(s), tendon(s), nerve(s), or blood vessel(s) with modifier -52 Reduced Services or 09952)

(20832 has been deleted. To report, see specific code(s) for repair of bone(s), ligament(s), tendon(s), nerve(s), or blood vessel(s) with modifier -52 Reduced Services or 09952)

(20834 has been deleted. To report, see specific code(s) for repair of bone(s), ligament(s), tendon(s), nerve(s), or blood vessel(s) with modifier -52 Reduced Services or 09952)

20838 Replantation, foot, complete amputation

(20840 has been deleted. To report, see specific code(s) for repair of bone(s), ligament(s), tendon(s), nerve(s), or blood vessel(s) with modifier -52 Reduced Services or 09952)

Grafts (or Implants)

Codes for obtaining autogenous bone, cartilage, tendon, fascia lata grafts, or other tissues, through separate incisions are to be used only when graft is not already listed as part of basic procedure.

(For spinal surgery bone graft(s) see codes 20930-20938)

20900 Bone graft, any donor area; minor or small (eg, dowel or button)

20902 major or large

20910 Cartilage graft; costochondral

20912 nasal septum

(For ear cartilage, see 21235)

20920 Fascia lata graft; by stripper

20922 by incision and area exposure, complex or sheet

20924 Tendon graft, from a distance (eg, palmaris, toe extensor, plantaris)

20926 Tissue grafts, other (eg, paratenon, fat, dermis)

Codes 20930-20938 are reported in addition to codes for the definitive procedure(s) without modifier '-51'. Report only one bone graft code per operative session.

● **20930** Allograft for spine surgery only; morselized

● **20931** structural

● **20936** Autograft for spine surgery only (includes harvesting the graft); local (eg, ribs, spinous process, or laminar fragments) obtained from same incision

● **20937** morselized (through separate skin or fascial incision)

● **20938** structural, bicortical or tricortical (through separate skin or fascial incision)

(For needle aspiration of bone marrow for the purpose of bone grafting, see 85095)

Other Procedures

20950 Monitoring of interstitial fluid pressure (includes insertion of device, eg, wick catheter technique, needle manometer technique) in detection of muscle compartment syndrome

20955 Bone graft with microvascular anastomosis; fibula

20960 rib

20962 other bone graft (specify)

20969 Free osteocutaneous flap with microvascular anastomosis; other than iliac crest, rib, metatarsal, or great toe

20970 Free osteocutaneous flap with microvascular anastomosis; iliac crest

20971 rib

20972 metatarsal

20973 great toe with web space

20974 Electrical stimulation to aid bone healing; noninvasive (nonoperative)

(Use 20974 in addition to code for appropriate bony procedure, when applicable)

20975 invasive (operative)

(Use 20975 in addition to code for appropriate bony procedure, when applicable)

(20976 has been deleted)

20999 Unlisted procedure, musculoskeletal system, general

Head

Skull, facial bones and temporomandibular joint.

Incision

(For drainage of superficial abscess and hematoma, see 20000)

(For removal of embedded foreign body from dentoalveolar structure, see 41805, 41806)

21010 Arthrotomy, temporomandibular joint

(21011 has been deleted. To report, use 21010 with modifier -50 or 09950)

Excision

(For biopsy, see 20220, 20240)

21015   Radical resection of tumor (eg, malignant neoplasm), soft tissue of face or scalp

(21020 has been deleted. To report, use 61501)

21025   Excision of bone (eg, for osteomyelitis or bone abscess); mandible

21026   facial bone(s)

21029   Removal by contouring of benign tumor of facial bone (eg, fibrous dysplasia)

21030   Excision of benign tumor or cyst of facial bone other than mandible

21031   Excision of torus mandibularis

21032   Excision of maxillary torus palatinus

21034   Excision of malignant tumor of facial bone other than mandible

21040   Excision of benign cyst or tumor of mandible; simple

21041   complex

21044   Excision of malignant tumor of mandible;

21045   radical resection

(For bone graft, see 21215)

21050   Condylectomy, temporomandibular joint (separate procedure)

(21051 has been deleted. To report, use 21050 with modifier -50 or 09950)

21060   Meniscectomy, partial or complete, temporomandibular joint (separate procedure)

(21061 has been deleted. To report, use 21060 with modifier -50 or 09950)

21070   Coronoidectomy (separate procedure)

(21071 has been deleted. To report, use 21070 with modifier -50 or 09950)

Introduction or Removal

(For application or removal of caliper or tongs, see 20660, 20665) 21076-21089 describe professional services for the rehabilitation of patients with oral, facial or other anatomical deficiencies by means of prostheses such as an artificial eye, ear, or nose or intraoral obturator to close a cleft. Codes 21076-21089 should only be used when the physician actually designs and prepares the prosthesis (ie, not prepared by an outside laboratory).

● **21076**   Impression and custom preparation; surgical obturator prosthesis

● **21077**   orbital prosthesis

21079   interim obturator prosthesis

21080   definitive obturator prosthesis

21081   mandibular resection prosthesis

21082   palatal augmentation prosthesis

21083   palatal lift prosthesis

21084   speech aid prosthesis

21085   oral surgical splint

21086   auricular prosthesis

21087   nasal prosthesis

21088   facial prosthesis

21089   Unlisted maxillofacial prosthetic procedure

21100*   Application of halo type appliance for maxillofacial fixation, includes removal (separate procedure)

21110   Application of interdental fixation device for conditions other than fracture or dislocation, includes removal

(For removal of interdental fixation by another physician, see 20670-20680)

21116   Injection procedure for temporomandibular joint arthrography

(For radiological supervision and interpretation, see 70332)

Repair, Revision, and/or Reconstruction

(For cranioplasty, see 21179, 21180 and 62116, 62120, 62140-62147)

21120 Genioplasty; augmentation (autograft, allograft, prosthetic material)

21121 sliding osteotomy, single piece

21122 sliding osteotomies, two or more osteotomies (eg, wedge excision or bone wedge reversal for asymmetrical chin)

21123 sliding, augmentation with interpositional bone grafts (includes obtaining autografts)

21125 Augmentation, mandibular body or angle; prosthetic material

21127 with bone graft, onlay or interpositional (includes obtaining autograft)

21137 Reduction forehead; contouring only

21138 contouring and application of prosthetic material or bone graft (includes obtaining autograft)

21139 contouring and setback of anterior frontal sinus wall

●**21141** Reconstruction midface, LeFort I; single piece, segment movement in any direction (eg, for Long Face Syndrome), without bone graft

●**21142** two pieces, segment movement in any direction, without bone graft

●**21143** three or more pieces, segment movement in any direction, without bone graft

(21144 has been deleted. To report, see 21141)

▲**21145** single piece, segment movement in any direction, requiring bone grafts (includes obtaining autografts)

▲**21146** two pieces, segment movement in any direction, requiring bone grafts (includes obtaining autografts) (eg, ungrafted unilateral alveolar cleft)

▲**21147** three or more pieces, segment movement in any direction, requiring bone grafts (includes obtaining autografts) (eg, ungrafted bilateral alveolar cleft or multiple osteotomies)

21150 Reconstruction midface, LeFort II; anterior intrusion (eg, Treacher-Collins Syndrome)

21151 any direction, requiring bone grafts (includes obtaining autografts)

21154 Reconstruction midface, LeFort III (extracranial), any type, requiring bone grafts (includes obtaining autografts); without LeFort I

21155 with LeFort I

21159 Reconstruction midface, LeFort III (extra and intracranial) with forehead advancement (eg, mono bloc), requiring bone grafts (includes obtaining autografts); without LeFort I

21160 with LeFort I

21172 Reconstruction superior-lateral orbital rim and lower forehead, advancement or alteration, with or without grafts (includes obtaining autografts)

(For frontal or parietal craniotomy performed for craniosynostosis, see 61556)

21175 Reconstruction, bifrontal, superior-lateral orbital rims and lower forehead, advancement or alteration (eg, plagiocephaly, trigonocephaly, brachycephaly), with or without grafts (includes obtaining autografts)

(For bifrontal craniotomy performed for craniosynostosis, see 61557)

21179 Reconstruction, entire or majority of forehead and/or supraorbital rims; with grafts (allograft or prosthetic material)

21180 with autograft (includes obtaining grafts)

(For extensive craniectomy for multiple suture craniosynostosis, use only 61558 or 61559)

21181 Reconstruction by contouring of benign tumor of cranial bones (eg, fibrous dysplasia), extracranial

21182 Reconstruction of orbital walls, rims, forehead, nasoethmoid complex following intra- and extracranial excision of benign tumor of cranial bone (eg, fibrous dysplasia), with multiple autografts (includes obtaining grafts); total area of bone grafting less than 40 cm^2

21183 total area of bone grafting greater than 40 cm^2 but less than 80 cm^2

21184 total area of bone grafting greater than 80 cm^2

(For excision of benign tumor of cranial bones, see 61563, 61564)

21188 Reconstruction midface, osteotomies (other than LeFort type) and bone grafts (includes obtaining autografts)

▲21193 Reconstruction of mandibular rami, horizontal, vertical, "C", or "L" osteotomy; without bone graft

21194 with bone graft (includes obtaining graft)

▲21195 Reconstruction of mandibular rami and/or body, sagittal split; without internal rigid fixation

21196 with internal rigid fixation

21198 Osteotomy, mandible, segmental

(21200, 21202, 21203 have been deleted. To report, see 21193-21198)

(21204 has been deleted. To report, see 21144-21160)

21206 Osteotomy, maxilla, segmental (eg, Wassmund or Schuchard)

(21207 has been deleted. To report, use 21209)

21208 Osteoplasty, facial bones; augmentation (autograft, allograft, or prosthetic implant)

21209 reduction

21210 Graft, bone; nasal, maxillary or malar areas (includes obtaining graft)

(For cleft palate repair, see 42200-42225)

21215 mandible (includes obtaining graft)

21230 Graft; rib cartilage, autogenous, to face, chin, nose or ear (includes obtaining graft)

21235 ear cartilage, autogenous, to nose or ear (includes obtaining graft)

(21239 has been deleted. To report, use 21208)

21240 Arthroplasty, temporomandibular joint, with or without autograft (includes obtaining graft)

(21241 has been deleted. To report, use 21240 with modifier -50 or 09950)

21242 Arthroplasty, temporomandibular joint, with allograft

21243 Arthroplasty, temporomandibular joint, with prosthetic joint replacement

21244 Reconstruction of mandible, extraoral, with transosteal bone plate (eg, mandibular staple bone plate)

21245 Reconstruction of mandible or maxilla, subperiosteal implant; partial

21246 complete

21247 Reconstruction of mandibular condyle with bone and cartilage autografts (includes obtaining grafts) (eg, for hemifacial microsomia)

21248 Reconstruction of mandible or maxilla, endosteal implant (eg, blade, cylinder); partial

21249 complete

(21250, 21254 have been deleted. To report, see 21144-21160)

21255 Reconstruction of zygomatic arch and glenoid fossa with bone and cartilage (includes obtaining autografts)

21256 Reconstruction of orbit with osteotomies (extracranial) and with bone grafts (includes obtaining autografts) (eg, micro-ophthalmia)

21260 Periorbital osteotomies for orbital hypertelorism, with bone grafts; extracranial approach

21261 combined intra- and extracranial approach

21263 with forehead advancement

21267 Orbital repositioning, periorbital osteotomies, unilateral, with bone grafts; extracranial approach

21268 combined intra- and extracranial approach

21270 Malar augmentation, prosthetic material

(For malar augmentation with bone graft, see 21210)

21275 Secondary revision of orbitocraniofacial reconstruction

21280 Medial canthopexy (separate procedure)

(For medial canthoplasty, see 67950)

21282 Lateral canthopexy

21295 Reduction of masseter muscle and bone (eg, for treatment of benign masseteric hypertrophy); extraoral approach

21296 intraoral approach

Other Procedures

21299 Unlisted craniofacial and maxillofacial procedure

Fracture and/or Dislocation

21300 Closed treatment of skull fracture without operation

(For operative repair, see 62000-62010)

21310 Closed treatment of nasal bone fracture without manipulation

21315* Closed treatment of nasal bone fracture; without stabilization

21320 with stabilization

21325 Open treatment of nasal fracture; uncomplicated

21330 complicated, with internal and/or external skeletal fixation

21335 with concomitant open treatment of fractured septum

21336 Open treatment of nasal septal fracture, with or without stabilization

21337 Closed treatment of nasal septal fracture, with or without stabilization

21338 Open treatment of nasoethmoid fracture; without external fixation

21339 with external fixation

21340 Percutaneous treatment of nasoethmoid complex fracture, with splint, wire or headcap fixation, including repair of canthal ligaments and/or the nasolacrimal apparatus

21343 Open treatment of depressed frontal sinus fracture

21344 Open treatment of complicated (eg, comminuted or involving posterior wall) frontal sinus fracture, via coronal or multiple approaches

21345 Closed treatment of nasomaxillary complex fracture (LeFort II type), with interdental wire fixation or fixation of denture or splint

21346 Open treatment of nasomaxillary complex fracture (LeFort II type); with wiring and/or local fixation

21347 requiring multiple open approaches

21348 with bone grafting (includes obtaining graft)

(21350 has been deleted. If necessary to report, use appropriate Evaluation and Management code)

21355* Percutaneous treatment of fracture of malar area, including zygomatic arch and malar tripod, with manipulation

21356 Open treatment of depressed zygomatic arch fracture (eg, Gilles approach)

21360 Open treatment of depressed malar fracture, including zygomatic arch and malar tripod

21365 Open treatment of complicated (eg, comminuted or involving cranial nerve foramina) fracture(s) of malar area, including zygomatic arch and malar tripod; with internal fixation and multiple surgical approaches

21366 with bone grafting (includes obtaining graft)

(21380 has been deleted. If necessary to report, use appropriate Evaluation and Management code)

21385 Open treatment of orbital floor "blowout" fracture; transantral approach (Caldwell-Luc type operation)

21386 periorbital approach

21387 combined approach

21390 periorbital approach, with alloplastic or other implant

21395 periorbital approach with bone graft (includes obtaining graft)

21400 Closed treatment of fracture of orbit, except "blowout"; without manipulation

21401 with manipulation

21406 Open treatment of fracture of orbit, except "blowout"; without implant

21407 with implant

21408 with bone grafting (includes obtaining graft)

(21420 has been deleted. If necessary to report, use appropriate Evaluation and Management code)

21421 Closed treatment of palatal or maxillary fracture (LeFort I type), with interdental wire fixation or fixation of denture or splint

21422 Open treatment of palatal or maxillary fracture (LeFort I type);

21423 complicated (comminuted or involving cranial nerve foramina), multiple approaches

21431 Closed treatment of craniofacial separation (LeFort III type) using interdental wire fixation of denture or splint

21432 Open treatment of craniofacial separation (LeFort III type); with wiring and/or internal fixation

21433 complicated (eg, comminuted or involving cranial nerve foramina), multiple surgical approaches

21435 complicated, utilizing internal and/or external fixation techniques (eg, head cap, halo device, and/or intermaxillary fixation)

(For removal of internal or external fixation device, see 20670)

21436 complicated, multiple surgical approaches, internal fixation, with bone grafting (includes obtaining graft)

21440 Closed treatment of mandibular or maxillary alveolar ridge fracture (separate procedure)

21445 Open treatment of mandibular or maxillary alveolar ridge fracture (separate procedure)

21450 Closed treatment of mandibular fracture; without manipulation

21451 with manipulation

21452 Percutaneous treatment of mandibular fracture, with external fixation

21453 Closed treatment of mandibular fracture with interdental fixation

21454 Open treatment of mandibular fracture with external fixation

(21455 has been deleted. To report, see 21453)

21461 Open treatment of mandibular fracture; without interdental fixation

21462 with interdental fixation

21465 Open treatment of mandibular condylar fracture

21470 Open treatment of complicated mandibular fracture by multiple surgical approaches including internal fixation, interdental fixation, and/or wiring of dentures or splints

21480 Closed treatment of temporomandibular dislocation; initial or subsequent

21485 complicated (eg, recurrent requiring intermaxillary fixation or splinting), initial or subsequent

21490 Open treatment of temporomandibular dislocation

(For interdental wire fixation, see 21497)

21493 Closed treatment of hyoid fracture; without manipulation

21494 with manipulation

21495 Open treatment of hyoid fracture

(For treatment of fracture of larynx, see 31584-31586)

21497   Interdental wiring, for condition other than fracture

Other Procedures

21499   Unlisted musculoskeletal procedure, head

(For unlisted craniofacial or maxillofacial procedure, use 21299)

Neck (Soft Tissues) and Thorax

(For cervical spine and back, see 21920 et seq)

(For injection of fracture site or trigger point, see 20550)

Incision

(For incision and drainage of abscess or hematoma, superficial, see 10060, 10140)

21501   Incision and drainage, deep abscess or hematoma, soft tissues of neck or thorax;

21502   with partial rib ostectomy

21510   Incision, deep, with opening of bone cortex (eg, for osteomyelitis or bone abscess), thorax

(21511 has been deleted)

Excision

(For bone biopsy, see 20220-20251)

21550   Biopsy, soft tissue of neck or thorax

(For needle biopsy of soft tissue, see 20206)

21555   Excision tumor, soft tissue of neck or thorax; subcutaneous

21556   deep, subfascial, intramuscular

21557   Radical resection of tumor (eg, malignant neoplasm), soft tissue of neck or thorax

21600   Excision of rib, partial

(For radical resection of chest wall and rib cage for tumor, see 19260)

(For radical debridement of chest wall and rib cage for injury, see 11040-11044)

21610   Costotransversectomy (separate procedure)

21615   Excision first and/or cervical rib;

21616   with sympathectomy

21620   Ostectomy of sternum, partial

21627   Sternal debridement

(For debridement and closure, see 21750)

21630   Radical resection of sternum;

21632   with mediastinal lymphadenectomy

(21633 has been deleted. To report, use 21630)

Repair, Revision, and/or Reconstruction

(For superficial wound, see Integumentary System section under Repair-Simple)

21700   Division of scalenus anticus; without resection of cervical rib

21705   with resection of cervical rib

21720   Division of sternocleidomastoid for torticollis, open operation; without cast application

(For transection of spinal accessory and cervical nerves, see 63191, 64722)

21725   with cast application

21740   Reconstructive repair of pectus excavatum or carinatum

(21741 has been deleted. To report, use 21899)

21750   Closure of sternotomy separation with or without debridement (separate procedure)

Fracture and/or Dislocation

21800   Closed treatment of rib fracture, uncomplicated, each

21805   Open treatment of rib fracture without fixation, each

21810 Treatment of rib fracture requiring external fixation ("flail chest")

21820 Closed treatment of sternum fracture

21825 Open treatment of sternum fracture with or without skeletal fixation

(For sternoclavicular dislocation, see 23520-23532)

Other Procedures

21899 Unlisted procedure, neck or thorax

Back and Flank

Excision

21920 Biopsy, soft tissue of back or flank; superficial

21925   deep

(For needle biopsy of soft tissue, use 20206)

21930 Excision, tumor, soft tissue of back or flank

21935 Radical resection of tumor (eg, malignant neoplasm), soft tissue of back or flank

Spine (Vertebral Column)

Cervical, thoracic, and lumbar spine.

Within the *SPINE* section, bone grafting procedures are reported separately and in addition to arthrodesis. For bone grafts in other Musculoskeletal sections, see specific code(s) descriptor(s) and/or accompanying guidelines.

To report bone grafts performed after arthrodesis, see codes 20930-20938. Bone graft codes are reported without modifier '-51' (multiple procedure).

Example:

Posterior arthrodesis of L4-S1 for degenerative disc disease utilizing morselized autogenous iliac bone graft harvested through a separate fascial incision.

Report as 22612 and 20937

Within the *SPINE* section, instrumentation is reported separately and in addition to arthrodesis. To report instrumentation procedures performed with definitive vertebral procedure(s), see codes

22840-22855. Instrumentation procedure codes are reported in addition to the definitive procedure(s) without modifier '-51'.

Example:

Posterior arthrodesis of L4-S1, utilizing morselized autogenous iliac bone graft harvested through separate fascial incision, and pedicle screw fixation.

Report as 22612, 22842 and 20937

Vertebral procedures are sometimes followed by arthrodesis and in addition may include bone grafts and instrumentation. When arthrodesis is performed in addition to another procedure, the arthrodesis should be reported in addition to the original procedure with a modifier '-51' (multiple procedures). Examples are after osteotomy, fracture care, vertebral corpectomy and laminectomy. Since bone grafts and instrumentation are never performed without arthrodesis, they are reported as add-on codes and modifier '-51' (multiple procedures) is not used. Arthrodesis, however, may be performed in the absence of other procedures and therefore when it is combined with another definitive procedure, modifier '-51' (multiple procedure) is appropriate.

Example:

Treatment of a burst fracture of L2 by corpectomy followed by arthrodesis of L1-L3, utilizing anterior instrumentation L1-L3 and structural allograft.

Report as 63090, 22558-51, 22845 and 20931

(For injection procedure for myelography, use 62284)

(For injection procedure for diskography, see 62290, 62291)

(For injection procedure, chemonucleolysis, single or multiple levels, use 62292)

(For injection procedure for facet joints, see 64442, 64443, 64622, 64623)

(For needle or trocar biopsy, see 20220-20225)

Excision

(For bone biopsy, see 20220-20251)

(22010 has been deleted. To report, use 21920)

(22011 has been deleted. To report, use 21925)

(22012 has been deleted. To report, use 20206)

(22030-22033 have been deleted. To report, use 21930)

▲**22100** Partial excision of posterior vertebral component (eg, spinous process, lamina or facet) for intrinsic bony lesion, single vertebral segment; cervical

22101 thoracic

22102 lumbar

●**22103** each additional segment (List separately in addition to code for primary procedure)

(Use 22103 only for codes 22100, 22101, 22102)

(22105 has been deleted. To report, see 22100)

(22106 has been deleted. To report, see 22101)

(22107 has been deleted. To report, see 22102)

▲**22110** Partial excision of vertebral body for intrinsic bony lesion, without decompression of spinal cord or nerve root(s), single vertebral segment; cervical

(22111 has been deleted)

22112 thoracic

(22113 has been deleted)

22114 lumbar

(22115 has been deleted)

●**22116** each additional vertebral segment (List separately in addition to code for primary procedure)

(Use 22116 only for codes 22110, 22112, 22114)

(22120-22130 have been deleted. For complete or near complete resection of vertebral body, see vertebral corpectomy, 63081-63091)

(22140 has been deleted. To report, use 63081 and 22554 and 20931 or 20938)

(22141 has been deleted. To report, use 63085 or 63087 and 22556 and 20931 or 20938)

(22142 has been deleted. To report, use 63087 or 63090 and 22558 and 20931 or 20938)

(22145 has been deleted. To report, use 63082 or 63086 or 63088 or 63091, and 22585)

(22148 has been deleted. To report, see 20931 or 20938)

(22150 has been deleted. To report, use 63081 and 22554 and 20931 or 20938 and 22851)

(22151 has been deleted. To report, use 63085 or 63087 and 22556 and 20931 or 20938 and 22851)

(22152 has been deleted. To report, use 63087 or 63090 and 22558, and 20931 or 20938 and 22851)

(22200-22207 have been deleted. For osteotomy of spine, see 22210-22226)

Osteotomy

To report arthrodesis, see codes 22590-22632. (Report in addition to code(s) for the definitive procedure with modifier '-51'.)

To report instrumentation procedures, see codes 22840-22855. (Report in addition to code(s) for the definitive procedure(s) without modifier '-51'.)

To report bone graft procedures, see codes 20930-20938. (Report in addition to code(s) for the definitive procedure(s) without modifier '-51'.)

▲**22210** Osteotomy of spine, posterior or posterolateral approach, one vertebral segment; cervical

22212 thoracic

22214 lumbar

●**22216** each additional vertebral segment (List separately in addition to primary procedure)

(Use 22216 only for codes 22210, 22212, 22214)

▲ **22220** Osteotomy of spine, including diskectomy, anterior approach, single vertebral segment; cervical

22222 thoracic

22224 lumbar

● **22226** each additional vertebral segment (List separately in addition to code for primary procedure)

(Use 22226 only for codes 22220, 22222, 22224)

(22230 has been deleted. To report, use 22216 or 22226)

(22250, 22251 have been deleted. For vertebral corpectomy, see 63081-63091)

Fracture and/or Dislocation

To report arthrodesis, see codes 22590-22632. (Report in addition to code(s) for the definitive procedure with modifier '-51'.)

To report instrumentation procedures, see codes 22840-22855. (Report in addition to code(s) for the definitive procedure(s) without modifier '-51'.)

To report bone graft procedures, see codes 20930-20938. (Report in addition to code(s) for the definitive procedure(s) without modifier '-51'.)

22305 Closed treatment of vertebral process fracture(s)

▲ **22310** Closed treatment of vertebral body fracture(s), without manipulation, requiring and including casting or bracing

▲ **22315** Closed treatment of vertebral fracture(s) and/or dislocation(s) requiring casting or bracing, with and including casting and/or bracing, with or without anesthesia, by manipulation or traction

(For spinal subluxation, see 97260, 97261)

▲ **22325** Open treatment and/or reduction of vertebral fracture(s) and/or dislocation(s); posterior approach, one fractured vertebrae or dislocated segment; lumbar

▲ **22326** cervical

▲ **22327** thoracic

● **22328** each additional fractured vertebrae or dislocated segment (List separately in addition to code for primary procedure)

(Use 22328 only for codes 22325, 22326, 22327)

(For treatment of vertebral fracture by the anterior approach, see corpectomy 63081-63091, and appropriate arthrodesis, bone graft and instrument codes)

(22330-22379 have been deleted. For decompression of spine following fracture, see 63001-63091; for arthrodesis of spine following fracture, see 22548-22632)

Manipulation

(22500 has been deleted. To report, use 97260)

22505 Manipulation of spine requiring anesthesia, any region

Arthrodesis

Arthrodesis may be performed in the absence of other procedures and therefore when it is combined with another definitive procedure (eg, osteotomy, fracture care, vertebral corpectomy or laminectomy), modifier '-51' is appropriate. However, arthrodesis codes 22585, 22614, and 22632 are considered add-on procedure codes and should not be used with modifier '-51'.

To report instrumentation procedures, see codes 22840-22855. (Report in addition to code(s) for the definitive procedure(s) without modifier '-51'.)

To report bone graft procedures, see codes 20930-20938. (Report in addition to code(s) for the definitive procedure(s) without modifier '-51'.)

Anterior or Anterolateral Approach Technique

Procedure codes 22554-22558 are for SINGLE interspace arthrodesis (2 adjacent vertebral segments); for additional interspaces or segments, use 22585.

▲**22548** Arthrodesis, anterior transoral or extraoral technique, clivus-C1-C2 (atlas-axis), with or without excision of odontoid process

(22550, 22552, 22555, 22560, 22561, 22565 have been deleted. For intervertebral disk excision by laminotomy or laminectomy, see 63020-63042. For arthrodesis, see 22548-22632)

▲**22554** Arthrodesis, anterior interbody technique, including minimal diskectomy to prepare interspace (other than for decompression); cervical below C2

▲**22556** thoracic

▲**22558** lumbar

▲**22585** each additional interspace (List separately in addition to code for primary procedure)

(Use 22585 only for codes 22554, 22556, 22558)

Posterior, Posterolateral or Lateral Transverse Process Technique

To report instrumentation procedures, see codes 22840-22855. (Report in addition to code(s) for the definitive procedure(s) without modifier '-51'.)

To report bone graft procedures, see codes 20930-20938. (Report in addition to code(s) for the definitive procedure(s) without modifier '-51'.)

▲**22590** Arthrodesis, posterior technique, craniocervical (occiput-C2)

▲**22595** Arthrodesis, posterior technique, atlas-axis (C1-C2)

▲**22600** Arthrodesis, posterior or posterolateral technique, single level; cervical below C2 segment

(22605 has been deleted. To report, use 22600)

▲**22610** thoracic (with or without lateral transverse technique)

▲**22612** lumbar (with or without lateral transverse technique)

●**22614** each additional vertebral segment (List separately in addition to code for primary procedure)

(Use 22614 only for codes 22600, 22610, 22612)

(22615 has been deleted. To report, use 22554 and 20930-20938)

(22617 has been deleted. To report, use 22548 and 20930-20938)

(22620 has been deleted. To report, use 22590 and 20930-20938)

(22625 has been deleted. To report, use 22612 and 22840-22855, and 20930-20938)

▲**22630** Arthrodesis, posterior interbody technique, single interspace; lumbar

●**22632** each additional interspace (List separately in addition to code for primary procedure)

(Use code 22632 only for code 22630)

(22640-22645 have been deleted. To report, see 22610, 22612, and 20930-20938)

(22650 has been deleted. To report, see 22614)

(22655 has been deleted. To report, see 22630, 22632 and 20930-20938)

(22670 has been deleted. To report, see 22610 or 22612 and 22840-22855, and 20930-20938)

(22680 has been deleted. To report, see 22556-22585 and 20930-20938)

(22700 has been deleted. To report, see 22558 and 20930-20938)

(22720 has been deleted. To report, see 22612 and 20930-20938)

(22730 has been deleted. To report, see 22585, 22614)

(22735 has been deleted. To report, see 22585, 22614)

Spine Deformity (eg, Scoliosis, Kyphosis)

To report instrumentation procedures, see codes 22840-22855. (Report in addition to code(s) for the definitive procedure(s) without modifier '-51'.)

To report bone graft procedures, see codes 20930-20938. (Report in addition to code(s) for the definitive procedure(s) without modifier '-51'.)

Report only one spine deformity arthrodesis code per operative session.

▲22800   Arthrodesis, posterior, for spinal deformity, with or without cast; up to 6 vertebral segments

(22801 has been deleted. To report, use 22800)

▲22802   7 to 12 vertebral segments

(22803 has been deleted. To report, use 22802)

●22804   13 or more vertebral segments

●22808   Arthrodesis, anterior, for spinal deformity, with or without cast; 2 to 3 vertebral segments

▲22810   4 to 7 vertebral segments

▲22812   8 or more vertebral segments

Exploration

(22820 has been deleted. To report, see 20930-20938)

22830   Exploration of spinal fusion

Spinal Instrumentation

Segmental instrumentation is defined as fixation at each end of the construct and at least one additional interposed bony attachment.

Non-segmental instrumentation is defined as fixation at each end of the construct and may span several vertebral segments without attachment to the intervening segments.

Instrumentation is reported separately and in addition to arthrodesis. Instrumentation procedure codes are reported in addition to the definitive procedure(s) without modifier '-51'.

To report bone graft procedures, see codes 20930-20938. (Report in addition to code(s) for definitive procedure(s) without modifier '-51'.)

List codes 22840-22848, 22851 separately, in addition to code for fracture, dislocation or arthrodesis of the spine, 22325, 22326, 22327, 22548-22812.

▲22840   Posterior non-segmental instrumentation (eg, single Harrington rod technique)

●22841   Internal spinal fixation by wiring of spinous processes

▲22842   Posterior segmental instrumentation (eg, pedicle fixation, dual rods with multiple hooks and sublaminal wires); 3 to 6 vertebral segments

●22843   7 to 12 vertebral segments

●22844   13 or more vertebral segments

▲22845   Anterior instrumentation; 3 vertebral segments

●22846   4 to 7 vertebral segments

●22847   8 or more vertebral segments

●22848   Pelvic fixation (attachment of caudal end of instrumentation to pelvic bony structures) other than sacrum

22849   Reinsertion of spinal fixation device

22850   Removal of posterior nonsegmental instrumentation (eg, Harrington rod)

●22851   Application of prosthetic device (eg, metal cages, methylmethacrylate) to vertebral defect or interspace

22852   Removal of posterior segmental instrumentation

22855   Removal of anterior instrumentation

Other Procedures

22899   Unlisted procedure, spine

Abdomen

Excision

22900   Excision, abdominal wall tumor, subfascial (eg, desmoid)

(22910 has been deleted. To report, use 22999)

Other Procedures

22999   Unlisted procedure, abdomen, musculoskeletal system

Shoulder

Clavicle, scapula, humerus head and neck, sterno-clavicular joint, acromioclavicular joint and shoulder joint.

Incision

23000   Removal of subdeltoid (or intratendinous) calcareous deposits, open method

23020   Capsular contracture release (Sever type procedure)

(For incision and drainage procedures, superficial, see 10040-10160)

23030   Incision and drainage, shoulder area; deep abscess or hematoma

23031   infected bursa

23035   Incision, deep, with opening of cortex (eg, for osteomyelitis or bone abscess), shoulder area

(23036 has been deleted)

23040   Arthrotomy, glenohumeral joint, for infection, with exploration, drainage or removal of foreign body

(23042 has been deleted)

23044   Arthrotomy, acromioclavicular, sternoclavicular joint, for infection, with exploration, drainage or removal of foreign body

Excision

23065   Biopsy, soft tissue of shoulder area; superficial

23066   deep

(For needle biopsy of soft tissue, use 20206)

23075   Excision, tumor, shoulder area; subcutaneous

23076   deep, subfascial or intramuscular

23077   Radical resection of tumor (eg, malignant neoplasm), soft tissue of shoulder area

23100   Arthrotomy with biopsy, glenohumeral joint

23101   Arthrotomy with biopsy, or with excision of torn cartilage, acromioclavicular, sternoclavicular joint

23105   Arthrotomy with synovectomy; glenohumeral joint

23106   sternoclavicular joint

23107   Arthrotomy, glenohumeral joint, with joint exploration, with or without removal of loose or foreign body

(23110 has been deleted. To report, use 23929)

23120   Claviculectomy; partial

23125   total

23130   Acromioplasty or acromionectomy, partial

23140   Excision or curettage of bone cyst or benign tumor of clavicle or scapula;

23145   with autograft (includes obtaining graft)

23146   with allograft

23150   Excision or curettage of bone cyst or benign tumor of proximal humerus;

23155   with autograft (includes obtaining graft)

23156   with allograft

23170   Sequestrectomy (eg, for osteomyelitis or bone abscess), clavicle

(23171 has been deleted)

23172   Sequestrectomy (eg, for osteomyelitis or bone abscess), scapula

(23173 has been deleted)

23174   Sequestrectomy (eg, for osteomyelitis or bone abscess), humeral head to surgical neck

(23175 has been deleted)

23180   Partial excision (craterization, saucerization, or diaphysectomy) of bone (eg, for osteomyelitis), clavicle

(23181 has been deleted)

23182 Partial excision (craterization, saucerization, or diaphysectomy) of bone (eg, for osteomyelitis), scapula

(23183 has been deleted)

23184 Partial excision (craterization, saucerization, or diaphysectomy) of bone (eg, for osteomyelitis), proximal humerus

(23185 has been deleted)

23190 Ostectomy of scapula, partial (eg, superior medial angle)

23195 Resection humeral head

(For replacement with implant, see 23470)

23200 Radical resection for tumor; clavicle

23210 scapula

23220 Radical resection for tumor, proximal humerus;

23221 with autograft (includes obtaining graft)

23222 with prosthetic replacement

Introduction or Removal

(For arthrocentesis or needling of bursa, see 20610)

(For K-wire or pin insertion or removal, see 20650, 20670, 20680)

23330 Removal of foreign body, shoulder; subcutaneous

23331 deep (eg, Neer prosthesis removal)

23332 complicated, including "total shoulder"

23350 Injection procedure for shoulder arthrography

(For radiological supervision and interpretation, see 73040)

(23355-23358 have been deleted. To report, see 29815-29825)

Repair, Revision, and/or Reconstruction

23395 Muscle transfer, any type, shoulder or upper arm; single

23397 multiple

23400 Scapulopexy (eg, Sprengel's deformity or for paralysis)

23405 Tenomyotomy, shoulder area; single

23406 multiple through same incision

23410 Repair of ruptured musculotendinous cuff (eg, rotator cuff); acute

23412 chronic

23415 Coracoacromial ligament release, with or without acromioplasty

23420 Repair of complete shoulder (rotator) cuff avulsion, chronic (includes acromioplasty)

23430 Tenodesis of long tendon of biceps

23440 Resection or transplantation of long tendon of biceps

23450 Capsulorrhaphy, anterior; Putti-Platt procedure or Magnuson type operation

23455 Bankart type operation with or without stapling

23460 Capsulorrhaphy, anterior, any type; with bone block

23462 with coracoid process transfer

23465 Capsulorrhaphy for recurrent dislocation, posterior, with or without bone block

(For sternoclavicular and acromioclavicular reconstruction, see 23530, 23550)

23466 Capsulorrhaphy with any type multi-directional instability

23470 Arthroplasty with proximal humeral implant (eg, Neer type operation)

23472 Arthroplasty with glenoid and proximal humeral replacement (eg, total shoulder)

(For removal of total shoulder implants, see 23331, 23332)

(For osteotomy, proximal humerus, see 24400)

23480 Osteotomy, clavicle, with or without internal fixation;

23485 with bone graft for nonunion or malunion (includes obtaining graft and/or necessary fixation)

23490 Prophylactic treatment (nailing, pinning, plating or wiring) with or without methylmethacrylate; clavicle

23491 proximal humerus and humeral head

Fracture and/or Dislocation

23500 Closed treatment of clavicular fracture; without manipulation

23505 with manipulation

(23510 has been deleted. To report, see 23500, 23505, 23515)

23515 Open treatment of clavicular fracture, with or without internal or external fixation

23520 Closed treatment of sternoclavicular dislocation; without manipulation

23525 with manipulation

23530 Open treatment of sternoclavicular dislocation, acute or chronic;

23532 with fascial graft (includes obtaining graft)

23540 Closed treatment of acromioclavicular dislocation; without manipulation

23545 with manipulation

23550 Open treatment of acromioclavicular dislocation, acute or chronic;

23552 with fascial graft (includes obtaining graft)

23570 Closed treatment of scapular fracture; without manipulation

23575 with manipulation, with or without skeletal traction (with or without shoulder joint involvement)

(23580 has been deleted. To report, see 23570, 23575, 23585)

23585 Open treatment of scapular fracture (body, glenoid or acromion) with or without internal fixation

23600 Closed treatment of proximal humeral (surgical or anatomical neck) fracture; without manipulation

23605 with manipulation, with or without skeletal traction

(23610 has been deleted. To report, see 23600, 23605, 23615)

23615 Open treatment of proximal humeral (surgical or anatomical neck) fracture, with or without internal or external fixation, with or without repair of tuberosity(-ies);

23616 with proximal humeral prosthetic replacement

23620 Closed treatment of greater tuberosity fracture; without manipulation

23625 with manipulation

23630 Open treatment of greater tuberosity fracture, with or without internal or external fixation

23650 Closed treatment of shoulder dislocation, with manipulation; without anesthesia

23655 requiring anesthesia

(23658 has been deleted. To report, see 23650, 23655, 23660, 23665, 23670)

23660 Open treatment of acute shoulder dislocation

(Repairs for recurrent dislocations, see 23450-23466)

23665 Closed treatment of shoulder dislocation, with fracture of greater tuberosity, with manipulation

23670 Open treatment of shoulder dislocation, with fracture of greater tuberosity, with or without internal or external fixation

23675 Closed treatment of shoulder dislocation, with surgical or anatomical neck fracture, with manipulation

23680 Open treatment of shoulder dislocation, with surgical or anatomical neck fracture, with or without internal or external fixation

Manipulation

23700* Manipulation under anesthesia, shoulder joint, including application of fixation apparatus (dislocation excluded)

Arthrodesis

23800 Arthrodesis, shoulder joint; with or without local bone graft

23802 with primary autogenous graft (includes obtaining graft)

Amputation

23900 Interthoracoscapular amputation (forequarter)

23920 Disarticulation of shoulder;

23921 secondary closure or scar revision

Other Procedures

23929 Unlisted procedure, shoulder

Humerus (Upper Arm) and Elbow

Elbow area includes head and neck of radius and olecranon process.

Incision

(For incision and drainage procedures, superficial, see 10040-10160)

23930 Incision and drainage, upper arm or elbow area; deep abscess or hematoma

23931 infected bursa

23935 Incision, deep, with opening of bone cortex (eg, for osteomyelitis or bone abscess), humerus or elbow

(23936 has been deleted)

24000 Arthrotomy, elbow, for infection, with exploration, drainage or removal of foreign body

(24001 has been deleted)

24006 Arthrotomy of the elbow, with capsular excision for capsular release (separate procedure)

Excision

24065 Biopsy, soft tissue of upper arm or elbow area; superficial

24066 deep

(For needle biopsy of soft tissue, use 20206)

24075 Excision, tumor, upper arm or elbow area; subcutaneous

24076 deep, subfascial or intramuscular

24077 Radical resection of tumor (eg, malignant neoplasm), soft tissue of upper arm or elbow area

24100 Arthrotomy, elbow; with synovial biopsy only

24101 with joint exploration, with or without biopsy, with or without removal of loose or foreign body

24102 with synovectomy

24105 Excision, olecranon bursa

24110 Excision or curettage of bone cyst or benign tumor, humerus;

24115 with autograft (includes obtaining graft)

24116 with allograft

24120 Excision or curettage of bone cyst or benign tumor of head or neck of radius or olecranon process;

24125 with autograft (includes obtaining graft)

24126 with allograft

24130 Excision, radial head

(For replacement with implant, see 24366)

24134 Sequestrectomy (eg, for osteomyelitis or bone abscess), shaft or distal humerus

(24135 has been deleted)

24136 Sequestrectomy (eg, for osteomyelitis or bone abscess), radial head or neck

---

(24137 has been deleted)

24138 Sequestrectomy (eg, for osteomyelitis or bone abscess), olecranon process

(24139 has been deleted)

24140 Partial excision (craterization, saucerization or diaphysectomy) of bone (eg, for osteomyelitis), humerus

(24144 has been deleted)

24145 Partial excision (craterization, saucerization or diaphysectomy) of bone (eg, for osteomyelitis), radial head or neck

(24146 has been deleted)

24147 Partial excision (craterization, saucerization or diaphysectomy) of bone (eg, for osteomyelitis), olecranon process

(24148 has been deleted)

24150 Radical resection for tumor, shaft or distal humerus;

24151   with autograft (includes obtaining graft)

24152 Radical resection for tumor, radial head or neck;

24153   with autograft (includes obtaining graft)

24155 Resection of elbow joint (arthrectomy)

Introduction or Removal

(For K-wire or pin insertion or removal, see 20650, 20670, 20680)

(For arthrocentesis or needling of bursa or joint, see 20605)

24160 Implant removal; elbow joint

24164   radial head

24200 Removal of foreign body, upper arm or elbow area; subcutaneous

24201   deep

24220 Injection procedure for elbow arthrography

(For radiological supervision and interpretation, see 73085)

(For injection of tennis elbow, see 20550)

Repair, Revision, and/or Reconstruction

24301 Muscle or tendon transfer, any type, upper arm or elbow, single (excluding 24320-24331)

24305 Tendon lengthening, upper arm or elbow, single, each

24310 Tenotomy, open, elbow to shoulder, single, each

24320 Tenoplasty, with muscle transfer, with or without free graft, elbow to shoulder, single (Seddon-Brookes type procedure)

24330 Flexor-plasty, elbow (eg, Steindler type advancement);

24331   with extensor advancement

24340 Tenodesis of biceps tendon at elbow (separate procedure)

24342 Reinsertion or repair of ruptured or lacerated biceps or triceps tendon, distal, with or without tendon graft

24350 Fasciotomy, lateral or medial (eg, "tennis elbow" or epicondylitis);

24351   with extensor origin detachment

24352   with annular ligament resection

24354   with stripping

24356   with partial ostectomy

24360 Arthroplasty, elbow; with membrane

24361   with distal humeral prosthetic replacement

24362   with implant and fascia lata ligament reconstruction

24363   with distal humerus and proximal ulnar prosthetic replacement ("total elbow")

24365 Arthroplasty, radial head;

24366   with implant

24400 Osteotomy, humerus, with or without internal fixation

24410 Multiple osteotomies with realignment on intramedullary rod, humeral shaft (Sofield type procedure)

24420 Osteoplasty, humerus (eg, shortening or lengthening) (excluding 64876)

24430 Repair of nonunion or malunion, humerus; without graft (eg, compression technique)

24435 with iliac or other autograft (includes obtaining graft)

(For proximal radius and/or ulna, see 25400-25420)

24470 Hemiepiphyseal arrest (eg, for cubitus varus or valgus, distal humerus)

24495 Decompression fasciotomy, forearm, with brachial artery exploration

24498 Prophylactic treatment (nailing, pinning, plating or wiring), with or without methylmethacrylate, humerus

Fracture and/or Dislocation

24500 Closed treatment of humeral shaft fracture; without manipulation

24505 with manipulation, with or without skeletal traction

(24506 has been deleted. To report, see 24516)

(24510 has been deleted. To report, see 24500, 24505, 24515, 24516)

24515 Open treatment of humeral shaft fracture with plate/screws, with or without cerclage

24516 Open treatment of humeral shaft fracture, with insertion of intramedullary implant, with or without cerclage and/or locking screws

24530 Closed treatment of supracondylar or transcondylar humeral fracture, with or without intercondylar extension; without manipulation

(24531 has been deleted. To report, see 24535)

24535 with manipulation, with or without skin or skeletal traction

(24536 has been deleted. To report, see 24535)

24538 Percutaneous skeletal fixation of supracondylar or transcondylar humeral fracture, with or without intercondylar extension

(24540 and 24542 have been deleted. To report, see 24530, 24535, 24538, 24545, 24546)

24545 Open treatment of humeral supracondylar or transcondylar fracture, with or without internal or external fixation; without intercondylar extension

24546 with intercondylar extension

24560 Closed treatment of humeral epicondylar fracture, medial or lateral; without manipulation

24565 with manipulation

24566 Percutaneous skeletal fixation of humeral epicondylar fracture, medial or lateral, with manipulation

(24570 has been deleted. To report, see 24560, 24565, 24575)

24575 Open treatment of humeral epicondylar fracture, medial or lateral, with or without internal or external fixation

24576 Closed treatment of humeral condylar fracture, medial or lateral; without manipulation

24577 with manipulation

(24578 has been deleted. To report, see 24576, 24577, 24579)

24579 Open treatment of humeral condylar fracture, medial or lateral, with or without internal or external fixation

(24580 has been deleted. To report, see 24530, 24560, 24576, 24650, 24670)

(24581 has been deleted. To report, see 24535, 24565, 24577, 24675)

24582 Percutaneous skeletal fixation of humeral condylar fracture, medial or lateral, with manipulation

(24583 has been deleted. To report, see 24535, 24538, 24545, 24560, 24565, 24577)

(24585 has been deleted. To report, see 24538, 24545, 24575, 24579, 24665, 24666, 24685)

24586 Open treatment of periarticular fracture and/or dislocation of the elbow (fracture distal humerus and proximal ulna and/or proximal radius);

24587   with implant arthroplasty

(See also 24361)

(24588 has been deleted. To report, see 24586, 24587)

24600 Treatment of closed elbow dislocation; without anesthesia

24605   requiring anesthesia

(24610 has been deleted. To report, see 24586, 24600, 24605, 24615)

24615 Open treatment of acute or chronic elbow dislocation

24620 Closed treatment of Monteggia type of fracture dislocation at elbow (fracture proximal end of ulna with dislocation of radial head), with manipulation

(24625 has been deleted. To report, see 24620, 24635)

24635 Open treatment of Monteggia type of fracture dislocation at elbow (fracture proximal end of ulna with dislocation of radial head), with or without internal or external fixation

24640* Closed treatment of radial head subluxation in child, "nursemaid elbow", with manipulation

24650 Closed treatment of radial head or neck fracture; without manipulation

24655   with manipulation

(24660 has been deleted. To report, see 24650, 24655, 24665, 24666)

24665 Open treatment of radial head or neck fracture, with or without internal fixation or radial head excision;

24666   with radial head prosthetic replacement

24670 Closed treatment of ulnar fracture, proximal end (olecranon process); without manipulation

24675   with manipulation

(24680 has been deleted. To report, see 24670, 24675, 24685)

24685 Open treatment of ulnar fracture proximal end (olecranon process), with or without internal or external fixation

(24700 has been deleted. To report, use 24999)

Arthrodesis

24800 Arthrodesis, elbow joint; with or without local autograft or allograft

24802   with autograft (includes obtaining graft other than locally obtained)

Amputation

24900 Amputation, arm through humerus; with primary closure

24920   open, circular (guillotine)

24925   secondary closure or scar revision

24930   re-amputation

24931   with implant

24935 Stump elongation, upper extremity

24940 Cineplasty, upper extremity, complete procedure

Other Procedures

24999 Unlisted procedure, humerus or elbow

Forearm and Wrist

Radius, ulna, carpal bones and joints.

Incision

25000 Tendon sheath incision; at radial styloid (eg, for deQuervain's disease)

(For decompression median nerve or for carpal tunnel syndrome, see 64721)

(25005 has been deleted. To report, use 25000)

25020 Decompression fasciotomy, forearm and/or wrist; flexor or extensor compartment

25023 with debridement of nonviable muscle and/or nerve

(For decompression fasciotomy with brachial artery exploration, see 24495)

(For incision and drainage procedures, superficial, see 10040-10160)

(For debridement, see also 11000-11044)

25028 Incision and drainage, forearm and/or wrist; deep abscess or hematoma

25031 infected bursa

25035 Incision, deep, with opening of bone cortex (eg, for osteomyelitis or bone abscess), forearm and/or wrist

(25036 has been deleted)

25040 Arthrotomy, radiocarpal or midcarpal joint, with exploration, drainage, or removal of foreign body

(25041 has been deleted)

Excision

25065 Biopsy, soft tissue of forearm and/or wrist; superficial

25066 deep

(For needle biopsy of soft tissue, use 20206)

25075 Excision, tumor, forearm and/or wrist area; subcutaneous

25076 deep, subfascial or intramuscular

25077 Radical resection of tumor (eg, malignant neoplasm), soft tissue of forearm and/or wrist area

25085 Capsulotomy, wrist (eg, for contracture)

25100 Arthrotomy, wrist joint; with biopsy

25101 with joint exploration, with or without biopsy, with or without removal of loose or foreign body

25105 with synovectomy

25107 Arthrotomy, distal radioulnar joint for repair of triangular cartilage complex

25110 Excision, lesion of tendon sheath, forearm and/or wrist

25111 Excision of ganglion, wrist (dorsal or volar); primary

25112 recurrent

(For hand or finger, see 26160)

25115 Radical excision of bursa, synovia of wrist, or forearm tendon sheaths (eg, tenosynovitis, fungus, Tbc, or other granulomas, rheumatoid arthritis); flexors

25116 extensors, with or without transposition of dorsal retinaculum

(For finger synovectomies, see 26145)

25118 Synovectomy, extensor tendon sheath, wrist, single compartment;

25119 with resection of distal ulna

25120 Excision or curettage of bone cyst or benign tumor of radius or ulna (excluding head or neck of radius and olecranon process);

(For head or neck of radius or olecranon process, see 24120-24126)

25125 with autograft (includes obtaining graft)

25126 with allograft

25130 Excision or curettage of bone cyst or benign tumor of carpal bones;

25135 with autograft (includes obtaining graft)

25136 with allograft

25145 Sequestrectomy (eg, for osteomyelitis or bone abscess), forearm and/or wrist

(25146 has been deleted)

25150 Partial excision (craterization, saucerization or diaphysectomy) of bone (eg, for osteomyelitis); ulna

25151 radius

(25153 has been deleted)

(For head or neck of radius or olecranon process, see 24145, 24147)

25170 Radical resection for tumor, radius or ulna

25210 Carpectomy; one bone

(For carpectomy with implant, see 25441-25445)

25215 all bones of proximal row

25230 Radial styloidectomy (separate procedure)

25240 Excision distal ulna partial or complete (eg, Darrach type or matched resection)

(For implant replacement, distal ulna, see 25442)

(For obtaining fascia for interposition, see 20920, 20922)

Introduction or Removal

(For K-wire, pin or rod insertion or removal, see 20650, 20670, 20680)

25246 Injection procedure for wrist arthrography

(For radiological supervision and interpretation, see 73115)

(For foreign body removal, superficial see 20520)

25248 Exploration with removal of deep foreign body, forearm or wrist

25250 Removal of wrist prosthesis; (separate procedure)

25251 complicated, including "total wrist"

Repair, Revision, and/or Reconstruction

25260 Repair, tendon or muscle, flexor, forearm and/or wrist; primary, single, each tendon or muscle

25263 secondary, single, each tendon or muscle

25265 secondary, with free graft (includes obtaining graft), each tendon or muscle

25270 Repair, tendon or muscle, extensor, forearm and/or wrist; primary, single, each tendon or muscle

25272 secondary, single, each tendon or muscle

25274 Repair, tendon or muscle, extensor, secondary, with tendon graft (includes obtaining graft), forearm and/or wrist, each tendon or muscle

25280 Lengthening or shortening of flexor or extensor tendon, forearm and/or wrist, single, each tendon

25290 Tenotomy, open, flexor or extensor tendon, forearm and/or wrist, single, each tendon

25295 Tenolysis, flexor or extensor tendon, forearm and/or wrist, single, each tendon

25300 Tenodesis at wrist; flexors of fingers

25301 extensors of fingers

25310 Tendon transplantation or transfer, flexor or extensor, forearm and/or wrist, single; each tendon

25312 with tendon graft(s) (includes obtaining graft), each tendon

25315 Flexor origin slide (eg, for cerebral palsy, Volkmann contracture), forearm and/or wrist;

25316 with tendon(s) transfer

(25317, 25318 have been deleted. To report, see 25315, 25316)

25320 Capsulorrhaphy or reconstruction, wrist, any method (eg, capsulodesis, ligament repair, tendon transfer or graft) (includes synovectomy, capsulotomy and open reduction) for carpal instability

25330 Arthroplasty, wrist;

25331 with implant

25332 pseudarthrosis type with internal fixation

(For obtaining fascia for interposition, see 20920, 20922)

25335 Centralization of wrist on ulna (eg, radial club hand)

25337   Reconstruction for stabilization of unstable distal ulna or distal radioulnar joint, secondary by soft tissue stabilization (eg, tendon transfer, tendon graft or weave, or tenodesis) with or without open reduction of distal radioulnar joint

(For harvesting of fascia lata graft, see 20920, 20922)

25350   Osteotomy, radius; distal third

25355   middle or proximal third

25360   Osteotomy; ulna

25365   radius and ulna

25370   Multiple osteotomies, with realignment on intramedullary rod (Sofield type procedure); radius OR ulna

25375   radius AND ulna

25390   Osteoplasty, radius OR ulna; shortening

25391   lengthening with autograft

25392   Osteoplasty, radius AND ulna; shortening (excluding 64876)

25393   lengthening with autograft

25400   Repair of nonunion or malunion, radius OR ulna; without graft (eg, compression technique)

25405   with iliac or other autograft (includes obtaining graft)

25415   Repair of nonunion or malunion, radius AND ulna; without graft (eg, compression technique)

25420   with iliac or other autograft (includes obtaining graft)

25425   Repair of defect with autograft; radius OR ulna

25426   radius AND ulna

25440   Repair of nonunion, scaphoid (navicular) bone, with or without radial styloidectomy (includes obtaining graft and necessary fixation)

25441   Arthroplasty with prosthetic replacement; distal radius

25442   distal ulna

25443   scaphoid (navicular)

25444   lunate

25445   trapezium

25446   distal radius and partial or entire carpus ("total wrist")

25447   Interposition arthroplasty, intercarpal or carpometacarpal joints

25449   Revision of arthroplasty, including removal of implant, wrist joint

25450   Epiphyseal arrest by epiphysiodesis or stapling; distal radius OR ulna

25455   distal radius AND ulna

25490   Prophylactic treatment (nailing, pinning, plating or wiring) with or without methylmethacrylate; radius

25491   ulna

25492   radius AND ulna

Fracture and/or Dislocation

25500   Closed treatment of radial shaft fracture; without manipulation

25505   with manipulation

(25510 has been deleted. To report, see 25500, 25505, 25515)

25515   Open treatment of radial shaft fracture, with or without internal or external fixation

25520   Closed treatment of radial shaft fracture, with dislocation of distal radio-ulnar joint (Galeazzi fracture/dislocation)

25525   Open treatment of radial shaft fracture, with internal and/or external fixation and closed treatment of dislocation of distal radio-ulnar joint (Galeazzi fracture/dislocation), with or without percutaneous skeletal fixation

25526   Open treatment of radial shaft fracture, with internal and/or external fixation and open treatment, with or without internal or external fixation of distal radio-ulnar joint (Galeazzi fracture/dislocation), includes repair of triangular cartilage

---

▲=Revised Code   ●=New Code   ✱=Service Includes Surgical Procedure Only

25530   Closed treatment of ulnar shaft fracture; without manipulation

25535   with manipulation

(25540 has been deleted. To report, see 25530, 25535, 25545)

25545   Open treatment of ulnar shaft fracture, with or without internal or external fixation

25560   Closed treatment of radial and ulnar shaft fractures; without manipulation

25565   with manipulation

(25570 has been deleted. To report, see 25560, 25565, 25574, 25575)

25574   Open treatment of radial AND ulnar shaft fractures, with internal or external fixation; of radius or ulna

25575   of radius AND ulna

25600   Closed treatment of distal radial fracture (eg, Colles or Smith type) or epiphyseal separation, with or without fracture of ulnar styloid; without manipulation

25605   with manipulation

(25610 has been deleted. To report, see 25605)

25611   Percutaneous skeletal fixation of distal radial fracture (eg, Colles or Smith type) or epiphyseal separation, with or without fracture of ulnar styloid, requiring manipulation, with or without external fixation

(25615 has been deleted. To report, see 25600, 25605, 25611, 25620)

25620   Open treatment of distal radial fracture (eg, Colles or Smith type) or epiphyseal separation, with or without fracture of ulnar styloid, with or without internal or external fixation

25622   Closed treatment of carpal scaphoid (navicular) fracture; without manipulation

25624   with manipulation

(25626 has been deleted. To report, see 25622, 25624, 25628)

25628   Open treatment of carpal scaphoid (navicular) fracture, with or without internal or external fixation

25630   Closed treatment of carpal bone fracture (excluding carpal scaphoid (navicular)); without manipulation, each bone

25635   with manipulation, each bone

(25640 has been deleted. To report, see 25630, 25635, 25645)

25645   Open treatment of carpal bone fracture (excluding carpal scaphoid (navicular)), each bone

25650   Closed treatment of ulnar styloid fracture

25660   Closed treatment of radiocarpal or intercarpal dislocation, one or more bones, with manipulation

(25665 has been deleted. To report, see 25650, 25660, 25670)

25670   Open treatment of radiocarpal or intercarpal dislocation, one or more bones

25675   Closed treatment of distal radioulnar dislocation with manipulation

25676   Open treatment of distal radioulnar dislocation, acute or chronic

25680   Closed treatment of trans-scaphoperilunar type of fracture dislocation, with manipulation

25685   Open treatment of trans-scaphoperilunar type of fracture dislocation

25690   Closed treatment of lunate dislocation, with manipulation

25695   Open treatment of lunate dislocation

(25700 has been deleted. To report, use 25999)

Arthrodesis

25800   Arthrodesis, wrist joint (including radiocarpal and/or ulnocarpal fusion); without bone graft

25805   with sliding graft

25810   with iliac or other autograft (includes obtaining graft)

(25815 has been deleted. To report, see 25820, 25825)

25820   Intercarpal fusion; without bone graft

25825   with autograft (includes obtaining graft)

25830   Distal radioulnar joint arthrodesis and segmental resection of ulna (eg, Sauvé-Kapandji procedure), with or without bone graft

Amputation

25900   Amputation, forearm, through radius and ulna;

25905   open, circular (guillotine)

25907   secondary closure or scar revision

25909   re-amputation

25915   Krukenberg procedure

25920   Disarticulation through wrist;

25922   secondary closure or scar revision

25924   re-amputation

25927   Transmetacarpal amputation;

25929   secondary closure or scar revision

25931   re-amputation

Other Procedures

25999   Unlisted procedure, forearm or wrist

Hand and Fingers

Incision

26010*   Drainage of finger abscess; simple

26011*   complicated (eg, felon)

26020   Drainage of tendon sheath, one digit and/or palm

26025   Drainage of palmar bursa; single, ulnar or radial

26030   multiple or complicated

(26032 has been deleted)

26034   Incision, deep, with opening of bone cortex (eg, for osteomyelitis or bone abscess), hand or finger

26035   Decompression fingers and/or hand, injection injury (eg, grease gun)

26037   Decompressive fasciotomy, hand (excludes 26035)

(For injection injury, see 26035)

26040   Fasciotomy, palmar, for Dupuytren's contracture; closed (subcutaneous)

26045   open, partial

(For fasciectomy, see 26121-26125)

26055   Tendon sheath incision (eg, for trigger finger)

26060   Tenotomy, subcutaneous, single, each digit

26070   Arthrotomy, for infection, with exploration, drainage or removal of foreign body; carpometacarpal joint

26075   metacarpophalangeal joint

26080   interphalangeal joint, each

Excision

26100   Arthrotomy with synovial biopsy; carpometacarpal joint

26105   metacarpophalangeal joint

26110   interphalangeal joint, each

26115   Excision, tumor or vascular malformation, hand or finger; subcutaneous

26116   deep, subfascial, intramuscular

26117   Radical resection of tumor (eg, malignant neoplasm), soft tissue of hand or finger

(26120 has been deleted. To report, use 26121-26125)

26121   Fasciectomy, palmar only, with or without Z-plasty, other local tissue rearrangement, or skin grafting (includes obtaining graft);

(26122 has been deleted. To report, use 26121-26125)

26123   partial palmar excision with release of single digit including proximal interphalangeal joint

(26124 has been deleted. To report, use 26121-26125)

26125   partial excision with release of each additional digit, including proximal interphalangeal joint

(26126, 26128 have been deleted. To report, use 26121-26125)

(For fasciotomy, see 26040, 26045)

26130 Synovectomy, carpometacarpal joint

26135 Synovectomy, metacarpophalangeal joint including intrinsic release and extensor hood reconstruction, each digit

26140 Synovectomy, proximal interphalangeal joint, including extensor reconstruction, each interphalangeal joint

26145 Synovectomy tendon sheath, radical (tenosynovectomy), flexor, palm or finger, single, each digit

(For tendon sheath synovectomies at wrist, see 25115, 25116)

26160 Excision of lesion of tendon sheath or capsule (eg, cyst, mucous cyst, or ganglion), hand or finger

(For wrist ganglion, see 25111, 25112)

(For trigger digit, see 26055)

26170 Excision of tendon, palm, flexor, single (separate procedure), each

26180 Excision of tendon, finger, flexor (separate procedure)

26200 Excision or curettage of bone cyst or benign tumor of metacarpal;

26205   with autograft (includes obtaining graft)

(26206 has been deleted. To report, use 26989)

26210 Excision or curettage of bone cyst or benign tumor of proximal, middle or distal phalanx of finger;

26215   with autograft (includes obtaining graft)

(26216 has been deleted. To report, use 26989)

26230 Partial excision (craterization, saucerization, or diaphysectomy) of bone (eg, for osteomyelitis); metacarpal

26235   proximal or middle phalanx of finger

26236   distal phalanx of finger

26250 Radical resection (ostectomy) for tumor, metacarpal;

26255   with autograft (includes obtaining graft)

26260 Radical resection (ostectomy) for tumor, proximal or middle phalanx of finger;

26261   with autograft (includes obtaining graft)

26262 Radical resection (ostectomy) for tumor, distal phalanx of finger

Introduction or Removal

26320 Removal of implant from finger or hand

(For removal of foreign body in hand or finger, see 20520, 20525)

Repair, Revision, and/or Reconstruction

26350 Flexor tendon repair or advancement, single, not in "no man's land"; primary or secondary without free graft, each tendon

26352   secondary with free graft (includes obtaining graft), each tendon

26356 Flexor tendon repair or advancement, single, in "no man's land"; primary, each tendon

26357   secondary, each tendon

26358   secondary with free graft (includes obtaining graft), each tendon

26370 Profundus tendon repair or advancement, with intact sublimis; primary

26372   secondary with free graft (includes obtaining graft)

26373   secondary without free graft

26390 Flexor tendon excision, implantation of plastic tube or rod for delayed tendon graft, hand or finger

26392 Removal of tube or rod and insertion of flexor tendon graft (includes obtaining graft), hand or finger

26410 Extensor tendon repair, dorsum of hand, single, primary or secondary; without free graft, each tendon

26412   with free graft (includes obtaining graft), each tendon

26415 Extensor tendon excision, implantation of plastic tube or rod for delayed extensor tendon graft, hand or finger

26416 Removal of tube or rod and insertion of extensor tendon graft (includes obtaining graft), hand or finger

26418 Extensor tendon repair, dorsum of finger, single, primary or secondary; without free graft, each tendon

26420   with free graft (includes obtaining graft) each tendon

26426 Extensor tendon repair, central slip repair, secondary (boutonniere deformity); using local tissues

26428   with free graft (includes obtaining graft)

26432 Extensor tendon repair, distal insertion ("mallet finger"), closed, splinting with or without percutaneous pinning

26433 Extensor tendon repair, distal insertion ("mallet finger"), open, primary or secondary repair; without graft

26434   with free graft (includes obtaining graft)

(For tenovaginotomy for trigger finger, see 26055)

26437 Extensor tendon realignment, hand

26440 Tenolysis, simple, flexor tendon; palm OR finger, single, each tendon

26442   palm AND finger, each tendon

26445 Tenolysis, extensor tendon, dorsum of hand or finger; each tendon

26449 Tenolysis, complex, extensor tendon, dorsum of hand or finger, including hand and forearm

26450 Tenotomy, flexor, single, palm, open, each

26455 Tenotomy, flexor, single, finger, open, each

26460 Tenotomy, extensor, hand or finger, single, open, each

26471 Tenodesis; for proximal interphalangeal joint stabilization

26474   for distal joint stabilization

26476 Tendon lengthening, extensor, hand or finger, single, each

26477 Tendon shortening, extensor, hand or finger, single, each

26478 Tendon lengthening, flexor, hand or finger, single, each

26479 Tendon shortening, flexor, hand or finger, single, each

26480 Tendon transfer or transplant, carpometacarpal area or dorsum of hand, single; without free graft, each

26483   with free tendon graft (includes obtaining graft), each tendon

26485 Tendon transfer or transplant, palmar, single, each tendon; without free tendon graft

26489   with free tendon graft (includes obtaining graft), each tendon

26490 Opponensplasty; sublimis tendon transfer type

26492   tendon transfer with graft (includes obtaining graft)

26494   hypothenar muscle transfer

26496   other methods

(For thumb fusion in opposition, see 26820)

26497 Tendon transfer to restore intrinsic function; ring and small finger

26498   all four fingers

26499 Correction claw finger, other methods

26500 Tendon pulley reconstruction; with local tissues (separate procedure)

26502 with tendon or fascial graft (includes obtaining graft) (separate procedure)

26504 with tendon prosthesis (separate procedure)

26508 Thenar muscle release for thumb contracture

26510 Cross intrinsic transfer

26516 Capsulodesis for M-P joint stabilization; single digit

26517 two digits

26518 three or four digits

26520 Capsulectomy or capsulotomy for contracture; metacarpophalangeal joint, single, each

26525 interphalangeal joint, single, each

(26527 has been deleted. To report, use 25447)

26530 Arthroplasty, metacarpophalangeal joint; single, each

26531 with prosthetic implant, single, each

26535 Arthroplasty interphalangeal joint; single, each

26536 with prosthetic implant, single, each

26540 Primary repair of collateral ligament, metacarpophalangeal joint;

26541 with tendon or fascial graft (includes obtaining graft)

26542 with local tissue (eg, adductor advancement)

26545 Reconstruction, collateral ligament, interphalangeal joint, single, including graft, each joint

26548 Repair and reconstruction, finger, volar plate, interphalangeal joint

26550 Pollicization of a digit

26552 Reconstruction thumb with toe

26555 Positional change of other finger

26557 Toe to finger transfer; first stage

26558 each delay

26559 second stage

26560 Repair of syndactyly (web finger) each web space; with skin flaps

26561 with skin flaps and grafts

26562 complex (eg, involving bone, nails)

26565 Osteotomy for correction of deformity; metacarpal

26567 phalanx of finger

26568 Osteoplasty for lengthening of metacarpal or phalanx

(26570, 26574 have been deleted. To report, use 26989)

26580 Repair cleft hand

26585 Repair bifid digit

26587 Reconstruction of supernumerary digit, soft tissue and bone

(For excision of supernumerary digit, soft tissue only, use 11200)

26590 Repair macrodactylia

26591 Repair, intrinsic muscles of hand (specify)

(For microsurgical technique, use modifier -20 or 09920)

26593 Release, intrinsic muscles of hand (specify)

(For microsurgical technique, use modifier -20 or 09920)

26596 Excision of constricting ring of finger, with multiple Z-plasties

26597 Release of scar contracture, flexor or extensor, with skin grafts, rearrangement flaps, or Z-plasties, hand and/or finger

Fracture and/or Dislocation

26600 Closed treatment of metacarpal fracture, single; without manipulation, each bone

26605 with manipulation, each bone

26607 Closed treatment of metacarpal fracture, with manipulation, with internal or external fixation, each bone

26608 Percutaneous skeletal fixation of metacarpal fracture, each bone

(26610 has been deleted. To report, see 26605, 26607, 26608)

26615 Open treatment of metacarpal fracture, single, with or without internal or external fixation, each bone

26641 Closed treatment of carpometacarpal dislocation, thumb, with manipulation

26645 Closed treatment of carpometacarpal fracture dislocation, thumb (Bennett fracture), with manipulation

26650 Percutaneous skeletal fixation of carpometacarpal fracture dislocation, thumb (Bennett fracture), with manipulation, with or without external fixation

(26655 has been deleted. To report, see 26645, 26650, 26665)

(26660 has been deleted. To report, see 26650, 26665)

26665 Open treatment of carpometacarpal fracture dislocation, thumb (Bennett fracture), with or without internal or external fixation

26670 Closed treatment of carpometacarpal dislocation, other than thumb (Bennett fracture), single, with manipulation; without anesthesia

26675 requiring anesthesia

26676 Percutaneous skeletal fixation of carpometacarpal dislocation, other than thumb (Bennett fracture), single, with manipulation

(26680 has been deleted. To report, see 26670, 26675, 26676, 26685)

26685 Open treatment of carpometacarpal dislocation, other than thumb (Bennett fracture); single, with or without internal or external fixation

26686 complex, multiple or delayed reduction

26700 Closed treatment of metacarpophalangeal dislocation, single, with manipulation; without anesthesia

26705 requiring anesthesia

26706 Percutaneous skeletal fixation of metacarpophalangeal dislocation, single, with manipulation

(26710 has been deleted. To report, see 26700, 26705, 26706, 26715)

26715 Open treatment of metacarpophalangeal dislocation, single, with or without internal or external fixation

26720 Closed treatment of phalangeal shaft fracture, proximal or middle phalanx, finger or thumb; without manipulation, each

26725 with manipulation, with or without skin or skeletal traction, each

26727 Percutaneous skeletal fixation of unstable phalangeal shaft fracture, proximal or middle phalanx, finger or thumb, with manipulation, each

(26730 has been deleted. To report, see 26720, 26725, 26727, 26735)

26735 Open treatment of phalangeal shaft fracture, proximal or middle phalanx, finger or thumb, with or without internal or external fixation, each

26740 Closed treatment of articular fracture, involving metacarpophalangeal or interphalangeal joint; without manipulation, each

26742 with manipulation, each

(26743 has been deleted. To report, use 26989)

(26744 has been deleted. To report, see 26740, 26742, 26746)

26746 Open treatment of articular fracture, involving metacarpophalangeal or interphalangeal joint, with or without internal or external fixation, each

26750 Closed treatment of distal phalangeal fracture, finger or thumb; without manipulation, each

26755 with manipulation, each

26756 Percutaneous skeletal fixation of distal phalangeal fracture, finger or thumb, each

(26760 has been deleted. To report, see 26750, 26755, 26756, 26765)

26765 Open treatment of distal phalangeal fracture, finger or thumb, with or without internal or external fixation, each

26770 Closed treatment of interphalangeal joint dislocation, single, with manipulation; without anesthesia

26775   requiring anesthesia

26776 Percutaneous skeletal fixation of interphalangeal joint dislocation, single, with manipulation

(26780 has been deleted. To report, see 26770, 26775, 26776, 26785)

26785 Open treatment of interphalangeal joint dislocation, with or without internal or external fixation, single

Arthrodesis

26820 Fusion in opposition, thumb, with autogenous graft (includes obtaining graft)

26841 Arthrodesis, carpometacarpal joint, thumb, with or without internal fixation;

26842   with autograft (includes obtaining graft)

26843 Arthrodesis, carpometacarpal joint, digits, other than thumb;

26844   with autograft (includes obtaining graft)

26850 Arthrodesis, metacarpophalangeal joint, with or without internal fixation;

26852   with autograft (includes obtaining graft)

26860 Arthrodesis, interphalangeal joint, with or without internal fixation;

26861   each additional interphalangeal joint

26862   with autograft (includes obtaining graft)

26863   with autograft (includes obtaining graft), each additional joint

Amputation

(For hand through metacarpal bones, see 25927)

26910 Amputation, metacarpal, with finger or thumb (ray amputation), single, with or without interosseous transfer

(For repositioning, see 26550, 26555)

26951 Amputation, finger or thumb, primary or secondary, any joint or phalanx, single, including neurectomies; with direct closure

26952   with local advancement flaps (V-Y, hood)

(For repair of soft tissue defect requiring split or full thickness graft or other pedicle flaps, see 15050-15755)

Other Procedures

26989 Unlisted procedure, hands or fingers

Pelvis and Hip Joint

Including head and neck of femur.

Incision

(For incision and drainage procedures, superficial, see 10040-10160)

26990 Incision and drainage, pelvis or hip joint area; deep abscess or hematoma

26991   infected bursa

26992 Incision, deep, with opening of bone cortex (eg, for osteomyelitis or bone abscess), pelvis and/or hip joint

(26995 has been deleted)

27000 Tenotomy, adductor of hip, subcutaneous, closed (separate procedure)

27001 Tenotomy, adductor of hip, subcutaneous, open

(27002 has been deleted. To report, use 27001 with modifier -50 or 09950)

27003 Tenotomy, adductor, subcutaneous, open, with obturator neurectomy

(27004 has been deleted. To report, use 27003 with modifier -50 or 09950)

27005 Tenotomy, iliopsoas, open (separate procedure)

27006 Tenotomy, abductors of hip, open (separate procedure)

(27010, 27015 have been deleted. To report, see 27025)

27025 Fasciotomy, hip or thigh, any type

(27026 has been deleted. To report, use 27025 with modifier -50 or 09950)

27030 Arthrotomy, hip, for infection, with drainage

(27031 has been deleted)

27033 Arthrotomy, hip, with exploration or removal of loose or foreign body

27035 Hip joint denervation, intrapelvic or extrapelvic intra-articular branches of sciatic, femoral or obturator nerves

(For obturator neurectomy, see 64763, 64766)

Excision

27040 Biopsy, soft tissue of pelvis and hip area; superficial

27041 deep

(For needle biopsy of soft tissue, use 20206)

27047 Excision, tumor, pelvis and hip area; subcutaneous

27048 deep, subfascial, intramuscular

27049 Radical resection of tumor (eg, malignant neoplasm), soft tissue of pelvis and hip area

27050 Arthrotomy, with biopsy; sacroiliac joint

27052 hip joint

27054 Arthrotomy with synovectomy, hip joint

27060 Excision; ischial bursa

27062 trochanteric bursa or calcification

(For arthrocentesis or needling of bursa, see 20610)

27065 Excision of bone cyst or benign tumor; superficial (wing of ilium, symphysis pubis, or greater trochanter of femur) with or without autograft

27066 deep, with or without autograft

27067 with autograft requiring separate incision

27070 Partial excision (craterization, saucerization) (eg, for osteomyelitis); superficial (eg, wing of ilium, symphysis pubis or greater trochanter of femur)

27071 deep

27075 Radical resection of tumor or infection; wing of ilium, one pubic or ischial ramus or symphysis pubis

27076 ilium, including acetabulum, both pubic rami, or ischium and acetabulum

27077 innominate bone, total

27078 ischial tuberosity and greater trochanter of femur

27079 ischial tuberosity and greater trochanter of femur, with skin flaps

27080 Coccygectomy, primary

(For pressure (decubitus) ulcer, see 15920, 15922 and 15931-15958)

Introduction or Removal

27086* Removal of foreign body, pelvis or hip; subcutaneous tissue

27087 deep

(27088 has been deleted. To report, use 27087)

27090 Removal of hip prosthesis; (separate procedure)

27091 complicated, including "total hip" and methylmethacrylate, when applicable

27093 Injection procedure for hip arthrography; without anesthesia

(For radiological supervision and interpretation, see 73525)

27095 with anesthesia

(For radiological supervision and interpretation, see 73525)

Repair, Revision, and/or Reconstruction

27097   Hamstring recession, proximal

27098   Adductor transfer to ischium

27100   Transfer external oblique muscle to greater trochanter including fascial or tendon extension (graft)

27105   Transfer paraspinal muscle to hip (includes fascial or tendon extension graft)

27110   Transfer iliopsoas; to greater trochanter

27111   to femoral neck

(27115 has been deleted. To report, use 27299)

27120   Acetabuloplasty; (eg, Whitman, Colonna, Haygroves, or cup type)

27122   resection femoral head (Girdlestone procedure)

27125   Partial hip replacement, prosthesis (eg, femoral stem prosthesis, bipolar arthroplasty)

(For prosthetic replacement following fracture of the hip, use 27236)

(27126, 27127 have been deleted. To report, use 27120)

27130   Arthroplasty, acetabular and proximal femoral prosthetic replacement (total hip replacement), with or without autograft or allograft

(27131 has been deleted. To report, use 27132)

27132   Conversion of previous hip surgery to total hip replacement, with or without autograft or allograft

27134   Revision of total hip arthroplasty; both components, with or without autograft or allograft

(27135 has been deleted. To report, see 27134, 27137, 27138)

27137   acetabular component only, with or without autograft or allograft

27138   femoral component only, with or without allograft

27140   Osteotomy and transfer of greater trochanter (separate procedure)

27146   Osteotomy, iliac, acetabular or innominate bone;

27147   with open reduction of hip

27151   with femoral osteotomy

27156   with femoral osteotomy and with open reduction of hip

(27157 has been deleted)

27158   Osteotomy, pelvis, bilateral (eg, for congenital malformation)

27161   Osteotomy, femoral neck (separate procedure)

27165   Osteotomy, intertrochanteric or subtrochanteric including internal or external fixation and/or cast

27170   Bone graft, femoral head, neck, intertrochanteric or subtrochanteric area (includes obtaining bone graft)

27175   Treatment of slipped femoral epiphysis; by traction, without reduction

27176   by single or multiple pinning, in situ

27177   Open treatment of slipped femoral epiphysis; single or multiple pinning or bone graft (includes obtaining graft)

27178   closed manipulation with single or multiple pinning

27179   osteoplasty of femoral neck (Heyman type procedure)

27181   osteotomy and internal fixation

27185   Epiphyseal arrest by epiphysiodesis or stapling, greater trochanter

27187   Prophylactic treatment (nailing, pinning, plating or wiring) with or without methylmethacrylate, femoral neck and proximal femur

Fracture and/or Dislocation

(27190, 27191 have been deleted. To report, see 27193, 27194)

(27192 has been deleted. To report, see 27215, 27216)

27193 Closed treatment of pelvic ring fracture, dislocation, diastasis or subluxation; without manipulation

27194 with manipulation, requiring more than local anesthesia

(27195 has been deleted. To report, see 27193)

(27196 has been deleted. To report, see 27194)

27200 Closed treatment of coccygeal fracture

(27201 has been deleted. To report, see 27200, 27202)

27202 Open treatment of coccygeal fracture

(27210, 27211, 27212 have been deleted. To report, see 27193, 27194, 27215, 27216, 27217, 27218)

(27214 has been deleted. To report, see 27215, 27216, 27217, 27218)

27215 Open treatment of iliac spine(s), tuberosity avulsion, or iliac wing fracture(s) (eg, pelvic fracture(s) which do not disrupt the pelvic ring), with internal fixation

27216 Percutaneous skeletal fixation of posterior pelvic ring fracture and/or dislocation (includes ilium, sacroiliac joint and/or sacrum)

27217 Open treatment of anterior ring fracture and/or dislocation with internal fixation (includes pubic symphysis and/or rami)

27218 Open treatment of posterior ring fracture and/or dislocation with internal fixation (includes ilium, sacroiliac joint and/or sacrum)

27220 Closed treatment of acetabulum (hip socket) fracture(s); without manipulation

27222 with manipulation, with or without skeletal traction

(27224 has been deleted. To report, see 27226, 27227)

(27225 has been deleted. To report, see 27227, 27228)

27226 Open treatment of posterior or anterior acetabular wall fracture, with internal fixation

27227 Open treatment of acetabular fracture(s) involving anterior or posterior (one) column, or a fracture running transversely across the acetabulum, with internal fixation

27228 Open treatment of acetabular fracture(s) involving anterior and posterior (two) columns, includes T-fracture and both column fracture with complete articular detachment, or single column or transverse fracture with associated acetabular wall fracture, with internal fixation

27230 Closed treatment of femoral fracture, proximal end, neck; without manipulation

27232 with manipulation, with or without skeletal traction

(27234 has been deleted. To report, see 27230, 27232, 27235, 27236)

27235 Percutaneous skeletal fixation of femoral fracture, proximal end, neck, undisplaced, mildly displaced, or impacted fracture

27236 Open treatment of femoral fracture, proximal end, neck, internal fixation or prosthetic replacement (direct fracture exposure)

27238 Closed treatment of intertrochanteric, pertrochanteric, or subtrochanteric femoral fracture; without manipulation

27240 with manipulation, with or without skin or skeletal traction

(27242 has been deleted. To report, see 27238, 27240, 27244, 27245)

27244 Open treatment of intertrochanteric, pertrochanteric or subtrochanteric femoral fracture; with plate/screw type implant, with or without cerclage

27245 with intramedullary implant, with or without interlocking screws and/or cerclage

27246 Closed treatment of greater trochanteric fracture, without manipulation

27248 Open treatment of greater trochanteric fracture, with or without internal or external fixation

27250 Closed treatment of hip dislocation, traumatic; without anesthesia

27252 requiring anesthesia

27253 Open treatment of hip dislocation, traumatic, without internal fixation

27254 Open treatment of hip dislocation, traumatic, with acetabular wall and femoral head fracture, with or without internal or external fixation

(27255 has been deleted. To report, see 27226, 27227, 27253, 27254)

27256* Treatment of spontaneous hip dislocation (developmental, including congenital or pathological), by abduction, splint or traction; without anesthesia, without manipulation

27257* with manipulation, requiring anesthesia

27258 Open treatment of spontaneous hip dislocation (developmental, including congenital or pathological), replacement of femoral head in acetabulum (including tenotomy, etc);

27259 with femoral shaft shortening

27265 Closed treatment of post hip arthroplasty dislocation; without anesthesia

27266 requiring regional or general anesthesia

Manipulation

27275* Manipulation, hip joint, requiring general anesthesia

Arthrodesis

27280 Arthrodesis, sacroiliac joint (including obtaining graft)

(27281 has been deleted. To report, use 27280 with modifier -50 or 09950)

27282 Arthrodesis, symphysis pubis (including obtaining graft)

27284 Arthrodesis, hip joint (includes obtaining graft);

27286 with subtrochanteric osteotomy

Amputation

27290 Interpelviabdominal amputation (hindquarter amputation)

27295 Disarticulation of hip

Other Procedures

27299 Unlisted procedure, pelvis or hip joint

Femur (Thigh Region) and Knee Joint

Including tibial plateaus.

Incision

(For incision and drainage of abscess or hematoma, superficial, see 10040-10160)

27301 Incision and drainage of deep abscess, infected bursa, or hematoma, thigh or knee region

27303 Incision, deep, with opening of bone cortex (eg, for osteomyelitis or bone abscess), femur or knee

(27304 has been deleted)

27305 Fasciotomy, iliotibial (tenotomy), open

(For combined Ober-Yount fasciotomy, see 27025)

27306 Tenotomy, subcutaneous, closed, adductor or hamstring, (separate procedure); single

27307 multiple

27310 Arthrotomy, knee, for infection, with exploration, drainage or removal of foreign body

(27311 has been deleted)

27315 Neurectomy, hamstring muscle

27320 Neurectomy, popliteal (gastrocnemius)

Excision

27323 Biopsy, soft tissue of thigh or knee area;
superficial

27324   deep

(For needle biopsy of soft tissue, use 20206)

27327 Excision, tumor, thigh or knee area;
subcutaneous

27328   deep, subfascial, or intramuscular

27329 Radical resection of tumor (eg, malignant
neoplasm), soft tissue of thigh or knee area

27330 Arthrotomy, knee; with synovial biopsy only

27331   with joint exploration, with or without
biopsy, with or without removal of loose or
foreign bodies

27332 Arthrotomy, knee, with excision of semilunar
cartilage (meniscectomy); medial OR lateral

27333   medial AND lateral

27334 Arthrotomy, knee, with synovectomy; anterior
OR posterior

27335   anterior AND posterior including popliteal
area

27340 Excision, prepatellar bursa

27345 Excision of synovial cyst of popliteal space
(Baker's cyst)

27350 Patellectomy or hemipatellectomy

27355 Excision or curettage of bone cyst or benign
tumor of femur;

27356   with allograft

27357   with autograft (includes obtaining graft)

27358   with internal fixation (list in addition to
27355, 27356, or 27357)

27360 Partial excision (craterization, saucerization,
or diaphysectomy) of bone (eg, for osteomyelitis), femur, proximal tibia and/or fibula

(27361 has been deleted)

27365 Radical resection of tumor, bone, femur or
knee

(For radical resection of tumor, soft tissue, use
27329)

Introduction or Removal

27370 Injection procedure for knee arthrography

(For radiological supervision and
interpretation, see 73580)

27372 Removal of foreign body, deep, thigh region or
knee area

(For removal of knee prosthesis including
"total knee", see 27488)

(27373-27379 have been deleted. To report,
see 29870-29887)

Repair, Revision, and/or Reconstruction

27380 Suture of infrapatellar tendon; primary

27381   secondary reconstruction, including fascial
or tendon graft

27385 Suture of quadriceps or hamstring muscle
rupture; primary

27386   secondary reconstruction, including fascial
or tendon graft

27390 Tenotomy, open, hamstring, knee to hip; single

27391   multiple, one leg

27392   multiple, bilateral

27393 Lengthening of hamstring tendon; single

27394   multiple, one leg

27395   multiple, bilateral

27396 Transplant, hamstring tendon to patella; single

27397   multiple

27400 Tendon or muscle transfer, hamstrings to
femur (Eggers type procedure)

27403 Arthrotomy with open meniscus repair

(For arthroscopic repair, use 29882)

27405 Repair, primary, torn ligament and/or capsule,
knee; collateral

27407   cruciate

(27408 has been deleted. To report, use 27427)

27409   collateral and cruciate ligaments

(27410-27416 have been deleted. To report, see 27427-27429)

27418   Anterior tibial tubercleplasty (eg, for chondromalacia patellae)

27420   Reconstruction for recurrent dislocating patella; (Hauser type procedure)

27422   with extensor realignment and/or muscle advancement or release (Campbell, Goldwaite type procedure)

27424   with patellectomy

27425   Lateral retinacular release (any method)

27427   Ligamentous reconstruction (augmentation), knee; extra-articular

27428   intra-articular (open)

27429   intra-articular (open) and extra-articular

(When performed with primary repair, use in addition to the code for the primary repair)

27430   Quadricepsplasty (Bennett or Thompson type)

27435   Capsulotomy, knee, posterior capsular release

(27436 has been deleted. To report, use 29887)

27437   Arthroplasty, patella; without prosthesis

27438   with prosthesis

27440   Arthroplasty, knee, tibial plateau;

27441   with debridement and partial synovectomy

27442   Arthroplasty, knee, femoral condyles or tibial plateaus;

27443   with debridement and partial synovectomy

(27444 has been deleted. To report, see 27445-27447)

27445   Arthroplasty, knee, constrained prosthesis (eg, Walldius type)

27446   Arthroplasty, knee, condyle and plateau; medial OR lateral compartment

27447   medial AND lateral compartments with or without patella resurfacing ("total knee replacement")

(For revision of total knee arthroplasty, see 27487)

(For removal of total knee prosthesis, see 27488)

27448   Osteotomy, femur, shaft or supracondylar; without fixation

(27449 has been deleted. To report, use 27448 with modifier -50 or 09950)

27450   with fixation

(27452 has been deleted. To report, use 27450 with modifier -50 or 09950)

27454   Osteotomy, multiple, femoral shaft, with realignment on intramedullary rod (Sofield type procedure)

27455   Osteotomy, proximal tibia, including fibular excision or osteotomy (includes correction of genu varus (bowleg) or genu valgus (knock-knee)); before epiphyseal closure

27457   after epiphyseal closure

(27460 has been deleted. To report, use 27455 with modifier -50 or 09950)

(27462 has been deleted. To report, use 27457 with modifier -50 or 09950)

27465   Osteoplasty, femur; shortening (excluding 64876)

27466   lengthening

27468   combined, lengthening and shortening with femoral segment transfer

27470   Repair, nonunion or malunion, femur, distal to head and neck; without graft (eg, compression technique)

27472   with iliac or other autogenous bone graft (includes obtaining graft)

27475   Epiphyseal arrest by epiphysiodesis or stapling; distal femur

27477   tibia and fibula, proximal

27479   combined distal femur, proximal tibia and fibula

27485   Arrest, hemiepiphyseal, distal femur or proximal leg (eg, for genu varus or valgus)

27486   Revision of total knee arthroplasty, with or without allograft; one component

27487   all components

27488   Removal of knee prosthesis, including "total knee," methylmethacrylate and insertion of spacer, when applicable

(27490 has been deleted. To report, use 29882)

27495   Prophylactic treatment (nailing, pinning, plating or wiring) with or without methylmethacrylate, femur

27496   Decompression fasciotomy, thigh and/or knee, one compartment (flexor or extensor or adductor);

27497   with debridement of nonviable muscle and/or nerve

27498   Decompression fasciotomy, thigh and/or knee, multiple compartments;

27499   with debridement of nonviable muscle and/or nerve

Fracture and/or Dislocation

(For arthroscopic treatment of intercondylar spine(s) and tuberosity fracture(s) of the knee, see 29850, 29851)

(For arthroscopic treatment of tibial fracture, see 29855, 29856)

27500   Closed treatment of femoral shaft fracture, without manipulation

27501   Closed treatment of supracondylar or transcondylar femoral fracture with or without intercondylar extension, without manipulation

27502   Closed treatment of femoral shaft fracture, with manipulation, with or without skin or skeletal traction

27503   Closed treatment of supracondylar or transcondylar femoral fracture with or without intercondylar extension, with manipulation, with or without skin or skeletal traction

(27504 has been deleted. To report, see 27500, 27501, 27502, 27503, 27506, 27507, 27509, 27511, 27513)

27506   Open treatment of femoral shaft fracture, with or without external fixation, with insertion of intramedullary implant, with or without cerclage and/or locking screws

27507   Open treatment of femoral shaft fracture with plate/screws, with or without cerclage

27508   Closed treatment of femoral fracture, distal end, medial or lateral condyle, without manipulation

27509   Percutaneous skeletal fixation of femoral fracture, distal end, medial or lateral condyle, or supracondylar or transcondylar, with or without intercondylar extension, or distal femoral epiphyseal separation

27510   Closed treatment of femoral fracture, distal end, medial or lateral condyle, with manipulation

27511   Open treatment of femoral supracondylar or transcondylar fracture without intercondylar extension, with or without internal or external fixation

(27512 has been deleted. To report, see 27508, 27510, 27514)

27513   Open treatment of femoral supracondylar or transcondylar fracture with intercondylar extension, with or without internal or external fixation

27514   Open treatment of femoral fracture, distal end, medial or lateral condyle, with or without internal or external fixation

27516   Closed treatment of distal femoral epiphyseal separation; without manipulation

27517   with manipulation, with or without skin or skeletal traction

(27518 has been deleted. To report, see 27516, 27517, 27519)

27519   Open treatment of distal femoral epiphyseal separation, with or without internal or external fixation

27520 Closed treatment of patellar fracture, without manipulation

(27522 has been deleted. To report, see 27520, 27524)

27524 Open treatment of patellar fracture, with internal fixation and/or partial or complete patellectomy and soft tissue repair

27530 Closed treatment of tibial fracture, proximal (plateau); without manipulation

27532 with or without manipulation, with skeletal traction

(27534 has been deleted. To report, see 27530, 27532, 27535, 27536)

(For arthroscopic treatment, see 29855, 29856)

27535 Open treatment of tibial fracture, proximal (plateau); unicondylar, with or without internal or external fixation

27536 bicondylar, with or without internal fixation

(For arthroscopic treatment, see 29855, 29856)

(27537 has been deleted. To report, see 27535, 27536)

27538 Closed treatment of intercondylar spine(s) and/or tuberosity fracture(s) of knee, with or without manipulation

(For arthroscopic treatment, see 29850, 29851)

27540 Open treatment of intercondylar spine(s) and/or tuberosity fracture(s) of the knee, with or without internal or external fixation

27550 Closed treatment of knee dislocation; without anesthesia

27552 requiring anesthesia

(27554 has been deleted. To report, see 27550, 27552, 27556, 27557, 27558)

27556 Open treatment of knee dislocation, with or without internal or external fixation; without primary ligamentous repair or augmentation/reconstruction

27557 with primary ligamentous repair

27558 with primary ligamentous repair, with augmentation/reconstruction

27560 Closed treatment of patellar dislocation; without anesthesia

(For recurrent dislocation, see 27420-27424)

27562 requiring anesthesia

(27564 has been deleted. To report, see 27560, 27562, 27566)

27566 Open treatment of patellar dislocation, with or without partial or total patellectomy

Manipulation

27570* Manipulation of knee joint under general anesthesia (includes application of traction or other fixation devices)

Arthrodesis

27580 Fusion of knee, any technique

Amputation

27590 Amputation, thigh, through femur, any level;

27591 immediate fitting technique including first cast

27592 open, circular (guillotine)

27594 secondary closure or scar revision

27596 re-amputation

27598 Disarticulation at knee

Other Procedures

27599 Unlisted procedure, femur or knee

Leg (Tibia and Fibula) and Ankle Joint

Incision

27600 Decompression fasciotomy, leg; anterior and/or lateral compartments only

27601 posterior compartment(s) only

27602   anterior and/or lateral, and posterior
             compartment(s)

             (For incision and drainage procedures,
             superficial, see 10040-10160)

             (For decompression fasciotomy with
             debridement, see 27892-27894)

27603 Incision and drainage, leg or ankle; deep
          abscess or hematoma

27604   infected bursa

27605* Tenotomy, Achilles tendon, subcutaneous
           (separate procedure); local anesthesia

27606   general anesthesia

27607 Incision, deep, with opening of bone cortex
          (eg, for osteomyelitis or bone abscess), leg
          or ankle

          (27608 has been deleted)

27610 Arthrotomy, ankle, for infection, with
          exploration, drainage or removal of foreign
          body

          (27611 has been deleted)

27612 Arthrotomy, ankle, posterior capsular release,
          with or without Achilles tendon lengthening

          (See also 27685)

Excision

27613 Biopsy, soft tissue of leg or ankle area;
          superficial

27614   deep

          (For needle biopsy of soft tissue, use 20206)

27615 Radical resection of tumor (eg, malignant
          neoplasm), soft tissue of leg or ankle area

27618 Excision, tumor, leg or ankle area;
          subcutaneous

27619   deep, subfascial or intramuscular

27620 Arthrotomy, ankle, with joint exploration, with
          or without biopsy, with or without removal of
          loose or foreign body

27625 Arthrotomy, ankle, with synovectomy;

27626   including tenosynovectomy

27630 Excision of lesion of tendon sheath or capsule
          (eg, cyst or ganglion), leg and/or ankle

27635 Excision or curettage of bone cyst or benign
          tumor, tibia or fibula;

27637   with autograft (includes obtaining graft)

27638   with allograft

27640 Partial excision (craterization, saucerization, or
          diaphysectomy) of bone (eg, for osteomyelitis
          or exostosis); tibia

27641   fibula

27645 Radical resection of tumor, bone; tibia

27646   fibula

27647   talus or calcaneus

Introduction or Removal

27648 Injection procedure for ankle arthrography

          (For radiological supervision and interpre-
          tation, see 73615)

          (For ankle arthroscopy, see 29894-29898)

Repair, Revision, and/or Reconstruction

27650 Repair, primary, open or percutaneous,
          ruptured Achilles tendon;

27652   with graft (includes obtaining graft)

27654 Repair, secondary, ruptured Achilles tendon,
          with or without graft

27656 Repair, fascial defect of leg

27658 Repair or suture of flexor tendon of leg;
          primary, without graft, single, each

27659   secondary with or without graft, single
             tendon, each

27664 Repair or suture of extensor tendon of leg;
          primary, without graft, single, each

27665   secondary with or without graft, single
             tendon, each

27675 Repair for dislocating peroneal tendons; without fibular osteotomy

27676 with fibular osteotomy

27680 Tenolysis, including tibia, fibula and ankle flexor; single

27681 multiple (through same incision), each

27685 Lengthening or shortening of tendon, leg or ankle; single (separate procedure)

27686 multiple (through same incision), each

27687 Gastrocnemius recession (eg, Strayer procedure)

(Toe extensors are considered as a group to be a single tendon when transplanted into midfoot)

27690 Transfer or transplant of single tendon (with muscle redirection or rerouting); superficial (eg, anterior tibial extensors into midfoot)

▲**27691** deep (eg, anterior tibial or posterior tibial through interosseous space, flexor digitorum longus, flexor hallucis longus, or peroneal tendon to midfoot or hindfoot)

27692 each additional tendon

27695 Suture, primary, torn, ruptured or severed ligament, ankle; collateral

27696 both collateral ligaments

27698 Suture, secondary repair, torn, ruptured or severed ligament, ankle, collateral (eg, Watson-Jones procedure)

27700 Arthroplasty, ankle;

27702 with implant ("total ankle")

27703 secondary reconstruction, total ankle

27704 Removal of ankle implant

27705 Osteotomy; tibia

27707 fibula

27709 tibia and fibula

27712 multiple, with realignment on intramedullary rod (Sofield type procedure)

(For osteotomy to correct genu varus (bowleg) or genu valgus (knock-knee), see 27455-27457)

27715 Osteoplasty, tibia and fibula, lengthening

27720 Repair of nonunion or malunion, tibia; without graft, (eg, compression technique)

27722 with sliding graft

27724 with iliac or other autograft (includes obtaining graft)

27725 by synostosis, with fibula, any method

27727 Repair of congenital pseudarthrosis, tibia

27730 Epiphyseal arrest by epiphysiodesis or stapling; distal tibia

27732 distal fibula

27734 distal tibia and fibula

27740 Epiphyseal arrest by epiphysiodesis or stapling, combined, proximal and distal tibia and fibula;

27742 and distal femur

(For epiphyseal arrest of proximal tibia and fibula, see 27477)

27745 Prophylactic treatment (nailing, pinning, plating or wiring) with or without methylmethacrylate, tibia

Fracture and/or Dislocation

27750 Closed treatment of tibial shaft fracture (with or without fibular fracture); without manipulation

27752 with manipulation, with or without skeletal traction

(27754 has been deleted. To report, see 27750, 27752, 27756, 27758)

27756 Percutaneous skeletal fixation of tibial shaft fracture (with or without fibular fracture) (eg, pins or screws)

27758 Open treatment of tibial shaft fracture, (with or without fibular fracture) with plate/screws, with or without cerclage

27759 Open treatment of tibial shaft fracture (with or without fibular fracture) by intramedullary implant, with or without interlocking screws and/or cerclage

27760 Closed treatment of medial malleolus fracture; without manipulation

27762 with manipulation, with or without skin or skeletal traction

(27764 has been deleted. To report, see 27762, 27766)

27766 Open treatment of medial malleolus fracture, with or without internal or external fixation

27780 Closed treatment of proximal fibula or shaft fracture; without manipulation

27781 with manipulation

(27782 has been deleted. To report, see 27780, 27781, 27784)

27784 Open treatment of proximal fibula or shaft fracture, with or without internal or external fixation

27786 Closed treatment of distal fibular fracture (lateral malleolus); without manipulation

27788 with manipulation

(27790 has been deleted. To report, see 27786, 27788, 27792)

27792 Open treatment of distal fibular fracture (lateral malleolus), with or without internal or external fixation

(27800 has been deleted. To report, see 27750)

(27802 has been deleted. To report, see 27752)

(27804 has been deleted. To report, see 27750, 27752, 27756, 27758, 27759)

(27806 has been deleted. To report, see 27756, 27758, 27759)

27808 Closed treatment of bimalleolar ankle fracture, (including Potts); without manipulation

27810 with manipulation

(27812 has been deleted. To report, see 27808, 27810, 27814)

27814 Open treatment of bimalleolar ankle fracture, with or without internal or external fixation

27816 Closed treatment of trimalleolar ankle fracture; without manipulation

27818 with manipulation

(27820 has been deleted. To report, see 27816, 27818, 27822, 27823)

27822 Open treatment of trimalleolar ankle fracture, with or without internal or external fixation, medial and/or lateral malleolus; without fixation of posterior lip

27823 with fixation of posterior lip

27824 Closed treatment of fracture of weight bearing articular portion of distal tibia (eg, pilon or tibial plafond), with or without anesthesia; without manipulation

27825 with skeletal traction and/or requiring manipulation

27826 Open treatment of fracture of weight bearing articular surface/portion of distal tibia (eg, pilon or tibial plafond), with internal or external fixation; of fibula only

27827 of tibia only

27828 of both tibia and fibula

27829 Open treatment of distal tibiofibular joint (syndesmosis) disruption, with or without internal or external fixation

27830 Closed treatment of proximal tibiofibular joint dislocation; without anesthesia

27831 requiring anesthesia

27832 Open treatment of proximal tibiofibular joint dislocation, with or without internal or external fixation, or with excision of proximal fibula

27840 Closed treatment of ankle dislocation; without anesthesia

27842 requiring anesthesia, with or without percutaneous skeletal fixation

(27844 has been deleted. To report, see 27840, 27842, 27846, 27848)

27846 Open treatment of ankle dislocation, with or without percutaneous skeletal fixation; without repair or internal fixation

27848 with repair or internal or external fixation

(27850-27853 have been deleted. To report, see 29894-29898)

Manipulation

27860* Manipulation of ankle under general anesthesia (includes application of traction or other fixation apparatus)

Arthrodesis

27870 Arthrodesis, ankle, any method

27871 Arthrodesis, tibiofibular joint, proximal or distal

Amputation

27880 Amputation, leg, through tibia and fibula;

27881 with immediate fitting technique including application of first cast

27882 open, circular (guillotine)

27884 secondary closure or scar revision

27886 re-amputation

27888 Amputation, ankle, through malleoli of tibia and fibula (Syme, Pirogoff type procedures), with plastic closure and resection of nerves

27889 Ankle disarticulation

Other Procedures

27892 Decompression fasciotomy, leg; anterior and/or lateral compartments only, with debridement of nonviable muscle and/or nerve

(For decompression fasciotomy of the leg without debridement, see 27600)

27893 posterior compartment(s) only, with debridement of nonviable muscle and/or nerve

(For decompression fasciotomy of the leg without debridement, see 27601)

27894 anterior and/or lateral, and posterior compartment(s), with debridement of nonviable muscle and/or nerve

(For decompression fasciotomy of the leg without debridement, see 27602)

27899 Unlisted procedure, leg or ankle

Foot and Toes

Incision

(For incision and drainage procedures, superficial, see 10040-10160)

28001* Incision and drainage, infected bursa, foot

28002* Deep dissection below fascia, for deep infection of foot, with or without tendon sheath involvement; single bursal space, specify

28003 multiple areas

(28004 has been deleted)

28005 Incision, deep, with opening of bone cortex (eg, for osteomyelitis or bone abscess), foot

(28006 has been deleted)

28008 Fasciotomy, foot and/or toe

(See also 28060, 28062, 28250)

28010 Tenotomy, subcutaneous, toe; single

28011 multiple

(For open tenotomy, see 28230-28234)

28020 Arthrotomy, with exploration, drainage or removal of loose or foreign body; intertarsal or tarsometatarsal joint

28022 metatarsophalangeal joint

28024 interphalangeal joint

28030 Neurectomy of intrinsic musculature of foot

28035 Tarsal tunnel release (posterior tibial nerve decompression)

(For other nerve entrapments, see 64704, 64722)

Excision

28043 Excision, tumor, foot; subcutaneous

28045   deep, subfascial, intramuscular

28046 Radical resection of tumor (eg, malignant neoplasm), soft tissue of foot

28050 Arthrotomy for synovial biopsy; intertarsal or tarsometatarsal joint

28052   metatarsophalangeal joint

28054   interphalangeal joint

28060 Fasciectomy, excision of plantar fascia; partial (separate procedure)

28062   radical (separate procedure)

(For plantar fasciotomy, see 28008, 28250)

28070 Synovectomy; intertarsal or tarsometatarsal joint, each

28072   metatarsophalangeal joint, each

28080 Excision of interdigital (Morton) neuroma, single, each

28086 Synovectomy, tendon sheath, foot; flexor

28088   extensor

28090 Excision of lesion of tendon or fibrous sheath or capsule (including synovectomy) (cyst or ganglion); foot

28092   toes

28100 Excision or curettage of bone cyst or benign tumor, talus or calcaneus;

28102   with iliac or other autograft (includes obtaining graft)

28103   with allograft

28104 Excision or curettage of bone cyst or benign tumor, tarsal or metatarsal bones, except talus or calcaneus;

28106   with iliac or other autograft (includes obtaining graft)

28107   with allograft

28108 Excision or curettage of bone cyst or benign tumor, phalanges of foot

(For ostectomy, partial (eg, hallux valgus, Silver type procedure), see 28290)

(28109 has been deleted. To report, use 28899)

28110 Ostectomy, partial excision, fifth metatarsal head (bunionette) (separate procedure)

28111 Ostectomy, complete excision; first metatarsal head

28112   other metatarsal head (second, third or fourth)

28113   fifth metatarsal head

28114   all metatarsal heads, with partial proximal phalangectomy, excluding first metatarsal (Clayton type procedure)

28116 Ostectomy, excision of tarsal coalition

28118 Ostectomy, calcaneus;

28119   for spur, with or without plantar fascial release

28120 Partial excision (craterization, saucerization, sequestrectomy, or diaphysectomy) of bone (eg, for osteomyelitis or talar bossing), talus or calcaneus

(28121 has been deleted)

28122 Partial excision (craterization, saucerization, or diaphysectomy) of bone (eg, for osteomyelitis or tarsal bossing), tarsal or metatarsal bone, except talus or calcaneus

(28123 has been deleted)

28124 Partial excision (craterization, saucerization, or diaphysectomy) of bone (eg, for osteomyelitis or dorsal bossing), phalanx of toe

28126 Resection, partial or complete, phalangeal base, single toe, each

28130 Talectomy (astragalectomy)

(28135 has been deleted. To report, use 28118)

28140 Metatarsectomy

28150 Phalangectomy of toe, single, each

28153 Resection, head of phalanx, toe

28160 Hemiphalangectomy or interphalangeal joint excision, toe, single, each

28171 Radical resection of tumor, bone; tarsal (except talus or calcaneus)

28173 metatarsal

28175 phalanx of toe

(For talus or calcaneus, see 27647)

Introduction or Removal

28190* Removal of foreign body, foot; subcutaneous

28192 deep

28193 complicated

Repair, Revision, and/or Reconstruction

28200 Repair or suture of tendon, foot, flexor, single; primary or secondary, without free graft, each tendon

28202 secondary with free graft, each tendon (includes obtaining graft)

28208 Repair or suture of tendon, foot, extensor, single; primary or secondary, each tendon

28210 secondary with free graft, each tendon (includes obtaining graft)

28220 Tenolysis, flexor, foot; single

28222 multiple (through same incision)

28225 Tenolysis, extensor, foot; single

28226 multiple (through same incision)

28230 Tenotomy, open, flexor; foot, single or multiple (separate procedure)

28232 toe, single (separate procedure)

28234 Tenotomy, open, extensor, foot or toe

(28236 has been deleted. To report, see 27690, 27691)

28238 Advancement of posterior tibial tendon with excision of accessory navicular bone (Kidner type procedure)

(For subcutaneous tenotomy, see 28010, 28011)

(For transfer or transplant of tendon with muscle redirection or rerouting, see 27690-27692)

(For extensor hallucis longus transfer with great toe IP fusion (Jones procedure), see 28760)

28240 Tenotomy, lengthening, or release, abductor hallucis muscle

28250 Division of plantar fascia and muscle ("Steindler stripping") (separate procedure)

28260 Capsulotomy, midfoot; medial release only (separate procedure)

28261 with tendon lengthening

28262 extensive, including posterior talotibial capsulotomy and tendon(s) lengthening as for resistant clubfoot deformity

28264 Capsulotomy, midtarsal (Heyman type procedure)

28270 Capsulotomy; metatarsophalangeal joint, with or without tenorrhaphy, single, each joint (separate procedure)

28272 interphalangeal joint, single, each joint (separate procedure)

28280 Webbing operation (create syndactylism of toes) (Kelikian type procedure)

28285 Hammertoe operation, one toe (eg, interphalangeal fusion, filleting, phalangectomy)

28286 Cock-up fifth toe operation with plastic skin closure (Ruiz-Mora type procedure)

28288 Ostectomy, partial, exostectomy or condylectomy, single, metatarsal head, first through fifth, each metatarsal head

28290 Hallux valgus (bunion) correction, with or without sesamoidectomy; simple exostectomy (Silver type procedure)

28292 Keller, McBride or Mayo type procedure

28293 resection of joint with implant

28294 with tendon transplants (Joplin type procedure)

28296 with metatarsal osteotomy (eg, Mitchell, Chevron, or concentric type procedures)

28297 Lapidus type procedure

28298 by phalanx osteotomy

28299 by other methods (eg, double osteotomy)

28300 Osteotomy; calcaneus (Dwyer or Chambers type procedure), with or without internal fixation

28302 talus

28304 Osteotomy, midtarsal bones, other than calcaneus or talus;

28305 with autograft (includes obtaining graft) (Fowler type)

28306 Osteotomy, metatarsal, base or shaft, single, with or without lengthening, for shortening or angular correction; first metatarsal

28307 first metatarsal with autograft

28308 other than first metatarsal

28309 Osteotomy, metatarsals, multiple, for cavus foot (Swanson type procedure)

28310 Osteotomy for shortening, angular or rotational correction; proximal phalanx, first toe (separate procedure)

28312 other phalanges, any toe

28313 Reconstruction, angular deformity of toe (overlapping second toe, fifth toe, curly toes), soft tissue procedures only

28315 Sesamoidectomy, first toe (separate procedure)

28320 Repair of nonunion or malunion; tarsal bones (eg, calcaneus, talus)

28322 metatarsal, with or without bone graft (includes obtaining graft)

28340 Reconstruction, toe, macrodactyly; soft tissue resection

28341 requiring bone resection

28344 Reconstruction, toe(s); polydactyly

28345 syndactyly, with or without skin graft(s), each web

28360 Reconstruction, cleft foot

Fracture and/or Dislocation

28400 Closed treatment of calcaneal fracture; without manipulation

28405 with manipulation

28406 Percutaneous skeletal fixation of calcaneal fracture, with manipulation

(28410 has been deleted. To report, see 28400, 28405, 28406, 28415, 28420)

28415 Open treatment of calcaneal fracture, with or without internal or external fixation;

28420 with primary iliac or other autogenous bone graft (includes obtaining graft)

28430 Closed treatment of talus fracture; without manipulation

28435 with manipulation

28436 Percutaneous skeletal fixation of talus fracture, with manipulation

(28440 has been deleted. To report, see 28430, 28435, 28436, 28445)

28445 Open treatment of talus fracture, with or without internal or external fixation

28450 Treatment of tarsal bone fracture (except talus and calcaneus); without manipulation, each

28455 with manipulation, each

28456 Percutaneous skeletal fixation of tarsal bone fracture (except talus and calcaneus), with manipulation, each

(28460 has been deleted. To report, see 28450, 28455, 28456, 28465)

28465 Open treatment of tarsal bone fracture (except talus and calcaneus), with or without internal or external fixation, each

28470 Closed treatment of metatarsal fracture; without manipulation, each

---

28475   with manipulation, each

28476   Percutaneous skeletal fixation of metatarsal fracture, with manipulation, each

(28480 has been deleted. To report, see 28470, 28475, 28476, 28485)

28485   Open treatment of metatarsal fracture, with or without internal or external fixation, each

28490   Closed treatment of fracture great toe, phalanx or phalanges; without manipulation

28495   with manipulation

28496   Percutaneous skeletal fixation of fracture great toe, phalanx or phalanges, with manipulation

(28500 has been deleted. To report, see 28490, 28495, 28496, 28505)

28505   Open treatment of fracture great toe, phalanx or phalanges, with or without internal or external fixation

28510   Closed treatment of fracture, phalanx or phalanges, other than great toe; without manipulation, each

28515   with manipulation, each

(28520 has been deleted. To report, see 28510, 28515, 28525)

28525   Open treatment of fracture, phalanx or phalanges, other than great toe, with or without internal or external fixation, each

28530   Closed treatment of sesamoid fracture

28531   Open treatment of sesamoid fracture, with or without internal fixation

28540   Closed treatment of tarsal bone dislocation, other than talotarsal; without anesthesia

28545   requiring anesthesia

28546   Percutaneous skeletal fixation of tarsal bone dislocation, other than talotarsal, with manipulation

(28550 has been deleted. To report, see 28540, 28545, 28546, 28555)

28555   Open treatment of tarsal bone dislocation, with or without internal or external fixation

28570   Closed treatment of talotarsal joint dislocation; without anesthesia

28575   requiring anesthesia

28576   Percutaneous skeletal fixation of talotarsal joint dislocation, with manipulation

(28580 has been deleted. To report, see 28570, 28575, 28576, 28585)

28585   Open treatment of talotarsal joint dislocation, with or without internal or external fixation

28600   Closed treatment of tarsometatarsal joint dislocation; without anesthesia

28605   requiring anesthesia

28606   Percutaneous skeletal fixation of tarsometatarsal joint dislocation, with manipulation

(28610 has been deleted. To report, see 28600, 28605, 28606, 28615)

28615   Open treatment of tarsometatarsal joint dislocation, with or without internal or external fixation

28630*   Closed treatment of metatarsophalangeal joint dislocation; without anesthesia

28635*   requiring anesthesia

28636   Percutaneous skeletal fixation of metatarsophalangeal joint dislocation, with manipulation

(28640 has been deleted. To report, see 28630, 28635, 28636, 28645)

28645   Open treatment of metatarsophalangeal joint dislocation, with or without internal or external fixation

28660*   Closed treatment of interphalangeal joint dislocation; without anesthesia

28665*   requiring anesthesia

28666   Percutaneous skeletal fixation of interphalangeal joint dislocation, with manipulation

(28670 has been deleted. To report, see 28660, 28665, 28666, 28675)

28675 Open treatment of interphalangeal joint dislocation, with or without internal or external fixation

Arthrodesis

28705 Pantalar arthrodesis

28715 Triple arthrodesis

28725 Subtalar arthrodesis

28730 Arthrodesis, midtarsal or tarsometatarsal, multiple or transverse;

28735   with osteotomy as for flatfoot correction

28737 Arthrodesis, midtarsal navicular-cuneiform, with tendon lengthening and advancement (Miller type procedure)

28740 Arthrodesis, midtarsal or tarsometatarsal, single joint

28750 Arthrodesis, great toe; metatarsophalangeal joint

28755   interphalangeal joint

28760 Arthrodesis, great toe, interphalangeal joint, with extensor hallucis longus transfer to first metatarsal neck (Jones type procedure)

(For hammertoe operation or interphalangeal fusion, see 28285)

Amputation

28800 Amputation, foot; midtarsal (Chopart type procedure)

28805   transmetatarsal

28810 Amputation, metatarsal, with toe, single

28820 Amputation, toe; metatarsophalangeal joint

28825   interphalangeal joint

(For amputation of tuft of distal phalanx, use 11752)

Other Procedures

28899 Unlisted procedure, foot or toes

Application of Casts and Strapping

The listed procedures apply when the cast application or strapping is a replacement procedure used during or after the period of follow-up care, or when the cast application or strapping is an initial service performed without a restorative treatment or procedure(s) to stabilize or protect a fracture, injury or dislocation and/or to afford comfort to a patient. Restorative treatment or procedure(s) rendered by another physician following the application of the initial cast/splint/strap may be reported with a treatment of fracture and/or dislocation code.

A physician who applies the initial cast, strap or splint and also assumes all of the subsequent fracture, dislocation or injury care cannot use the application of casts and strapping codes as an initial service, since the first cast/splint or strap application is included in the treatment of fracture and/or dislocation codes. (See notes under Musculoskeletal System, page 73). A temporary cast/splint/strap is not considered to be part of the preoperative care, and the use of the modifier '-56' is not applicable. Additional evaluation and management services are reportable only if significant identifiable further services are provided at the time of the cast application or strapping.

If cast application or strapping is provided as an initial service (eg, casting of a sprained ankle or knee) in which no other procedure or treatment (eg, surgical repair, reduction of a fracture or joint dislocation) is performed or is expected to be performed by a physician rendering the initial care only, use the casting, strapping and/or supply code (99070) in addition to an evaluation and management code as appropriate.

Listed procedures include removal of cast or strapping.

Body and Upper Extremity

Casts

29000 Application of halo type body cast (see 20661-20663 for insertion)

29010 Application of Risser jacket, localizer, body; only

29015   including head

29020 Application of turnbuckle jacket, body; only

29025   including head

29035 Application of body cast, shoulder to hips;

29040   including head, Minerva type

29044   including one thigh

29046   including both thighs

29049 Application; plaster figure-of-eight

29055   shoulder spica

29058   plaster Velpeau

29065   shoulder to hand (long arm)

29075   elbow to finger (short arm)

29085   hand and lower forearm (gauntlet)

Splints

29105 Application of long arm splint (shoulder to hand)

29125 Application of short arm splint (forearm to hand); static

29126   dynamic

29130 Application of finger splint; static

29131   dynamic

Strapping—Any Age

29200 Strapping; thorax

29220   low back

29240   shoulder (eg, Velpeau)

29260   elbow or wrist

29280   hand or finger

Lower Extremity
Casts

29305 Application of hip spica cast; one leg

29325   one and one-half spica or both legs

(For hip spica (body) cast, including thighs only, see 29046)

29345 Application of long leg cast (thigh to toes);

29355   walker or ambulatory type

29358 Application of long leg cast brace

29365 Application of cylinder cast (thigh to ankle)

29405 Application of short leg cast (below knee to toes);

29425   walking or ambulatory type

29435 Application of patellar tendon bearing (PTB) cast

29440 Adding walker to previously applied cast

29445 Application of rigid total contact leg cast

29450 Application of clubfoot cast with molding or manipulation, long or short leg

(29455 has been deleted. To report, use 29450 with modifier -50 or 09950)

Splints

29505 Application of long leg splint (thigh to ankle or toes)

29515 Application of short leg splint (calf to foot)

Strapping—Any Age

29520 Strapping; hip

29530   knee

29540   ankle

29550   toes

29580   Unna boot

29590 Denis-Browne splint strapping

Removal or Repair

Codes for cast removals should be employed only for casts applied by another physician.

29700 Removal or bivalving; gauntlet, boot or body cast

29705   full arm or full leg cast

29710   shoulder or hip spica, Minerva, or Risser jacket, etc.

29715   turnbuckle jacket

29720   Repair of spica, body cast or jacket

29730   Windowing of cast

29740   Wedging of cast (except clubfoot casts)

29750   Wedging of clubfoot cast

     (29751 has been deleted. To report, use 29750 with modifier -50 or 09950)

Other Procedures

29799   Unlisted procedure, casting or strapping

Arthroscopy

Surgical arthroscopy always includes a diagnostic arthroscopy.

When arthroscopy is performed in conjunction with arthrotomy, add modifier '-51' or 09951.

29800   Arthroscopy, temporomandibular joint, diagnostic, with or without synovial biopsy (separate procedure)

29804   Arthroscopy, temporomandibular joint, surgical

29815   Arthroscopy, shoulder, diagnostic, with or without synovial biopsy (separate procedure)

29819   Arthroscopy, shoulder, surgical; with removal of loose body or foreign body

29820   synovectomy, partial

29821   synovectomy, complete

29822   debridement, limited

29823   debridement, extensive

29825   with lysis and resection of adhesions, with or without manipulation

29826   decompression of subacromial space with partial acromioplasty, with or without coracoacromial release

29830   Arthroscopy, elbow, diagnostic, with or without synovial biopsy (separate procedure)

29834   Arthroscopy, elbow, surgical; with removal of loose body or foreign body

29835   synovectomy, partial

29836   synovectomy, complete

29837   debridement, limited

29838   debridement, extensive

29840   Arthroscopy, wrist, diagnostic, with or without synovial biopsy (separate procedure)

29843   Arthroscopy, wrist, surgical; for infection, lavage and drainage

29844   synovectomy, partial

29845   synovectomy, complete

29846   excision and/or repair of triangular fibrocartilage and/or joint debridement

29847   internal fixation for fracture or instability

29848   with release of transverse carpal ligament

     (For open procedure, see 64721)

29850   Arthroscopically aided treatment of intercondylar spine(s) and/or tuberosity fracture(s) of the knee, with or without manipulation; without internal or external fixation (includes arthroscopy)

29851   with internal or external fixation (includes arthroscopy)

     (For bone graft, use 20900, 20902)

29855   Arthroscopically aided treatment of tibial fracture, proximal (plateau); unicondylar, with or without internal or external fixation (includes arthroscopy)

29856   bicondylar, with or without internal or external fixation (includes arthroscopy)

     (For bone graft, use 20900, 20902)

29870   Arthroscopy, knee, diagnostic, with or without synovial biopsy (separate procedure)

29871   Arthroscopy, knee, surgical; for infection, lavage and drainage

     (29872 has been deleted)

29874   for removal of loose body or foreign body (eg, osteochondritis dissecans fragmentation, chondral fragmentation)

29875   synovectomy, limited (eg, plica or shelf resection) (separate procedure)

29876   synovectomy, major, two or more compartments (eg, medial or lateral)

29877   debridement/shaving of articular cartilage (chondroplasty)

29879   abrasion arthroplasty (includes chondro- plasty where necessary) or multiple drilling

29880   with meniscectomy (medial AND lateral, including any meniscal shaving)

29881   with meniscectomy (medial OR lateral, including any meniscal shaving)

29882   with meniscus repair (medial OR lateral)

29883   with meniscus repair (medial AND lateral)

29884   with lysis of adhesions, with or without manipulation (separate procedure)

29885   drilling for osteochondritis dissecans with bone grafting, with or without internal fixation (including debridement of base of lesion)

29886   drilling for intact osteochondritis dissecans lesion

29887   drilling for intact osteochondritis dissecans lesion with internal fixation

29888   Arthroscopically aided anterior cruciate ligament repair/augmentation or reconstruction

29889   Arthroscopically aided posterior cruciate ligament repair/augmentation or reconstruction

(Procedures 29888 and 29889 should not be used with reconstruction procedures 27427- 27429)

(29890 has been deleted)

29894   Arthroscopy, ankle (tibiotalar and fibulotalar joints), surgical; with removal of loose body or foreign body

29895   synovectomy, partial

(29896 has been deleted)

29897   debridement, limited

29898   debridement, extensive

29909   Unlisted procedure, arthroscopy

Respiratory System

Nose

Incision

30000* Drainage abscess or hematoma, nasal, internal approach

(For external approach, see 10060, 10140)

30020* Drainage abscess or hematoma, nasal septum

(For lateral rhinotomy, see specific application (eg, 30118, 30320))

Excision

30100 Biopsy, intranasal

(For biopsy skin of nose, see 11100, 11101)

30110 Excision, nasal polyp(s), simple

(30110 would normally be completed in an office setting)

(30111 has been deleted. To report, use 30110 with modifier -50 or 09950)

30115 Excision, nasal polyp(s), extensive

(30115 would normally require the facilities available in a hospital setting)

(30116 has been deleted. To report, use 30115 with modifier -50 or 09950)

30117 Excision or destruction, any method (including laser), intranasal lesion; internal approach

30118 external approach (lateral rhinotomy)

30120 Excision or surgical planing of skin of nose for rhinophyma

30124 Excision dermoid cyst, nose; simple, skin, subcutaneous

30125 complex, under bone or cartilage

30130 Excision turbinate, partial or complete

30140 Submucous resection turbinate, partial or complete

(For submucous resection of nasal septum, use 30520)

(For reduction of turbinates, use 30140 with modifier -52)

30150 Rhinectomy; partial

30160 total

(For closure and/or reconstruction, primary or delayed, see Integumentary System, 13150-13152, 14060-14300, 15120, 15121, 15260, 15261, 15760, 20900-20912)

Introduction

30200* Injection into turbinate(s), therapeutic

30210* Displacement therapy (Proetz type)

30220 Insertion, nasal septal prosthesis (button)

Removal of Foreign Body

30300* Removal foreign body, intranasal; office type procedure

30310 requiring general anesthesia

30320 by lateral rhinotomy

Repair

(For obtaining tissues for graft, see 20900-20926, 21210)

30400 Rhinoplasty, primary; lateral and alar cartilages and/or elevation of nasal tip

(For columellar reconstruction, see 13150 et seq)

30410 complete, external parts including bony pyramid, lateral and alar cartilages, and/or elevation of nasal tip

30420 including major septal repair

30430 Rhinoplasty, secondary; minor revision (small amount of nasal tip work)

30435 intermediate revision (bony work with osteotomies)

30450 major revision (nasal tip work and osteotomies)

Respiratory 30000–32999

30460 Rhinoplasty for nasal deformity secondary to congenital cleft lip and/or palate, including columellar lengthening; tip only

30462 tip, septum, osteotomies

(30500 has been deleted. To report, use 30520)

30520 Septoplasty or submucous resection, with or without cartilage scoring, contouring or replacement with graft

(For submucous resection of turbinates, use 30140)

30540 Repair choanal atresia; intranasal

30545 transpalatine

30560* Lysis intranasal synechia

30580 Repair fistula; oromaxillary (combine with 31030 if antrotomy is included)

30600 oronasal

30620 Septal or other intranasal dermatoplasty (does not include obtaining graft)

30630 Repair nasal septal perforations

Destruction

(30800 has been deleted. To report, see 30801 and 30802)

30801* Cauterization and/or ablation, mucosa of turbinates, unilateral or bilateral, any method, (separate procedure); superficial

30802 intramural

(30805, 30820 have been deleted. To report, see 30801 and 30802)

Other Procedures

(30900 has been deleted. To report, see 30901, 30903)

30901* Control nasal hemorrhage, anterior, simple (limited cautery and/or packing) any method

(30902 has been deleted. To report, use 30901 with modifier -50 or 09950)

30903* Control nasal hemorrhage, anterior, complex (extensive cautery and/or packing) any method

(30904 has been deleted. To report, use 30903 with modifier -50 or 09950)

30905* Control nasal hemorrhage, posterior, with posterior nasal packs and/or cauterization, any method; initial

30906* subsequent

30915 Ligation arteries; ethmoidal

30920 internal maxillary artery, transantral

(For ligation external carotid artery, see 37600)

30930 Fracture nasal turbinate(s), therapeutic

30999 Unlisted procedure, nose

Accessory Sinuses

Incision

31000* Lavage by cannulation; maxillary sinus (antrum puncture or natural ostium)

(31001 has been deleted. To report, use 31000 with modifier -50 or 09950)

31002* sphenoid sinus

31020 Sinusotomy, maxillary (antrotomy); intranasal

(31021 has been deleted. To report, use 31020 with modifier -50 or 09950)

31030 radical (Caldwell-Luc) without removal of antrochoanal polyps

(31031 has been deleted. To report, use 31030 with modifier -50 or 09950)

31032 radical (Caldwell-Luc) with removal of antrochoanal polyps

(31033 has been deleted. To report, use 31032 with modifier -50 or 09950)

31040 Pterygomaxillary fossa surgery, any approach

(For transantral ligation of internal maxillary artery, see 30920)

31050 Sinusotomy, sphenoid, with or without biopsy;

31051   with mucosal stripping or removal of polyp(s)

31070   Sinusotomy frontal; external, simple (trephine operation)

(31071 has been deleted. To report, use 31276)

31075   transorbital, unilateral (for mucocele or osteoma, Lynch type)

31080   obliterative without osteoplastic flap, brow incision (includes ablation)

31081   obliterative, without osteoplastic flap, coronal incision (includes ablation)

31084   obliterative, with osteoplastic flap, brow incision

31085   obliterative, with osteoplastic flap, coronal incision

31086   nonobliterative, with osteoplastic flap, brow incision

31087   nonobliterative, with osteoplastic flap, coronal incision

31090   Sinusotomy combined, three or more sinuses

Excision

31200   Ethmoidectomy; intranasal, anterior

31201   intranasal, total

31205   extranasal, total

31225   Maxillectomy; without orbital exenteration

31230   with orbital exenteration (en bloc)

(For orbital exenteration only, see 65110 et seq)

(For skin grafts, see 15120 et seq)

Endoscopy

A surgical sinus endoscopy always includes a sinusotomy and diagnostic endoscopy.

Codes 31231-31294 are used to report unilateral procedures unless otherwise specified.

The codes 31231-31235 for diagnostic evaluation refer to employing a nasal/sinus endoscope to inspect the interior of the nasal cavity and the middle and superior meatus, the turbinates, and the spheno-ethmoid recess. Any time a diagnostic evaluation is performed all these areas would be inspected and a separate code is not reported for each area.

31231   Nasal endoscopy, diagnostic, unilateral or bilateral (separate procedure)

31233   Nasal/sinus endoscopy, diagnostic with maxillary sinusoscopy (via inferior meatus or canine fossa puncture)

31235   Nasal/sinus endoscopy, diagnostic with sphenoid sinusoscopy (via puncture of sphenoidal face or cannulation of ostium)

31237   Nasal/sinus endoscopy, surgical; with biopsy, polypectomy or debridement (separate procedure)

31238   with control of epistaxis

31239   with dacryocystorhinostomy

31240   with concha bullosa resection

(31245 has been deleted. To report, use 31254)

(31246 has been deleted. To report, use 31254 and 31256)

(31247 has been deleted. To report, use 31254 and 31267)

(31248 has been deleted. To report, use 31254 and 31276)

(31249 has been deleted. To report, use 31254, 31256, and 31276)

(31250 has been deleted. To report, see 31231-31235)

(31251 has been deleted. To report, use 31254, 31267, and 31276)

(31252 has been deleted. To report, use 31237)

31254   Nasal/sinus endoscopy, surgical; with ethmoidectomy, partial (anterior)

31255   with ethmoidectomy, total (anterior and posterior)

31256 Nasal/sinus endoscopy, surgical, with maxillary antrostomy;

(31258 has been deleted. To report, use 31237)

(31260 has been deleted. To report, use 31233)

(31261 has been deleted. To report, use 31255)

(31262 has been deleted. To report, use 31255 and 31256)

(31263 has been deleted. To report, use 31267)

(31264 has been deleted. To report, use 31255 and 31267)

(31265 has been deleted. To report, use 31267)

(31266 has been deleted. To report, use 31255 and 31276)

31267　　with removal of tissue from maxillary sinus

(31268 has been deleted. To report, use 31267)

(31269 has been deleted. To report, use 31255, 31256, and 31276)

(31270 has been deleted. To report, use 31235)

(31271 has been deleted. To report, use 31255, 31267, and 31276)

(31275 has been deleted. To report, use 31287)

31276 Nasal/sinus endoscopy, surgical with frontal sinus exploration, with or without removal of tissue from frontal sinus

(31277 has been deleted. To report, use 31288)

(31280 has been deleted. To report, use 31255, and 31287 or 31288)

(31281 has been deleted. To report, use 31255, 31256, and 31287 or 31288)

(31282 has been deleted. To report, use 31255, 31267, and 31287 or 31288)

(31283 has been deleted. To report, use 31255, 31287 or 31288, and 31276)

(31284 has been deleted. To report, use 31255, 31256, 31287 or 31288, and 31276)

(31285 has been deleted. To report, use 31231-31235)

(31286 has been deleted. To report, use 31255, 31267, 31287 or 31288, and 31276)

31287 Nasal/sinus endoscopy, surgical, with sphenoidotomy;

31288　　with removal of tissue from the sphenoid sinus

31290 Nasal/sinus endoscopy, surgical, with repair of cerebrospinal fluid leak; ethmoid region

31291　　sphenoid region

31292 Nasal/sinus endoscopy, surgical; with medial or inferior orbital wall decompression

31293　　with medial orbital wall and inferior orbital wall decompression

31294　　with optic nerve decompression

Other Procedures

(For hypophysectomy, transantral or transeptal approach, see 61548)

(For transcranial hypophysectomy, see 61546)

31299 Unlisted procedure, accessory sinuses

Larynx

Excision

31300 Laryngotomy (thyrotomy, laryngofissure); with removal of tumor or laryngocele, cordectomy

31320　　diagnostic

31360 Laryngectomy; total, without radical neck dissection

31365　　total, with radical neck dissection

31367　　subtotal supraglottic, without radical neck dissection

31368   subtotal supraglottic, with radical neck dissection

31370   Partial laryngectomy (hemilaryngectomy); horizontal

31375   laterovertical

31380   anterovertical

31382   antero-latero-vertical

31390   Pharyngolaryngectomy, with radical neck dissection; without reconstruction

31395   with reconstruction

31400   Arytenoidectomy or arytenoidopexy, external approach

(For endoscopic arytenoidectomy, see 31560)

31420   Epiglottidectomy

Introduction

31500   Intubation, endotracheal, emergency procedure

(For injection procedure for bronchography, see 31656, 31708, 31710)

31502   Tracheotomy tube change prior to establishment of fistula tract

Endoscopy

For endoscopic procedures, code appropriate endoscopy of each anatomic site examined.

31505   Laryngoscopy, indirect (separate procedure); diagnostic

31510   with biopsy

31511   with removal of foreign body

31512   with removal of lesion

31513   with vocal cord injection

31515   Laryngoscopy direct, with or without tracheoscopy; for aspiration

31520   diagnostic, newborn

31525   diagnostic, except newborn

31526   diagnostic, with operating microscope

31527   with insertion of obturator

31528   with dilatation, initial

31529   with dilatation, subsequent

31530   Laryngoscopy, direct, operative, with foreign body removal;

31531   with operating microscope

31535   Laryngoscopy, direct, operative, with biopsy;

31536   with operating microscope

31540   Laryngoscopy, direct, operative, with excision of tumor and/or stripping of vocal cords or epiglottis;

31541   with operating microscope

31560   Laryngoscopy, direct, operative, with arytenoidectomy;

31561   with operating microscope

31570   Laryngoscopy, direct, with injection into vocal cord(s), therapeutic;

31571   with operating microscope

31575   Laryngoscopy, flexible fiberoptic; diagnostic

31576   with biopsy

31577   with removal of foreign body

31578   with removal of lesion

▲**31579**   Laryngoscopy, flexible or rigid fiberoptic, with stroboscopy

Repair

31580   Laryngoplasty; for laryngeal web, two stage, with keel insertion and removal

31582   for laryngeal stenosis, with graft or core mold, including tracheotomy

31584   with open reduction of fracture

31585   Treatment of closed laryngeal fracture; without manipulation

31586   with closed manipulative reduction

31587   Laryngoplasty, cricoid split

31588 Laryngoplasty, not otherwise specified (eg, for burns, reconstruction after partial laryngectomy)

31590 Laryngeal reinnervation by neuromuscular pedicle

Destruction

31595 Section recurrent laryngeal nerve, therapeutic (separate procedure), unilateral

Other Procedures

31599 Unlisted procedure, larynx

Trachea and Bronchi

Incision

31600 Tracheostomy, planned (separate procedure);

31601   under two years

31603 Tracheostomy, emergency procedure; transtracheal

31605   cricothyroid membrane

31610 Tracheostomy, fenestration procedure with skin flaps

(For endotracheal intubation, see 31500)

(For tracheal aspiration under direct vision, see 31515)

31611 Construction of tracheoesophageal fistula and subsequent insertion of an alaryngeal speech prosthesis (eg, voice button, Blom-Singer prosthesis)

31612 Tracheal puncture, percutaneous with transtracheal aspiration and/or injection

31613 Tracheostoma revision; simple, without flap rotation

31614   complex, with flap rotation

Endoscopy

(For endoscopic procedures, code appropriate endoscopy of each anatomic site examined)

(For tracheoscopy, see laryngoscopy codes 31515-31578)

31615 Tracheobronchoscopy through established tracheostomy incision

(31620, 31621 have been deleted. To report, use 31622)

31622 Bronchoscopy; diagnostic, (flexible or rigid), with or without cell washing or brushing

31625   with biopsy

(31626 has been deleted. To report, use 31625)

(31627 has been deleted. To report, use 31622)

31628   with transbronchial lung biopsy, with or without fluoroscopic guidance

31629   with transbronchial needle aspiration biopsy

31630   with tracheal or bronchial dilation or closed reduction of fracture

31631   with tracheal dilation and placement of tracheal stent

31635   with removal of foreign body

31640   with excision of tumor

31641   with destruction of tumor or relief of stenosis by any method other than excision (eg, laser)

31645   with therapeutic aspiration of tracheo-bronchial tree, initial (eg, drainage of lung abscess)

31646   with therapeutic aspiration of tracheo-bronchial tree, subsequent

(For catheter aspiration of tracheobronchial tree at bedside, use 31725)

(31650, 31651 have been deleted. To report, see 31645, 31646)

31656   with injection of contrast material for segmental bronchography (fiberscope only)

(For radiological supervision and interpretation, see 71040, 71060)

(31659 has been deleted)

Introduction

(For endotracheal intubation, see 31500)

(For tracheal aspiration under direct vision, see 31515)

31700 Catheterization, transglottic (separate procedure)

31708 Instillation of contrast material for laryngography or bronchography, without catheterization

(For radiological supervision and interpretation, see 70373, 71040, 71060)

31710 Catheterization for bronchography, with or without instillation of contrast material

(For bronchoscopic catheterization for bronchography, fiberscope only, see 31656)

(For radiological supervision and interpretation, see 71040, 71060)

31715 Transtracheal injection for bronchography

(For radiological supervision and interpretation, see 71040, 71060)

(For prolonged services, see 99354-99360)

31717 Catheterization with bronchial brush biopsy

(31719 has been deleted. To report, use 31730)

31720 Catheter aspiration (separate procedure); nasotracheal

31725   tracheobronchial with fiberscope, bedside

31730 Transtracheal (percutaneous) introduction of needle wire dilator/stent or indwelling tube for oxygen therapy

Repair

31750 Tracheoplasty; cervical

31755   tracheopharyngeal fistulization, each stage

31760   intrathoracic

31766 Carinal reconstruction

31770 Bronchoplasty; graft repair

31775   excision stenosis and anastomosis

(For lobectomy and bronchoplasty, see 32485)

31780 Excision tracheal stenosis and anastomosis; cervical

31781   cervicothoracic

31785 Excision of tracheal tumor or carcinoma; cervical

31786   thoracic

31800 Suture of tracheal wound or injury; cervical

31805   intrathoracic

31820 Surgical closure tracheostomy or fistula; without plastic repair

31825   with plastic repair

(For repair tracheoesophageal fistula, see 43305, 43312)

31830 Revision of tracheostomy scar

Other Procedures

31899 Unlisted procedure, trachea, bronchi

Lungs and Pleura

Incision

32000* Thoracentesis, puncture of pleural cavity for aspiration, initial or subsequent

(For radiological supervision and interpretation, see 76003, 76360, 76934)

32002 Thoracentesis with insertion of tube with or without water seal (eg, for pneumothorax) (separate procedure)

32005 Chemical pleurodesis (eg, for recurrent or persistent pneumothorax)

32020 Tube thoracostomy with or without water seal (eg, for abscess, hemothorax, empyema) (separate procedure)

32035 Thoracostomy; with rib resection for empyema

32036   with open flap drainage for empyema

32095   Thoracotomy, limited, for biopsy of lung or pleura

(To report wound exploration due to penetrating trauma without thoractomy, use 20102)

32100   Thoracotomy, major; with exploration and biopsy

32110   with control of traumatic hemorrhage and/ or repair of lung tear

32120   for postoperative complications

32124   with open intrapleural pneumonolysis

32140   with cyst(s) removal, with or without a pleural procedure

32141   with excision-plication of bullae, with or without any pleural procedure

32150   with removal of intrapleural foreign body or fibrin deposit

32151   with removal of intrapulmonary foreign body

32160   with cardiac massage

(For segmental or other resections of lung, see 32480-32525)

32200   Pneumonostomy, with open drainage of abscess or cyst

32215   Pleural scarification for repeat pneumothorax

32220   Decortication, pulmonary (separate procedure); total

32225   partial

Excision

32310   Pleurectomy, parietal (separate procedure)

(32315 has been deleted. To report, use 32310)

32320   Decortication and parietal pleurectomy

32400*   Biopsy, pleura; percutaneous needle

(For radiological supervision and interpretation, see 71036, 76360, 76942)

(For fine needle aspiration, preparation, and interpretation of smears, see 88170-88173)

32402   open

32405   Biopsy, lung or mediastinum, percutaneous needle

(For radiological supervision and interpretation, see 71036, 76360, 76942)

(For fine needle aspiration, preparation, and interpretation of smears, see 88170-88173)

32420*   Pneumonocentesis, puncture of lung for aspiration

32440   Removal of lung, total pneumonectomy;

32442   with resection of segment of trachea followed by broncho-tracheal anastomosis (sleeve pneumonectomy)

32445   extrapleural

(32450 has been deleted. To report, use 32445 and 32540)

32480   Removal of lung, other than total pneumonectomy; single lobe (lobectomy)

32482   two lobes (bilobectomy)

32484   single segment (segmentectomy)

(32485 has been deleted. To report, use 32501)

32486   with circumferential resection of segment of bronchus followed by broncho-bronchial anastomosis (sleeve lobectomy)

32488   all remaining lung following previous removal of a portion of lung (completion pneumonectomy)

(32490 has been deleted. To report, use 32320 and the appropriate removal of lung code)

32500   wedge resection, single or multiple

● **32501** Resection and repair of portion of bronchus (bronchoplasty) when performed at time of lobectomy or segmentectomy (List separately in addition to code for primary procedure)

(Use 32501 only for codes 32480, 32482, 32484)

(32501 is to be used when a portion of the bronchus to preserved lung is removed and requires plastic closure to preserve function of that preserved lung. It is not to be used for closure for the proximal end of a resected bronchus)

32520 Resection of lung; with resection of chest wall

32522 with reconstruction of chest wall, without prosthesis

32525 with major reconstruction of chest wall, with prosthesis

32540 Extrapleural enucleation of empyema (empyemectomy)

(32545 has been deleted. To report, use 32540 and the appropriate removal of lung code)

Endoscopy

Surgical thoracoscopy always includes diagnostic thoracoscopy.

For endoscopic procedures, code appropriate endoscopy of each anatomic site examined.

32601 Thoracoscopy, diagnostic (separate procedure); lungs and pleural space, without biopsy

32602 lungs and pleural space, with biopsy

32603 pericardial sac, without biopsy

32604 pericardial sac, with biopsy

32605 mediastinal space, without biopsy

32606 mediastinal space, with biopsy

(Surgical thoracoscopy always includes diagnostic thoracoscopy)

32650 Thoracoscopy, surgical; with pleurodesis, any method

32651 with partial pulmonary decortication

32652 with total pulmonary decortication, including intrapleural pneumonolysis

32653 with removal of intrapleural foreign body or fibrin deposit

32654 with control of traumatic hemorrhage

32655 with excision-plication of bullae, including any pleural procedure

32656 with parietal pleurectomy

32657 with wedge resection of lung, single or multiple

32658 with removal of clot or foreign body from pericardial sac

32659 with creation of pericardial window or partial resection of pericardial sac for drainage

32660 with total pericardiectomy

32661 with excision of pericardial cyst, tumor, or mass

32662 with excision of mediastinal cyst, tumor, or mass

32663 with lobectomy, total or segmental

32664 with thoracic sympathectomy

32665 with esophagomyotomy (Heller type)

(32700 and 32705 have been deleted. To report, see 32601-32606)

Repair

32800 Repair lung hernia through chest wall

32810 Closure of chest wall following open flap drainage for empyema (Clagett type procedure)

32815 Open closure of major bronchial fistula

32820 Major reconstruction, chest wall (post-traumatic)

Lung Transplantation

32850 Donor pneumonectomy(ies) with preparation and maintenance of allograft (cadaver)

32851 Lung transplant, single; without cardiopulmonary bypass

32852   with cardiopulmonary bypass

32853 Lung transplant, double (bilateral sequential or en bloc); without cardiopulmonary bypass

32854   with cardiopulmonary bypass

Surgical Collapse Therapy; Thoracoplasty

(See also 32520-32525)

32900 Resection of ribs, extrapleural, all stages

32905 Thoracoplasty, Schede type or extrapleural (all stages);

32906   with closure of bronchopleural fistula

(For open closure of major bronchial fistula, see 32815)

(For resection of first rib for thoracic outlet compression, see 21615, 21616)

32940 Pneumonolysis, extraperiosteal, including filling or packing procedures

32960* Pneumothorax, therapeutic, intrapleural injection of air

Other Procedures

32999 Unlisted procedure, lungs and pleura

Cardiovascular System

Selective vascular catheterizations should be coded to include introduction and all lesser order selective catheterizations used in the approach (eg, the description for a selective right middle cerebral artery catheterization includes the introduction and placement catheterization of the right common and internal carotid arteries).

Additional second and/or third order arterial catheterizations within the same family of arteries supplied by a single first order artery should be expressed by 36218 or 36248. Additional first order or higher catheterizations in vascular families supplied by a first order vessel different from a previously selected and coded family should be separately coded using the conventions described above.

> (For monitoring, operation of pump and other nonsurgical services, see 99190-99192, 99291, 99292, 99354-99360)

> (For other medical or laboratory related services, see appropriate section)

> (For radiological supervision and interpretation, see 75600-75978)

Heart and Pericardium

Pericardium

33010* Pericardiocentesis; initial

> (For radiological supervision and interpretation, see 76930)

33011* subsequent

> (For radiological supervision and interpretation, see 76930)

33015 Tube pericardiostomy

33020 Pericardiotomy for removal of clot or foreign body (primary procedure)

33025 Creation of pericardial window or partial resection for drainage

33030 Pericardiectomy, subtotal or complete; without cardiopulmonary bypass

33031 with cardiopulmonary bypass

> (33035 has been deleted. To report, use 33031)

33050 Excision of pericardial cyst or tumor

> (33100 has been deleted. To report, see 33030, 33031)

Cardiac Tumor

33120 Excision of intracardiac tumor, resection with cardiopulmonary bypass

33130 Resection of external cardiac tumor

Pacemaker or Defibrillator

A pacemaker system includes a pulse generator containing electronics and a battery, and one or more electrodes (leads) inserted one of several ways. Pulse generators may be placed in a subcutaneous "pocket" created in either a subclavicular or intra-abdominal site. Electrodes may be inserted through a vein (transvenous) or on the surface of the heart (epicardial).

A single chamber system includes a pulse generator and one electrode inserted in either the atrium or ventricle. A dual chamber system includes a pulse generator and one electrode inserted in the atrium and one electrode inserted in the ventricle.

Similarly, a defibrillator system also includes a pulse generator and electrodes. The pulse generator may also be placed in subcutaneous subclavicular or intra-abdominal pocket. These electrodes may also be inserted transvenously or epicardially.

When the "battery" is changed, it is actually the pulse generator that is changed. Replacement of a pulse generator for either a pacemaker or defibrillator system requires selection of a code for removal of the pulse generator and another code for the insertion of a pulse generator.

These procedures include repositioning or replacement in the first 14 days after the insertion (or replacement) of the device. Modifiers '-76' and '-77' are not reported with pacemaker or defibrillator codes after 14 days as these are considered new, not repeat, services.

> (For electronic, telephonic analysis of internal pacemaker system, see 93731-93736)

> (For radiological supervision and interpretation with insertion of pacemaker, see 71090)

33200   Insertion of permanent pacemaker with epicardial electrode(s); by thoracotomy

33201   by xiphoid approach

   (33205 has been deleted. To report, see 33206-33208)

33206   Insertion or replacement of permanent pacemaker with transvenous electrode(s); atrial

33207   ventricular

33208   atrial and ventricular

33210   Insertion or replacement of temporary transvenous single chamber cardiac electrode or pacemaker catheter (separate procedure)

33211   Insertion or replacement of temporary transvenous dual chamber pacing electrodes (separate procedure)

33212   Insertion or replacement of pacemaker pulse generator only; single chamber, atrial or ventricular

33213   dual chamber

33214   Upgrade of implanted pacemaker system, conversion of single chamber system to dual chamber system (includes removal of previously placed pulse generator, testing of existing lead, insertion of new lead, insertion of new pulse generator)

33216   Insertion, replacement or repositioning of permanent transvenous electrode(s) only (15 days or more after initial insertion); single chamber, atrial or ventricular

33217   dual chamber

33218   Repair of pacemaker electrode(s) only; single chamber, atrial or ventricular

   (33219 has been deleted. To report, see 33212 or 33213 and 33218 or 33220)

33220   dual chamber

33222   Revision or relocation of skin pocket for pacemaker

33223   Revision or relocation of skin pocket for implantable cardioverter-defibrillator

   (33232 has been deleted. To report, see 33233, 33234, 33236)

33233   Removal of permanent pacemaker pulse generator;

33234   with transvenous electrode(s), single lead system, atrial or ventricular

33235   with transvenous electrode(s), dual lead system

33236   Removal of permanent epicardial pacemaker and electrodes by thoracotomy; single lead system, atrial or ventricular

33237   dual lead system

33238   Removal of permanent transvenous electrode(s) by thoracotomy

33240   Insertion or replacement of implantable cardioverter-defibrillator pulse generator only

33241   Removal of implantable cardioverter-defibrillator pulse generator only

33242   Repair of implantable cardioverter-defibrillator pulse generator and/or leads

33243   Removal of implantable cardioverter-defibrillator pulse generator and/or lead system; by thoracotomy

33244   by other than thoracotomy

33245   Implantation or replacement of implantable cardioverter-defibrillator pads by thoracotomy, with or without sensing electrodes;

33246   with insertion of implantable cardioverter-defibrillator pulse generator

33247   Insertion or replacement of implantable cardioverter-defibrillator lead(s), by other than thoracotomy;

   (33248 has been deleted. To report, see 33242, 33243, 33244)

33249   with insertion of cardio-defibrillator pulse generator

33250   Operative ablation of supraventricular arrhythmogenic focus or pathway (eg, Wolff-Parkinson-White, A-V node re-entry), tract(s) and/or focus (foci); without cardiopulmonary bypass

33251   with cardiopulmonary bypass

● **33253** Operative incisions and reconstruction of atria for treatment of atrial fibrillation or atrial flutter (eg, maze procedure)

(33260 has been deleted. To report, use 33261)

▲ **33261** Operative ablation of ventricular arrhythmogenic focus with cardiopulmonary bypass

Wounds of the Heart and Great Vessels

33300 Repair of cardiac wound; without bypass

33305 with cardiopulmonary bypass

33310 Cardiotomy, exploratory (includes removal of foreign body); without bypass

33315 with cardiopulmonary bypass

33320 Suture repair of aorta or great vessels; without shunt or cardiopulmonary bypass

33321 with shunt bypass

33322 with cardiopulmonary bypass

33330 Insertion of graft, aorta or great vessels; without shunt, or cardiopulmonary bypass

33332 with shunt bypass

33335 with cardiopulmonary bypass

(33350 has been deleted)

Cardiac Valves

Aortic Valve

33400 Valvuloplasty, aortic valve; open, with cardiopulmonary bypass

33401 open, with inflow occlusion

33403 using transventricular dilation, with cardiopulmonary bypass

33404 Construction of apical-aortic conduit

33405 Replacement, aortic valve, with cardiopulmonary bypass; with prosthetic valve other than homograft

33406 with homograft valve (freehand)

(33407 has been deleted. To report, use 33403)

(33408 has been deleted. To report, use 33401)

33411 Replacement, aortic valve; with aortic annulus enlargement, noncoronary cusp

33412 with transventricular aortic annulus enlargement (Konno procedure)

33413 by translocation of autologous pulmonary valve with homograft replacement of pulmonary valve (Ross procedure)

33414 Repair of left ventricular outflow tract obstruction by patch enlargement of the outflow tract

33415 Resection or incision of subvalvular tissue for discrete subvalvular aortic stenosis

33416 Ventriculomyotomy (-myectomy) for idiopathic hypertrophic subaortic stenosis (eg, asymmetric septal hypertrophy)

33417 Aortoplasty (gusset) for supravalvular stenosis

Mitral Valve

33420 Valvotomy, mitral valve; closed heart

33422 open heart, with cardiopulmonary bypass

33425 Valvuloplasty, mitral valve, with cardiopulmonary bypass;

33426 with prosthetic ring

33427 radical reconstruction, with or without ring

33430 Replacement, mitral valve, with cardiopulmonary bypass

Tricuspid Valve

(33450 has been deleted. To report, see 33463, 33464)

(33452 has been deleted. To report, see 33463, 33464)

33460 Valvectomy, tricuspid valve, with cardiopulmonary bypass

33463 Valvuloplasty, tricuspid valve; without ring insertion

33464   with ring insertion

33465   Replacement, tricuspid valve, with cardio-pulmonary bypass

33468   Tricuspid valve repositioning and plication for Ebstein anomaly

Pulmonary Valve

33470   Valvotomy, pulmonary valve, closed heart; transventricular

33471   via pulmonary artery

(To report percutaneous valvuloplasty of pulmonary valve, use 92990)

33472   Valvotomy, pulmonary valve, open heart; with inflow occlusion

33474   with cardiopulmonary bypass

33475   Replacement, pulmonary valve

33476   Right ventricular resection for infundibular stenosis, with or without commissurotomy

33478   Outflow tract augmentation (gusset), with or without commissurotomy or infundibular resection

(33480-33492 have been deleted. To report, see 33400-33478 and add modifier -51 to the secondary valve procedure code when multiple valve procedures are performed.)

Coronary Artery Anomalies

Basic procedures include endarterectomy or angioplasty.

33500   Repair of coronary arteriovenous or arteriocardiac chamber fistula; with cardiopulmonary bypass

33501   without cardiopulmonary bypass

33502   Repair of anomalous coronary artery; by ligation

33503   by graft, without cardiopulmonary bypass

33504   by graft, with cardiopulmonary bypass

33505   with construction of intrapulmonary artery tunnel (Takeuchi procedure)

33506   by translocation from pulmonary artery to aorta

Venous Grafting Only for Coronary Artery Bypass

The following codes are used to report coronary artery bypass procedures using venous grafts only. These codes should NOT be used to report the performance of coronary artery bypass procedures using arterial grafts and venous grafts during the same procedure. See 33517-33523 and 33533-33536 for reporting combined arterial-venous grafts.

Procurement of the saphenous vein graft is included in the description of the work for 33510-33516 and should not be reported as a separate service or co-surgery. When graft procurement is performed by surgical assistant, add modifier '-80' to 33510-33516.

33510   Coronary artery bypass, vein only; single coronary venous graft

33511   two coronary venous grafts

33512   three coronary venous grafts

33513   four coronary venous grafts

33514   five coronary venous grafts

33516   six or more coronary venous grafts

Combined Arterial-Venous Grafting for Coronary Bypass

The following codes are used to report coronary artery bypass procedures using venous grafts and arterial grafts during the same procedure. These codes may NOT be used alone.

To report combined arterial-venous grafts it is necessary to report two codes: 1) the appropriate combined arterial-venous graft code (33517-33523); and, 2) the appropriate arterial graft code (33533-33536).

Procurement of the saphenous vein graft is included in the description of the work for 33517-33523 and should not be reported as a separate service or co-surgery. When graft procurement is performed by surgical assistant, add modifier '-80' to 33517-33523.

33517   Coronary artery bypass, using venous graft(s) and arterial graft(s); single vein graft (list separately in addition to code for arterial graft)

33518   two venous grafts (list separately in addition to code for arterial graft)

33519   three venous grafts (list separately in addition to code for arterial graft)

(33520 has been deleted)

33521   four venous grafts (list separately in addition to code for arterial graft)

33522   five venous grafts (list separately in addition to code for arterial graft)

33523   six or more venous grafts (list separately in addition to code for arterial graft)

(33525, 33528 have been deleted)

33530   Reoperation, coronary artery bypass procedure or valve procedure, more than one month after original operation (list separately in addition to code for primary procedure)

(Use 33530 only for codes 33400-33478; 33510-33536)

(33532 has been deleted. To report, use 33999)

Arterial Grafting for Coronary Artery Bypass

The following codes are used to report coronary artery bypass procedures using either arterial grafts only or a combination of arterial-venous grafts. The codes include the use of the internal mammary artery, gastroepiploic artery, epigastric artery, radial artery, and arterial conduits procured from other sites.

To report combined arterial-venous grafts it is necessary to report two codes: 1) the appropriate arterial graft code (33533-33536); and, 2) the appropriate combined arterial-venous graft code (33517-33523).

33533   Coronary artery bypass, using arterial graft(s); single arterial graft

33534   two coronary arterial grafts

33535   three coronary arterial grafts

33536   four or more coronary arterial grafts

33542   Myocardial resection (eg, ventricular aneurysmectomy)

33545   Repair of postinfarction ventricular septal defect, with or without myocardial resection

(33560 has been deleted)

Coronary Endarterectomy

(33570 has been deleted. To report, see 33510-33536 and 33572)

33572   Coronary endarterectomy, open, any method, of left anterior descending, circumflex, or right coronary artery performed in conjunction with coronary artery bypass graft procedure, each vessel (list separately in addition to primary procedure)

(Use 33572 only with 33510-33516, 33533-33536)

(33575 has been deleted. To report, see 33510-33536 and 33572)

Single Ventricle and Other Complex Cardiac Anomalies

33600   Closure of atrioventricular valve (mitral or tricuspid) by suture or patch

33602   Closure of semilunar valve (aortic or pulmonary) by suture or patch

33606   Anastomosis of pulmonary artery to aorta (Damus-Kaye-Stansel procedure)

33608   Repair of complex cardiac anomaly other than pulmonary atresia with ventricular septal defect by construction or replacement of conduit from right or left ventricle to pulmonary artery

(For repair of pulmonary atresia with ventricular septal defect, see 33918, 33919, 33920)

33610   Repair of complex cardiac anomalies (eg, single ventricle with subaortic obstruction) by surgical enlargement of interventricular septal defect

33611   Repair of double outlet right ventricle with intraventricular tunnel repair;

33612   with repair of right ventricular outflow tract obstruction

33615 Repair of complex cardiac anomalies (eg, tricuspid atresia) by closure of atrial septal defect and anastomosis of atria or vena cava to pulmonary artery (simple Fontan procedure)

33617 Repair of complex cardiac anomalies (eg, single ventricle) by modified Fontan procedure

33619 Repair of single ventricle with aortic outflow obstruction and aortic arch hypoplasia (hypoplastic left heart syndrome) (eg, Norwood procedure)

Septal Defect

(33640 has been deleted. To report, use 33641)

33641 Repair atrial septal defect, secundum, with cardiopulmonary bypass, with or without patch

(33643 has been deleted. To report, use 33641)

33645 Direct or patch closure, sinus venosus, with or without anomalous pulmonary venous drainage

33647 Repair of atrial septal defect and ventricular septal defect, with direct or patch closure

(33649 has been deleted. To report, use 33615)

33660 Repair of incomplete or partial atrioventricular canal (ostium primum atrial septal defect), with or without atrioventricular valve repair

33665 Repair of intermediate or transitional atrioventricular canal, with or without atrioventricular valve repair

33670 Repair of complete atrioventricular canal, with or without prosthetic valve

33681 Closure of ventricular septal defect, with or without patch

(33682 has been deleted. To report, use 33681)

33684 with pulmonary valvotomy or infundibular resection (acyanotic)

33688 with removal of pulmonary artery band, with or without gusset

33690 Banding of pulmonary artery

33692 Complete repair tetralogy of Fallot without pulmonary atresia;

33694 with transannular patch

(33696 has been deleted. To report, see 33924)

33697 Complete repair tetralogy of Fallot with pulmonary atresia including construction of conduit from right ventricle to pulmonary artery and closure of ventricular septal defect

(33698 has been deleted. To report, see 33924)

Sinus of Valsalva

33702 Repair sinus of Valsalva fistula, with cardiopulmonary bypass;

33710 with repair of ventricular septal defect

33720 Repair sinus of Valsalva aneurysm, with cardiopulmonary bypass

33722 Closure of aortico-left ventricular tunnel

Total Anomalous Pulmonary Venous Drainage

33730 Complete repair of anomalous venous return (supracardiac, intracardiac, or infracardiac types)

(For partial anomalous return, see atrial septal defect)

33732 Repair of cor triatriatum or supravalvular mitral ring by resection of left atrial membrane

Shunting Procedures

33735 Atrial septectomy or septostomy; closed heart (Blalock-Hanlon type operation)

33736 open heart with cardiopulmonary bypass

33737 open heart, with inflow occlusion

(33738 has been deleted. To report, use 92992)

(33739 has been deleted. To report, use 92993)

33750 Shunt; subclavian to pulmonary artery (Blalock-Taussig type operation)

33755   ascending aorta to pulmonary artery (Waterston type operation)

33762   descending aorta to pulmonary artery (Potts-Smith type operation)

33764   central, with prosthetic graft

33766   superior vena cava to pulmonary artery for flow to one lung (classical Glenn procedure)

33767   superior vena cava to pulmonary artery for flow to both lungs (bidirectional Glenn procedure)

Transposition of the Great Vessels

33770 Repair of transposition of the great arteries with ventricular septal defect and subpulmonary stenosis; without surgical enlargement of ventricular septal defect

33771   with surgical enlargement of ventricular septal defect

33774 Repair of transposition of the great arteries, atrial baffle procedure (eg, Mustard or Senning type) with cardiopulmonary bypass;

33775   with removal of pulmonary band

33776   with closure of ventricular septal defect

33777   with repair of subpulmonic obstruction

33778 Repair of transposition of the great arteries, aortic pulmonary artery reconstruction (eg, Jatene type);

33779   with removal of pulmonary band

33780   with closure of ventricular septal defect

33781   with repair of subpulmonic obstruction

(33782, 33783, 33784, 33785 have been deleted. To report, see 33774-33781)

Truncus Arteriosus

33786 Total repair, truncus arteriosus (Rastelli type operation)

33788 Reimplantation of an anomalous pulmonary artery

(For pulmonary artery band, see 33690)

Aortic Anomalies

33800 Aortic suspension (aortopexy) for tracheal decompression (eg, for tracheomalacia) (separate procedure)

33802 Division of aberrant vessel (vascular ring);

33803   with reanastomosis

(33810, 33812 have been deleted)

33813 Obliteration of aortopulmonary septal defect; without cardiopulmonary bypass

33814   with cardiopulmonary bypass

33820 Repair of patent ductus arteriosus; by ligation

33822   by division, under 18 years

33824   by division, 18 years and older

(33830 has been deleted. To report, see 33820-33824)

33840 Excision of coarctation of aorta, with or without associated patent ductus arteriosus; with direct anastomosis

33845   with graft

(33850 has been deleted. To report, use 33999)

33851   repair using either left subclavian artery or prosthetic material as gusset for enlargement

33852 Repair of hypoplastic or interrupted aortic arch using autogenous or prosthetic material; without cardiopulmonary bypass

33853   with cardiopulmonary bypass

(33855 has been deleted. To report, use 33619)

Thoracic Aortic Aneurysm

33860 Ascending aorta graft, with cardiopulmonary bypass, with or without valve suspension;

33861   with coronary reconstruction

33863 with aortic root replacement using composite prosthesis and coronary reconstruction

(33865 has been deleted. To report, see 33860 or 33861 and 33405 or 33406)

33870 Transverse arch graft, with cardiopulmonary bypass

33875 Descending thoracic aorta graft, with or without bypass

33877 Repair of thoracoabdominal aortic aneurysm with graft, with or without cardiopulmonary bypass

Pulmonary Artery

33910 Pulmonary artery embolectomy; with cardiopulmonary bypass

33915 without cardiopulmonary bypass

33916 Pulmonary endarterectomy, with or without embolectomy, with cardiopulmonary bypass

33917 Repair of pulmonary artery stenosis by reconstruction with patch or graft

33918 Repair of pulmonary atresia with ventricular septal defect, by unifocalization of pulmonary arteries; without cardiopulmonary bypass

33919 with cardiopulmonary bypass

33920 Repair of pulmonary atresia with ventricular septal defect, by construction or replacement of conduit from right or left ventricle to pulmonary artery

(For repair of other complex cardiac anomalies by construction or replacement of right or left ventricle to pulmonary artery conduit, see 33608)

33922 Transection of pulmonary artery with cardiopulmonary bypass

●**33924** Ligation and takedown of a systemic-to-pulmonary artery shunt, performed in conjunction with a congenital heart procedure (List separately in addition to code for primary procedure)

(Use 33924 only with 33470-33475, 33600-33619, 33684-33688, 33692-33697, 33735-33767, 33770-33781, 33786, 33918-33922)

Heart/Lung Transplantation

33930 Donor cardiectomy-pneumonectomy, with preparation and maintenance of allograft

33935 Heart-lung transplant with recipient cardiectomy-pneumonectomy

33940 Donor cardiectomy, with preparation and maintenance of allograft

33945 Heart transplant, with or without recipient cardiectomy

(33950 has been deleted. To report, see 33940, 33945)

Cardiac Assist

33960 Prolonged extracorporeal circulation for cardiopulmonary insufficiency; initial 24 hours

33961 each additional 24 hours

(For insertion of cannula for prolonged extracorporeal circulation, use 36822)

33970 Insertion of intra-aortic balloon assist device through the femoral artery, open approach

(For percutaneous insertion, use 93536)

33971 Removal of intra-aortic balloon assist device including repair of femoral artery, with or without graft

(33972 has been deleted. To report, use appropriate E/M code)

33973 Insertion of intra-aortic balloon assist device through the ascending aorta

33974 Removal of intra-aortic balloon assist device from the ascending aorta, including repair of the ascending aorta, with or without graft

33975 Implantation of ventricular assist device; single ventricle support

33976 biventricular support

33977 Removal of ventricular assist device; single ventricle support

33978 biventricular support

Other Procedures

33999   Unlisted procedure, cardiac surgery

Arteries and Veins

Primary vascular procedure listings include establishing both inflow and outflow by whatever procedures necessary. Also included is that portion of the operative arteriogram performed by the surgeon, as indicated. Sympathectomy, when done, is included in the listed aortic procedures. For unlisted vascular procedure, use 37799.

Embolectomy/Thrombectomy

Arterial, With or Without Catheter

34001   Embolectomy or thrombectomy, with or without catheter; carotid, subclavian or innominate artery, by neck incision

34051   innominate, subclavian artery, by thoracic incision

34101   axillary, brachial, innominate, subclavian artery, by arm incision

34111   radial or ulnar artery, by arm incision

34151   renal, celiac, mesentery, aortoiliac artery, by abdominal incision

34201   femoropopliteal, aortoiliac artery, by leg incision

34203   popliteal-tibio-peroneal artery, by leg incision

Venous, Direct or With Catheter

34401   Thrombectomy, direct or with catheter; vena cava, iliac vein, by abdominal incision

34421   vena cava, iliac, femoropopliteal vein, by leg incision

34451   vena cava, iliac, femoropopliteal vein, by abdominal and leg incision

34471   subclavian vein, by neck incision

34490   axillary and subclavian vein, by arm incision

Venous Reconstruction

34501   Valvuloplasty, femoral vein

34502   Reconstruction of vena cava, any method

34510   Venous valve transposition, any vein donor

34520   Cross-over vein graft to venous system

34530   Saphenopopliteal vein anastomosis

Direct Repair of Aneurysm or Excision (Partial or Total) and Graft Insertion for Aneurysm, False Aneurysm, Ruptured Aneurysm, and Associated Occlusive Disease

Procedures 35001-35162 include preparation of artery for anastomosis including endarterectomy.

> (For direct repairs associated with occlusive disease only, see 35201-35286)
>
> (For intracranial aneurysm, see 61700 et seq)
>
> (For thoracic aortic aneurysm, see 33860-33875)

35001   Direct repair of aneurysm, false aneurysm, or excision (partial or total) and graft insertion, with or without patch graft; for aneurysm and associated occlusive disease, carotid, subclavian artery, by neck incision

35002   for ruptured aneurysm, carotid, subclavian artery, by neck incision

35005   for aneurysm, false aneurysm, and associated occlusive disease, vertebral artery

35011   for aneurysm and associated occlusive disease, axillary-brachial artery, by arm incision

35013   for ruptured aneurysm, axillary-brachial artery, by arm incision

35021   for aneurysm, false aneurysm, and associated occlusive disease, innominate, subclavian artery, by thoracic incision

35022   for ruptured aneurysm, innominate, subclavian artery, by thoracic incision

35045   for aneurysm, false aneurysm, and associated occlusive disease, radial or ulnar artery

35081 for aneurysm, false aneurysm, and associated occlusive disease, abdominal aorta

35082 for ruptured aneurysm, abdominal aorta

35091 for aneurysm, false aneurysm, and associated occlusive disease, abdominal aorta involving visceral vessels (mesenteric, celiac, renal)

35092 for ruptured aneurysm, abdominal aorta involving visceral vessels (mesenteric, celiac, renal)

35102 for aneurysm, false aneurysm, and associated occlusive disease, abdominal aorta involving iliac vessels (common, hypogastric, external)

35103 for ruptured aneurysm, abdominal aorta involving iliac vessels (common, hypogastric, external)

35111 for aneurysm, false aneurysm, and associated occlusive disease, splenic artery

35112 for ruptured aneurysm, splenic artery

35121 for aneurysm, false aneurysm, and associated occlusive disease, hepatic, celiac, renal, or mesenteric artery

35122 for ruptured aneurysm, hepatic, celiac, renal, or mesenteric artery

35131 for aneurysm, false aneurysm, and associated occlusive disease, iliac artery (common, hypogastric, external)

35132 for ruptured aneurysm, iliac artery (common, hypogastric, external)

35141 for aneurysm, false aneurysm, and associated occlusive disease, common femoral artery (profunda femoris, superficial femoral)

35142 for ruptured aneurysm, common femoral artery (profunda femoris, superficial femoral)

35151 for aneurysm, false aneurysm, and associated occlusive disease, popliteal artery

35152 for ruptured aneurysm, popliteal artery

35161 for aneurysm, false aneurysm, and associated occlusive disease, other arteries

35162 for ruptured aneurysm, other arteries

Repair Arteriovenous Fistula

35180 Repair, congenital arteriovenous fistula; head and neck

35182 thorax and abdomen

35184 extremities

35188 Repair, acquired or traumatic arteriovenous fistula; head and neck

35189 thorax and abdomen

35190 extremities

Repair Blood Vessel Other Than for Fistula, With or Without Patch Angioplasty

(For AV fistula repair, see 35180-35190)

35201 Repair blood vessel, direct; neck

35206 upper extremity

35207 hand, finger

35211 intrathoracic, with bypass

35216 intrathoracic, without bypass

35221 intra-abdominal

35226 lower extremity

35231 Repair blood vessel with vein graft; neck

35236 upper extremity

35241 intrathoracic, with bypass

35246 intrathoracic, without bypass

35251 intra-abdominal

35256 lower extremity

35261 Repair blood vessel with graft other than vein; neck

35266 upper extremity

35271	intrathoracic, with bypass	**35452**	aortic
35276	intrathoracic, without bypass	**35454**	iliac
35281	intra-abdominal	**35456**	femoral-popliteal
35286	lower extremity	**35458**	brachiocephalic trunk or branches, each vessel

Thromboendarterectomy

(For coronary artery, see 33570, 33575)

35301 Thromboendarterectomy, with or without patch graft; carotid, vertebral, subclavian, by neck incision

35311 subclavian, innominate, by thoracic incision

35321 axillary-brachial

35331 abdominal aorta

35341 mesenteric, celiac, or renal

35351 iliac

35355 iliofemoral

35361 combined aortoiliac

35363 combined aortoiliofemoral

35371 common femoral

35372 deep (profunda) femoral

35381 femoral and/or popliteal, and/or tibioperoneal

35390 Reoperation, carotid, thromboendarterectomy, more than one month after original operation (List separately in addition to code for primary procedure) (Use 35390 only with 35301)

Transluminal Angioplasty

(If done as part of another operation, use modifier -51 or 09951 or use modifier -52 or 09952)

(For radiological supervision and interpretation, see 75962-75968 and 75978)

Open

35450 Transluminal balloon angioplasty, open; renal or other visceral artery

35459 tibioperoneal trunk and branches

35460 venous

Percutaneous

35470 Transluminal balloon angioplasty, percutaneous; tibioperoneal trunk or branches, each vessel

35471 renal or visceral artery

35472 aortic

35473 iliac

35474 femoral-popliteal

35475 brachiocephalic trunk or branches, each vessel

35476 venous

(For radiological supervision and interpretation, see 75978)

Transluminal Atherectomy

(If done as part of another operation, use modifier -51 or 09951 or use modifier -52 or 09952)

(For radiological supervision and interpretation, see 75992-75996)

Open

35480 Transluminal peripheral atherectomy, open; renal or other visceral artery

35481 aortic

35482 iliac

35483 femoral-popliteal

35484 brachiocephalic trunk or branches, each vessel

35485 tibioperoneal trunk and branches

Percutaneous

35490 Transluminal peripheral atherectomy, percutaneous; renal or other visceral artery

35491   aortic

35492   iliac

35493   femoral-popliteal

35494   brachiocephalic trunk or branches, each vessel

35495   tibioperoneal trunk and branches

Bypass Graft

Vein

35501 Bypass graft, with vein; carotid

35506   carotid-subclavian

35507   subclavian-carotid

35508   carotid-vertebral

35509   carotid-carotid

35511   subclavian-subclavian

35515   subclavian-vertebral

35516   subclavian-axillary

35518   axillary-axillary

35521   axillary-femoral

(For bypass graft performed with synthetic graft, see 35621)

35526   aortosubclavian or carotid

(For bypass graft performed with synthetic graft, see 35626)

35531   aortoceliac or aortomesenteric

35533   axillary-femoral-femoral

(For bypass graft performed with synthetic graft, see 35654)

35536   splenorenal

35541   aortoiliac or bi-iliac

(For bypass graft performed with synthetic graft, see 35641)

35546   aortofemoral or bifemoral

(For bypass graft performed with synthetic graft, see 35646)

35548   aortoiliofemoral, unilateral

(For bypass graft performed with synthetic graft, see 37799)

35549   aortoiliofemoral, bilateral

(For bypass graft performed with synthetic graft, see 37799)

35551   aortofemoral-popliteal

35556   femoral-popliteal

35558   femoral-femoral

35560   aortorenal

35563   ilioiliac

35565   iliofemoral

35566   femoral-anterior tibial, posterior tibial, peroneal artery or other distal vessels

35571   popliteal-tibial, -peroneal artery or other distal vessels

In-Situ Vein

35582 In-situ vein bypass; aortofemoral-popliteal (only femoral-popliteal portion in-situ)

35583   femoral-popliteal

35585   femoral-anterior tibial, posterior tibial, or peroneal artery

35587   popliteal-tibial, peroneal

Other Than Vein

35601 Bypass graft, with other than vein; carotid

35606   carotid-subclavian

35612   subclavian-subclavian

35616   subclavian-axillary

35621   axillary-femoral

35623   axillary-popliteal or -tibial

35626   aortosubclavian or carotid

35631   aortoceliac, aortomesenteric, aortorenal

35636   splenorenal (splenic to renal arterial anastomosis)

(35637 has been deleted. To report, use 35691)

(35638 has been deleted. To report, use 35693)

35641   aortoiliac or bi-iliac

35642   carotid-vertebral

35645   subclavian-vertebral

35646   aortofemoral or bifemoral

35650   axillary-axillary

35651   aortofemoral-popliteal

35654   axillary-femoral-femoral

35656   femoral-popliteal

35661   femoral-femoral

35663   ilioiliac

35665   iliofemoral

35666   femoral-anterior tibial, posterior tibial, or peroneal artery

35671   popliteal-tibial or -peroneal artery

35681   Bypass graft, composite

(List procedure 35681 separately in addition to code for primary procedure)

Arterial Transposition

35691   Transposition and/or reimplantation; vertebral to carotid artery

35693   vertebral to subclavian artery

35694   subclavian to carotid artery

35695   carotid to subclavian artery

Exploration

35700   Reoperation, femoral-popliteal or femoral (popliteal) -anterior tibial, posterior tibial, peroneal artery or other distal vessels, more than one month after original operation (List separately in addition to code for primary procedure)

(Use 35700 only for codes 35556, 35566, 35571, 35583, 35585, 35587, 35656, 35666, 35671)

35701   Exploration (not followed by surgical repair), with or without lysis of artery; carotid artery

35721   femoral artery

35741   popliteal artery

35761   other vessels

35800   Exploration for postoperative hemorrhage, thrombosis or infection; neck

35820   chest

35840   abdomen

35860   extremity

35870   Repair of graft-enteric fistula

35875   Thrombectomy of arterial or venous graft;

35876   with revision of arterial or venous graft

(35880 has been deleted. To report, use 35875)

(35900 has been deleted. To report, see 35901-35907 and appropriate revascularization code)

35901   Excision of infected graft; neck

35903   extremity

35905   thorax

35907   abdomen

(35910 has been deleted. To report, see 35901-35907 and appropriate revascularization code)

Vascular Injection Procedures

Listed services for injection procedures include necessary local anesthesia, introduction of needles or catheter, injection of contrast media with or without automatic power injection, and/or necessary pre- and postinjection care specifically related to the injection procedure.

Catheters, drugs, and contrast media are not included in the listed service for the injection procedures.

Selective vascular catheterization should be coded to include introduction and all lesser order selective catheterization used in the approach (eg, the description for a selective right middle cerebral artery catheterization includes the introduction and placement catheterization of the right common and internal carotid arteries).

Additional second and/or third order arterial catheterization within the same family of arteries or veins supplied by a single first order vessel should be expressed by 36012, 36218 or 36248. Additional first order or higher catheterization in vascular families supplied by a first order vessel different from a previously selected and coded family should be separately coded using the conventions described above.

(For radiological supervision and interpretation, see **Radiology**)

(For injection procedures in conjunction with cardiac catheterization, see 93541-93545)

(For chemotherapy of malignant disease, see 96400-96549)

Intravenous

(An intracatheter is a sheathed combination of needle and short catheter)

36000* Introduction of needle or intracatheter, vein

(36001 has been deleted. To report, use 36000 with modifier -50 or 09950)

36005 Injection procedure for contrast venography (including introduction of needle or intracatheter)

36010 Introduction of catheter, superior or inferior vena cava

36011 Selective catheter placement, venous system; first order branch (eg, renal vein, jugular vein)

36012 second order, or more selective, branch (eg, left adrenal vein, petrosal sinus)

36013 Introduction of catheter, right heart or main pulmonary artery

36014 Selective catheter placement, left or right pulmonary artery

36015 Selective catheter placement, segmental or subsegmental pulmonary artery

(For insertion of flow directed catheter (eg, Swan-Ganz), see 93503)

(For venous catheterization for selective organ blood sampling, see 36500)

Intra-Arterial—Intra-Aortic

(For radiological supervision and interpretation, see **Radiology**)

36100 Introduction of needle or intracatheter, carotid or vertebral artery

(36101 has been deleted. To report, use 36100 with modifier -50 or 09950)

36120 Introduction of needle or intracatheter; retrograde brachial artery

36140 extremity artery

36145 arteriovenous shunt created for dialysis (cannula, fistula, or graft)

(For insertion of arteriovenous cannula, see 36810-36821)

36160 Introduction of needle or intracatheter, aortic, translumbar

36200 Introduction of catheter, aorta

(36210 has been deleted. To report, see 36215-36218)

36215 Selective catheter placement, arterial system; each first order thoracic or brachiocephalic branch, within a vascular family

36216 initial second order thoracic or brachiocephalic branch, within a vascular family

36217 initial third order or more selective thoracic or brachiocephalic branch, within a vascular family

36218 additional second order, third order, and beyond, thoracic or brachiocephalic branch, within a vascular family (use in addition to 36216 or 36217 as appropriate)

(36220 has been deleted. To report, see 36215-36218)

(36230 has been deleted. When coronary artery, arterial conduit (eg, internal mammary, inferior epigastric or free radical artery) or venous bypass graft angiography is performed in conjunction with cardiac catheterization, see the appropriate cardiac catheterization, injection procedure, and imaging supervision code(s) (93501-93556) in the **Medicine** Section of *CPT*. When coronary artery, internal mammary artery or venous bypass graft angiography is performed without a concomitant cardiac catheterization, use 36215, 36216 or 36217 as appropriate).

(36240 has been deleted. To report, use 36248)

36245 Selective catheter placement, arterial system; each first order abdominal, pelvic, or lower extremity artery branch, within a vascular family

36246 initial second order abdominal, pelvic, or lower extremity artery branch, within a vascular family

36247 initial third order or more selective abdominal, pelvic, or lower extremity artery branch, within a vascular family

36248 additional second order, third order, and beyond, abdominal, pelvic, or lower extremity artery branch, within a vascular family (use in addition to 36246 or 36247 as appropriate)

(36250 has been deleted. To report, use 36248)

36260 Insertion of implantable intra-arterial infusion pump (eg, for chemotherapy of liver)

36261 Revision of implanted intra-arterial infusion pump

36262 Removal of implanted intra-arterial infusion pump

36299 Unlisted procedure, vascular injection

Venous

Venipuncture, needle or catheter for diagnostic study or intravenous therapy, percutaneous.

36400 Venipuncture, under age 3 years; femoral, jugular or sagittal sinus

36405* scalp vein

36406 other vein

36410* Venipuncture, child over age 3 years or adult, necessitating physician's skill (separate procedure), for diagnostic or therapeutic purposes. Not to be used for routine venipuncture.

36415* Routine venipuncture or finger/heel/ear stick for collection of specimen(s)

36420 Venipuncture, cutdown; under age 1 year

36425 age 1 or over

36430 Transfusion, blood or blood components

(36431 has been deleted)

36440* Push transfusion, blood, 2 years or under

36450 Exchange transfusion, blood; newborn

36455 other than newborn

36460 Transfusion, intrauterine, fetal

(For radiological supervision and interpretation, see 76941)

36468 Single or multiple injections of sclerosing solutions, spider veins (telangiectasia); limb or trunk

36469 face

36470* Injection of sclerosing solution; single vein

36471* multiple veins, same leg

(36480 has been deleted. To report, use 36488 or 36489)

36481 Percutaneous portal vein catheterization by any method

(36485 has been deleted. To report, use 36490 or 36491)

▲=Revised Code   ●=New Code   ✱=Service Includes Surgical Procedure Only

36488* Placement of central venous catheter (subclavian, jugular, or other vein) (eg, for central venous pressure, hyperalimentation, hemodialysis, or chemotherapy); percutaneous, age 2 years or under

36489*   percutaneous, over age 2

36490*   cutdown, age 2 years or under

36491*   cutdown, over age 2

(For examination of patient and instruction to patient, review of prescription of fluids for long-term or permanent hyperalimentation, use Evaluation and Management codes for office or hospital inpatient category or follow-up inpatient consultation codes as appropriate)

36493 Repositioning of previously placed central venous catheter under fluoroscopic guidance

(36495-36497 have been deleted. To report, see 36530-36535)

36500 Venous catheterization for selective organ blood sampling

(For catheterization in superior or inferior vena cava, see 36010)

(For radiological supervision and interpretation, see 75893)

36510* Catheterization of umbilical vein for diagnosis or therapy, newborn

36520 Therapeutic apheresis (plasma and/or cell exchange)

36522 Photopheresis, extracorporeal

36530 Insertion of implantable intravenous infusion pump

36531 Revision of implantable intravenous infusion pump

36532 Removal of implantable intravenous infusion pump

36533 Insertion of implantable venous access port, with or without subcutaneous reservoir

36534 Revision of implantable venous access port and/or subcutaneous reservoir

36535 Removal of implantable venous access port and/or subcutaneous reservoir

Arterial

36600* Arterial puncture, withdrawal of blood for diagnosis

36620 Arterial catheterization or cannulation for sampling, monitoring or transfusion (separate procedure); percutaneous

36625   cutdown

36640 Arterial catheterization for prolonged infusion therapy (chemotherapy), cutdown

(See also 96420-96425)

(For arterial catheterization for occlusion therapy, see 75894)

36660* Catheterization, umbilical artery, newborn, for diagnosis or therapy

Intraosseous

36680 Placement of needle for intraosseous infusion

Intervascular Cannulization or Shunt

36800 Insertion of cannula for hemodialysis, other purpose (separate procedure); vein to vein

36810   arteriovenous, external (Scribner type)

36815   arteriovenous, external revision, or closure

(36820 has been deleted. To report, use 36821)

36821 Arteriovenous anastomosis, direct, any site (eg, Cimino type) (separate procedure)

36822 Insertion of cannula(s) for prolonged extracorporeal circulation for cardiopulmonary insufficiency (ECMO) (separate procedure)

(For maintenance of prolonged extracorporal circulation, use 33960)

36825 Creation of arteriovenous fistula by other than direct arteriovenous anastomosis (separate procedure); autogenous graft

(For direct arteriovenous anastomosis, use 36821)

36830   nonautogenous graft

(For direct arteriovenous anastomosis, use 36821)

36832 Revision of an arteriovenous fistula, with or without thrombectomy, autogenous or nonautogenous graft (separate procedure)

36834 Plastic repair of arteriovenous aneurysm (separate procedure)

36835 Insertion of Thomas shunt (separate procedure)

(36840 has been deleted)

(36845 has been deleted)

36860 Cannula declotting (separate procedure); without balloon catheter

36861 with balloon catheter

Portal Decompression Procedures

37140 Venous anastomosis; portocaval

(For peritoneal-venous shunt, see 49425)

37145 renoportal

37160 caval-mesenteric

37180 splenorenal, proximal

37181 splenorenal, distal (selective decompression of esophagogastric varices, any technique)

(37190 has been renumbered to 36834 without change in terminology)

Transcatheter Therapy and Biopsy

(For radiological supervision and interpretation, see **Radiology**)

37200 Transcatheter biopsy

(For radiological supervision and interpretation, see 75970)

37201 Transcatheter therapy, infusion for thrombolysis other than coronary

37202 Transcatheter therapy, infusion other than for thrombolysis, any type (eg, spasmolytic, vasoconstrictive)

(For thrombolysis of coronary vessels, see 92975, 92977)

37203 Transcatheter retrieval, percutaneous, of intravascular foreign body (eg, fractured venous or arterial catheter)

(For radiological supervision and interpretation, see 75961)

37204 Transcatheter occlusion or embolization (eg, for tumor destruction, to achieve hemostasis, to occlude a vascular malformation), percutaneous, any method, non-central nervous system, non-head or neck

(See also 61624, 61626)

(For radiological supervision and interpretation, see 75894)

37205 Transcatheter placement of an intravascular stent(s), (non-coronary vessel), percutaneous; initial vessel

37206 each additional vessel

37207 Transcatheter placement of an intravascular stent(s), (non-coronary vessel), open; initial vessel

37208 each additional vessel

(For transcatheter placement of intracoronary stent(s), see 92980, 92981)

37209 Exchange of a previously placed arterial catheter during thrombolytic therapy

(For radiological supervision and interpretation, see 75900)

Ligation and Other Procedures

(37400-37560 have been deleted. To report, see 35201-35286)

37565 Ligation, internal jugular vein

37600 Ligation; external carotid artery

37605 internal or common carotid artery

37606 internal or common carotid artery, with gradual occlusion, as with Selverstone or Crutchfield clamp

(For ligation treatment of intracranial aneurysm, see 61703)

37607 Ligation or banding of angioaccess arteriovenous fistula

37609 Ligation or biopsy, temporal artery

37615 Ligation, major artery (eg, post-traumatic, rupture); neck

37616   chest

37617   abdomen

37618   extremity

37620 Interruption, partial or complete, of inferior vena cava by suture, ligation, plication, clip, extravascular, intravascular (umbrella device)

(For radiological supervision and interpretation, see 75940)

37650 Ligation of femoral vein

(37651 has been deleted. To report, use 37650 with modifier -50 or 09950)

37660 Ligation of common iliac vein

37700 Ligation and division of long saphenous vein at saphenofemoral junction, or distal interruptions

(37701 has been deleted. To report, use 37700 with modifier -50 or 09950)

37720 Ligation and division and complete stripping of long or short saphenous veins

(37721 has been deleted. To report, use 37720 with modifier -50 or 09950)

37730 Ligation and division and complete stripping of long and short saphenous veins

(37731 has been deleted. To report, use 37730 with modifier -50 or 09950)

37735 Ligation and division and complete stripping of long or short saphenous veins with radical excision of ulcer and skin graft and/or interruption of communicating veins of lower leg, with excision of deep fascia

(37737 has been deleted. To report, use 37735 with modifier -50 or 09950)

37760 Ligation of perforators, subfascial, radical (Linton type), with or without skin graft

37780 Ligation and division of short saphenous vein at saphenopopliteal junction (separate procedure)

(37781 has been deleted. To report, use 37780 with modifier -50 or 09950)

37785 Ligation, division, and/or excision of recurrent or secondary varicose veins (clusters), one leg

(37787 has been deleted. To report, use 37785 with modifier -50 or 09950)

37788 Penile revascularization, artery, with or without vein graft

37790 Penile venous occlusive procedure

37799 Unlisted procedure, vascular surgery

Hemic and Lymphatic Systems

Spleen

Excision

(38090 has been deleted. To report, use 38999)

38100 Splenectomy; total (separate procedure)

38101 partial (separate procedure)

38102 total, en bloc for extensive disease, in conjunction with other procedure (Report in addition to code for primary procedure)

Repair

38115 Repair of ruptured spleen (splenorrhaphy) with or without partial splenectomy

Introduction

38200 Injection procedure for splenoportography

(For radiological supervision and interpretation, see 75810)

Bone Marrow or Stem Cell Transplantation Services

38230 Bone marrow harvesting for transplantation

●**38231** Blood-derived peripheral stem cell harvesting for transplantation, per collection

▲**38240** Bone marrow or blood-derived peripheral stem cell transplantation; allogenic

38241 autologous

(For harvesting of bone marrow specimen, use 85095)

(For modification, treatment, and processing of bone marrow specimens for transplantation, use code 86915)

(For collection of blood specimen, modification, treatment, and processing of autologous blood specimens for transplantation, use 86890, 86985)

(For compatibility studies, see 86812-86822)

Lymph Nodes and Lymphatic Channels

Incision

38300* Drainage of lymph node abscess or lymphadenitis; simple

38305 extensive

38308 Lymphangiotomy or other operations on lymphatic channels

38380 Suture and/or ligation of thoracic duct; cervical approach

38381 thoracic approach

38382 abdominal approach

Excision

38500 Biopsy or excision of lymph node(s); superficial (separate procedure)

38505 by needle, superficial (eg, cervical, inguinal, axillary)

(For fine needle aspiration, use 88170)

38510 deep cervical node(s)

38520 deep cervical node(s) with excision scalene fat pad

38525 deep axillary node(s)

38530 internal mammary node(s) (separate procedure)

(For percutaneous needle biopsy, retroperitoneal lymph node or mass, see 49180; for fine needle aspiration, use 88171)

(38540 has been deleted. To report, see 38510, 38520)

38542 Dissection, deep jugular node(s)

(For radical cervical neck dissection, see 38720)

38550 Excision of cystic hygroma, axillary or cervical; without deep neurovascular dissection

Lymphatic 38100–38999

38555   with deep neurovascular dissection

Limited Lymphadenectomy for Staging

38562 Limited lymphadenectomy for staging (separate procedure); pelvic and para-aortic

(When combined with prostatectomy, use 55812 or 55842)

(When combined with insertion of radioactive substance into prostate, use 55862)

38564   retroperitoneal (aortic and/or splenic)

Radical Lymphadenectomy (Radical Resection of Lymph Nodes)

(For limited pelvic and retroperitoneal lymphadenectomies, see 38562, 38564)

38700 Suprahyoid lymphadenectomy

(38701 has been deleted. To report, use 38700 with modifier -50 or 09950)

38720 Cervical lymphadenectomy (complete)

(38721 has been deleted. To report, use 38720 with modifier -50 or 09950)

38724 Cervical lymphadenectomy (modified radical neck dissection)

38740 Axillary lymphadenectomy; superficial

38745   complete

38746 Thoracic lymphadenectomy, regional, including mediastinal and peritracheal nodes (Report in addition to code for primary procedure)

38747 Abdominal lymphadenectomy, regional, including celiac, para-aortic and vena caval nodes (Report in addition to code for primary procedure)

38760 Inguinofemoral lymphadenectomy, superficial, including Cloquet's node (separate procedure)

(38761 has been deleted. To report, use 38760 with modifier -50 or 09950)

38765 Inguinofemoral lymphadenectomy, superficial, in continuity with pelvic lymphadenectomy, including external iliac, hypogastric, and obturator nodes (separate procedure)

(38766 has been deleted. To report, use 38765 with modifier -50 or 09950)

38770 Pelvic lymphadenectomy, including external iliac, hypogastric, and obturator nodes (separate procedure)

(38771 has been deleted. To report, use 38770 with modifier -50 or 09950)

38780 Retroperitoneal transabdominal lymphadenectomy, extensive, including pelvic, aortic, and renal nodes (separate procedure)

(For excision and repair of lymphedematous skin and subcutaneous tissue, see 15000, 15570-15650)

Introduction

38790 Injection procedure for lymphangiography

(For radiological supervision and interpretation, see 75801-75807)

(38791 has been deleted. To report, use 38790 with modifier -50 or 09950)

38794 Cannulation, thoracic duct

Other Procedures

38999 Unlisted procedure, hemic or lymphatic system

Mediastinum and Diaphragm

Mediastinum

Incision

39000   Mediastinotomy with exploration, drainage, removal of foreign body, or biopsy; cervical approach

39010   transthoracic approach, including either transthoracic or median sternotomy

(39020 has been deleted. To report, use 39010)

(39050-39070 have been deleted. To report, see 39000-39020)

Excision

39200   Excision of mediastinal cyst

39220   Excision of mediastinal tumor

(For substernal thyroidectomy, see 60270)

(For thymectomy, see 60520)

Endoscopy

39400   Mediastinoscopy, with or without biopsy

Other Procedures

39499   Unlisted procedure, mediastinum

Diaphragm

Repair

(39500 has been deleted. To report, see 43324, 43325)

39501   Repair, laceration of diaphragm, any approach

39502   Repair, paraesophageal hiatus hernia, transabdominal, with or without fundoplasty, vagotomy, and/or pyloroplasty, except neonatal

39503   Repair, neonatal diaphragmatic hernia, with or without chest tube insertion and with or without creation of ventral hernia

(39510 has been deleted. To report, see 43324, 43325)

39520   Repair, diaphragmatic hernia (esophageal hiatal); transthoracic

39530   combined, thoracoabdominal

39531   combined, thoracoabdominal, with dilation of stricture (with or without gastroplasty)

39540   Repair, diaphragmatic hernia (other than neonatal), traumatic; acute

39541   chronic

39545   Imbrication of diaphragm for eventration, transthoracic or transabdominal, paralytic or nonparalytic

(39547 has been deleted. To report, use 39545)

Other Procedures

39599   Unlisted procedure, diaphragm

Notes

Digestive System

Lips

(For procedures on skin of lips, see 10040 et seq)

Excision

40490   Biopsy of lip

40500   Vermilionectomy (lip shave), with mucosal advancement

40510   Excision of lip; transverse wedge excision with primary closure

40520   V-excision with primary direct linear closure

(For excision of mucous lesions, see 40810-40816)

40525   full thickness, reconstruction with local flap (eg, Estlander or fan)

40527   full thickness, reconstruction with cross lip flap (Abbe-Estlander)

40530   Resection of lip, more than one-fourth, without reconstruction

(For reconstruction, see 13131 et seq)

Repair (Cheiloplasty)

40650   Repair lip, full thickness; vermilion only

40652   up to half vertical height

40654   over one-half vertical height, or complex

40700   Plastic repair of cleft lip/nasal deformity; primary, partial or complete, unilateral

40701   primary bilateral, one stage procedure

40702   primary bilateral, one of two stages

40720   secondary, by recreation of defect and reclosure

(To report rhinoplasty only for nasal deformity secondary to congenital cleft lip, see 30460, 30462)

(40740 has been deleted. To report, use 40720 with modifier -50 or 09950)

(40760 has been deleted. To report, use 40527)

40761   with cross lip pedicle flap (Abbe-Estlander type), including sectioning and inserting of pedicle

(For repair cleft palate, see 42200 et seq)

(For other reconstructive procedures, see 14060, 14061, 15120-15261, 15574, 15576, 15630)

Other Procedures

40799   Unlisted procedure, lips

Vestibule of Mouth

The vestibule is the part of the oral cavity outside the dentoalveolar structures; it includes the mucosal and submucosal tissue of lips and cheeks.

Incision

40800* Drainage of abscess, cyst, hematoma, vestibule of mouth; simple

40801   complicated

40804* Removal of embedded foreign body, vestibule of mouth; simple

40805   complicated

40806   Incision of labial frenum (frenotomy)

Excision, Destruction

40808   Biopsy, vestibule of mouth

40810   Excision of lesion of mucosa and submucosa, vestibule of mouth; without repair

40812   with simple repair

40814   with complex repair

40816   complex, with excision of underlying muscle

40818   Excision of mucosa of vestibule of mouth as donor graft

40819   Excision of frenum, labial or buccal (frenumectomy, frenulectomy, frenectomy)

**Digestive System
40490–49999**

40820   Destruction of lesion or scar of vestibule of mouth by physical methods (eg, laser, thermal, cryo, chemical)

Repair

40830   Closure of laceration, vestibule of mouth; 2.5 cm or less

40831   over 2.5 cm or complex

40840   Vestibuloplasty; anterior

40842   posterior, unilateral

40843   posterior, bilateral

40844   entire arch

40845   complex (including ridge extension, muscle repositioning)

(For skin grafts, see 15000 et seq)

Other Procedures

40899   Unlisted procedure, vestibule of mouth

Tongue and Floor of Mouth

Incision

41000*   Intraoral incision and drainage of abscess, cyst, or hematoma of tongue or floor of mouth; lingual

41005*   sublingual, superficial

41006   sublingual, deep, supramylohyoid

41007   submental space

41008   submandibular space

41009   masticator space

41010   Incision of lingual frenum (frenotomy)

41015   Extraoral incision and drainage of abscess, cyst, or hematoma of floor of mouth; sublingual

41016   submental

41017   submandibular

41018   masticator space

(For frenoplasty, see 41520)

Excision

41100   Biopsy of tongue; anterior two-thirds

41105   posterior one-third

41108   Biopsy of floor of mouth

41110   Excision of lesion of tongue without closure

41112   Excision of lesion of tongue with closure; anterior two-thirds

41113   posterior one-third

41114   with local tongue flap

(List 41114 in addition to code 41112 or 41113)

41115   Excision of lingual frenum (frenectomy)

41116   Excision, lesion of floor of mouth

41120   Glossectomy; less than one-half tongue

41130   hemiglossectomy

41135   partial, with unilateral radical neck dissection

41140   complete or total, with or without tracheostomy, without radical neck dissection

41145   complete or total, with or without tracheostomy, with unilateral radical neck dissection

41150   composite procedure with resection floor of mouth and mandibular resection, without radical neck dissection

41153   composite procedure with resection floor of mouth, with suprahyoid neck dissection

41155   composite procedure with resection floor of mouth, mandibular resection, and radical neck dissection (Commando type)

Repair

41250*   Repair of laceration 2.5 cm or less; floor of mouth and/or anterior two-thirds of tongue

41251*   posterior one-third of tongue

41252* Repair of laceration of tongue, floor of mouth, over 2.6 cm or complex

Other Procedures

41500 Fixation of tongue, mechanical, other than suture (eg, K-wire)

41510 Suture of tongue to lip for micrognathia (Douglas type procedure)

41520 Frenoplasty (surgical revision of frenum, eg, with Z-plasty)

(For frenotomy, see 40806, 41010)

41599 Unlisted procedure, tongue, floor of mouth

Dentoalveolar Structures

Incision

41800* Drainage of abscess, cyst, hematoma from dentoalveolar structures

41805 Removal of embedded foreign body from dentoalveolar structures; soft tissues

41806 bone

Excision, Destruction

41820 Gingivectomy, excision gingiva, each quadrant

41821 Operculectomy, excision pericoronal tissues

41822 Excision of fibrous tuberosities, dentoalveolar structures

41823 Excision of osseous tuberosities, dentoalveolar structures

41825 Excision of lesion or tumor (except listed above), dentoalveolar structures; without repair

41826 with simple repair

41827 with complex repair

(For nonexcisional destruction, see 41850)

41828 Excision of hyperplastic alveolar mucosa, each quadrant (specify)

41830 Alveolectomy, including curettage of osteitis or sequestrectomy

41850 Destruction of lesion (except excision), dentoalveolar structures

Other Procedures

41870 Periodontal mucosal grafting

41872 Gingivoplasty, each quadrant (specify)

41874 Alveoloplasty, each quadrant (specify)

(For closure of lacerations, see 40830, 40831)

(For segmental osteotomy, see 21206)

(For reduction of fractures, see 21421-21490)

41899 Unlisted procedure, dentoalveolar structures

Palate and Uvula

Incision

42000* Drainage of abscess of palate, uvula

Excision, Destruction

42100 Biopsy of palate, uvula

42104 Excision, lesion of palate, uvula; without closure

42106 with simple primary closure

42107 with local flap closure

(For skin graft, see 14040-14300)

(For mucosal graft, see 40818)

42120 Resection of palate or extensive resection of lesion

(For reconstruction of palate with extraoral tissue, see 14040-14300, 15050, 15120, 15240, 15576)

42140 Uvulectomy, excision of uvula

42145 Palatopharyngoplasty (eg, uvulopalatopharyngoplasty, uvulopharyngoplasty)

(42150 has been deleted. To report, see 21031, 21032)

42160 Destruction of lesion, palate or uvula (thermal, cryo or chemical)

Repair

42180 Repair, laceration of palate; up to 2 cm

42182 over 2 cm or complex

42200 Palatoplasty for cleft palate, soft and/or hard palate only

42205 Palatoplasty for cleft palate, with closure of alveolar ridge; soft tissue only

42210 with bone graft to alveolar ridge (includes obtaining graft)

42215 Palatoplasty for cleft palate; major revision

42220 secondary lengthening procedure

42225 attachment pharyngeal flap

42226 Lengthening of palate, and pharyngeal flap

42227 Lengthening of palate, with island flap

42235 Repair of anterior palate, including vomer flap

(42250 has been deleted. To report, use 30600)

42260 Repair of nasolabial fistula

(For repair of cleft lip, see 40700 et seq)

42280 Maxillary impression for palatal prosthesis

42281 Insertion of pin-retained palatal prosthesis

Other Procedures

42299 Unlisted procedure, palate, uvula

Salivary Gland and Ducts

Incision

42300* Drainage of abscess; parotid, simple

42305 parotid, complicated

42310* Drainage of abscess; submaxillary or sublingual, intraoral

42320* submaxillary, external

42325 Fistulization of sublingual salivary cyst (ranula);

42326 with prosthesis

42330 Sialolithotomy; submandibular (submaxillary), sublingual or parotid, uncomplicated, intraoral

42335 submandibular (submaxillary), complicated, intraoral

42340 parotid, extraoral or complicated intraoral

Excision

42400* Biopsy of salivary gland; needle

42405 incisional

42408 Excision of sublingual salivary cyst (ranula)

42409 Marsupialization of sublingual salivary cyst (ranula)

(For fistulization of sublingual salivary cyst, see 42325)

42410 Excision of parotid tumor or parotid gland; lateral lobe, without nerve dissection

42415 lateral lobe, with dissection and preservation of facial nerve

42420 total, with dissection and preservation of facial nerve

42425 total, en bloc removal with sacrifice of facial nerve

42426 total, with unilateral radical neck dissection

(For suture or grafting of facial nerve, see 64864, 64865, 69740, 69745)

42440 Excision of submandibular (submaxillary) gland

42450 Excision of sublingual gland

Repair

42500 Plastic repair of salivary duct, sialodochoplasty; primary or simple

42505 secondary or complicated

42507 Parotid duct diversion, bilateral (Wilke type procedure);

42508 with excision of one submandibular gland

42509 with excision of both submandibular glands

42510 with ligation of both submandibular (Wharton's) ducts

Other Procedures

42550 Injection procedure for sialography

(For radiological supervision and interpretation, see 70390)

42600 Closure salivary fistula

42650* Dilation salivary duct

42660* Dilation and catheterization of salivary duct, with or without injection

42665 Ligation salivary duct, intraoral

42699 Unlisted procedure, salivary glands or ducts

Pharynx, Adenoids, and Tonsils

Incision

42700* Incision and drainage abscess; peritonsillar

42720 retropharyngeal or parapharyngeal, intraoral approach

42725 retropharyngeal or parapharyngeal, external approach

Excision, Destruction

42800 Biopsy; oropharynx

42802 hypopharynx

42804 nasopharynx, visible lesion, simple

42806 nasopharynx, survey for unknown primary lesion

(For laryngoscopic biopsy, see 31510, 31535, 31536)

42808 Excision or destruction of lesion of pharynx, any method

42809 Removal of foreign body from pharynx

42810 Excision branchial cleft cyst or vestige, confined to skin and subcutaneous tissues

42815 Excision branchial cleft cyst, vestige, or fistula, extending beneath subcutaneous tissues and/or into pharynx

42820 Tonsillectomy and adenoidectomy; under age 12

42821 age 12 or over

42825 Tonsillectomy, primary or secondary; under age 12

42826 age 12 or over

42830 Adenoidectomy, primary; under age 12

42831 age 12 or over

42835 Adenoidectomy, secondary; under age 12

42836 age 12 or over

42842 Radical resection of tonsil, tonsillar pillars, and/or retromolar trigone; without closure

42844 closure with local flap (eg, tongue, buccal)

42845 closure with other flap

(For closure with other flap(s), use appropriate number for flap(s))

(When combined with radical neck dissection, use also 38720)

42860 Excision of tonsil tags

42870 Excision or destruction lingual tonsil, any method (separate procedure)

42880 Excision nasopharyngeal lesion (eg, fibroma)

(For excision and repair of hypopharyngeal diverticulum, cervical approach, see 43130)

42890 Limited pharyngectomy

42892 Resection of lateral pharyngeal wall or pyriform sinus, direct closure by advancement of lateral and posterior pharyngeal walls

(When combined with radical neck dissection, use also 38720)

42894 Resection of pharyngeal wall requiring closure with myocutaneous flap

(When combined with radical neck dissection, use also 38720)

(42895 has been deleted. To report, use 38720 with 42890)

Repair

42900 Suture pharynx for wound or injury

42950 Pharyngoplasty (plastic or reconstructive operation on pharynx)

(For pharyngeal flap, see 42225)

42953 Pharyngoesophageal repair

(For closure with myocutaneous or other flap, use appropriate number in addition)

Other Procedures

42955 Pharyngostomy (fistulization of pharynx, external for feeding)

42960 Control oropharyngeal hemorrhage, primary or secondary (eg, post-tonsillectomy); simple

42961   complicated, requiring hospitalization

42962   with secondary surgical intervention

42970 Control of nasopharyngeal hemorrhage, primary or secondary (eg, postadenoidectomy); simple, with posterior nasal packs, with or without anterior packs and/or cauterization

42971   complicated, requiring hospitalization

42972   with secondary surgical intervention

42999 Unlisted procedure, pharynx, adenoids, or tonsils

Esophagus

Incision

(For esophageal intubation with laparotomy, see 43510)

(43000 has been deleted)

43020 Esophagotomy, cervical approach, with removal of foreign body

43030 Cricopharyngeal myotomy

(43040 has been deleted)

43045 Esophagotomy, thoracic approach, with removal of foreign body

Excision

(For gastrointestinal reconstruction for previous esophagectomy, see 43360, 43361)

43100 Excision of lesion, esophagus, with primary repair; cervical approach

43101   thoracic or abdominal approach

(43105 has been deleted. To report, see 43107, 43116, 43124, and 31360)

(43106 has been deleted. To report, see 43107, 43116, 43124, and 31365)

43107 Total or near total esophagectomy, without thoracotomy; with pharyngogastrostomy or cervical esophagogastrostomy, with or without pyloroplasty (transhiatal)

43108   with colon interposition or small bowel reconstruction, including bowel mobilization, preparation and anastomosis(es)

(43110 has been deleted. To report, see 43107-43113)

(43111 has been deleted. To report, see 43107-43113)

43112 Total or near total esophagectomy, with thoracotomy; with pharyngogastrostomy or cervical esophagogastrostomy, with or without pyloroplasty

43113   with colon interposition or small bowel reconstruction, including bowel mobilization, preparation, and anastomosis(es)

(43115 has been deleted. To report, see 43116-43118)

43116 Partial esophagectomy, cervical, with free intestinal graft, including microvascular anastomosis, obtaining the graft and intestinal reconstruction

43117 Partial esophagectomy, distal two-thirds, with thoracotomy and separate abdominal incision, with or without proximal gastrectomy; with thoracic esophagogastrostomy, with or without pyloroplasty (Ivor Lewis)

43118   with colon interposition or small bowel reconstruction, including bowel mobilization, preparation, and anastomosis(es)

(43119 has been deleted. To report, see 43107, 43124)

(43120 has been deleted. To report, see 43122)

43121   Partial esophagectomy, distal two-thirds, with thoracotomy only, with or without proximal gastrectomy, with thoracic esophagogastrostomy, with or without pyloroplasty

43122   Partial esophagectomy, thoracoabdominal or abdominal approach, with or without proximal gastrectomy; with esophagogastrostomy, with or without pyloroplasty

43123   with colon interposition or small bowel reconstruction, including bowel mobilization, preparation, and anastomosis(es)

43124   Total or partial esophagectomy, without reconstruction (any approach), with cervical esophagostomy

43130   Diverticulectomy of hypopharynx or esophagus, with or without myotomy; cervical approach

43135   thoracic approach

(43136 has been deleted. To report, use 43499)

Endoscopy

For endoscopic procedures, code appropriate endoscopy of each anatomic site examined.

Surgical endoscopy always includes diagnostic endoscopy.

43200   Esophagoscopy, rigid or flexible; diagnostic, with or without collection of specimen(s) by brushing or washing (separate procedure)

43202   with biopsy, single or multiple

43204   with injection sclerosis of esophageal varices

43205   with band ligation of esophageal varices

43215   with removal of foreign body

(For radiological supervision and interpretation, see 74235)

43216   with removal of tumor(s), polyp(s), or other lesion(s) by hot biopsy forceps or bipolar cautery

43217   with removal of tumor(s), polyp(s), or other lesion(s) by snare technique

(43218 has been deleted. To report, use 43499)

43219   with insertion of plastic tube or stent

43220   with balloon dilation (less than 30 mm diameter)

(For endoscopic dilation with balloon 30 mm diameter or larger, use 43458)

(For dilation without visualization, see 43450-43453)

(43221 has been deleted. To report, use 43200 or 43235)

(43222 has been deleted. To report, use 43200, 43202, 43235, or 43236)

(43223 has been deleted. To report, use 43215 or 43247)

(43224 has been deleted. To report, use 43217 or 43251)

(43225 has been deleted. To report, use 43499)

43226   with insertion of guide wire followed by dilation over guide wire

(For radiological supervision and interpretation, see 74360)

43227   with control of bleeding, any method

43228   with ablation of tumor(s), polyp(s), or other lesion(s), not amenable to removal by hot biopsy forceps, bipolar cautery or snare technique

(Surgical endoscopy always includes diagnostic endoscopy)

43234   Upper gastrointestinal endoscopy, simple primary examination (eg, with small diameter flexible endoscope) (separate procedure)

43235 Upper gastrointestinal endoscopy including esophagus, stomach, and either the duodenum and/or jejunum as appropriate; diagnostic, with or without collection of specimen(s) by brushing or washing (separate procedure)

43239 with biopsy, single or multiple

43241 with transendoscopic tube or catheter placement

43243 with injection sclerosis of esophageal and/or gastric varices

43244 with band ligation of esophageal and/or gastric varices

43245 with dilation of gastric outlet for obstruction, any method

43246 with directed placement of percutaneous gastrostomy tube

(For radiological supervision and interpretation, see 74350)

43247 with removal of foreign body

(For radiological supervision and interpretation, see 74235)

43248 with insertion of guide wire followed by dilation of esophagus over guide wire

43249 with balloon dilation of esophagus (less than 30 mm diameter)

43250 with removal of tumor(s), polyp(s), or other lesion(s) by hot biopsy forceps or bipolar cautery

43251 with removal of tumor(s), polyp(s), or other lesion(s) by snare technique

43255 with control of bleeding, any method

43258 with ablation of tumor(s), polyp(s), or other lesion(s) not amenable to removal by hot biopsy forceps, bipolar cautery or snare technique

(For injection sclerosis of esophageal varices, use 43204 or 43243)

43259 with endoscopic ultrasound examination

(For radiological supervision and interpretation, see 76975)

(Surgical endoscopy always includes diagnostic endoscopy)

43260 Endoscopic retrograde cholangio-pancreatography (ERCP); diagnostic, with or without collection of specimen(s) by brushing or washing (separate procedure)

(For radiological supervision and interpretation, see 74328, 74329, 74330)

43261 with biopsy, single or multiple

43262 with sphincterotomy/papillotomy

(For radiological supervision and interpretation, see 74328, 74329, 74330)

43263 with pressure measurement of sphincter of Oddi (pancreatic duct or common bile duct)

(For radiological supervision and interpretation, see 74328, 74329, 74330)

43264 with endoscopic retrograde removal of stone(s) from biliary and/or pancreatic ducts

(When done with sphincterotomy, also use 43262)

(For radiological supervision and interpretation, see 74328, 74329, 74330)

43265 with endoscopic retrograde destruction, lithotripsy of stone(s), any method

(When done with sphincterotomy, also use 43262)

(For radiological supervision and interpretation, see 74328, 74329, 74330)

43267 with endoscopic retrograde insertion of nasobiliary or nasopancreatic drainage tube

(When done with sphincterotomy, also use 43262)

(For radiological supervision and interpretation, see 74328, 74329, 74330)

43268 with endoscopic retrograde insertion of tube or stent into bile or pancreatic duct

(When done with sphincterotomy, also use 43262)

(For radiological supervision and interpretation, see 74328, 74329, 74330)

43269 with endoscopic retrograde removal of foreign body and/or change of tube or stent

(When done with sphincterotomy, also use 43262)

(For radiological supervision and interpretation, see 74328, 74329, 74330)

43271 with endoscopic retrograde balloon dilation of ampulla, biliary and/or pancreatic duct(s)

(When done with sphincterotomy, also use 43262)

(For radiological supervision and interpretation, see 74328, 74329, 74330)

43272 with ablation of tumor(s), polyp(s), or other lesion(s) not amenable to removal by hot biopsy forceps, bipolar cautery or snare technique

(For radiological supervision and interpretation, see 74328, 74329, 74330)

Repair

43300 Esophagoplasty, (plastic repair or reconstruction), cervical approach; without repair of tracheoesophageal fistula

43305 with repair of tracheoesophageal fistula

43310 Esophagoplasty, (plastic repair or reconstruction), thoracic approach; without repair of tracheoesophageal fistula

43312 with repair of tracheoesophageal fistula

43320 Esophagogastrostomy (cardioplasty), with or without vagotomy and pyloroplasty, transabdominal or transthoracic approach

(43321 has been deleted. To report, use 43320)

43324 Esophagogastric fundoplasty (eg, Nissen, Belsey IV, Hill procedures)

43325 Esophagogastric fundoplasty; with fundic patch (Thal-Nissen procedure)

(For cricopharyngeal myotomy, see 43030)

43326 with gastroplasty (eg, Collis)

43330 Esophagomyotomy (Heller type); abdominal approach

43331 thoracic approach

43340 Esophagojejunostomy (without total gastrectomy); abdominal approach

43341 thoracic approach

43350 Esophagostomy, fistulization of esophagus, external; abdominal approach

43351 thoracic approach

43352 cervical approach

43360 Gastrointestinal reconstruction for previous esophagectomy, for obstructing esophageal lesion or fistula, or for previous esophageal exclusion; with stomach, with or without pyloroplasty

43361 with colon interposition or small bowel reconstruction, including bowel mobilization, preparation, and anastomosis(es)

43400 Ligation, direct, esophageal varices

43401 Transection of esophagus with repair, for esophageal varices

43405 Ligation or stapling at gastroesophageal junction for pre-existing esophageal perforation

43410 Suture of esophageal wound or injury; cervical approach

43415 transthoracic or transabdominal approach

43420 Closure of esophagostomy or fistula; cervical approach

43425 transthoracic or transabdominal approach

(For repair of esophageal hiatal hernia, see 39520 et seq)

Manipulation

(For associated esophagogram, use 74220)

43450* Dilation of esophagus, by unguided sound or bougie, single or multiple passes

(43451 has been deleted. To report, use 43450)

43453 Dilation of esophagus, over guide wire

(For dilation with direct visualization, see 43220)

(43455 has been deleted. To report, see 43220, 43458, 74360)

43456 Dilation of esophagus, by balloon or dilator, retrograde

43458 Dilation of esophagus with balloon (30 mm diameter or larger) for achalasia

(For dilation with balloon less than 30 mm diameter, use 43220)

(For radiological supervision and interpretation, see 74360)

43460 Esophagogastric tamponade, with balloon (Sengstaaken type)

(For removal of esophageal foreign body by balloon catheter, see 43215, 43247, 74235)

Other Procedures

43499 Unlisted procedure, esophagus

Stomach

Incision

43500 Gastrotomy; with exploration or foreign body removal

43501 with suture repair of bleeding ulcer

43502 with suture repair of pre-existing esophagogastric laceration (eg, Mallory-Weiss)

43510 with esophageal dilation and insertion of permanent intraluminal tube (eg, Celestin or Mousseaux-Barbin)

43520 Pyloromyotomy, cutting of pyloric muscle (Fredet-Ramstedt type operation)

Excision

43600 Biopsy of stomach; by capsule, tube, peroral (one or more specimens)

43605 by laparotomy

43610 Excision, local; ulcer or benign tumor of stomach

43611 malignant tumor of stomach

43620 Gastrectomy, total; with esophagoenterostomy

43621 with Roux-en-Y reconstruction

43622 with formation of intestinal pouch, any type

(43625 has been deleted. To report, use 43622)

(43630 has been deleted. To report, see 43631-43634)

43631 Gastrectomy, partial, distal; with gastroduodenostomy

43632 with gastrojejunostomy

43633 with Roux-en-Y reconstruction

43634 with formation of intestinal pouch

43635 Vagotomy with partial distal gastrectomy (List separately in addition to code(s) for primary procedure) (Use 43635 only with 43631, 43632, 43633, 43634)

43638 Gastrectomy, partial, proximal, thoracic or abdominal approach including esophagogastrostomy, with vagotomy;

43639 with pyloroplasty or pyloromyotomy

(For regional thoracic lymphadenectomy, use 38746)

(For regional abdominal lymphadenectomy, use 38747)

43640 Vagotomy including pyloroplasty, with or without gastrostomy; truncal or selective

(For pyloroplasty, see 43800)

(For vagotomy, see 64752-64760)

43641 parietal cell (highly selective)

(For upper gastrointestinal endoscopy, see 43234-43259)

(43700 has been deleted. To report, use 43235)

(43702 has been deleted. To report, use 43239)

(43709 has been deleted. To report, use 43247)

(43711 has been deleted. To report, use 43251)

(43712 has been deleted. To report, use 43255)

(43714 has been deleted. To report, use 43258)

Introduction

43750   Percutaneous placement of gastrostomy tube

(For radiological supervision and interpretation, see 74350)

43760*   Change of gastrostomy tube

(For endoscopic placement of gastrostomy tube, use 43246)

(For radiological supervision and interpretation, see 75984)

43761   Repositioning of the gastric feeding tube through the duodenum for enteric nutrition

(43765 has been deleted. To report, use 43760)

Other Procedures

43800   Pyloroplasty

(For pyloroplasty and vagotomy, see 43640)

43810   Gastroduodenostomy

43820   Gastrojejunostomy; without vagotomy

43825   with vagotomy, any type

43830   Gastrostomy, temporary (tube, rubber or plastic) (separate procedure);

43831   neonatal, for feeding

(For change of gastrostomy tube, see 43760)

43832   Gastrostomy, permanent, with construction of gastric tube

(43834 has been deleted. To report, use 43246)

43840   Gastrorrhaphy, suture of perforated duodenal or gastric ulcer, wound, or injury

43842   Gastric restrictive procedure, without gastric bypass, for morbid obesity; vertical-banded gastroplasty

43843   other than vertical-banded gastroplasty

(43844 has been deleted. To report, use 43847)

(43845 has been deleted. To report, see 43842, 43843)

43846   Gastric restrictive procedure, with gastric bypass for morbid obesity; with short limb (less than 100 cm) Roux-en-Y gastroenterostomy

43847   with small bowel reconstruction to limit absorption

43848   Revision of gastric restrictive procedure for morbid obesity (separate procedure)

43850   Revision of gastroduodenal anastomosis (gastroduodenostomy) with reconstruction; without vagotomy

43855   with vagotomy

43860   Revision of gastrojejunal anastomosis (gastrojejunostomy) with reconstruction, with or without partial gastrectomy or bowel resection; without vagotomy

43865   with vagotomy

43870   Closure of gastrostomy, surgical

43880   Closure of gastrocolic fistula

(43885 has been deleted)

43999   Unlisted procedure, stomach

Intestines (Except Rectum)

Incision

(44000 has been deleted)

44005   Enterolysis (freeing of intestinal adhesion) (separate procedure)

44010   Duodenotomy, for exploration, biopsy(s), or foreign body removal

44015   Tube or needle catheter jejunostomy for enteral alimentation, intraoperative, any method (List separately in addition to primary procedure)

44020   Enterotomy, small bowel, other than duodenum; for exploration, biopsy(s), or foreign body removal

44021   for decompression (eg, Baker tube)

44025   Colotomy, for exploration, biopsy(s), or foreign body removal

(44040 has been deleted. To report, see 44602-44605)

44050   Reduction of volvulus, intussusception, internal hernia, by laparotomy

44055   Correction of malrotation by lysis of duodenal bands and/or reduction of midgut volvulus (eg, Ladd procedure)

(44060 has been deleted. To report, use 44799)

Excision

44100   Biopsy of intestine by capsule, tube, peroral (one or more specimens)

44110   Excision of one or more lesions of small or large bowel not requiring anastomosis, exteriorization, or fistulization; single enterotomy

44111   multiple enterotomies

(44115 has been deleted. To report, use 44799)

44120   Enterectomy, resection of small intestine; single resection and anastomosis

44121   each additional resection and anastomosis

44125   with enterostomy

44130   Enteroenterostomy, anastomosis of intestine, with or without cutaneous enterostomy (separate procedure)

(44131 has been deleted)

44139   Mobilization (take-down) of splenic flexure performed in conjunction with partial colectomy (List separately in addition to primary procedure)

(Use 44139 only for codes 44140-44147)

44140   Colectomy, partial; with anastomosis

44141   with skin level cecostomy or colostomy

44143   with end colostomy and closure of distal segment (Hartmann type procedure)

44144   with resection, with colostomy or ileostomy and creation of mucofistula

44145   with coloproctostomy (low pelvic anastomosis)

44146   with coloproctostomy (low pelvic anastomosis), with colostomy

44147   abdominal and transanal approach

44150   Colectomy, total, abdominal, without proctectomy; with ileostomy or ileoproctostomy

44151   with continent ileostomy

44152   with rectal mucosectomy, ileoanal anastomosis, with or without loop ileostomy

44153   with rectal mucosectomy, ileoanal anastomosis, creation of ileal reservoir (S or J), with or without loop ileostomy

44155   Colectomy, total, abdominal, with proctectomy; with ileostomy

44156   with continent ileostomy

44160   Colectomy with removal of terminal ileum and ileocolostomy

Enterostomy—External Fistulization of Intestines

44300   Enterostomy or cecostomy, tube (eg, for decompression or feeding) (separate procedure)

(44305 has been deleted)

(44308 has been deleted. To report, use 44799)

44310   Ileostomy or jejunostomy, non-tube (separate procedure)

44312   Revision of ileostomy; simple (release of superficial scar) (separate procedure)

44314   complicated (reconstruction in-depth) (separate procedure)

44316   Continent ileostomy (Kock procedure) (separate procedure)

(For fiberoptic evaluation, see 44385)

44320   Colostomy or skin level cecostomy; (separate procedure)

44322   with multiple biopsies (eg, for Hirschsprung disease) (separate procedure)

44340   Revision of colostomy; simple (release of superficial scar) (separate procedure)

44345   complicated (reconstruction in-depth) (separate procedure)

44346   with repair of paracolostomy hernia (separate procedure)

Endoscopy, Small Bowel and Stomal

Surgical endoscopy always includes diagnostic endoscopy.

(For upper gastrointestinal endoscopy, see 43234-43258)

44360   Small intestinal endoscopy, enteroscopy beyond second portion of duodenum, not including ileum; diagnostic, with or without collection of specimen(s) by brushing or washing (separate procedure)

44361   with biopsy, single or multiple

44363   with removal of foreign body

44364   with removal of tumor(s), polyp(s), or other lesion(s) by snare technique

44365   with removal of tumor(s), polyp(s), or other lesion(s) by hot biopsy forceps or bipolar cautery

44366   with control of bleeding, any method

44369   with ablation of tumor(s), polyp(s), or other lesion(s) not amenable to removal by hot biopsy forceps, bipolar cautery or snare technique

44372   with placement of percutaneous jejunostomy tube

44373   with conversion of percutaneous gastrostomy tube to percutaneous jejunostomy tube

(44375 has been deleted. To report, use 43235)

(Surgical endoscopy always includes diagnostic endoscopy)

44376   Small intestinal endoscopy, enteroscopy beyond second portion of duodenum, including ileum; diagnostic, with or without collection of specimen(s) by brushing or washing (separate procedure)

44377   with biopsy, single or multiple

44378   with control of bleeding, any method

(Surgical endoscopy always includes diagnostic endoscopy)

44380   Ileoscopy, through stoma; diagnostic, with or without collection of specimen(s) by brushing or washing (separate procedure)

44382   with biopsy, single or multiple

44385   Endoscopic evaluation of small intestinal (abdominal or pelvic) pouch; diagnostic, with or without collection of specimen(s) by brushing or washing (separate procedure)

44386   with biopsy, single or multiple

(Surgical endoscopy always includes diagnostic endoscopy)

44388   Colonoscopy through stoma; diagnostic, with or without collection of specimen(s) by brushing or washing (separate procedure)

44389   with biopsy, single or multiple

44390   with removal of foreign body

44391   with control of bleeding, any method

44392   with removal of tumor(s), polyp(s), or other lesion(s) by hot biopsy forceps or bipolar cautery

44393   with ablation of tumor(s), polyp(s), or other lesion(s) not amenable to removal by hot biopsy forceps, bipolar cautery or snare technique

44394   with removal of tumor(s), polyp(s), or other lesion(s) by snare technique

---

(For colonoscopy per rectum, see 45330-45385)

(44400, 44405 have been deleted. To report, use 44799)

Introduction

44500 Introduction of long gastrointestinal tube (eg, Miller-Abbott) (separate procedure)

(For radiological supervision and interpretation, see 74340)

Repair

(44600 has been deleted. To report, see 44602, 44604)

44602 Suture of small intestine (enterorrhaphy) for perforated ulcer, diverticulum, wound, injury or rupture; single perforation

44603 multiple perforations

44604 Suture of large intestine (colorrhaphy) for perforated ulcer, diverticulum, wound, injury or rupture (single or multiple perforations); without colostomy

44605 with colostomy

(44610 has been deleted. To report, see 44603, 44604)

44615 Intestinal stricturoplasty (enterotomy and enterorrhaphy) with or without dilation, for intestinal obstruction

44620 Closure of enterostomy, large or small intestine;

44625 with resection and anastomosis

44640 Closure of intestinal cutaneous fistula

44650 Closure of enteroenteric or enterocolic fistula

44660 Closure of enterovesical fistula; without intestinal or bladder resection

44661 with bowel and/or bladder resection

(For closure of renocolic fistula, see 50525, 50526)

(For closure of gastrocolic fistula, see 43880)

(For closure of rectovesical fistula, see 45800, 45805)

44680 Intestinal plication (separate procedure)

Other Procedures

44799 Unlisted procedure, intestine

Meckel's Diverticulum and the Mesentery

Excision

44800 Excision of Meckel's diverticulum (diverticulectomy) or omphalomesenteric duct

44820 Excision of lesion of mesentery (separate procedure)

(With bowel resection, see 44120 or 44140 et seq)

Suture

44850 Suture of mesentery (separate procedure)

(For reduction and repair of internal hernia, see 44050)

Other Procedures

44899 Unlisted procedure, Meckel's diverticulum and the mesentery

Appendix

Incision

44900 Incision and drainage of appendiceal abscess, transabdominal

Excision

44950 Appendectomy;

(Incidental appendectomy during intra-abdominal surgery does not usually warrant a separate identification. If necessary to report, add modifier -52 or 09952)

44955 when done for indicated purpose at time of other major procedure (not as separate procedure)

44960 for ruptured appendix with abscess or generalized peritonitis

Rectum

Incision

45000 Transrectal drainage of pelvic abscess

45005 Incision and drainage of submucosal abscess, rectum

45020 Incision and drainage of deep supralevator, pelvirectal, or retrorectal abscess

(See also 46050, 46060)

Excision

45100 Biopsy of anorectal wall, anal approach (eg, congenital megacolon)

(45105 has been deleted. To report, use 45100)

(For endoscopic biopsy, see 45305)

45108 Anorectal myomectomy

45110 Proctectomy; complete, combined abdominoperineal, with colostomy

45111 partial resection of rectum, transabdominal approach

45112 Proctectomy, combined abdominoperineal, pull-through procedure (eg, colo-anal anastomosis)

45113 Proctectomy, partial, with rectal mucosectomy, ileoanal anastomosis, creation of ileal reservoir (S or J), with or without loop ileostomy

45114 Proctectomy, partial, with anastomosis; abdominal and transsacral approach

45116 transsacral approach only (Kraske type)

45120 Proctectomy, complete (for congenital megacolon), abdominal and perineal approach; with pull-through procedure and anastomosis (eg, Swenson, Duhamel, or Soave type operation)

45121 with subtotal or total colectomy, with multiple biopsies

45123 Proctectomy, partial, without anastomosis, perineal approach

45130 Excision of rectal procidentia, with anastomosis; perineal approach

45135 abdominal and perineal approach

45150 Division of stricture of rectum

45160 Excision of rectal tumor by proctotomy, transacral or transcoccygeal approach

45170 Excision of rectal tumor, transanal approach

(45180, 45181 have been deleted. To report, see 45170, 45190)

Destruction

45190 Destruction of rectal tumor, any method (eg, electrodesiccation) transanal approach

Endoscopy

Definitions

Proctosigmoidoscopy is the examination of the rectum and sigmoid colon.

Sigmoidoscopy is the examination of the entire rectum, sigmoid colon and may include examination of a portion of the descending colon.

Colonoscopy is the examination of the entire colon, from the rectum to the cecum, and may include the examination of the terminal ileum.

For an incomplete colonoscopy, with full preparation for a colonoscopy, use a colonoscopy code with the modifier -52 or 09952 and provide documentation.

Surgical endoscopy always includes diagnostic endoscopy.

45300 Proctosigmoidoscopy, rigid; diagnostic, with or without collection of specimen(s) by brushing or washing (separate procedure)

(45302 has been deleted. To report, use 45300)

45303 with dilation, any method

(For radiological supervision and interpretation, see 74360)

45305 with biopsy, single or multiple

45307 with removal of foreign body

45308   with removal of single tumor, polyp, or other lesion by hot biopsy forceps or bipolar cautery

45309   with removal of single tumor, polyp, or other lesion by snare technique

(45310 has been deleted. To report, see 45308, 45309)

45315   with removal of multiple tumors, polyps, or other lesions by hot biopsy forceps, bipolar cautery or snare technique

45317   with control of bleeding, any method

(45319 has been deleted. To report, use 45999)

45320   with ablation of tumor(s), polyp(s), or other lesion(s) not amenable to removal by hot biopsy forceps, bipolar cautery or snare technique (eg, laser)

45321   with decompression of volvulus

(45325 colonoscopy has been renumbered 45355 without change in terminology)

(Surgical endoscopy always includes diagnostic endoscopy)

45330 Sigmoidoscopy, flexible; diagnostic, with or without collection of specimen(s) by brushing or washing (separate procedure)

45331   with biopsy, single or multiple

45332   with removal of foreign body

45333   with removal of tumor(s), polyp(s), or other lesion(s) by hot biopsy forceps or bipolar cautery

45334   with control of bleeding, any method

(45336 has been deleted. To report, use 45339)

45337   with decompression of volvulus, any method

45338   with removal of tumor(s), polyp(s), or other lesion(s) by snare technique

45339   with ablation of tumor(s), polyp(s), or other lesion(s) not amenable to removal by hot biopsy forceps, bipolar cautery or snare technique

45355 Colonoscopy, rigid or flexible, transabdominal via colotomy, single or multiple

(45360-45372 have been deleted. To report, see 45330-45337)

(Surgical endoscopy always includes diagnostic endoscopy)

45378 Colonoscopy, flexible, proximal to splenic flexure; diagnostic, with or without collection of specimen(s) by brushing or washing, with or without colon decompression (separate procedure)

45379   with removal of foreign body

45380   with biopsy, single or multiple

45382   with control of bleeding, any method

45383   with ablation of tumor(s), polyp(s), or other lesion(s) not amenable to removal by hot biopsy forceps, bipolar cautery or snare technique

45384   with removal of tumor(s), polyp(s), or other lesion(s) by hot biopsy forceps or bipolar cautery

45385   with removal of tumor(s), polyp(s), or other lesion(s) by snare technique

(45386 has been deleted. To report, use 44799)

(For small bowel and stomal endoscopy, see 44360-44393)

Repair

45500 Proctoplasty; for stenosis

45505   for prolapse of mucous membrane

45520 Perirectal injection of sclerosing solution for prolapse

(45521 has been deleted)

45540 Proctopexy for prolapse; abdominal approach

45541   perineal approach

45550 Proctopexy combined with sigmoid resection, abdominal approach

45560 Repair of rectocele (separate procedure)

(For repair of rectocele with posterior colporrhaphy, see 57250)

45562 Exploration, repair, and presacral drainage for rectal injury;

45563   with colostomy

45800 Closure of rectovesical fistula;

45805   with colostomy

45820 Closure of rectourethral fistula;

45825   with colostomy

(For rectovaginal fistula closure, see 57300-57307)

Manipulation

45900* Reduction of procidentia (separate procedure) under anesthesia

45905* Dilation of anal sphincter (separate procedure) under anesthesia other than local

45910 Dilation of rectal stricture (separate procedure) under anesthesia other than local

45915* Removal of fecal impaction or foreign body (separate procedure) under anesthesia

Other Procedures

45999 Unlisted procedure, rectum

Anus

Incision

(46000 has been deleted. To report, use 46270)

46030* Removal of anal seton, other marker

(46032 has been deleted. To report, use 46999)

46040 Incision and drainage of ischiorectal and/or perirectal abscess (separate procedure)

46045 Incision and drainage of intramural, intramuscular, or submucosal abscess, transanal, under anesthesia

46050* Incision and drainage, perianal abscess, superficial

(See also 45020, 46060)

46060 Incision and drainage of ischiorectal or intramural abscess, with fistulectomy or fistulotomy, submuscular, with or without placement of seton

(See also 45020)

46070 Incision, anal septum (infant)

(For anoplasty, see 46700-46705)

46080* Sphincterotomy, anal, division of sphincter (separate procedure)

46083 Incision of thrombosed hemorrhoid, external

Excision

46200 Fissurectomy, with or without sphincterotomy

46210 Cryptectomy; single

46211   multiple (separate procedure)

46220 Papillectomy or excision of single tag, anus (separate procedure)

46221 Hemorrhoidectomy, by simple ligature (eg, rubber band)

46230 Excision of external hemorrhoid tags and/or multiple papillae

46250 Hemorrhoidectomy, external, complete

46255 Hemorrhoidectomy, internal and external, simple;

46257   with fissurectomy

46258   with fistulectomy, with or without fissurectomy

46260 Hemorrhoidectomy, internal and external, complex or extensive;

46261   with fissurectomy

46262   with fistulectomy, with or without fissurectomy

46270 Surgical treatment of anal fistula (fistulectomy/fistulotomy); subcutaneous

46275   submuscular

46280   complex or multiple, with or without placement of seton

(46281 has been renumbered to 46288 without change in terminology)

46285 second stage

46288 Closure of anal fistula with rectal advancement flap

46320* Enucleation or excision of external thrombotic hemorrhoid

Introduction

46500* Injection of sclerosing solution, hemorrhoids

(46510, 46530 have been deleted. To report, use 46999)

Endoscopy

(Surgical endoscopy always includes diagnostic endoscopy)

46600 Anoscopy; diagnostic, with or without collection of specimen(s) by brushing or washing (separate procedure)

(46602 has been deleted. To report, use 46600)

46604 with dilation, any method

46606 with biopsy, single or multiple

46608 with removal of foreign body

46610 with removal of single tumor, polyp, or other lesion by hot biopsy forceps or bipolar cautery

46611 with removal of single tumor, polyp, or other lesion by snare technique

46612 with removal of multiple tumors, polyps, or other lesions by hot biopsy forceps, bipolar cautery or snare technique

46614 with control of bleeding, any method

46615 with ablation of tumor(s), polyp(s), or other lesion(s) not amenable to removal by hot biopsy forceps, bipolar cautery or snare technique

Repair

46700 Anoplasty, plastic operation for stricture; adult

46705 infant

(For simple incision of anal septum, see 46070)

46715 Repair of low imperforate anus; with anoperineal fistula ("cut-back" procedure)

46716 with transposition of anoperineal or anovestibular fistula

46730 Repair of high imperforate anus without fistula; perineal or sacroperineal approach

46735 combined transabdominal and sacroperineal approaches

46740 Repair of high imperforate anus with rectourethral or rectovaginal fistula; perineal or sacroperineal approach

46742 combined transabdominal and sacroperineal approaches

46744 Repair of cloacal anomaly by anorectovaginoplasty and urethroplasty, sacroperineal approach

46746 Repair of cloacal anomaly by anorectovaginoplasty and urethroplasty, combined abdominal and sacroperineal approach;

46748 with vaginal lengthening by intestinal graft or pedicle flaps

46750 Sphincteroplasty, anal, for incontinence or prolapse; adult

46751 child

46753 Graft (Thiersch operation) for rectal incontinence and/or prolapse

46754 Removal of Thiersch wire or suture, anal canal

46760 Sphincteroplasty, anal, for incontinence, adult; muscle transplant

46761 levator muscle imbrication (Park posterior anal repair)

46762 implantation artificial sphincter

Destruction

46900* Destruction of lesion(s), anus (eg, condyloma, papilloma, molluscum contagiosum, herpetic vesicle), simple; chemical

46910*   electrodesiccation

46916   cryosurgery

46917   laser surgery

(46920 has been deleted. To report, use 46922)

46922   surgical excision

46924   Destruction of lesion(s), anus (eg, condyloma, papilloma, molluscum contagiosum, herpetic vesicle), extensive, any method

(46930 has been deleted. To report, use 46924)

(46932 has been deleted. To report, use 46916)

(46933 has been deleted. To report, use 46924)

46934   Destruction of hemorrhoids, any method; internal

46935   external

46936   internal and external

46937   Cryosurgery of rectal tumor; benign

46938   malignant

46940   Curettage or cauterization of anal fissure, including dilation of anal sphincter (separate procedure); initial

46942   subsequent

Suture

46945   Ligation of internal hemorrhoids; single procedure

46946   multiple procedures

Other Procedures

46999   Unlisted procedure, anus

Liver

Incision

47000*   Biopsy of liver, needle; percutaneous

(For radiological supervision and interpretation, see 76003, 76360, 76942)

47001   when done for indicated purpose at time of other major procedure

(For radiological supervision and interpretation, see 76003, 76360, 76942)

(For fine needle aspiration, preparation, and interpretation of smears, see 88170-88173)

47010   Hepatotomy for drainage of abscess or cyst, one or two stages

47015   Laparotomy, with aspiration and/or injection of hepatic parasitic (eg, amoebic or echinococcal) cyst(s) or abscess(es)

Excision

47100   Biopsy of liver, wedge

47120   Hepatectomy, resection of liver; partial lobectomy

47122   trisegmentectomy

47125   total left lobectomy

47130   total right lobectomy

47133   Donor hepatectomy, with preparation and maintenance of allograft; from cadaver donor

47134   partial, from living donor

47135   Liver allotransplantation; orthotopic, partial or whole, from cadaver or living donor, any age

47136   heterotopic, partial or whole, from cadaver or living donor, any age

Repair

47300   Marsupialization of cyst or abscess of liver

▲**47350**   Management of liver hemorrhage; simple suture of liver wound or injury

(47355 has been deleted)

▲**47360**   complex suture of liver wound or injury, with or without hepatic artery ligation

●**47361**   exploration of hepatic wound, extensive debridement, coagulation and/or suture, with or without packing of liver

---

▲=Revised Code   ●=New Code   *=Service Includes Surgical Procedure Only

● **47362**   re-exploration of hepatic wound for removal of packing

Other Procedures

47399   Unlisted procedure, liver

Biliary Tract

Incision

47400   Hepaticotomy or hepaticostomy with exploration, drainage, or removal of calculus

47420   Choledochotomy or choledochostomy with exploration, drainage, or removal of calculus, with or without cholecystotomy; without transduodenal sphincterotomy or sphincteroplasty

47425   with transduodenal sphincterotomy or sphincteroplasty

(47440 has been deleted)

47460   Transduodenal sphincterotomy or sphincteroplasty, with or without transduodenal extraction of calculus (separate procedure)

47480   Cholecystotomy or cholecystostomy with exploration, drainage, or removal of calculus (separate procedure)

47490   Percutaneous cholecystostomy

(For radiological supervision and interpretation, see 75989)

Introduction

47500   Injection procedure for percutaneous transhepatic cholangiography

(For radiological supervision and interpretation, see 74320)

47505   Injection procedure for cholangiography through an existing catheter (eg, percutaneous transhepatic or T-tube)

47510   Introduction of percutaneous transhepatic catheter for biliary drainage

(For radiological supervision and interpretation, see 75980)

47511   Introduction of percutaneous transhepatic stent for internal and external biliary drainage

(For radiological supervision and interpretation, see 75982)

47525   Change of percutaneous biliary drainage catheter

(For radiological supervision and interpretation, see 75984)

47530   Revision and/or reinsertion of transhepatic tube

(For radiological supervision and interpretation, see 75984)

Endoscopy

Surgical endoscopy always includes diagnostic endoscopy.

47550   Biliary endoscopy, intraoperative (choledochoscopy)

(Use 47550 with either 47420 or 47610)

47552   Biliary endoscopy, percutaneous via T-tube or other tract; diagnostic, with or without collection of specimen(s) by brushing and/or washing (separate procedure)

47553   with biopsy, single or multiple

47554   with removal of stone(s)

47555   with dilation of biliary duct stricture(s) without stent

(For ERCP, see 43260-43272, 74363)

47556   with dilation of biliary duct stricture(s) with stent

(For radiological supervision and interpretation, see 75982)

Excision

47600   Cholecystectomy;

47605   with cholangiography

(For laparoscopic cholecystectomy, see 56340-56342)

47610   Cholecystectomy with exploration of common duct;

(47611 has been deleted. To report, use 47610 with 47550)

47612 with choledochoenterostomy

47620 with transduodenal sphincterotomy or sphincteroplasty, with or without cholangiography

47630 Biliary duct stone extraction, percutaneous via T-tube tract, basket, or snare (eg, Burhenne technique)

(For radiological supervision and interpretation, see 74327)

47700 Exploration for congenital atresia of bile ducts, without repair, with or without liver biopsy, with or without cholangiography

47701 Portoenterostomy (eg, Kasai procedure)

(47710 has been deleted. To report, see 47711, 47712)

47711 Excision of bile duct tumor, with or without primary repair of bile duct; extrahepatic

47712 intrahepatic

(For anastomosis, see 47760-47800)

47715 Excision of choledochal cyst

47716 Anastomosis, choledochal cyst, without excision

Repair

47720 Cholecystoenterostomy; direct

47721 with gastroenterostomy

47740 Roux-en-Y

47741 Roux-en-Y with gastroenterostomy

47760 Anastomosis, of extrahepatic biliary ducts and gastrointestinal tract

47765 Anastomosis, of intrahepatic ducts and gastrointestinal tract

47780 Anastomosis, Roux-en-Y, of extrahepatic biliary ducts and gastrointestinal tract

47785 Anastomosis, Roux-en-Y, of intrahepatic biliary ducts and gastrointestinal tract

47800 Reconstruction, plastic, of extrahepatic biliary ducts with end-to-end anastomosis

47801 Placement of choledochal stent

47802 U-tube hepaticoenterostomy

(47810 has been deleted. To report, use 47999)

(47850, 47855 have been deleted. To report, use 47999)

47900 Suture of extrahepatic biliary duct for pre-existing injury (separate procedure)

Other Procedures

47999 Unlisted procedure, biliary tract

Pancreas

(For peroral pancreatic endoscopic procedures, see 43260-43272)

Incision

48000 Placement of drains, peripancreatic, for acute pancreatitis;

48001 with cholecystostomy, gastrostomy, and jejunostomy

48005 Resection or debridement of pancreas and peripancreatic tissue for acute necrotizing pancreatitis

48020 Removal of pancreatic calculus

Excision

48100 Biopsy of pancreas, open, any method (eg, fine needle aspiration, needle core biopsy, wedge biopsy)

48102* Biopsy of pancreas, percutaneous needle

(For radiological supervision and interpretation, see 76003, 76360, 76942)

(For fine needle aspiration, preparation, and interpretation of smears, see 88170-88173)

48120 Excision of lesion of pancreas (eg, cyst, adenoma)

48140 Pancreatectomy, distal subtotal, with or without splenectomy; without pancreaticojejunostomy

48145   with pancreaticojejunostomy

48146 Pancreatectomy, distal, near-total with preservation of duodenum (Child-type procedure)

48148 Excision of ampulla of Vater

48150 Pancreatectomy, proximal subtotal with total duodenectomy, partial gastrectomy, choledochoenterostomy and gastrojejunostomy (Whipple-type procedure); with pancreatojejunostomy

(48151 has been deleted. To report, use 48146)

48152   without pancreatojejunostomy

48153 Pancreatectomy, proximal subtotal with near-total duodenectomy, choledochoenterostomy and duodenojejunostomy (pylorus-sparing, Whipple-type procedure); with pancreatojejunostomy

48154   without pancreatojejunostomy

48155 Pancreatectomy, total

48160 Pancreatectomy, total or subtotal, with autologous transplantation of pancreas or pancreatic islets

48180 Pancreaticojejunostomy, side-to-side anastomosis (Puestow-type operation)

Introduction

48400 Injection procedure for intraoperative pancreatography

(For radiological supervision and interpretation, see 74300-74305)

Repair

48500 Marsupialization of cyst of pancreas

48510 External drainage, pseudocyst of pancreas

48520 Internal anastomosis of pancreatic cyst to gastrointestinal tract; direct

48540   Roux-en-Y

48545 Pancreatorrhaphy for trauma

48547 Duodenal exclusion with gastrojejunostomy for pancreatic trauma

Pancreas Transplantation

48550 Donor pancreatectomy, with preparation and maintenance of allograft from cadaver donor, with or without duodenal segment for transplantation

48554 Transplantation of pancreatic allograft

48556 Removal of transplanted pancreatic allograft

Other Procedures

48999 Unlisted procedure, pancreas

Abdomen, Peritoneum, and Omentum

Incision

49000 Exploratory laparotomy, exploratory celiotomy with or without biopsy(s) (separate procedure)

(To report wound exploration due to penetrating trauma without laparotomy, use 20102)

49002 Reopening of recent laparotomy

(To report re-exploration of hepatic wound for removal of packing, use 47362)

49010 Exploration, retroperitoneal area with or without biopsy(s) (separate procedure)

(To report wound exploration due to penetrating trauma without laparotomy, use 20102)

49020 Drainage of peritoneal abscess or localized peritonitis, exclusive of appendiceal abscess, transabdominal

(For appendiceal abscess, see 44900)

49040 Drainage of subdiaphragmatic or subphrenic abscess

49060 Drainage of retroperitoneal abscess

49080* Peritoneocentesis, abdominal paracentesis, or peritoneal lavage (diagnostic or therapeutic); initial

49081* subsequent

49085 Removal of peritoneal foreign body from peritoneal cavity

(For lysis of intestinal adhesions, see 44005)

Excision, Destruction

49180* Biopsy, abdominal or retroperitoneal mass, percutaneous needle

(For radiological supervision and interpretation, see 76003, 76360, 76365, 76942)

(For fine needle aspiration, preparation, and interpretation of smears, see 88170-88173)

49200 Excision or destruction by any method of intra-abdominal or retroperitoneal tumors or cysts or endometriomas;

49201 extensive

49215 Excision of presacral or sacrococcygeal tumor

49220 Staging celiotomy (laparotomy) for Hodgkin's disease or lymphoma (includes splenectomy, needle or open biopsies of both liver lobes, possibly also removal of abdominal nodes, abdominal node and/or bone marrow biopsies, ovarian repositioning)

49250 Umbilectomy, omphalectomy, excision of umbilicus (separate procedure)

49255 Omentectomy, epiploectomy, resection of omentum (separate procedure)

(49300 has been deleted. To report, use 56360)

(49301 has been deleted. To report, use 56361)

(49302 has been deleted. To report, use 56362)

(49303 has been deleted. To report, use 56363)

(49310 has been deleted. To report, use 56340)

(49311 has been deleted. To report, use 56341)

(49315 has been deleted. To report, use 56315)

Introduction, Revision, and/or Removal

49400* Injection of air or contrast into peritoneal cavity (separate procedure)

(For radiological supervision and interpretation, see 74190)

(49401 has been deleted. To report, use 49400)

49420* Insertion of intraperitoneal cannula or catheter for drainage or dialysis; temporary

49421 permanent

49422 Removal of permanent intraperitoneal cannula or catheter

(For removal of a temporary catheter/cannula, use appropriate E/M code)

49425 Insertion of peritoneal-venous shunt

49426 Revision of peritoneal-venous shunt

(For shunt patency test, see 78291)

49427 Injection procedure (eg, contrast media) for evaluation of previously placed peritoneal-venous shunt

(For radiological supervision and interpretation, see 75809)

49428 Ligation of peritoneal-venous shunt

49429 Removal of peritoneal-venous shunt

(49430, 49440 have been deleted. To report, use 49999)

Repair

Hernioplasty, Herniorrhaphy, Herniotomy

The hernia repair codes in this section are categorized primarily by the type of hernia (inguinal, femoral, incisional, etc.). Some types of hernias are further categorized as "initial" or "recurrent" based on whether or not the hernia has required previous repair(s).

Additional variables accounted for by some of the codes include patient age and clinical presentation (reducible vs. incarcerated or strangulated).

With the exception of the incisional hernia repairs (see 49560-49566) the use of mesh or other prostheses is not separately reported.

The excision/repair of strangulated organs or structures such as testicle(s), intestine, ovaries are reported by using the appropriate code for the excision/repair (eg, 44120, 54520, and 58940) in addition to the appropriate code for the repair of the strangulated hernia.

(For reduction and repair of intra-abdominal hernia, see 44050)

(For debridement of abdominal wall, see 11042, 11043)

(All codes for bilateral procedures in hernia repair have been deleted. To report, add modifier -50 or 09950)

49495   Repair initial inguinal hernia, under age 6 months, with or without hydrocelectomy; reducible

49496   incarcerated or strangulated

49500   Repair initial inguinal hernia, age 6 months to under 5 years, with or without hydrocelectomy; reducible

49501   incarcerated or strangulated

49505   Repair initial inguinal hernia, age 5 years or over; reducible

49507   incarcerated or strangulated

(49510 has been deleted. To report, see 49505 or 49507 and 54520)

(49515 has been deleted. To report, see 49505 or 49507 and 54840 or 55040)

49520   Repair recurrent inguinal hernia, any age; reducible

49521   incarcerated or strangulated

49525   Repair inguinal hernia, sliding, any age

(49530 has been deleted. To report, see 49496, 49501, 49507, 49521)

(49535 has been deleted. To report, see 49496, 49501, 49507, 49521)

49540   Repair lumbar hernia

49550   Repair initial femoral hernia, any age, reducible;

(49552 has been deleted. To report, see 49550 or 49553)

49553   incarcerated or strangulated

49555   Repair recurrent femoral hernia; reducible

49557   incarcerated or strangulated

49560   Repair initial incisional hernia; reducible

49561   incarcerated or strangulated

49565   Repair recurrent incisional hernia; reducible

49566   incarcerated or strangulated

49568   Implantation of mesh or other prosthesis for incisional hernia repair (list separately in addition to code for the incisional hernia repair)

49570   Repair epigastric hernia (eg, preperitoneal fat); reducible (separate procedure)

49572   incarcerated or strangulated

(49575 has been deleted. To report, use 49572)

49580   Repair umbilical hernia, under age 5 years; reducible

(49581 has been deleted. To report, see 49585 or 49587)

49582   incarcerated or strangulated

49585   Repair umbilical hernia, age 5 years or over; reducible

49587   incarcerated or strangulated

49590   Repair spigelian hernia

49600   Repair of small omphalocele, with primary closure

49605   Repair of large omphalocele or gastroschisis; with or without prosthesis

49606   with removal of prosthesis, final reduction and closure, in operating room

49610   Repair of omphalocele (Gross type operation); first stage

49611   second stage

(For diaphragmatic or hiatal hernia repair, see 39502-39541)

(49630-49640 have been deleted. For surgical repair of omentum, use 49999)

Suture

49900   Suture, secondary, of abdominal wall for evisceration or dehiscence

(For suture of ruptured diaphragm, see 39540, 39541)

(For debridement of abdominal wall, see 11042, 11043)

Other Procedures

49905   Omental flap (eg, for reconstruction of sternal and chest wall defects) (list separately in addition to code for primary procedure)

(49910 has been deleted. To report, use 49999)

49999   Unlisted procedure, abdomen, peritoneum and omentum

Notes

Urinary System

(For provision of chemotherapeutic agents, use 96545 in addition to primary procedure)

Kidney

Incision

(For retroperitoneal exploration, abscess, tumor, or cyst, see 49010, 49060, 49200, 49201)

50010   Renal exploration, not necessitating other specific procedures

50020   Drainage of perirenal or renal abscess (separate procedure)

50040   Nephrostomy, nephrotomy with drainage

50045   Nephrotomy, with exploration

(For renal endoscopy performed in conjunction with this procedure, see 50570-50580)

50060   Nephrolithotomy; removal of calculus

50065   secondary surgical operation for calculus

50070   complicated by congenital kidney abnormality

50075   removal of large staghorn calculus filling renal pelvis and calyces (including anatrophic pyelolithotomy)

50080   Percutaneous nephrostolithotomy or pyelostolithotomy, with or without dilation, endoscopy, lithotripsy, stenting, or basket extraction; up to 2 cm

50081   over 2 cm

(For establishment of nephrostomy without nephrostolithotomy, see 50040, 50395, 52334)

(For fluoroscopic guidance, see 76000, 76001)

50100   Transection or repositioning of aberrant renal vessels (separate procedure)

50120   Pyelotomy; with exploration

(For renal endoscopy performed in conjunction with this procedure, see 50570-50580)

50125   with drainage, pyelostomy

50130   with removal of calculus (pyelolithotomy, pelviolithotomy, including coagulum pyelolithotomy)

50135   complicated (eg, secondary operation, congenital kidney abnormality)

(For supply of anticarcinogenic agents, use 99070 in addition to primary procedure)

Excision

(For excision of retroperitoneal tumor or cyst, see 49200, 49201)

50200*   Renal biopsy; percutaneous, by trocar or needle

(For radiological supervision and interpretation, see 76003, 76360, 76942)

(For fine needle aspiration, preparation, and interpretation of smears, see 88170-88173)

50205   by surgical exposure of kidney

50220   Nephrectomy, including partial ureterectomy, any approach including rib resection;

50225   complicated because of previous surgery on same kidney

50230   radical, with regional lymphadenectomy and/or vena caval thrombectomy

(When vena caval resection with reconstruction is necessary, use 37799)

50234   Nephrectomy with total ureterectomy and bladder cuff; through same incision

50236   through separate incision

50240   Nephrectomy, partial

50280   Excision or unroofing of cyst(s) of kidney

50290   Excision of perinephric cyst

Renal Transplantation

(For dialysis, see 90935-90999)

**Urinary
50010—53899**

▲=Revised Code   ●=New Code   ✳=Service Includes Surgical Procedure Only

50300 Donor nephrectomy, with preparation and maintenance of allograft; from cadaver donor, unilateral or bilateral

50320   from living donor

50340 Recipient nephrectomy (separate procedure)

(50341 has been deleted. To report, use 50340 with modifier -50 or 09950)

50360 Renal allotransplantation, implantation of graft; excluding donor and recipient nephrectomy

50365   with recipient nephrectomy

(50366 has been deleted. To report, use 50365 with modifier -50 or 09950)

50370 Removal of transplanted renal allograft

50380 Renal autotransplantation, reimplantation of kidney

(For extra-corporeal "bench" surgery, use autotransplantation as the primary procedure and add the secondary procedure (eg, partial nephrectomy, nephrolithotomy), and use the modifier -51 or 09951)

Introduction

50390* Aspiration and/or injection of renal cyst or pelvis by needle, percutaneous

(For radiological supervision and interpretation, see 74425, 74470, 76003, 76365, 76938)

(For fine needle aspiration, preparation, and interpretation of smears, see 88170-88173)

50392 Introduction of intracatheter or catheter into renal pelvis for drainage and/or injection, percutaneous

(For radiological supervision and interpretation, see 74475, 76365, 76938)

50393 Introduction of ureteral catheter or stent into ureter through renal pelvis for drainage and/or injection, percutaneous

(For radiological supervision and interpretation, see 74480, 76003, 76365, 76938)

50394 Injection procedure for pyelography (as nephrostogram, pyelostogram, antegrade pyeloureterograms) through nephrostomy or pyelostomy tube, or indwelling ureteral catheter

(For radiological supervision and interpretation, see 74425)

50395 Introduction of guide into renal pelvis and/or ureter with dilation to establish nephrostomy tract, percutaneous

(For radiological supervision and interpretation, see 74475, 74480, 74485)

(For nephrostolithotomy, see 50080, 50081)

(For retrograde percutaneous nephrostomy, use 52334)

(For endoscopic surgery, see 50551-50561)

50396 Manometric studies through nephrostomy or pyelostomy tube, or indwelling ureteral catheter

(For radiological supervision and interpretation, see 74425, 74475, 74480)

50398* Change of nephrostomy or pyelostomy tube

(For fluoroscopic guidance, use 76000)

(For radiological supervision and interpretation, see 75984)

Repair

50400 Pyeloplasty (Foley Y-pyeloplasty), plastic operation on renal pelvis, with or without plastic operation on ureter, nephropexy, nephrostomy, pyelostomy, or ureteral splinting; simple

50405   complicated (congenital kidney abnormality, secondary pyeloplasty, solitary kidney, calycoplasty)

(50420 has been deleted)

50500 Nephrorrhaphy, suture of kidney wound or injury

50520 Closure of nephrocutaneous or pyelocutaneous fistula

50525 Closure of nephrovisceral fistula (eg, renocolic), including visceral repair; abdominal approach

50526   thoracic approach

50540 Symphysiotomy for horseshoe kidney with or without pyeloplasty and/or other plastic procedure, unilateral or bilateral (one operation)

Endoscopy

(For supplies and materials, use 99070)

(References to office and hospital have been deleted)

50551 Renal endoscopy through established nephrostomy or pyelostomy, with or without irrigation, instillation, or ureteropyelography, exclusive of radiologic service;

50553   with ureteral catheterization, with or without dilation of ureter

50555   with biopsy

50557   with fulguration and/or incision, with or without biopsy

50559   with insertion of radioactive substance with or without biopsy and/or fulguration

50561   with removal of foreign body or calculus

(When procedures 50570-50580 provide a significant identifiable service, they may be added to 50045 and 50120)

50570 Renal endoscopy through nephrotomy or pyelotomy, with or without irrigation, instillation, or ureteropyelography, exclusive of radiologic service;

(For nephrotomy, see 50045)

(For pyelotomy, see 50120)

50572   with ureteral catheterization, with or without dilation of ureter

50574   with biopsy

50575   with endopyelotomy (includes cystoscopy, ureteroscopy, dilation of ureter and ureteral pelvic junction, incision of ureteral pelvic junction and insertion of endopyelotomy stent)

50576   with fulguration and/or incision, with or without biopsy

50578   with insertion of radioactive substance, with or without biopsy and/or fulguration

50580   with removal of foreign body or calculus

Other Procedures

50590 Lithotripsy, extracorporeal shock wave

Ureter

Incision

50600 Ureterotomy with exploration or drainage (separate procedure)

(For ureteral endoscopy performed in conjunction with this procedure, see 50970-50980)

50605 Ureterotomy for insertion of indwelling stent, all types

50610 Ureterolithotomy; upper one-third of ureter

50620   middle one-third of ureter

50630   lower one-third of ureter

(For transvesical ureterolithotomy, see 51060)

(For cystotomy with stone basket extraction of ureteral calculus, see 51065)

(For endoscopic extraction or manipulation of ureteral calculus, see 50080, 50081, 50561, 50961, 50980, 52320-52330, 52336, 52337)

Excision

(For ureterocele, see 51535, 52300)

50650 Ureterectomy, with bladder cuff (separate procedure)

50660   Ureterectomy, total, ectopic ureter, combination abdominal, vaginal and/or perineal approach

Introduction

50684   Injection procedure for ureterography or ureteropyelography through ureterostomy or indwelling ureteral catheter

(For radiological supervision and interpretation, see 74425)

50686   Manometric studies through ureterostomy or indwelling ureteral catheter

50688*   Change of ureterostomy tube

(For radiological supervision and interpretation, see 74425)

50690   Injection procedure for visualization of ileal conduit and/or ureteropyelography, exclusive of radiologic service

(For radiological supervision and interpretation, see 74425)

Repair

50700   Ureteroplasty, plastic operation on ureter (eg, stricture)

50715   Ureterolysis, with or without repositioning of ureter for retroperitoneal fibrosis

(50716 has been deleted. To report, use 50715 with modifier -50 or 09950)

50722   Ureterolysis for ovarian vein syndrome

50725   Ureterolysis for retrocaval ureter, with reanastomosis of upper urinary tract or vena cava

50727   Revision of urinary-cutaneous anastomosis (any type urostomy);

50728   with repair of fascial defect and hernia

50740   Ureteropyelostomy, anastomosis of ureter and renal pelvis

50750   Ureterocalycostomy, anastomosis of ureter to renal calyx

50760   Ureteroureterostomy

50770   Transureteroureterostomy, anastomosis of ureter to contralateral ureter

(Codes 50780-50785 include minor procedures to prevent vesicoureteral reflux)

50780   Ureteroneocystostomy; anastomosis of single ureter to bladder

(50781 has been deleted. To report, use 50780 with modifier -50 or 09950)

(When combined with cystourethroplasty or vesical neck revision, see 51820)

50782   anastomosis of duplicated ureter to bladder

50783   with extensive ureteral tailoring

50785   with vesico-psoas hitch or bladder flap

(50786 has been deleted. To report, use 50785 with modifier -50 or 09950)

50800   Ureteroenterostomy, direct anastomosis of ureter to intestine

(50801 has been deleted. To report, use 50800 with modifier -50 or 09950)

50810   Ureterosigmoidostomy, with creation of sigmoid bladder and establishment of abdominal or perineal colostomy, including bowel anastomosis

50815   Ureterocolon conduit, including bowel anastomosis

(50816 has been deleted. To report, use 50815 with modifier -50 or 09950)

50820   Ureteroileal conduit (ileal bladder), including bowel anastomosis (Bricker operation)

(50821 has been deleted. To report, use 50820 with modifier -50 or 09950)

(For combination of 50800-50820 with cystectomy, see 51580-51595)

50825   Continent diversion, including bowel anastomosis using any segment of small and/or large bowel (Kock pouch or Camey enterocystoplasty)

50830   Urinary undiversion (eg, taking down of ureteroileal conduit, ureterosigmoidostomy or ureteroenterostomy with ureteroureterostomy or ureteroneocystostomy)

50840   Replacement of all or part of ureter by bowel segment, including bowel anastomosis

(50841 has been deleted. To report, use 50840 with modifier -50 or 09950)

50845   Cutaneous appendico-vesicostomy

50860   Ureterostomy, transplantation of ureter to skin

(50861 has been deleted. To report, use 50860 with modifier -50 or 09950)

50900   Ureterorrhaphy, suture of ureter (separate procedure)

50920   Closure of ureterocutaneous fistula

50930   Closure of ureterovisceral fistula (including visceral repair)

50940   Deligation of ureter

(For ureteroplasty, ureterolysis, see 50700-50860)

Endoscopy

(References to office and hospital have been deleted)

50951   Ureteral endoscopy through established ureterostomy, with or without irrigation, instillation, or ureteropyelography, exclusive of radiologic service;

50953   with ureteral catheterization, with or without dilation of ureter

50955   with biopsy

50957   with fulguration and/or incision, with or without biopsy

50959   with insertion of radioactive substance, with or without biopsy and/or fulguration (not including provision of material)

50961   with removal of foreign body or calculus

(When procedures 50970-50980 provide a significant identifiable service, they may be added to 50600)

50970   Ureteral endoscopy through ureterotomy, with or without irrigation, instillation, or ureteropyelography, exclusive of radiologic service;

(For ureterotomy, see 50600)

50972   with ureteral catheterization, with or without dilation of ureter

50974   with biopsy

50976   with fulguration and/or incision, with or without biopsy

50978   with insertion of radioactive substance, with or without biopsy and/or fulguration (not including provision of material)

50980   with removal of foreign body or calculus

Bladder

Incision

51000*   Aspiration of bladder by needle

51005*   Aspiration of bladder; by trocar or intracatheter

51010   with insertion of suprapubic catheter

51020   Cystotomy or cystostomy; with fulguration and/or insertion of radioactive material

51030   with cryosurgical destruction of intravesical lesion

51040   Cystostomy, cystotomy with drainage

51045   Cystotomy, with insertion of ureteral catheter or stent (separate procedure)

51050   Cystolithotomy, cystotomy with removal of calculus, without vesical neck resection

51060   Transvesical ureterolithotomy

51065   Cystotomy, with stone basket extraction and/or ultrasonic or electrohydraulic fragmentation of ureteral calculus

51080   Drainage of perivesical or prevesical space abscess

Excision

51500 Excision of urachal cyst or sinus, with or without umbilical hernia repair

51520 Cystotomy; for simple excision of vesical neck (separate procedure)

51525 for excision of bladder diverticulum, single or multiple (separate procedure)

51530 for excision of bladder tumor

(For transurethral resection, see 52234-52240, 52305)

51535 Cystotomy for excision, incision, or repair of ureterocele

(For transurethral excision, see 52300)

(51536 has been deleted. To report, use 51535 with modifier -50 or 09950)

51550 Cystectomy, partial; simple

51555 complicated (eg, postradiation, previous surgery, difficult location)

51565 Cystectomy, partial, with reimplantation of ureter(s) into bladder (ureteroneocystostomy)

51570 Cystectomy, complete; (separate procedure)

51575 with bilateral pelvic lymphadenectomy, including external iliac, hypogastric, and obturator nodes

51580 Cystectomy, complete, with uretero-sigmoidostomy or ureterocutaneous transplantations;

51585 with bilateral pelvic lymphadenectomy, including external iliac, hypogastric, and obturator nodes

51590 Cystectomy, complete, with ureteroileal conduit or sigmoid bladder, including bowel anastomosis;

51595 with bilateral pelvic lymphadenectomy, including external iliac, hypogastric, and obturator nodes

51596 Cystectomy, complete, with continent diversion, any technique, using any segment of small and/or large bowel to construct neobladder

51597 Pelvic exenteration, complete, for vesical, prostatic or urethral malignancy, with removal of bladder and ureteral transplantations, with or without hysterectomy and/or abdominoperineal resection of rectum and colon and colostomy, or any combination thereof

(For pelvic exenteration for gynecologic malignancy, use 58240)

Introduction

(For bladder catheterization, see 53670, 53675)

51600* Injection procedure for cystography or voiding urethrocystography

(For radiological supervision and interpretation, see 74430, 74455)

51605 Injection procedure and placement of chain for contrast and/or chain urethrocystography

(For radiological supervision and interpretation, see 74430)

51610 Injection procedure for retrograde urethrocystography

(For radiological supervision and interpretation, see 74450)

51700* Bladder irrigation, simple, lavage and/or instillation

51705* Change of cystostomy tube; simple

51710* complicated

51715 Endoscopic injection of implant material into the submucosal tissues of the urethra and/or bladder neck

51720 Bladder instillation of anticarcinogenic agent (including detention time)

Urodynamics

The following section (51725-51797) lists procedures that may be used separately or in many and varied combinations. When multiple procedures are performed in the same investigative session, either modifier '-51' or code 09951 should be employed.

All procedures in this section imply that these services are performed by, or are under the direct supervision of, a physician and that all instruments, equipment, fluids, gases, probes, catheters, technician's fees, medications, gloves, trays, tubing and other sterile supplies be provided by the physician. When the physician only interprets the results and/or operates the equipment, a professional component, modifier '-26' or code 09926, should be used to identify physicians' services.

51725   Simple cystometrogram (CMG) (eg, spinal manometer)

51726   Complex cystometrogram (eg, calibrated electronic equipment)

   (51727-51733 have been deleted. To report, use 51726)

51736   Simple uroflowmetry (UFR) (eg, stop-watch flow rate, mechanical uroflowmeter)

   (51737, 51738 have been deleted. To report, use 51736)

   (51739 has been deleted)

51741   Complex uroflowmetry (eg, calibrated electronic equipment)

   (51742-51749 have been deleted. To report, use 51741)

   (51751-51769 have been deleted. To report, use 53899)

51772   Urethral pressure profile studies (UPP) (urethral closure pressure profile), any technique

   (51773-51783 have been deleted. To report, use 51772)

51784   Electromyography studies (EMG) of anal or urethral sphincter, other than needle, any technique

51785   Needle electromyography studies (EMG) of anal or urethral sphincter, any technique

   (51786-51791 have been deleted. To report, use 51785)

51792   Stimulus evoked response (eg, measurement of bulbocavernosus reflex latency time)

51795   Voiding pressure studies (VP); bladder voiding pressure, any technique

   (51796 has been deleted. To report, use 51795)

51797   intra-abdominal voiding pressure (AP) (rectal, gastric, intraperitoneal)

Repair

51800   Cystoplasty or cystourethroplasty, plastic operation on bladder and/or vesical neck (anterior Y-plasty, vesical fundus resection), any procedure, with or without wedge resection of posterior vesical neck

51820   Cystourethroplasty with unilateral or bilateral ureteroneocystostomy

51840   Anterior vesicourethropexy, or urethropexy (Marshall-Marchetti-Krantz type); simple

51841   complicated (eg, secondary repair)

   (For urethropexy (Pereyra type), see 57289)

51845   Abdomino-vaginal vesical neck suspension, with or without endoscopic control (eg, Stamey, Raz, modified Pereyra)

51860   Cystorrhaphy, suture of bladder wound, injury or rupture; simple

51865   complicated

51880   Closure of cystostomy (separate procedure)

51900   Closure of vesicovaginal fistula, abdominal approach

   (For vaginal approach, see 57320-57330)

51920   Closure of vesicouterine fistula;

51925   with hysterectomy

   (For closure of vesicoenteric fistula, see 44660, 44661)

   (For closure of rectovesical fistula, see 45800-45805)

51940   Closure of bladder exstrophy

   (See also 54390)

51960 Enterocystoplasty, including bowel anastomosis

51980 Cutaneous vesicostomy

Endoscopy—Cystoscopy, Urethroscopy, Cystourethroscopy

Endoscopic descriptions are listed so that the main procedure can be identified without having to list all the minor related functions performed at the same time. For example: meatotomy, urethral calibration and/or dilation, urethroscopy, and cystoscopy prior to a transurethral resection of prostate; ureteral catheterization following extraction of ureteral calculus; internal urethrotomy and bladder neck fulguration when performing a cystourethroscopy for the female urethral syndrome. When the secondary procedure requires significant additional time and effort, it may be identified by the addition of either modifier '-22' or 09922. For example: urethrotomy performed for a documented pre-existing stricture or bladder neck contracture.

(References to office and hospital have been deleted)

52000 Cystourethroscopy (separate procedure)

52005 Cystourethroscopy, with ureteral catheterization, with or without irrigation, instillation, or ureteropyelography, exclusive of radiologic service;

52007 with brush biopsy of ureter and/or renal pelvis

52010 Cystourethroscopy, with ejaculatory duct catheterization, with or without irrigation, instillation, or duct radiography, exclusive of radiologic service

(For radiological supervision and interpretation, see 74440)

(52190 has been deleted)

Transurethral Surgery

Urethra and Bladder

(References to office and hospital have been deleted)

52204 Cystourethroscopy, with biopsy

52214 Cystourethroscopy, with fulguration (including cryosurgery or laser surgery) of trigone, bladder neck, prostatic fossa, urethra, or periurethral glands

52224 Cystourethroscopy, with fulguration (including cryosurgery or laser surgery) or treatment of MINOR (less than 0.5 cm) lesion(s) with or without biopsy

52234 Cystourethroscopy, with fulguration (including cryosurgery or laser surgery) and/or resection of; SMALL bladder tumor(s) (0.5 to 2.0 cm)

52235 MEDIUM bladder tumor(s) (2.0 to 5.0 cm)

52240 LARGE bladder tumor(s)

52250 Cystourethroscopy with insertion of radioactive substance, with or without biopsy or fulguration

52260 Cystourethroscopy, with dilation of bladder for interstitial cystitis; general or conduction (spinal) anesthesia

52265 local anesthesia

52270 Cystourethroscopy, with internal urethrotomy; female

52275 male

52276 Cystourethroscopy with direct vision internal urethrotomy

52277 Cystourethroscopy, with resection of external sphincter (sphincterotomy)

52281 Cystourethroscopy, with calibration and/or dilation of urethral stricture or stenosis, with or without meatotomy and injection procedure for cystography, male or female

52283 Cystourethroscopy, with steroid injection into stricture

52285 Cystourethroscopy for treatment of the female urethral syndrome with any or all of the following: urethral meatotomy, urethral dilation, internal urethrotomy, lysis of urethrovaginal septal fibrosis, lateral incisions of the bladder neck, and fulguration of polyp(s) of urethra, bladder neck, and/or trigone

52290 Cystourethroscopy; with ureteral meatotomy, unilateral or bilateral

52300 with resection or fulguration of ureterocele(s), unilateral or bilateral

52305 with incision or resection of orifice of bladder diverticulum, single or multiple

52310 Cystourethroscopy, with removal of foreign body, calculus, or ureteral stent from urethra or bladder (separate procedure); simple

52315 complicated

52317 Litholapaxy: crushing or fragmentation of calculus by any means in bladder and removal of fragments; simple or small (less than 2.5 cm)

52318 complicated or large (over 2.5 cm)

Ureter and Pelvis

The insertion of a stent is included in 52320-52339 when done and should not be reported separately.

52320 Cystourethroscopy (including ureteral catheterization); with removal of ureteral calculus

52325 with fragmentation of ureteral calculus (eg, ultrasonic or electro-hydraulic technique)

52327 with subureteric injection of implant material

52330 with manipulation, without removal of ureteral calculus

52332 Cystourethroscopy, with insertion of indwelling ureteral stent (eg, Gibbons or double-J type)

52334 Cystourethroscopy with insertion of ureteral guide wire through kidney to establish a percutaneous nephrostomy, retrograde

(For percutaneous nephrostolithotomy, see 50080, 50081; for establishment of nephrostomy tract only, see 50395)

52335 Cystourethroscopy, with ureteroscopy and/or pyeloscopy (includes dilation of the ureter and/or pyeloureteral junction by any method);

(For radiological supervision and interpretation, see 74485)

52336 with removal or manipulation of calculus (ureteral catheterization is included)

52337 with lithotripsy (ureteral catheterization is included)

52338 with biopsy and/or fulguration of lesion

52339 with resection of tumor

Vesical Neck and Prostate

52340 Cystourethroscopy with incision, fulguration, or resection of bladder neck and/or posterior urethra (congenital valves, obstructive hypertrophic mucosal folds)

52450 Transurethral incision of prostate

52500 Transurethral resection of bladder neck (separate procedure)

52510 Transurethral balloon dilation of the prostatic urethra, any method

52601 Transurethral electrosurgical resection of prostate, including control of postoperative bleeding, complete (vasectomy, meatotomy, cystourethroscopy, urethral calibration and/or dilation, and internal urethrotomy are included)

(For other approaches, see 55801-55845)

(52605 has been deleted. To report, use 52606)

52606 Transurethral fulguration for postoperative bleeding occurring after the usual follow-up time

52612 Transurethral resection of prostate; first stage of two-stage resection (partial resection)

52614 second stage of two-stage resection (resection completed)

52620 Transurethral resection; of residual obstructive tissue after 90 days postoperative

52630 of regrowth of obstructive tissue longer than one year postoperative

52640 of postoperative bladder neck contracture

52647 Non-contact laser coagulation of prostate, including control of postoperative bleeding, complete (vasectomy, meatotomy, cystourethroscopy, urethral calibration and/or dilation, and internal urethrotomy are included)

52648 Contact laser vaporization with or without transurethral resection of prostate, including control of postoperative bleeding, complete (vasectomy, meatotomy, cystourethroscopy, urethral calibration and/or dilation, and internal urethrotomy are included)

(52650 has been deleted)

52700 Transurethral drainage of prostatic abscess

(52800, 52805 have been deleted. To report, use 52317, 52318)

Urethra

(For endoscopy, see cystoscopy, urethroscopy, cystourethroscopy, 52000-52700)

(For injection procedure for urethrocystography, see 51600-51610)

Incision

53000 Urethrotomy or urethrostomy, external (separate procedure); pendulous urethra

53010 perineal urethra, external

53020 Meatotomy, cutting of meatus (separate procedure); except infant

(53021 has been deleted. To report, use 53020)

53025 infant

53040 Drainage of deep periurethral abscess

(For subcutaneous abscess, see 10060, 10061)

53060 Drainage of Skene's gland abscess or cyst

53080 Drainage of perineal urinary extravasation; uncomplicated (separate procedure)

53085 complicated

Excision

53200 Biopsy of urethra

53210 Urethrectomy, total, including cystostomy; female

53215 male

53220 Excision or fulguration of carcinoma of urethra

53230 Excision of urethral diverticulum (separate procedure); female

53235 male

53240 Marsupialization of urethral diverticulum, male or female

53250 Excision of bulbourethral gland (Cowper's gland)

53260 Excision or fulguration; urethral polyp(s), distal urethra

(For endoscopic approach, see 52214, 52224)

53265 urethral caruncle

53270 Skene's glands

53275 urethral prolapse

Repair

(For hypospadias, see 54300-54352)

53400 Urethroplasty; first stage, for fistula, diverticulum, or stricture (eg, Johannsen type)

53405 second stage (formation of urethra), including urinary diversion

53410 Urethroplasty, one-stage reconstruction of male anterior urethra

53415 Urethroplasty, transpubic or perineal, one stage, for reconstruction or repair of prostatic or membranous urethra

53420 Urethroplasty, two-stage reconstruction or repair of prostatic or membranous urethra; first stage

53425 second stage

53430 Urethroplasty, reconstruction of female urethra

53440 Operation for correction of male urinary incontinence, with or without introduction of prosthesis

53442 Removal of perineal prosthesis introduced for continence

53443 Urethroplasty with tubularization of posterior urethra and/or lower bladder for incontinence (eg, Tenago, Leadbetter procedure)

53445 Operation for correction of urinary incontinence with placement of inflatable urethral or bladder neck sphincter, including placement of pump and/or reservoir

53447 Removal, repair, or replacement of inflatable sphincter including pump and/or reservoir and/or cuff

53449 Surgical correction of hydraulic abnormality of inflatable sphincter device

53450 Urethromeatoplasty, with mucosal advancement

(For meatotomy, see 53020, 53025)

53460 Urethromeatoplasty, with partial excision of distal urethral segment (Richardson type procedure)

53502 Urethrorrhaphy, suture of urethral wound or injury, female

53505 Urethrorrhaphy, suture of urethral wound or injury; penile

53510   perineal

53515   prostatomembranous

53520 Closure of urethrostomy or urethrocutaneous fistula, male (separate procedure)

(For closure of urethrovaginal fistula, see 57310)

(For closure of urethrorectal fistula, see 45820, 45825)

Manipulation

(For radiological supervision and interpretation, see 74485)

53600* Dilation of urethral stricture by passage of sound or urethral dilator, male; initial

53601*   subsequent

53605 Dilation of urethral stricture or vesical neck by passage of sound or urethral dilator, male, general or conduction (spinal) anesthesia

53620* Dilation of urethral stricture by passage of filiform and follower, male; initial

53621*   subsequent

53640* Passage of filiform and follower for acute vesical retention, male

53660* Dilation of female urethra including suppository and/or instillation; initial

53661*   subsequent

53665 Dilation of female urethra, general or conduction (spinal) anesthesia

53670* Catheterization, urethra; simple

53675*   complicated (may include difficult removal of balloon catheter)

Other Procedures

(53800 has been deleted. To report, use 81020)

53899 Unlisted procedure, urinary system

Notes

Male Genital System

Penis

Incision

54000   Slitting of prepuce, dorsal or lateral (separate procedure); newborn

54001   except newborn

54015   Incision and drainage of penis, deep

    (For skin and subcutaneous abscess, see 10060-10160)

Destruction

54050*   Destruction of lesion(s), penis (eg, condyloma, papilloma, molluscum contagiosum, herpetic vesicle), simple; chemical

54055*   electrodesiccation

54056   cryosurgery

54057   laser surgery

54060   surgical excision

54065   Destruction of lesion(s), penis (eg, condyloma, papilloma, molluscum contagiosum, herpetic vesicle), extensive, any method

    (For destruction or excision of other lesions, see Integumentary System)

Excision

54100   Biopsy of penis; cutaneous (separate procedure)

54105   deep structures

54110   Excision of penile plaque (Peyronie disease);

54111   with graft to 5 cm in length

54112   with graft greater than 5 cm in length

54115   Removal foreign body from deep penile tissue (eg, plastic implant)

54120   Amputation of penis; partial

54125   complete

54130   Amputation of penis, radical; with bilateral inguinofemoral lymphadenectomy

54135   in continuity with bilateral pelvic lymphadenectomy, including external iliac, hypogastric and obturator nodes

    (For lymphadenectomy (separate procedure), see 38760-38770)

54150   Circumcision, using clamp or other device; newborn

54152   except newborn

    (54154 has been deleted. To report, use 54152)

54160   Circumcision, surgical excision other than clamp, device or dorsal slit; newborn

54161   except newborn

Introduction

54200*   Injection procedure for Peyronie disease;

54205   with surgical exposure of plaque

54220   Irrigation of corpora cavernosa for priapism

54230   Injection procedure for corpora cavernosography

    (For radiological supervision and interpretation, see 74445)

54231   Dynamic cavernosometry, including intra-cavernosal injection of vasoactive drugs (eg, papaverine, phentolamine)

54235   Injection of corpora cavernosa with pharmacologic agent(s) (eg, papaverine, phentolamine)

54240   Penile plethysmography

54250   Nocturnal penile tumescence and/or rigidity test

Repair

    (For other urethroplasties, see 53400-53430)

    (For penile revascularization, see 37788)

▲=Revised Code   ●=New Code   ✱=Service Includes Surgical Procedure Only

54300   Plastic operation of penis for straightening of chordee (eg, hypospadias), with or without mobilization of urethra

54304   Plastic operation on penis for correction of chordee or for first stage hypospadias repair with or without transplantation of prepuce and/or skin flaps

(54305 has been deleted. To report, see 54304 et seq)

54308   Urethroplasty for second stage hypospadias repair (including urinary diversion); less than 3 cm

54312   greater than 3 cm

54316   Urethroplasty for second stage hypospadias repair (including urinary diversion) with free skin graft obtained from site other than genitalia

54318   Urethroplasty for third stage hypospadias repair to release penis from scrotum (eg, third stage Cecil repair)

(54320 has been deleted. To report, see 54308 et seq)

54322   One stage distal hypospadias repair (with or without chordee or circumcision); with simple meatal advancement (eg, Magpi, V-flap)

54324   with urethroplasty by local skin flaps (eg, flip-flap, prepucial flap)

(54325 has been deleted. To report, see 54308 et seq)

54326   with urethroplasty by local skin flaps and mobilization of urethra

54328   with extensive dissection to correct chordee and urethroplasty with local skin flaps, skin graft patch, and/or island flap

(54330 has been deleted. To report, see 54308)

54332   One stage proximal penile or penoscrotal hypospadias repair requiring extensive dissection to correct chordee and urethroplasty by use of skin graft tube and/or island flap

54336   One stage perineal hypospadias repair requiring extensive dissection to correct chordee and urethroplasty by use of skin graft tube and/or island flap

54340   Repair of hypospadias complications (ie, fistula, stricture, diverticula); by closure, incision, or excision, simple

54344   requiring mobilization of skin flaps and urethroplasty with flap or patch graft

54348   requiring extensive dissection and urethroplasty with flap, patch or tubed graft (includes urinary diversion)

54352   Repair of hypospadias cripple requiring extensive dissection and excision of previously constructed structures including re-release of chordee and reconstruction of urethra and penis by use of local skin as grafts and island flaps and skin brought in as flaps or grafts

54360   Plastic operation on penis to correct angulation

54380   Plastic operation on penis for epispadias distal to external sphincter;

54385   with incontinence

54390   with exstrophy of bladder

54400   Insertion of penile prosthesis; non-inflatable (semi-rigid)

54401   inflatable (self-contained)

54402   Removal or replacement of non-inflatable (semi-rigid) or inflatable (self-contained) penile prosthesis

54405   Insertion of inflatable (multi-component) penile prosthesis, including placement of pump, cylinders, and/or reservoir

54407   Removal, repair, or replacement of inflatable (multi-component) penile prosthesis, including pump and/or reservoir and/or cylinders

54409   Surgical correction of hydraulic abnormality of inflatable (multi-component) prosthesis including pump and/or reservoir and/or cylinders

54420   Corpora cavernosa-saphenous vein shunt (priapism operation), unilateral or bilateral

54430   Corpora cavernosa-corpus spongiosum shunt (priapism operation), unilateral or bilateral

54435 Corpora cavernosa-glans penis fistulization (eg, biopsy needle, Winter procedure, rongeur, or punch) for priapism

54440 Plastic operation of penis for injury

Manipulation

54450 Foreskin manipulation including lysis of preputial adhesions and stretching

Testis

Excision

54500 Biopsy of testis, needle (separate procedure)

(For fine needle aspiration, preparation, and interpretation of smears, see 88170-88173)

54505 Biopsy of testis, incisional (separate procedure)

(When combined with vasogram, seminal vesiculogram, or epididymogram, see 55300)

(54506 has been deleted. To report, use 54505 with modifier -50 or 09950)

54510 Excision of local lesion of testis

54520 Orchiectomy, simple (including subcapsular), with or without testicular prosthesis, scrotal or inguinal approach

(54521 has been deleted. To report, use 54520 with modifier -50 or 09950)

54530 Orchiectomy, radical, for tumor; inguinal approach

54535 with abdominal exploration

(For orchiectomy with repair of hernia, see 49505 or 49507 and 54520)

(For radical retroperitoneal lymphadenectomy, see 38780)

54550 Exploration for undescended testis (inguinal or scrotal area)

(54555 has been deleted. To report, use 54550 with modifier -50 or 09950)

54560 Exploration for undescended testis with abdominal exploration

(54565 has been deleted. To report, use 54560 with modifier -50 or 09950)

Repair

54600 Reduction of torsion of testis, surgical, with or without fixation of contralateral testis

54620 Fixation of contralateral testis (separate procedure)

54640 Orchiopexy, inguinal approach, with or without hernia repair

(54641 has been deleted. To report, use 54640 with modifier -50 or 09950)

(54645 has been deleted)

54650 Orchiopexy, abdominal approach, for intra-abdominal testis (eg, Fowler-Stephens)

54660 Insertion of testicular prosthesis (separate procedure)

(54661 has been deleted. To report, use 54660 with modifier -50 or 09950)

54670 Suture or repair of testicular injury

54680 Transplantation of testis(es) to thigh (because of scrotal destruction)

Epididymis

Incision

54700 Incision and drainage of epididymis, testis and/or scrotal space (eg, abscess or hematoma)

Excision

54800 Biopsy of epididymis, needle

(For fine needle aspiration, preparation, and interpretation of smears, see 88170-88173)

54820 Exploration of epididymis, with or without biopsy

54830 Excision of local lesion of epididymis

54840 Excision of spermatocele, with or without epididymectomy

54860 Epididymectomy; unilateral

54861   bilateral

Repair

54900 Epididymovasostomy, anastomosis of epididymis to vas deferens; unilateral

54901   bilateral

(For microsurgical repair with use of operating microscope, add modifier -20 or 09920)

Tunica Vaginalis

Incision

55000* Puncture aspiration of hydrocele, tunica vaginalis, with or without injection of medication

Excision

55040 Excision of hydrocele; unilateral

55041   bilateral

(With hernia repair, see 49495-49501)

Repair

55060 Repair of tunica vaginalis hydrocele (Bottle type)

Scrotum

Incision

55100* Drainage of scrotal wall abscess

(See also 54700)

55110 Scrotal exploration

55120 Removal of foreign body in scrotum

Excision

(For excision of local lesion of skin of scrotum, see Integumentary System)

55150 Resection of scrotum

Repair

(55170 has been deleted. To report, see 55175, 55180)

55175 Scrotoplasty; simple

55180   complicated

Vas Deferens

Incision

55200 Vasotomy, cannulization with or without incision of vas, unilateral or bilateral (separate procedure)

Excision

55250 Vasectomy, unilateral or bilateral (separate procedure), including postoperative semen examination(s)

Introduction

55300 Vasotomy for vasograms, seminal vesiculograms, or epididymograms, unilateral or bilateral

(For radiological supervision and interpretation, see 74440)

(When combined with biopsy of testis, see 54505 and use modifier -51 or 09951)

Repair

55400 Vasovasostomy, vasovasorrhaphy

(55401 has been deleted. To report, use 55400 with modifier -50 or 09950)

(For microsurgical repair with use of operating microscope, add modifier -20 or 09920)

Suture

55450   Ligation (percutaneous) of vas deferens, unilateral or bilateral (separate procedure)

Spermatic Cord

Excision

55500   Excision of hydrocele of spermatic cord, unilateral (separate procedure)

55520   Excision of lesion of spermatic cord (separate procedure)

55530   Excision of varicocele or ligation of spermatic veins for varicocele; (separate procedure)

55535   abdominal approach

55540   with hernia repair

Seminal Vesicles

Incision

55600   Vesiculotomy;

(55601 has been deleted. To report, use 55600 with modifier -50 or 09950)

55605   complicated

Excision

55650   Vesiculectomy, any approach

(55651 has been deleted. To report, use 55650 with modifier -50 or 09950)

55680   Excision of Mullerian duct cyst

(For injection procedure, see 52010, 55300)

Prostate

Incision

55700   Biopsy, prostate; needle or punch, single or multiple, any approach

(For fine needle aspiration, preparation, and interpretation of smears, see 88170-88173)

55705   incisional, any approach

55720   Prostatotomy, external drainage of prostatic abscess, any approach; simple

55725   complicated

(For transurethral drainage, see 52700)

(55740 has been deleted. To report, use 55899)

Excision

(For transurethral removal of prostate, see 52601-52640)

(For limited pelvic lymphadenectomy for staging (separate procedure), use 38562)

(For independent node dissection, see 38770-38780)

55801   Prostatectomy, perineal, subtotal (including control of postoperative bleeding, vasectomy, meatotomy, urethral calibration and/or dilation, and internal urethrotomy)

55810   Prostatectomy, perineal radical;

55812   with lymph node biopsy(s) (limited pelvic lymphadenectomy)

55815   with bilateral pelvic lymphadenectomy, including external iliac, hypogastric and obturator nodes

(If 55815 is carried out on separate days, use 38770 with modifier -50 and 55810)

55821   Prostatectomy (including control of post-operative bleeding, vasectomy, meatotomy, urethral calibration and/or dilation, and internal urethrotomy); suprapubic, subtotal, one or two stages

55831   retropubic, subtotal

55840   Prostatectomy, retropubic radical, with or without nerve sparing;

55842   with lymph node biopsy(s) (limited pelvic lymphadenectomy)

55845   with bilateral pelvic lymphadenectomy, including external iliac, hypogastric, and obturator nodes

---

(If 55845 is carried out on separate days, use 38770 with modifier -50 and 55840)

●**55859**   Transperineal placement of needles or catheters into prostate for interstitial radioelement application, with or without cystoscopy

(For interstitial radioelement application, see 77776-77778)

(For ultrasonic guidance for interstitial radioelement application, see 76965)

55860   Exposure of prostate, any approach, for insertion of radioactive substance;

(For application of interstital radioelement, see 77776-77778)

55862   with lymph node biopsy(s) (limited pelvic lymphadenectomy)

55865   with bilateral pelvic lymphadenectomy, including external iliac, hypogastric and obturator nodes

Other Procedures

(For artificial insemination, see 58310, 58311)

55870   Electroejaculation

55899   Unlisted procedure, male genital system

Intersex Surgery

55970   Intersex surgery; male to female

55980   female to male

Laparoscopy/ Peritoneoscopy/ Hysteroscopy

The endoscopic descriptors in this publication are listed so that the main procedure can easily be identified without having to list all the minor related procedures that may be performed at the same time (such as lysis of adhesions and fulguration of bleeding points during laparoscopy with fulguration transection of the oviducts). When the laparoscopy requires mini-laparotomy (Hasson technique) or when secondary procedures involve significant additonal time and effort, they may be reported by using either modifier '-22' or code 09922.

Operative laparoscopy and hysteroscopy may utilize many methods to accomplish the same result (eg, hot cautry, CO_2 laser, ND-YAG laser, pelvioscopy). The CPT code is the same regardless of which technique is employed to achieve the desired result.

The use of these codes is not restricted to female patients. Certain procedures (eg, laparoscopy with biopsy) may be performed on either male or female patients.

For peritoneoscopy, see 56360-56363.

56300	Laparoscopy, diagnostic (separate procedure)
56301	Laparoscopy, surgical; with fulguration of oviducts (with or without transection)
56302	with occlusion of oviducts by device (eg, band, clip, or Falope ring)
56303	with fulguration or excision of lesions of the ovary, pelvic viscera, or peritoneal surface by any method
56304	with lysis of adhesions
56305	with biopsy of peritoneal surface(s), single or multiple
56306	with aspiration (single or multiple)
56307	with removal of adnexal structures (partial or total oophorectomy and/or salpingectomy)

56308	with vaginal hysterectomy with or without removal of tube(s), with or without removal of ovary(s) (laparoscopic assisted vaginal hysterectomy)
56309	with removal of leiomyomata, subserosal (single or multiple)
56311	with retroperitoneal lymph node sampling (biopsy), single or multiple
56312	with bilateral total pelvic lymphadenectomy
56313	with bilateral total pelvic lymphadenectomy and peri-aortic lymph node sampling (biopsy), single or multiple
56315	appendectomy
56316	repair of initial inguinal hernia
56317	repair of recurrent inguinal hernia
56320	with ligation of spermatic veins for varicocele
56322	transection of vagus nerves, truncal
56323	transection of vagus nerves, selective or highly selective
56324	cholecystoenterostomy
56340	cholecystectomy (any method)
56341	cholecystectomy with cholangiography
56342	cholecystectomy with exploration of common duct
●56343	with salpingostomy (salpingoneostomy)
●56344	with fimbrioplasty

(Codes 56343 and 56344 are used to report unilateral procedures unless otherwise specified)

56350	Hysteroscopy, diagnostic (separate procedure)
56351	Hysteroscopy, surgical; with sampling (biopsy) of endometrium and/or polypectomy, with or without D & C
56352	with lysis of intrauterine adhesions (any method)

56353   with division or resection of intrauterine septum (any method)

56354   with removal of leiomyomata

56355   with removal of impacted foreign body

56356   with endometrial ablation (any method)

56360   Peritoneoscopy; without biopsy

56361   with biopsy

56362   Peritoneoscopy with guided transhepatic cholangiography; without biopsy

56363   with biopsy

Other Procedures

56399   Unlisted procedure, laparoscopy, peritoneoscopy, hysteroscopy

Female Genital System

(For pelvic laparotomy, see 49000)

(For excision or destruction of endometriomas, open method, see 49200, 49201)

(For paracentesis, see 49080, 49081)

(For secondary closure of abdominal wall evisceration or disruption, see 49900)

(For fulguration or excision of lesions, laparoscopic approach, see 56303)

(For chemotherapy, see 96400-96549)

(56000 has been deleted. To report, see 56405)

(56100 has been deleted. To report, see 56605)

(56200 has been deleted. To report, see 56810)

Vulva, Perineum and Introitus

Definitions

The following definitions apply to the vulvectomy codes (56620-56640).

A simple procedure is the removal of skin and superficial subcutaneous tissues.

A radical procedure is the removal of skin and deep subcutaneous tissue.

A partial procedure is the removal of less than 80% of the vulvar area.

A complete procedure is the removal of greater than 80% of the vulvar area.

Incision

(For incision and drainage of sebaceous cyst, furuncle, or abscess, see 10040, 10060, 10061)

(56400 has been deleted. To report, see 56405)

56405* Incision and drainage of vulva or perineal abscess

56420* Incision and drainage of Bartholin's gland abscess

(For incision and drainage of Skene's gland abscess or cyst, see 53060)

56440 Marsupialization of Bartholin's gland cyst

56441 Lysis of labial adhesions

Destruction

(56500 has been deleted. To report, use 56501)

56501 Destruction of lesion(s), vulva; simple, any method

(56505-56507, 56510 have been deleted. To report, use 56501)

56515 extensive, any method

(56520, 56521 have been deleted. To report, use 56501 or 56515)

(For destruction of Skene's gland cyst or abscess, see 53270)

(For cautery destruction of urethral caruncle, see 53265)

Excision

(56600 has been deleted. To report, see 56605)

56605* Biopsy of vulva or perineum (separate procedure); one lesion

56606* each separate additional lesion

(For excision of local lesion, see 11420-11426, 11620-11626)

56620 Vulvectomy simple; partial

56625 complete

(For skin graft, see 15000 et seq)

56630 Vulvectomy, radical, partial;

(For skin graft, if used, see 15000, 15120, 15121, 15240, 15241)

▲=Revised Code   ●=New Code   ✱=Service Includes Surgical Procedure Only

Female Genital
56405—58999

56631   with unilateral inguinofemoral lymphadenectomy

56632   with bilateral inguinofemoral lymphadenectomy

56633   Vulvectomy, radical, complete;

56634   with unilateral inguinofemoral lymphadenectomy

(56635 has been deleted. To report, see 56634, 56637)

(56636 has been deleted. To report, see 56634, 56637)

56637   with bilateral inguinofemoral lymphadenectomy

56640   Vulvectomy, radical, complete, with inguinofemoral, iliac, and pelvic lymphadenectomy

(56641 has been deleted. To report, use 56640 with modifier -50 or 09950)

(For lymphadenectomy, see 38760-38780)

(56680, 56685 have been deleted)

56700   Partial hymenectomy or revision of hymenal ring

(56710 has been deleted. To report, see 56700)

56720*   Hymenotomy, simple incision

56740   Excision of Bartholin's gland or cyst

(For excision of Skene's gland, see 53270)

(For excision of urethral caruncle, see 53265)

(For excision or fulguration of urethral carcinoma, see 53220)

(For excision or marsupialization of urethral diverticulum, see 53230, 53240)

Repair

(For repair of urethra for mucosal prolapse, see 53275)

56800   Plastic repair of introitus

56805   Clitoroplasty for intersex state

56810   Perineoplasty, repair of perineum, nonobstetrical (separate procedure)

(See also 56800)

(For repair of wounds to genitalia, see 12001-12007, 12041-12047, 13131, 13132)

(For repair of recent injury of vagina and perineum, nonobstetrical, see 57210)

(For anal sphincteroplasty, see 46750, 46751)

(For episiorrhaphy, episioperineorrhaphy for recent injury of vulva and/or perineum, nonobstetrical, see 57210)

Vagina

Incision

57000   Colpotomy; with exploration

57010   with drainage of pelvic abscess

57020*   Colpocentesis (separate procedure)

Destruction

(57050, 57057, 57060 have been deleted. To report, use 57061 or 57065)

57061   Destruction of vaginal lesion(s); simple, any method

(57063 has been deleted. To report, use 57061 or 57065)

57065   extensive, any method

Excision

57100*   Biopsy of vaginal mucosa; simple (separate procedure)

57105   extensive, requiring suture (including cysts)

57108   Colpectomy, obliteration of vagina; partial

57110   complete

57120   Colpocleisis (Le Fort type)

57130   Excision of vaginal septum

57135   Excision of vaginal cyst or tumor

Introduction

57150*   Irrigation of vagina and/or application of medicament for treatment of bacterial, parasitic, or fungoid disease

57160*   Insertion of pessary

57170   Diaphragm or cervical cap fitting with instructions

57180   Introduction of any hemostatic agent or pack for spontaneous or traumatic nonobstetrical vaginal hemorrhage (separate procedure)

Repair

(For urethral suspension, Marshall-Marchetti-Krantz type, abdominal approach, see 51840, 51841)

57200   Colporrhaphy, suture of injury of vagina (nonobstetrical)

57210   Colpoperineorrhaphy, suture of injury of vagina and/or perineum (nonobstetrical)

57220   Plastic operation on urethral sphincter, vaginal approach (eg, Kelly urethral plication)

57230   Plastic repair of urethrocele

57240   Anterior colporrhaphy, repair of cystocele with or without repair of urethrocele

57250   Posterior colporrhaphy, repair of rectocele with or without perineorrhaphy

(For repair of rectocele (separate procedure) without posterior colporrhaphy, see 45560)

57260   Combined anteroposterior colporrhaphy;

57265   with enterocele repair

57268   Repair of enterocele, vaginal approach (separate procedure)

57270   Repair of enterocele, abdominal approach (separate procedure)

57280   Colpopexy, abdominal approach

57282   Sacrospinous ligament fixation for prolapse of vagina

●**57284**   Paravaginal defect repair (including repair of cystocele, stress urinary incontinence, and/or incomplete vaginal prolapse)

57288   Sling operation for stress incontinence (eg, fascia or synthetic)

57289   Pereyra procedure, including anterior colporrhaphy

(57290 has been deleted. To report, use 57291, 57292)

57291   Construction of artificial vagina; without graft

57292   with graft

57300   Closure of rectovaginal fistula; vaginal or transanal approach

57305   abdominal approach

57307   abdominal approach, with concomitant colostomy

57310   Closure of urethrovaginal fistula;

57311   with bulbocavernosus transplant

57320   Closure of vesicovaginal fistula; vaginal approach

(For concomitant cystostomy, see 51005-51040)

57330   transvesical and vaginal approach

(For abdominal approach, see 51900)

57335   Vaginoplasty for intersex state

Manipulation

57400*   Dilation of vagina under anesthesia

57410*   Pelvic examination under anesthesia

57415   Removal of impacted vaginal foreign body (separate procedure) under anesthesia

(For removal without anesthesia of an impacted vaginal foreign body, use the appropriate evaluation and management code)

Endoscopy

(57450, 57451 have been deleted)

57452* Colposcopy (vaginoscopy); (separate procedure)

57454* with biopsy(s) of the cervix and/or endocervical curettage

57460 with loop electrode excision procedure of the cervix

Cervix Uteri

Excision

(For radical surgical procedures, see 58200-58240)

57500* Biopsy, single or multiple, or local excision of lesion, with or without fulguration (separate procedure)

57505 Endocervical curettage (not done as part of a dilation and curettage)

57510 Cauterization of cervix; electro or thermal

57511* cryocautery, initial or repeat

57513 laser ablation

57520 Conization of cervix, with or without fulguration, with or without dilation and curettage, with or without repair; cold knife or laser

(See also 58120)

57522 loop electrode excision

57530 Trachelectomy (cervicectomy), amputation of cervix (separate procedure)

57540 Excision of cervical stump, abdominal approach;

57545 with pelvic floor repair

57550 Excision of cervical stump, vaginal approach;

57555 with anterior and/or posterior repair

57556 with repair of enterocele

(For insertion of intrauterine device, see 58300)

(57600-57620 have been deleted. For insertion of any hemostatic agent or pack for control of spontaneous non-obstetrical hemorrhage, see 57180)

Repair

57700 Cerclage of uterine cervix, nonobstetrical

57720 Trachelorrhaphy, plastic repair of uterine cervix, vaginal approach

Manipulation

57800* Dilation of cervical canal, instrumental (separate procedure)

57820 Dilation and curettage of cervical stump

Corpus Uteri

Excision

▲**58100*** Endometrial sampling (biopsy) with or without endocervical sampling (biopsy), without cervical dilation, any method (separate procedure)

(For endocervical curettage only, see 57505)

(58101, 58102, 58103 have been deleted)

58120 Dilation and curettage, diagnostic and/or therapeutic (nonobstetrical)

(For postpartum hemorrhage, see 59160)

58140 Myomectomy, excision of fibroid tumor of uterus, single or multiple (separate procedure); abdominal approach

58145 vaginal approach

58150 Total abdominal hysterectomy (corpus and cervix), with or without removal of tube(s), with or without removal of ovary(s);

58152 with colpo-urethrocystopexy (Marshall-Marchetti-Krantz type)

(For urethrocystopexy without hysterectomy, see 51840, 51841)

58180 Supracervical abdominal hysterectomy (subtotal hysterectomy), with or without removal of tube(s), with or without removal of ovary(s)

58200 Total abdominal hysterectomy, including partial vaginectomy, with para-aortic and pelvic lymph node sampling, with or without removal of tube(s), with or without removal of ovary(s)

(58205 has been deleted. For hysterectomy with pelvic lymphadenectomy, use 58210)

58210 Radical abdominal hysterectomy, with bilateral total pelvic lymphadenectomy and para-aortic lymph node sampling (biopsy), with or without removal of tube(s), with or without removal of ovary(s)

(For radical hysterectomy with ovarian transposition, use also 58825)

58240 Pelvic exenteration for gynecologic malignancy, with total abdominal hysterectomy or cervicectomy, with or without removal of tube(s), with or without removal of ovary(s), with removal of bladder and ureteral transplantations, and/or abdominoperineal resection of rectum and colon and colostomy, or any combination thereof

(For pelvic exenteration for lower urinary tract or male genital malignancy, use 51597)

58260 Vaginal hysterectomy;

58262 with removal of tube(s), and/or ovary(s)

58263 with removal of tube(s), and/or ovary(s), with repair of enterocele

(58265 has been deleted. To report, see 57240, 57250, 57260, 57265)

58267 with colpo-urethrocystopexy (Marshall-Marchetti-Krantz type, Pereyra type, with or without endoscopic control)

58270 with repair of enterocele

(For repair of enterocele with removal of tubes and/or ovaries, see 58263)

58275 Vaginal hysterectomy, with total or partial colpectomy;

58280 with repair of enterocele

58285 Vaginal hysterectomy, radical (Schauta type operation)

Introduction

(For insertion/removal of implantable contraceptive capsules, see 11975, 11976, 11977)

58300* Insertion of intrauterine device (IUD)

58301 Removal of intrauterine device (IUD)

(58310 has been deleted. To report, see 58321, 58322)

(58311 has been deleted. To report, see 58323)

(58320 has been deleted)

58321 Artificial insemination; intra-cervical

58322 intra-uterine

58323 Sperm washing for artificial insemination

58340* Injection procedure for hysterosalpingography

(For radiological supervision and interpretation, see 74740)

58345 Transcervical introduction of fallopian tube catheter for diagnosis and/or re-establishing patency (any method), with or without hysterosalpingography

(For radiological supervision and interpretation, see 74742)

58350* Chromotubation of oviduct, including materials

(For materials supplied by physician, see 99070)

Repair

58400 Uterine suspension, with or without shortening of round ligaments, with or without shortening of sacrouterine ligaments; (separate procedure)

58410 with presacral sympathectomy

(58430 has been deleted. To report, use 58999)

▲=Revised Code   ●=New Code   *=Service Includes Surgical Procedure Only

(58500 has been deleted. To report, use 58752)

58520   Hysterorrhaphy, repair of ruptured uterus (nonobstetrical)

58540   Hysteroplasty, repair of uterine anomaly (Strassman type)

(For closure of vesicouterine fistula, see 51920)

Oviduct

Incision

58600   Ligation or transection of fallopian tube(s), abdominal or vaginal approach, unilateral or bilateral

58605   Ligation or transection of fallopian tube(s), abdominal or vaginal approach, postpartum, unilateral or bilateral, during same hospitalization (separate procedure)

(For laparoscopic procedures, see 56301, 56302)

(58610 has been deleted. To report, see 58600-58611)

58611   Ligation or transection of fallopian tube(s) when done at the time of cesarean section or intra-abdominal surgery (not a separate procedure)

58615   Occlusion of fallopian tube(s) by device (eg, band, clip, Falope ring) vaginal or suprapubic approach

(For laparoscopic approach, see 56302)

(58618 has been deleted. To report, use 58740)

Excision

58700   Salpingectomy, complete or partial, unilateral or bilateral (separate procedure)

58720   Salpingo-oophorectomy, complete or partial, unilateral or bilateral (separate procedure)

Repair

58740   Lysis of adhesions (salpingolysis, ovariolysis)

(For laparascopic approach, see 56304)

(For excision or destruction of endometriomas, open method, see 49200, 49201)

(For fulguration or excision of lesions, laparoscopic approach, see 56303)

58750   Tubotubal anastomosis

58752   Tubouterine implantation

58760   Fimbrioplasty

58770   Salpingostomy (salpingoneostomy)

Ovary

Incision

58800   Drainage of ovarian cyst(s), unilateral or bilateral, (separate procedure); vaginal approach

58805   abdominal approach

58820   Drainage of ovarian abscess; vaginal approach

58822   abdominal approach

58825   Transposition, ovary(s)

Excision

58900   Biopsy of ovary, unilateral or bilateral (separate procedure)

58920   Wedge resection or bisection of ovary, unilateral or bilateral

58925   Ovarian cystectomy, unilateral or bilateral

58940   Oophorectomy, partial or total, unilateral or bilateral;

(58942 has been deleted. To report, use 58952)

58943   for ovarian malignancy, with para-aortic
            and pelvic lymph node biopsies, peritoneal
            washings, peritoneal biopsies, diaphrag-
            matic assessments, with or without
            salpingectomy(s), with or without
            omentectomy

            (58945 has been deleted. To report, use
            58950)

58950   Resection of ovarian malignancy with bilateral
            salpingo-oophorectomy and omentectomy;

58951   with total abdominal hysterectomy, pelvic
            and limited para-aortic lymphadenectomy

58952   with radical dissection for debulking

58960   Laparotomy, for staging or restaging of ovarian
            malignancy ("second look"), with or without
            omentectomy, peritoneal washing, biopsy of
            abdominal and pelvic peritoneum, diaphrag-
            matic assessment with pelvic and limited
            para-aortic lymphadenectomy

In Vitro Fertilization

58970   Follicle puncture for oocyte retrieval, any
            method

            (For radiological supervision and
            interpretation, see 76948)

            (58972 has been deleted. To report, see
            89250)

▲**58974**   Embryo transfer, intrauterine

▲**58976**   Gamete, zygote, or embryo intrafallopian
            transfer, any method

            (58980 has been deleted. To report, see
            56300)

            (58982 has been deleted. To report, see
            56301)

            (58983 has been deleted. To report, see
            56302)

            (58984 has been deleted. To report, see
            56303)

            (58985 has been deleted. To report, see
            56304)

            (58986 has been deleted. To report, see
            56305)

            (58987 has been deleted. To report, see
            56306)

            (58988 has been deleted. To report, see
            56307)

            (58990 has been deleted. To report, see
            56350)

            (58992 has been deleted. To report, see
            56352 and 56353)

            (58994 has been deleted. To report, see
            56354)

            (58995 has been deleted. To report, see
            56352, 56354, 56356)

            (58996 has been deleted. To report, see
            56356)

Other Procedures

58999   Unlisted procedure, female genital system
            (nonobstetrical)

▲=Revised Code   ●=New Code   ✱=Service Includes Surgical Procedure Only

Maternity Care and Delivery

The services normally provided in uncomplicated maternity cases include antepartum care, delivery, and postpartum care.

Antepartum care includes the initial and subsequent history, physical examinations, recording of weight, blood pressures, fetal heart tones, routine chemical urinalysis, and monthly visits up to 28 weeks gestation, biweekly visits to 36 weeks gestation, and weekly visits until delivery. Any other visits or services within this time period should be coded separately.

Delivery services include admission to the hospital, the admission history and physical examination, management of uncomplicated labor, vaginal delivery (with or without episiotomy, with or without forceps), or cesarean delivery. Medical problems complicating labor and delivery management may require additional resources and should be identified by utilizing the codes in the **Medicine** and **Evaluation and Management Services** section in addition to codes for maternity care.

Postpartum care includes hospital and office visits following vaginal or cesarean section delivery.

For medical complications of pregnancy (eg, cardiac problems, neurological problems, diabetes, hypertension, toxemia, hyperemesis, pre-term labor, premature rupture of membranes), see services in the **Medicine** and **Evaluation and Management Services** section. For surgical complications of pregnancy (eg, appendectomy, hernia, ovarian cyst, Bartholin cyst), see services in the **Surgery** section.

If a physician provides all or part of the antepartum and/or postpartum patient care but does not perform delivery due to termination of pregnancy by abortion or referral to another physician for delivery, see the antepartum and postpartum care codes 59425-59426 and 59430.

(For circumcision of newborn, see 54150, 54160)

Incision

59000* Amniocentesis, any method

(For radiological supervision and interpretation, see 76946)

(59010, 59011 have been deleted)

59012 Cordocentesis (intrauterine), any method

(For radiological supervision and interpretation, see 76941)

59015 Chorionic villus sampling, any method

(For radiological supervision and interpretation, see 76945)

59020* Fetal contraction stress test

59025 Fetal non-stress test

59030* Fetal scalp blood sampling

(59031 has been deleted. To report, use 59030 and see modifiers -76 and -77)

59050 Fetal monitoring during labor by consulting physician (ie, non-attending physician) with written report (separate procedure); supervision and interpretation

59051 interpretation only

59100 Hysterotomy, abdominal (eg, for hydatidiform mole, abortion)

(When tubal ligation is performed at the same time as hysterotomy, use 58611 in addition to 59100)

(59101, 59105, 59106 have been deleted. To report, see 59100, 58611)

Excision

59120 Surgical treatment of ectopic pregnancy; tubal or ovarian, requiring salpingectomy and/or oophorectomy, abdominal or vaginal approach

59121 tubal or ovarian, without salpingectomy and/or oophorectomy

(59125, 59126 have been deleted. To report, see 59120, 59121)

59130 abdominal pregnancy

59135 interstitial, uterine pregnancy requiring total hysterectomy

59136   interstitial, uterine pregnancy with partial resection of uterus

59140   cervical, with evacuation

59150   Laparoscopic treatment of ectopic pregnancy; without salpingectomy and/or oophorectomy

59151   with salpingectomy and/or oophorectomy

59160   Curettage, postpartum (separate procedure)

Introduction

(For intrauterine fetal transfusion, see 36460)

(For introduction of hypertonic solution and/or prostaglandins to initiate labor, see 59850–59857)

59200   Insertion of cervical dilator (eg, laminaria, prostaglandin) (separate procedure)

Repair

(For tracheloplasty, see 57700)

59300   Episiotomy or vaginal repair, by other than attending physician

(59305 has been deleted)

59320   Cerclage of cervix, during pregnancy; vaginal

59325   abdominal

59350   Hysterorrhaphy of ruptured uterus

(59351 has been deleted)

Vaginal Delivery, Antepartum and Postpartum Care

59400   Routine obstetric care including antepartum care, vaginal delivery (with or without episiotomy, and/or forceps) and postpartum care

59409   Vaginal delivery only (with or without episiotomy and/or forceps);

59410   including postpartum care

59412   External cephalic version, with or without tocolysis (list in addition to code(s) for delivery)

59414   Delivery of placenta (separate procedure)

(59420 has been deleted. To report, see 59425, 59426 or appropriate **Evaluation and Management** code(s))

(For 1-3 antepartum care visits, see appropriate **Evaluation and Management** code(s))

59425   Antepartum care only; 4-6 visits

59426   7 or more visits

59430   Postpartum care only (separate procedure)

Cesarean Delivery

(For standby attendance for infant, use 99360)

(59500, 59501 have been deleted. To report, see 59510, 59515, 59525)

59510   Routine obstetric care including antepartum care, cesarean delivery, and postpartum care

59514   Cesarean delivery only;

59515   including postpartum care

(59520, 59521 have been deleted. To report, see 59510, 59515, 59525)

59525   Subtotal or total hysterectomy after cesarean delivery (list in addition to 59510 or 59515)

(59540, 59541, 59560, 59561, 59580, 59581 have been deleted. To report, see 59510, 59515, 59525)

Delivery After Previous Cesarean Delivery

Patients who have had a previous cesarean delivery and now present with the expectation of a vaginal delivery are coded using codes 59610-59622. If the patient has a successful vaginal delivery after a previous cesarean delivery (VBAC), use codes 59610-59614. If the attempt is unsuccessful and another cesarean delivery is carried out, use codes 59618-59622. To report elective cesarean deliveries use code 59510, 59514 or 59515.

●**59610**   Routine obstetric care including antepartum care, vaginal delivery (with or without episiotomy, and/or forceps) and postpartum care, after previous cesarean delivery

● **59612**   Vaginal delivery only, after previous cesarean delivery (with or without episiotomy and/or forceps);

● **59614**   including postpartum care

● **59618**   Routine obstetric care including antepartum care, cesarean delivery, and postpartum care, following attempted vaginal delivery after previous cesarean delivery

● **59620**   Cesarean delivery only, following attempted vaginal delivery after previous cesarean delivery;

● **59622**   including postpartum care

Abortion

(For medical treatment of spontaneous complete abortion, any trimester, use Evaluation and Management codes 99201-99233)

(59800, 59810 have been deleted. To report, see 99201-99233)

(59801, 59811 have been deleted. To report, see 59812)

59812   Treatment of incomplete abortion, any trimester, completed surgically

59820   Treatment of missed abortion, completed surgically; first trimester

59821   second trimester

59830   Treatment of septic abortion, completed surgically

59840   Induced abortion, by dilation and curettage

59841   Induced abortion, by dilation and evacuation

59850   Induced abortion, by one or more intra-amniotic injections (amniocentesis-injections), including hospital admission and visits, delivery of fetus and secundines;

59851   with dilation and curettage and/or evacuation

59852   with hysterotomy (failed intra-amniotic injection)

(For insertion of cervical dilator, see 59200)

59855   Induced abortion, by one or more vaginal suppositories (eg, prostaglandin) with or without cervical dilation (eg, laminaria), including hospital admission and visits, delivery of fetus and secundines;

59856   with dilation and curettage and/or evacuation

59857   with hysterotomy (failed medical evacuation)

Other Procedures

59870   Uterine evacuation and curettage for hydatidiform mole

59899   Unlisted procedure, maternity care and delivery

Endocrine System

(For pituitary and pineal surgery, see Nervous System)

Thyroid Gland

Incision

60000* Incision and drainage of thyroglossal cyst, infected

Excision

60001 Aspiration and/or injection, thyroid cyst

(For fine needle aspiration, see 88170, 88171)

60100* Biopsy thyroid, percutaneous core needle

(For radiological supervision and interpretation, see 76360, 76942)

(For fine needle aspiration, preparation, and interpretation of smears, see 88170-88173)

60200 Excision of cyst or adenoma of thyroid, or transection of isthmus

60210 Partial thyroid lobectomy, unilateral; with or without isthmusectomy

(For fine needle aspiration, see 88170, 88171)

60212 with contralateral subtotal lobectomy, including isthmusectomy

(For fine needle aspiration, see 88170, 88171)

60220 Total thyroid lobectomy, unilateral; with or without isthmusectomy

60225 with contralateral subtotal lobectomy, including isthmusectomy

60240 Thyroidectomy, total or complete

(60242 has been deleted. To report, see 60210-60225)

(60245 has been deleted. To report, see 60210-60225)

(60246 has been deleted. To report, use 60271)

60252 Thyroidectomy, total or subtotal for malignancy; with limited neck dissection

60254 with radical neck dissection

60260 Thyroidectomy, removal of all remaining thyroid tissue following previous removal of a portion of thyroid

(60261 has been deleted. To report, use 60260 with modifier -50 or 09950)

60270 Thyroidectomy, including substernal thyroid gland; sternal split or transthoracic approach

60271 cervical approach

60280 Excision of thyroglossal duct cyst or sinus;

60281 recurrent

(For thyroid ultrasonography, see 76536)

Parathyroid, Thymus, Adrenal Glands, and Carotid Body

Excision

(For pituitary and pineal surgery, see Nervous System)

60500 Parathyroidectomy or exploration of parathyroid(s);

60502 re-exploration

60505 with mediastinal exploration, sternal split or transthoracic approach

(60510 has been deleted)

60512 Parathyroid autotransplantation

60520 Thymectomy, partial or total; transcervical approach (separate procedure)

60521 sternal split or transthoracic approach, without radical mediastinal dissection (separate procedure)

60522 sternal split or transthoracic approach, with radical mediastinal dissection (separate procedure)

Endocrine/Nervous 60000–64999

60540 Adrenalectomy, partial or complete, or exploration of adrenal gland with or without biopsy, transabdominal, lumbar or dorsal (separate procedure);

60545   with excision of adjacent retroperitoneal tumor

(For excision of remote or disseminated pheochromocytoma, see 49200, 49201)

(60550, 60555 have been deleted. To report, use 60540 with modifier -50 or 09950)

60600 Excision of carotid body tumor; without excision of carotid artery

60605   with excision of carotid artery

Other Procedures

60699 Unlisted procedure, endocrine system

Nervous System

Skull, Meninges, and Brain

(For injection procedure for cerebral angiography, see 36100-36218)

(For injection procedure for ventriculography, see 61026, 61120, 61130)

(For injection procedure for pneumo-encephalography, see 61055)

Injection, Drainage, or Aspiration

61000* Subdural tap through fontanelle, or suture, infant, unilateral or bilateral; initial

61001* subsequent taps

61020* Ventricular puncture through previous burr hole, fontanelle, suture, or implanted ventricular catheter/reservoir; without injection

(61025 has been deleted. To report, use 61026)

61026* with injection of drug or other substance for diagnosis or treatment

(61030, 61045 have been deleted. To report, use 61026)

61050* Cisternal or lateral cervical (C1-C2) puncture; without injection (separate procedure)

(61051, 61052, 61053 have been deleted. To report, use 61055)

61055* with injection of drug or other substance for diagnosis or treatment (eg, C1-C2)

(For radiological supervision and interpretation, see Radiology)

61070* Puncture of shunt tubing or reservoir for aspiration or injection procedure

(For radiological supervision and interpretation, see 75809)

Twist Drill, Burr Hole(s), or Trephine

61105* Twist drill hole for subdural or ventricular puncture; not followed by other surgery

61106 followed by other surgery

61107* for implanting ventricular catheter or pressure recording device

61108 for evacuation and/or drainage of subdural hematoma

61120 Burr hole(s) for ventricular puncture (including injection of gas, contrast media, dye, or radioactive material); not followed by other surgery

61130 followed by other surgery

61140 Burr hole(s) or trephine; with biopsy of brain or intracranial lesion

61150 with drainage of brain abscess or cyst

61151 with subsequent tapping (aspiration) of intracranial abscess or cyst

61154 Burr hole(s) with evacuation and/or drainage of hematoma, extradural or subdural

(61155 has been deleted. To report, use 61154 with modifier -50 or 09950)

61156 Burr hole(s); with aspiration of hematoma or cyst, intracerebral

61210* for implanting ventricular catheter, reservoir, EEG electrode(s) or pressure recording device (separate procedure)

61215 Insertion of subcutaneous reservoir, pump or continuous infusion system for connection to ventricular catheter

(For chemotherapy, see 96450)

61250 Burr hole(s) or trephine, supratentorial, exploratory, not followed by other surgery

(61251 has been deleted. To report, use 61250 with modifier -50 or 09950)

61253 Burr hole(s) or trephine, infratentorial, unilateral or bilateral

(If burr hole(s) or trephine are followed by craniotomy at same operative session, use 61304-61321; do not use 61250 or 61253)

Craniectomy or Craniotomy

61304 Craniectomy or craniotomy, exploratory; supratentorial

61305 infratentorial (posterior fossa)

(61310, 61311 have been deleted. To report, see 61312-61315)

61312 Craniectomy or craniotomy for evacuation of hematoma, supratentorial; extradural or subdural

61313 intracerebral

61314 Craniectomy or craniotomy for evacuation of hematoma, infratentorial; extradural or subdural

61315 intracerebellar

61320 Craniectomy or craniotomy, drainage of intracranial abscess; supratentorial

61321 infratentorial

61330 Decompression of orbit only, transcranial approach

(61331 has been deleted. To report, use 61330 with modifier -50 or 09950)

61332 Exploration of orbit (transcranial approach); with biopsy

61333 with removal of lesion

61334 with removal of foreign body

61340 Other cranial decompression (eg, subtemporal), supratentorial

(61341 has been deleted. To report, use 61340 with modifier -50 or 09950)

61343 Craniectomy, suboccipital with cervical laminectomy for decompression of medulla and spinal cord, with or without dural graft (eg, Arnold-Chiari malformation)

61345 Other cranial decompression, posterior fossa

(For orbital decompression by lateral wall approach, Kroenlein type, see 67445)

61440 Craniotomy for section of tentorium cerebelli (separate procedure)

61450 Craniectomy, subtemporal, for section, compression, or decompression of sensory root of gasserian ganglion

61458 Craniectomy, suboccipital; for exploration or decompression of cranial nerves

61460 for section of one or more cranial nerves

61470 for medullary tractotomy

61480 for mesencephalic tractotomy or pedunculotomy

61490 Craniotomy for lobotomy, including cingulotomy

(61491 has been deleted. To report, use 61490 with modifier -50 or 09950)

61500 Craniectomy; with excision of tumor or other bone lesion of skull

61501 for osteomyelitis

61510 Craniectomy, trephination, bone flap craniotomy; for excision of brain tumor, supratentorial, except meningioma

61512 for excision of meningioma, supratentorial

61514 for excision of brain abscess, supratentorial

61516 for excision or fenestration of cyst, supratentorial

(For excision of pituitary tumor or craniopharyngioma, see 61545, 61546, 61548)

61518 Craniectomy for excision of brain tumor, infratentorial or posterior fossa; except meningioma, cerebellopontine angle tumor, or midline tumor at base of skull

61519 meningioma

61520 cerebellopontine angle tumor

61521 midline tumor at base of skull

61522 Craniectomy, infratentorial or posterior fossa; for excision of brain abscess

61524   for excision or fenestration of cyst

61526   Craniectomy, bone flap craniotomy, transtemporal (mastoid) for excision of cerebellopontine angle tumor;

61530   combined with middle/posterior fossa craniotomy/craniectomy

61531   Subdural implantation of strip electrodes through one or more burr or trephine hole(s) for long term seizure monitoring

(For stereotactic implantation of electrodes, see 61760)

(61532 has been deleted. To report, see 61680-61692)

61533   Craniotomy with elevation of bone flap; for subdural implantation of an electrode array, for long term seizure monitoring

(For continuous EEG monitoring, see 95950-95954)

61534   for excision of epileptogenic focus without electrocorticography during surgery

61535   for removal of epidural or subdural electrode array, without excision of cerebral tissue (separate procedure)

61536   for excision of cerebral epileptogenic focus, with electrocorticography during surgery (includes removal of electrode array)

61538   for lobectomy with electrocorticography during surgery, temporal lobe

61539   for lobectomy with electrocorticography during surgery, other than temporal lobe, partial or total

61541   for transection of corpus callosum

61542   for total hemispherectomy

61543   for partial or subtotal hemispherectomy

61544   for excision or coagulation of choroid plexus

61545   for excision of craniopharyngioma

61546   Craniotomy for hypophysectomy or excision of pituitary tumor, intracranial approach

61548   Hypophysectomy or excision of pituitary tumor, transnasal or transseptal approach, nonstereotactic

61550   Craniectomy for craniosynostosis; single cranial suture

61552   multiple cranial sutures

(61553 has been deleted. To report, see 61552, 61558, 61559)

(61555 has been deleted. To report, see 21172-21180, 61552, 61558, 61559)

(For cranial reconstruction for orbital hypertelorism, see 21260-21263)

61556   Craniotomy for craniosynostosis; frontal or parietal bone flap

61557   bifrontal bone flap

61558   Extensive craniectomy for multiple cranial suture craniosynostosis (eg, cloverleaf skull); not requiring bone grafts

61559   recontouring with multiple osteotomies and bone autografts (eg, barrel-stave procedure) (includes obtaining grafts)

(61561 has been deleted. To report, see 21172-21180)

61563   Excision, intra and extracranial, benign tumor of cranial bone (eg, fibrous dysplasia); without optic nerve decompression

61564   with optic nerve decompression

(For reconstruction, see 21181-21183)

61570   Craniectomy or craniotomy; with excision of foreign body from brain

61571   with treatment of penetrating wound of brain

(For sequestrectomy for osteomyelitis, see 61501)

61575   Transoral approach to skull base, brain stem or upper spinal cord for biopsy, decompression or excision of lesion;

61576   requiring splitting of tongue and/or mandible (including tracheostomy)

(For arthrodesis, use 22548)

Surgery of Skull Base

The surgical management of lesions involving the skull base (base of anterior, middle, and posterior cranial fossae) often requires the skills of several surgeons of different surgical specialties working together or in tandem during the operative session. These operations are usually not staged because of the need for definitive closure of dura, subcutaneous tissues, and skin to avoid serious infections such as osteomyelitis and/or meningitis.

The procedures are categorized according to:
1) *approach procedure* necessary to obtain adequate exposure to the lesion (pathologic entity),
2) *definitive procedure(s)* necessary to biopsy, excise or otherwise treat the lesion, and
3) *repair/reconstruction* of the defect present following the definitive procedure(s).

The *approach procedure* is described according to anatomical area involved, ie, anterior cranial fossa, middle cranial fossa, posterior cranial fossa, and brain stem or upper spinal cord.

The *definitive procedure(s)* describes the repair, biopsy, resection, or excision of various lesions of the skull base and, when appropriate, primary closure of the dura, mucous membranes, and skin.

The *repair/reconstruction procedure(s)* is reported separately if extensive dural grafting, cranioplasty, local or regional myocutaneous pedicle flaps, or extensive skin grafts are required.

For primary closure, see the appropriate codes, ie, 15732, 15755.

When one surgeon performs the approach procedure, another surgeon performs the definitive procedure, and another surgeon performs the repair/reconstruction procedure, each surgeon reports only the code for the specific procedure performed. If one surgeon performs more than one procedure (ie, approach procedure and definitive procedure), then both codes are reported, adding modifier '-51' to the secondary, additional procedure(s).

Approach Procedures

Anterior Cranial Fossa

61580 Craniofacial approach to anterior cranial fossa; extradural, including lateral rhinotomy, ethmoidectomy, sphenoidectomy, without maxillectomy or orbital exenteration

61581 extradural, including lateral rhinotomy, orbital exenteration, ethmoidectomy, sphenoidectomy and/or maxillectomy

61582 extradural, including unilateral or bifrontal craniotomy, elevation of frontal lobe(s), osteotomy of base of anterior cranial fossa

61583 intradural, including unilateral or bifrontal craniotomy, elevation or resection of frontal lobe, osteotomy of base of anterior cranial fossa

61584 Orbitocranial approach to anterior cranial fossa, extradural, including supraorbital ridge osteotomy and elevation of frontal and/or temporal lobe(s); without orbital exenteration

61585 with orbital exenteration

Middle Cranial Fossa

61590 Infratemporal pre-auricular approach to middle cranial fossa (parapharyngeal space, infratemporal and midline skull base, nasopharynx), with or without disarticulation of the mandible, including parotidectomy, craniotomy, decompression and/or mobilization of the facial nerve and/or petrous carotid artery

61591 Infratemporal post-auricular approach to middle cranial fossa (internal auditory meatus, petrous apex, tentorium, cavernous sinus, parasellar area, infratemporal fossa) including mastoidectomy, resection of sigmoid sinus, with or without decompression and/or mobilization of contents of auditory canal or petrous carotid artery

61592 Orbitocranial zygomatic approach to middle cranial fossa (cavernous sinus and carotid artery, clivus, basilar artery or petrous apex) including osteotomy of zygoma, craniotomy, extra- or intradural elevation of temporal lobe

Posterior Cranial Fossa

61595 Transtemporal approach to posterior cranial fossa, jugular foramen or midline skull base, including mastoidectomy, decompression of sigmoid sinus and/or facial nerve, with or without mobilization

61596 Transcochlear approach to posterior cranial fossa, jugular foramen or midline skull base, including labyrinthectomy, decompression, with or without mobilization of facial nerve and/or petrous carotid artery

61597 Transcondylar (far lateral) approach to posterior cranial fossa, jugular foramen or midline skull base, including occipital condylectomy, mastoidectomy, resection of C1-C3 vertebral body(s), decompression of vertebral artery, with or without mobilization

61598 Transpetrosal approach to posterior cranial fossa, clivus or foramen magnum, including ligation of superior petrosal sinus and/or sigmoid sinus

Definitive Procedures

Base of Anterior Cranial Fossa

61600 Resection or excision of neoplastic, vascular or infectious lesion of base of anterior cranial fossa; extradural

61601 intradural, including dural repair, with or without graft

Base of Middle Cranial Fossa

61605 Resection or excision of neoplastic, vascular or infectious lesion of infratemporal fossa, parapharyngeal space, petrous apex; extradural

61606 intradural, including dural repair, with or without graft

61607 Resection or excision of neoplastic, vascular or infectious lesion of parasellar area, cavernous sinus, clivus or midline skull base; extradural

61608 intradural, including dural repair, with or without graft

(Report procedures 61609-61612 as "add-on" to primary definitive procedures 61605, 61606, 61607 or 61608)

61609 Transection or ligation, carotid artery in cavernous sinus; without repair

61610 with repair by anastomosis or graft

61611 Transection or ligation, carotid artery in petrous canal; without repair

61612 with repair by anastomosis or graft

61613 Obliteration of carotid aneurysm, arteriovenous malformation, or carotid-cavernous fistula by dissection within cavernous sinus

Base of Posterior Cranial Fossa

61615 Resection or excision of neoplastic, vascular or infectious lesion of base of posterior cranial fossa, jugular foramen, foramen magnum, or C1-C3 vertebral bodies; extradural

61616 intradural, including dural repair, with or without graft

Repair and/or Reconstruction of Surgical Defects of Skull Base

61618 Secondary repair of dura for CSF leak, anterior, middle or posterior cranial fossa following surgery of the skull base; by free tissue graft (eg, pericranium, fascia, tensor fascia lata, adipose tissue, homologous or synthetic grafts)

61619 by local or regionalized vascularized pedicle flap or myocutaneous flap (including galea, temporalis, frontalis or occipitalis muscle)

Endovascular Therapy

61624 Transcatheter occlusion or embolization (eg, for tumor destruction, to achieve hemostasis, to occlude a vascular malformation), percutaneous, any method; central nervous system (intracranial, spinal cord)

(See also 37204)

(For radiological supervision and interpretation, see 75894)

61626 non-central nervous system, head or neck (extracranial, brachiocephalic branch)

(See also 37204)

(For radiological supervision and interpretation, see 75894)

Surgery for Aneurysm, Arteriovenous Malformation or Vascular Disease

Includes craniotomy when appropriate for procedure.

61680 Surgery of intracranial arteriovenous malformation; supratentorial, simple

61682 supratentorial, complex

61684   infratentorial, simple

61686   infratentorial, complex

61690   dural, simple

61692   dural, complex

61700   Surgery of intracranial aneurysm, intracranial approach; carotid circulation

61702   vertebral-basilar circulation

61703   Surgery of intracranial aneurysm, cervical approach by application of occluding clamp to cervical carotid artery (Selverstone-Crutchfield type)

(For cervical approach for direct ligation of carotid artery, see 37600-37606)

61705   Surgery of aneurysm, vascular malformation or carotid-cavernous fistula; by intracranial and cervical occlusion of carotid artery

61708   by intracranial electrothrombosis

(For ligation or gradual occlusion of internal/common carotid artery, see 37605, 37606)

61710   by intra-arterial embolization, injection procedure, or balloon catheter

61711   Anastomosis, arterial, extracranial-intracranial (eg, middle cerebral/cortical) arteries

(For carotid or vertebral thrombo-endarterectomy, see 35301)

61712   Microdissection, intracranial or spinal procedure (list separately in addition to code for primary procedure)

(Use 61712 when the surgical microscope is employed for the microdissection and the anatomical structures or pathology present are too small for adequate visualization with magnifying loupes or normal/corrected vision)

(Use 61712 only with codes 61304-61711, 62010-62100, 63081-63308, 63704-63710)

Stereotaxis

61720   Creation of lesion by stereotactic method, including burr hole(s) and localizing and recording techniques, single or multiple stages; globus pallidus or thalamus

61735   subcortical structure(s) other than globus pallidus or thalamus

61750   Stereotactic biopsy, aspiration, or excision, including burr hole(s), for intracranial lesion;

61751   with computerized axial tomography

61760   Stereotactic implantation of depth electrodes into the cerebrum for long term seizure monitoring

61770   Stereotactic localization, any method, including burr hole(s), with insertion of catheter(s) for brachytherapy

(61780 has been deleted. To report, see 61760)

61790   Creation of lesion by stereotactic method, percutaneous, by neurolytic agent (eg, alcohol, thermal, electrical, radiofrequency); gasserian ganglion

61791   trigeminal medullary tract

61793   Stereotactic focused proton beam or gamma radiosurgery

61795   Stereotactic computer assisted volumetric intracranial procedure (list separately in addition to code for primary procedure)

Neurostimulators (Intracranial)

61850   Twist drill or burr hole(s) for implantation of neurostimulator electrodes; cortical

61855   subcortical

61860   Craniectomy or craniotomy for implantation of neurostimulator electrodes, cerebral; cortical

61865   subcortical

61870   Craniectomy for implantation of neuro-stimulator electrodes, cerebellar; cortical

61875   subcortical

61880   Revision or removal of intracranial neurostimulator electrodes

61885   Incision and subcutaneous placement of cranial neurostimulator pulse generator or receiver, direct or inductive coupling

61888   Revision or removal of cranial neurostimulator pulse generator or receiver

Repair

62000   Elevation of depressed skull fracture; simple, extradural

62005   compound or comminuted, extradural

62010   with repair of dura and/or debridement of brain

62100   Craniotomy for repair of dural/CSF leak, including surgery for rhinorrhea/otorrhea

(For repair of spinal dural/CSF leak, see 63707, 63709)

62115   Reduction of craniomegalic skull (eg, treated hydrocephalus); not requiring bone grafts or cranioplasty

62116   with simple cranioplasty

62117   requiring craniotomy and reconstruction with or without bone graft (includes obtaining grafts)

62120   Repair of encephalocele, skull vault, including cranioplasty

62121   Craniotomy for repair of encephalocele, skull base

62140   Cranioplasty for skull defect; up to 5 cm diameter

62141   larger than 5 cm diameter

62142   Removal of bone flap or prosthetic plate of skull

62143   Replacement of bone flap or prosthetic plate of skull

62145   Cranioplasty for skull defect with reparative brain surgery

62146   Cranioplasty with autograft (includes obtaining bone grafts); up to 5 cm diameter

62147   larger than 5 cm diameter

CSF Shunt

62180   Ventriculocisternostomy (Torkildsen type operation)

62190   Creation of shunt; subarachnoid/subdural-atrial, -jugular, -auricular

62192   subarachnoid/subdural-peritoneal, -pleural, other terminus

62194   Replacement or irrigation, subarachnoid/subdural catheter

62200   Ventriculocisternostomy, third ventricle;

62201   stereotactic method

62220   Creation of shunt; ventriculo-atrial, -jugular, -auricular

62223   ventriculo-peritoneal, -pleural, other terminus

62225   Replacement or irrigation, ventricular catheter

62230   Replacement or revision of CSF shunt, obstructed valve, or distal catheter in shunt system

62256   Removal of complete CSF shunt system; without replacement

62258   with replacement by similar or other shunt at same operation

(For percutaneous irrigation or aspiration of shunt reservoir, see 61070)

Spine and Spinal Cord

(For application of caliper or tongs, see 20660)

(For treatment of fracture or dislocation of spine, see 22305-22327)

Injection, Drainage, or Aspiration

62268*   Percutaneous aspiration, spinal cord cyst or syrinx

(For radiological supervision and interpretation, see 76003, 76365, 76938)

62269*   Biopsy of spinal cord, percutaneous needle

(For radiological supervision and interpretation, see 76003, 76360, 76942)

62270* Spinal puncture, lumbar, diagnostic

62272* Spinal puncture, therapeutic, for drainage of spinal fluid (by needle or catheter)

62273* Injection, lumbar epidural, of blood or clot patch

▲**62274*** Injection of diagnostic or therapeutic anesthetic or antispasmodic substance (including narcotics); subarachnoid or subdural, single

62275* epidural, cervical or thoracic, single

62276* subarachnoid or subdural, differential

62277* subarachnoid or subdural, continuous

62278* epidural, lumbar or caudal, single

62279* epidural, lumbar or caudal, continuous

62280* Injection of neurolytic substance (eg, alcohol, phenol, iced saline solutions); subarachnoid

62281* epidural, cervical or thoracic

62282* epidural, lumbar or caudal

62284* Injection procedure for myelography and/or computerized axial tomography, spinal (other than C1-C2 and posterior fossa)

(For injection procedure at C1-C2, see 61055)

(For radiological supervision and interpretation, see **Radiology**)

(62286 has been deleted. To report, use 64999)

62287 Aspiration procedure, percutaneous, of nucleus pulposus of intervertebral disk, any method, single or multiple levels, lumbar

▲**62288*** Injection of substance other than anesthetic, antispasmodic, contrast, or neurolytic solutions; subarachnoid (separate procedure)

62289* lumbar or caudal epidural (separate procedure)

62290* Injection procedure for diskography, each level; lumbar

62291* cervical

(For radiological supervision and interpretation, see 72285, 72295)

62292 Injection procedure for chemonucleolysis, including diskography, intervertebral disk, single or multiple levels, lumbar

(62293 has been deleted)

62294 Injection procedure, arterial, for occlusion of arteriovenous malformation, spinal

(62295-62297 have been deleted. To report, see 63001-63017)

62298* Injection of substance other than anesthetic, contrast, or neurolytic solutions, epidural, cervical or thoracic (separate procedure)

Catheter Implantation

(For percutaneous placement of intrathecal or epidural catheter, see codes 62274-62284, 62288, 62289, 62298)

●**62350** Implantation, revision or repositioning of intrathecal or epidural catheter, for implantable reservoir or implantable infusion pump; without laminectomy

●**62351** with laminectomy

●**62355** Removal of previously implanted intrathecal or epidural catheter

Reservoir/Pump Implantation

●**62360** Implantation or replacement of device for intrathecal or epidural drug infusion; subcutaneous reservoir

●**62361** non-programmable pump

●**62362** programmable pump, including preparation of pump, with or without programming

●**62365** Removal of subcutaneous reservoir or pump, previously implanted for intrathecal or epidural infusion

●**62367** Electronic analysis of programmable, implanted pump for intrathecal or epidural drug infusion (includes evaluation of reservoir status, alarm status, drug prescription status); without reprogramming

●**62368**   with reprogramming

(To report implantable pump or reservoir refill, use 96530)

Posterior Extradural Laminotomy or Laminectomy for Exploration/ Decompression of Neural Elements or Excision of Herniated Intervertebral Disks

(When 63001-63048 are followed by arthrodesis, see 22590-22650)

(62301-62303 have been deleted. To report, see 63001-63017)

63001   Laminectomy with exploration and/or decompression of spinal cord and/or cauda equina, without facetectomy, foraminotomy or diskectomy, (eg, spinal stenosis), one or two vertebral segments; cervical

63003   thoracic

63005   lumbar, except for spondylolisthesis

(63010 has been deleted. To report, use 63012)

63011   sacral

63012   Laminectomy with removal of abnormal facets and/or pars inter-articularis with decompression of cauda equina and nerve roots for spondylolisthesis, lumbar (Gill type procedure)

63015   Laminectomy with exploration and/or decompression of spinal cord and/or cauda equina, without facetectomy, foraminotomy or diskectomy, (eg, spinal stenosis), more than 2 vertebral segments; cervical

63016   thoracic

63017   lumbar

63020   Laminotomy (hemilaminectomy), with decompression of nerve root(s), including partial facetectomy, foraminotomy and/or excision of herniated intervertebral disk; one interspace, cervical

(63021 has been deleted. To report, use 63020 with modifier -50 or 09950)

63030   one interspace, lumbar

(63031 has been deleted. To report, use 63030 with modifier -50 or 09950)

63035   each additional interspace, cervical or lumbar

(Use 63035 only for procedures 63020-63030)

63040   Laminotomy (hemilaminectomy), with decompression of nerve root(s), including partial facetectomy, foraminotomy and/or excision of herniated intervertebral disk, re-exploration; cervical

(63041 has been deleted)

63042   lumbar

63045   Laminectomy, facetectomy and foraminotomy (unilateral or bilateral with decompression of spinal cord, cauda equina and/or nerve root(s), (eg, spinal or lateral recess stenosis)), single vertebral segment; cervical

63046   thoracic

63047   lumbar

63048   each additional segment, cervical, thoracic or lumbar

(Use 63048 only for procedures 63045-63047)

Transpedicular or Costovertebral Approach for Posterolateral Extradural Exploration/Decompression

63055   Transpedicular approach with decompression of spinal cord, equina and/or nerve root(s) (eg, herniated intervertebral disk), single segment; thoracic

63056   lumbar

63057   each additional segment, thoracic or lumbar

(63060 has been deleted)

63064   Costovertebral approach with decompression of spinal cord or nerve root(s), (eg, herniated intervertebral disk), thoracic; single segment

(63065 has been deleted)

63066   each additional segment

(For excision of thoracic intraspinal lesions by laminectomy, see 63266, 63271, 63276, 63281, 63286)

Anterior or Anterolateral Approach for Extradural Exploration/Decompression

63075 Diskectomy, anterior, with decompression of spinal cord and/or nerve root(s), including osteophytectomy; cervical, single interspace

63076   cervical, each additional interspace

63077   thoracic, single interspace

63078   thoracic, each additional interspace

63081 Vertebral corpectomy (vertebral body resection), partial or complete, anterior approach with decompression of spinal cord and/or nerve root(s); cervical, single segment

63082   cervical, each additional segment

(For transoral approach, see 61575, 61576)

63085 Vertebral corpectomy (vertebral body resection), partial or complete, transthoracic approach with decompression of spinal cord and/or nerve root(s); thoracic, single segment

63086   thoracic, each additional segment

63087 Vertebral corpectomy (vertebral body resection), partial or complete, combined thoracolumbar approach with decompression of spinal cord, cauda equina or nerve root(s), lower thoracic or lumbar; single segment

63088   each additional segment

63090 Vertebral corpectomy (vertebral body resection), partial or complete, transperitoneal or retroperitoneal approach with decompression of spinal cord, cauda equina or nerve root(s), lower thoracic, lumbar, or sacral; single segment

63091   each additional segment

(Procedures 63081-63091 include diskectomy above and/or below vertebral segment)

(If followed by arthrodesis, see 22554-22585)

(If followed by reconstruction of spine, see 22140-22152)

Incision

63170 Laminectomy with myelotomy (eg, Bischof or DREZ type), cervical, thoracic or thoracolumbar

63172 Laminectomy with drainage of intramedullary cyst/syrinx; to subarachnoid space

63173   to peritoneal space

63180 Laminectomy and section of dentate ligaments, with or without dural graft, cervical; one or two segments

63182   more than two segments

63185 Laminectomy with rhizotomy; one or two segments

63190   more than two segments

63191 Laminectomy with section of spinal accessory nerve

(63192 has been deleted. To report, use 63191 with modifier -50 or 09950)

(For resection of sternocleidomastoid muscle, use 21720)

63194 Laminectomy with cordotomy, with section of one spinothalamic tract, one stage; cervical

63195   thoracic

63196 Laminectomy with cordotomy, with section of both spinothalamic tracts, one stage; cervical

63197   thoracic

63198 Laminectomy with cordotomy with section of both spinothalamic tracts, two stages within 14 days; cervical

63199   thoracic

63200 Laminectomy, with release of tethered spinal cord, lumbar

Excision by Laminectomy of Lesion Other Than Herniated Disk

(63210-63242 have been deleted. To report, see 63265-63290)

63250 Laminectomy for excision or occlusion of arteriovenous malformation of spinal cord; cervical

63251 thoracic

63252 thoracolumbar

63265 Laminectomy for excision or evacuation of intraspinal lesion other than neoplasm, extradural; cervical

63266 thoracic

63267 lumbar

63268 sacral

63270 Laminectomy for excision of intraspinal lesion other than neoplasm, intradural; cervical

63271 thoracic

63272 lumbar

63273 sacral

63275 Laminectomy for biopsy/excision of intraspinal neoplasm; extradural, cervical

63276 extradural, thoracic

63277 extradural, lumbar

63278 extradural, sacral

63280 intradural, extramedullary, cervical

63281 intradural, extramedullary, thoracic

63282 intradural, extramedullary, lumbar

63283 intradural, sacral

63285 intradural, intramedullary, cervical

63286 intradural, intramedullary, thoracic

63287 intradural, intramedullary, thoracolumbar

63290 combined extradural-intradural lesion, any level

(For drainage of intramedullary cyst/syrinx, use 63172, 63173)

Excision, Anterior or Anterolateral Approach, Intraspinal Lesion

(For arthrodesis, see 22548-22650)

(For reconstruction of spine, see 22140-22152)

63300 Vertebral corpectomy (vertebral body resection), partial or complete, for excision of intraspinal lesion, single segment; extradural, cervical

63301 extradural, thoracic by transthoracic approach

63302 extradural, thoracic by thoracolumbar approach

63303 extradural, lumbar or sacral by trans-peritoneal or retroperitoneal approach

63304 intradural, cervical

63305 intradural, thoracic by transthoracic approach

63306 intradural, thoracic by thoracolumbar approach

63307 intradural, lumbar or sacral by trans-peritoneal or retroperitoneal approach

63308 each additional segment (list separately in addition to codes for single segment 63300-63307)

Stereotaxis

63600 Creation of lesion of spinal cord by stereotactic method, percutaneous, any modality (including stimulation and/or recording)

63610 Stereotactic stimulation of spinal cord, percutaneous, separate procedure not followed by other surgery

63615 Stereotactic biopsy, aspiration, or excision of lesion, spinal cord

Neurostimulators (Spinal)

63650 Percutaneous implantation of neurostimulator electrodes; epidural

(63652 has been deleted)

63655 Laminectomy for implantation of neurostimulator electrodes; epidural

(63656 has been deleted)

(63657 and 63658 have been deleted)

63660 Revision or removal of spinal neurostimulator electrodes

63685 Incision and subcutaneous placement of spinal neurostimulator pulse generator or receiver, direct or inductive coupling

63688 Revision or removal of implanted spinal neurostimulator pulse generator or receiver

63690 Electronic analysis of implanted neuro-stimulator pulse generator system (may include rate, pulse amplitude and duration, configuration of wave form, battery status, electrode selectability, output modulation, cycling, impedance and patient compliance measurements); without reprogramming of pulse generator

63691   with reprogramming of pulse generator

Repair

63700 Repair of meningocele; less than 5 cm diameter

63702   larger than 5 cm diameter

63704 Repair of myelomeningocele; less than 5 cm diameter

63706   larger than 5 cm diameter

(For complex skin closure, see Integumentary System)

63707 Repair of dural/CSF leak, not requiring laminectomy

(63708 has been deleted. To report, see 63707, 63709)

63709 Repair of dural/CSF leak or pseudo-meningocele, with laminectomy

63710 Dural graft, spinal

(For laminectomy and section of dentate ligaments, with or without dural graft, cervical, see 63180, 63182)

Shunt, Spinal CSF

63740 Creation of shunt, lumbar, subarachnoid-peritoneal, -pleural, or other; including laminectomy

63741   percutaneous, not requiring laminectomy

63744 Replacement, irrigation or revision of lumbosubarachnoid shunt

63746 Removal of entire lumbosubarachnoid shunt system without replacement

(63750 has been deleted. To report, see 62351 and 62360, 62361 or 62362)

(63780 has been deleted. To report, see 62350 and 62360, 62361 or 62362)

Extracranial Nerves, Peripheral Nerves, and Autonomic Nervous System

(For intracranial surgery on cranial nerves, see 61450, 61460, 61790)

Introduction/Injection of Anesthetic Agent (Nerve Block), Diagnostic or Therapeutic

Somatic Nerves

64400* Injection, anesthetic agent; trigeminal nerve, any division or branch

64402*   facial nerve

64405*   greater occipital nerve

64408*   vagus nerve

64410*   phrenic nerve

64412*   spinal accessory nerve

64413* cervical plexus

64415* brachial plexus

64417* axillary nerve

64418* suprascapular nerve

64420* intercostal nerve, single

64421* intercostal nerves, multiple, regional block

64425* ilioinguinal, iliohypogastric nerves

64430* pudendal nerve

64435* paracervical (uterine) nerve

64440* paravertebral nerve (thoracic, lumbar, sacral, coccygeal), single vertebral level

64441* paravertebral nerves, multiple levels (eg, regional block)

64442* paravertebral facet joint nerve, lumbar, single level

64443* paravertebral facet joint nerve, lumbar, each additional level

64445* sciatic nerve

64450* other peripheral nerve or branch

(For phenol destruction, see 64600-64640)

(For subarachnoid or subdural injection, see 62274-62277)

(For epidural or caudal injection, see 62278, 62279)

Sympathetic Nerves

64505* Injection, anesthetic agent; sphenopalatine ganglion

64508* carotid sinus (separate procedure)

64510* stellate ganglion (cervical sympathetic)

64520* lumbar or thoracic (paravertebral sympathetic)

64530* celiac plexus, with or without radiologic monitoring

Neurostimulators (Peripheral Nerve)

64550 Application of surface (transcutaneous) neurostimulator

64553 Percutaneous implantation of neurostimulator electrodes; cranial nerve

64555 peripheral nerve

64560 autonomic nerve

64565 neuromuscular

64573 Incision for implantation of neurostimulator electrodes; cranial nerve

64575 peripheral nerve

64577 autonomic nerve

64580 neuromuscular

64585 Revision or removal of peripheral neurostimulator electrodes

64590 Incision and subcutaneous placement of peripheral neurostimulator pulse generator or receiver, direct or inductive coupling

64595 Revision or removal of peripheral neurostimulator pulse generator or receiver

Destruction by Neurolytic Agent (eg, Chemical, Thermal, Electrical, Radiofrequency)

Somatic Nerves

64600 Destruction by neurolytic agent, trigeminal nerve; supraorbital, infraorbital, mental, or inferior alveolar branch

64605 second and third division branches at foramen ovale

64610 second and third division branches at foramen ovale under radiologic monitoring

64612 Destruction by neurolytic agent (chemodenervation of muscle endplate); muscles enervated by facial nerve (eg, for blepharospasm, hemifacial spasm)

64613 cervical spinal muscles (eg, for spasmodic torticollis)

(For chemodenervation for strabismus involving the extraocular muscles, see 67345)

64620 Destruction by neurolytic agent; intercostal nerve

64622 paravertebral facet joint nerve, lumbar, single level

64623 paravertebral facet joint nerve, lumbar, each additional level

64630 pudendal nerve

64640 other peripheral nerve or branch

Sympathetic Nerves

64680 Destruction by neurolytic agent, celiac plexus, with or without radiologic monitoring

Neuroplasty (Exploration, Neurolysis or Nerve Decompression)

Neuroplasty is the decompression or freeing of intact nerve from scar tissue, including external neurolysis and/or transposition.

(For internal neurolysis requiring use of operating microscope, use 64727)

(For facial nerve decompression, see 69720)

64702 Neuroplasty; digital, one or both, same digit

64704 nerve of hand or foot

64708 Neuroplasty, major peripheral nerve, arm or leg; other than specified

64712 sciatic nerve

64713 brachial plexus

64714 lumbar plexus

64716 Neuroplasty and/or transposition; cranial nerve (specify)

64718 ulnar nerve at elbow

64719 ulnar nerve at wrist

64721 median nerve at carpal tunnel

(For arthroscopic procedure, see 29848)

64722 Decompression; unspecified nerve(s) (specify)

64726 plantar digital nerve

64727 Internal neurolysis, requiring use of operating microscope (list separately in addition to code for neuroplasty) (Neuroplasty includes external neurolysis)

Transection or Avulsion

(For stereotactic lesion of gasserian ganglion, see 61790)

64732 Transection or avulsion of; supraorbital nerve

64734 infraorbital nerve

64736 mental nerve

64738 inferior alveolar nerve by osteotomy

64740 lingual nerve

64742 facial nerve, differential or complete

64744 greater occipital nerve

64746 phrenic nerve

(For section of recurrent laryngeal nerve, see 31595)

64752 vagus nerve (vagotomy), transthoracic

64755 vagi limited to proximal stomach (selective proximal vagotomy, proximal gastric vagotomy, parietal cell vagotomy, supra- or highly selective vagotomy)

64760 vagus nerve (vagotomy), abdominal

64761 pudendal nerve

(64762 has been deleted. To report, use 64761 with modifier -50 or 09950)

64763 Transection or avulsion of obturator nerve, extrapelvic, with or without adductor tenotomy

(64764 has been deleted. To report, use 64763 with modifier -50 or 09950)

64766 Transection or avulsion of obturator nerve, intrapelvic, with or without adductor tenotomy

(64768 has been deleted. To report, use 64766 with modifier -50 or 09950)

64771 Transection or avulsion of other cranial nerve, extradural

64772 Transection or avulsion of other spinal nerve, extradural

(For excision of tender scar, skin and subcutaneous tissue, with or without tiny neuroma, see 11400-11446, 13100-13300)

Excision

Somatic Nerves

(For Morton neurectomy, see 28080)

64774 Excision of neuroma; cutaneous nerve, surgically identifiable

64776 digital nerve, one or both, same digit

64778 digital nerve, each additional digit (list separately by this number)

64782 hand or foot, except digital nerve

64783 hand or foot, each additional nerve, except same digit (list separately by this number)

64784 major peripheral nerve, except sciatic

64786 sciatic nerve

64787 Implantation of nerve end into bone or muscle (list separately in addition to neuroma excision)

64788 Excision of neurofibroma or neurolemmoma; cutaneous nerve

64790 major peripheral nerve

64792 extensive (including malignant type)

64795 Biopsy of nerve

Sympathetic Nerves

64802 Sympathectomy, cervical

(64803 has been deleted. To report, use 64802 with modifier -50 or 09950)

64804 Sympathectomy, cervicothoracic

(64806 has been deleted. To report, use 64804 with modifier -50 or 09950)

64809 Sympathectomy, thoracolumbar

(64811 has been deleted. To report, use 64809 with modifier -50 or 09950)

(64814 has been deleted. To report, use 64999)

64818 Sympathectomy, lumbar

(64819 has been deleted. To report, use 64818 with modifier -50 or 09950)

64820 Sympathectomy, digital arteries, with magnification, each digit

(64824 has been deleted. To report, use 64999)

Neurorrhaphy

64830 Microdissection and/or microrepair of nerve (list separately in addition to code for nerve repair)

64831 Suture of digital nerve, hand or foot; one nerve

64832 each additional digital nerve

64834 Suture of one nerve, hand or foot; common sensory nerve

64835 median motor thenar

64836 ulnar motor

64837 Suture of each additional nerve, hand or foot

64840 Suture of posterior tibial nerve

64856 Suture of major peripheral nerve, arm or leg, except sciatic; including transposition

64857 without transposition

64858 Suture of sciatic nerve

64859 Suture of each additional major peripheral nerve

64861 Suture of; brachial plexus

64862 lumbar plexus

64864 Suture of facial nerve; extracranial

64865 infratemporal, with or without grafting

64866 Anastomosis; facial-spinal accessory

64868   facial-hypoglossal

64870   facial-phrenic

64872 Suture of nerve; requiring secondary or delayed suture (list separately in addition to code for primary neurorrhaphy)

64874   requiring extensive mobilization, or transposition of nerve (list separately in addition to code for nerve suture)

64876   requiring shortening of bone of extremity (list separately in addition to code for nerve suture)

Neurorrhaphy With Nerve Graft

64885 Nerve graft (includes obtaining graft), head or neck; up to 4 cm in length

64886   more than 4 cm length

64890 Nerve graft (includes obtaining graft), single strand, hand or foot; up to 4 cm length

64891   more than 4 cm length

64892 Nerve graft (includes obtaining graft), single strand, arm or leg; up to 4 cm length

64893   more than 4 cm length

64895 Nerve graft (includes obtaining graft), multiple strands (cable), hand or foot; up to 4 cm length

64896   more than 4 cm length

64897 Nerve graft (includes obtaining graft), multiple strands (cable), arm or leg; up to 4 cm length

64898   more than 4 cm length

64901 Nerve graft, each additional nerve; single strand

64902   multiple strands (cable)

64905 Nerve pedicle transfer; first stage

64907   second stage

Other Procedures

64999 Unlisted procedure, nervous system

Eye and Ocular Adnexa

(For diagnostic and treatment ophthalmological services, see **Medicine,** Ophthalmology, and 92002 et seq)

Eyeball

Removal of Eye

65091   Evisceration of ocular contents; without implant

65093   with implant

65101   Enucleation of eye; without implant

65103   with implant, muscles not attached to implant

65105   with implant, muscles attached to implant

(For conjunctivoplasty after enucleation, see 68320 et seq)

65110   Exenteration of orbit (does not include skin graft), removal of orbital contents; only

65112   with therapeutic removal of bone

65114   with muscle or myocutaneous flap

(For skin graft to orbit (split skin), see 15120, 15121; free, full thickness, see 15260, 15261)

(For eyelid repair involving more than skin, see 67930 et seq)

Secondary Implant(s) Procedures

An ocular implant is an implant inside muscular cone; an orbital implant is an implant outside muscular cone.

65125   Modification of ocular implant with placement or replacement of pegs (eg, drilling receptacle for prosthesis appendage) (separate procedure)

65130   Insertion of ocular implant secondary; after evisceration, in scleral shell

65135   after enucleation, muscles not attached to implant

65140   after enucleation, muscles attached to implant

65150   Reinsertion of ocular implant; with or without conjunctival graft

65155   with use of foreign material for reinforcement and/or attachment of muscles to implant

65175   Removal of ocular implant

(For orbital implant (implant outside muscle cone) insertion, see 67550; removal, see 67560)

Removal of Foreign Body

(For removal of implanted material: ocular implant, see 65175; anterior segment implant, see 65920; posterior segment implant, see 67120; orbital implant, see 67560)

(For diagnostic x-ray for foreign body, see 70030)

(For diagnostic echography for foreign body, see 76529)

(For removal of foreign body from orbit: frontal approach, see 67413; lateral approach, see 67430; transcranial approach, see 61334)

(For removal of foreign body from eyelid, embedded, see 67938)

(For removal of foreign body from lacrimal system, see 68530)

65205*   Removal of foreign body, external eye; conjunctival superficial

65210*   conjunctival embedded (includes concretions), subconjunctival, or scleral nonperforating

65220*   corneal, without slit lamp

65222*   corneal, with slit lamp

(For repair of corneal laceration with foreign body, see 65275)

(65230 has been deleted. To report, use 65235)

65235   Removal of foreign body, intraocular; from anterior chamber or lens

Eye 65091—68899

(65240, 65245 have been deleted. To report, use 65235)

(For removal of implanted material from anterior segment, see 65920)

65260 from posterior segment, magnetic extraction, anterior or posterior route

65265 from posterior segment, nonmagnetic extraction

(For removal of implanted material from posterior segment, see 67120)

Repair of Laceration

(For fracture of orbit, see 21385 et seq)

(For repair of wound of eyelid, skin, linear, simple, see 12011-12018; intermediate, layered closure, see 12051-12057; linear, complex, see 13150-13300; other, see 67930, 67935)

(For repair of wound of lacrimal system, see 68700)

(For repair of operative wound, see 66250)

65270* Repair of laceration; conjunctiva, with or without nonperforating laceration sclera, direct closure

65272 conjunctiva, by mobilization and rearrangement, without hospitalization

65273 conjunctiva, by mobilization and rearrangement, with hospitalization

65275 cornea, nonperforating, with or without removal foreign body

65280 cornea and/or sclera, perforating, not involving uveal tissue

65285 cornea and/or sclera, perforating, with reposition or resection of uveal tissue

65286 application of tissue glue, wounds of cornea and/or sclera

(Repair of laceration includes use of conjunctival flap and restoration of anterior chamber, by air or saline injection when indicated)

(For repair of iris or ciliary body, see 66680)

65290 Repair of wound, extraocular muscle, tendon and/or Tenon's capsule

Anterior Segment

Cornea

Excision

(65300 has been deleted)

65400 Excision of lesion, cornea (keratectomy, lamellar, partial), except pterygium

65410* Biopsy of cornea

65420 Excision or transposition of pterygium; without graft

65426 with graft

Removal or Destruction

65430* Scraping of cornea, diagnostic, for smear and/or culture

65435* Removal of corneal epithelium; with or without chemocauterization (abrasion, curettage)

65436 with application of chelating agent (eg, EDTA)

(65445 has been deleted. To report, use 65450)

65450 Destruction of lesion of cornea by cryotherapy, photocoagulation or thermocauterization

(65455 has been deleted. To report, use 65450)

65600 Multiple punctures of anterior cornea (eg, for corneal erosion, tattoo)

Keratoplasty

Corneal transplant includes use of fresh or preserved grafts, and preparation of donor material.

(Keratoplasty excludes refractive keratoplasty procedures, 65760, 65765, and 65767)

65710 Keratoplasty (corneal transplant); lamellar

Eye 65091–68899

(65720, 65725 have been deleted. To report, see 65710)

65730   penetrating (except in aphakia)

(65740, 65745 have been deleted. To report, see 65730)

65750   penetrating (in aphakia)

65755   penetrating (in pseudophakia)

Other Procedures

65760   Keratomileusis

65765   Keratophakia

65767   Epikeratoplasty

65770   Keratoprosthesis

65771   Radial keratotomy

65772   Corneal relaxing incision for correction of surgically induced astigmatism

65775   Corneal wedge resection for correction of surgically induced astigmatism

(For fitting of contact lens for treatment of disease, see 92070)

(For unlisted procedures on cornea, see 66999)

Anterior Chamber

Incision

65800*   Paracentesis of anterior chamber of eye (separate procedure); with diagnostic aspiration of aqueous

65805*   with therapeutic release of aqueous

65810   with removal of vitreous and/or discission of anterior hyaloid membrane, with or without air injection

65815   with removal of blood, with or without irrigation and/or air injection

(For injection, see 66020-66030)

(For removal of blood clot, see 65930)

65820   Goniotomy

(65825, 65830 have been deleted)

65850   Trabeculotomy ab externo

65855   Trabeculoplasty by laser surgery, one or more sessions (defined treatment series)

(If re-treatment is necessary after several months because of disease progression, a new treatment or treatment series should be reported with a modifier, if necessary, to indicate lesser or greater complexity)

(For trabeculectomy, see 66170)

65860   Severing adhesions of anterior segment, laser technique (separate procedure)

Other Procedures

65865   Severing adhesions of anterior segment of eye, incisional technique (with or without injection of air or liquid) (separate procedure); goniosynechiae

(For trabeculoplasty by laser surgery, use 65855)

65870   anterior synechiae, except goniosynechiae

65875   posterior synechiae

65880   corneovitreal adhesions

(For laser surgery, use 66821)

65900   Removal of epithelial downgrowth, anterior chamber eye

65920   Removal of implanted material, anterior segment eye

65930   Removal of blood clot, anterior segment eye

66020   Injection, anterior chamber (separate procedure); air or liquid

66030*   medication

(For unlisted procedures on anterior segment, see 66999)

▲=Revised Code   ●=New Code   ✱=Service Includes Surgical Procedure Only

Anterior Sclera

Excision

(For removal of intraocular foreign body, see 65235)

(For operations on posterior sclera, see 67250, 67255)

66130 Excision of lesion, sclera

66150 Fistulization of sclera for glaucoma; trephination with iridectomy

66155 thermocauterization with iridectomy

66160 sclerectomy with punch or scissors, with iridectomy

66165 iridencleisis or iridotasis

66170 trabeculectomy ab externo in absence of previous surgery

(For trabeculotomy ab externo, see 65850)

(For repair of operative wound, see 66250)

66172 trabeculectomy ab externo with scarring from previous ocular surgery or trauma (includes injection of antifibrotic agents)

66180 Aqueous shunt to extraocular reservoir (eg, Molteno, Schocket, Denver-Krupin)

66185 Revision of aqueous shunt to extraocular reservoir

(For removal of implanted shunt, use 67120)

Repair or Revision

(For scleral procedures in retinal surgery, see 67101 et seq)

66220 Repair of scleral staphyloma; without graft

66225 with graft

(For scleral reinforcement, see 67250, 67255)

66250 Revision or repair of operative wound of anterior segment, any type, early or late, major or minor procedure

(For unlisted procedures on anterior sclera, see 66999)

Iris, Ciliary Body

Incision

66500 Iridotomy by stab incision (separate procedure); except transfixion

66505 with transfixion as for iris bombe

(For "iridotomy" by photocoagulation, see 66761)

Excision

66600 Iridectomy, with corneoscleral or corneal section; for removal of lesion

66605 with cyclectomy

66625 peripheral for glaucoma (separate procedure)

66630 sector for glaucoma (separate procedure)

66635 "optical" (separate procedure)

(For "coreoplasty" by photocoagulation, see 66762)

Repair

66680 Repair of iris, ciliary body (as for iridodialysis)

(For reposition or resection of uveal tissue with perforating wound of cornea or sclera, see 65285)

66682 Suture of iris, ciliary body (separate procedure) with retrieval of suture through small incision (eg, McCannel suture)

Destruction

66700 Ciliary body destruction; diathermy

(66701, 66702 have been deleted. To report, see 66700, 66710, 66720, 66740)

66710 cyclophotocoagulation

66720 cryotherapy

(66721 has been deleted. To report, see 66700, 66710, 66720, 66740)

66740   cyclodialysis

(66741 has been deleted. To report, see 66700, 66710, 66720, 66740)

66761   Iridotomy/iridectomy by laser surgery (eg, for glaucoma) (one or more sessions)

66762   Iridoplasty by photocoagulation (one or more sessions) (eg, for improvement of vision, for widening of anterior chamber angle)

66770   Destruction of cyst or lesion iris or ciliary body (nonexcisional procedure)

(For excision lesion iris, ciliary body, see 66600, 66605; for removal of epithelial downgrowth, see 65900)

(For unlisted procedures on iris, ciliary body, see 66999)

Lens

Incision

(66800, 66801 have been deleted. To report, use 66999)

(66802 has been deleted)

66820   Discission of secondary membranous cataract (opacified posterior lens capsule and/or anterior hyaloid); stab incision technique (Ziegler or Wheeler knife)

66821   laser surgery (eg, YAG laser) (one or more stages)

66825   Repositioning of intraocular lens prosthesis, requiring an incision (separate procedure)

Removal Cataract

Lateral canthotomy, iridectomy, iridotomy, anterior capsulotomy, posterior capsulotomy, the use of viscoelastic agents, enzymatic zonulysis, use of other pharmacologic agents, and subconjunctival or sub-tenon injections are included as part of the code for the extraction of lens.

66830   Removal of secondary membranous cataract (opacified posterior lens capsule and/or anterior hyaloid) with corneo-scleral section, with or without iridectomy (iridocapsulotomy, iridocapsulectomy)

66840   Removal of lens material; aspiration technique, one or more stages

66850   phacofragmentation technique (mechanical or ultrasonic) (eg, phacoemulsification), with aspiration

66852   pars plana approach, with or without vitrectomy

(66915 has been deleted)

66920   intracapsular

66930   intracapsular, for dislocated lens

66940   extracapsular (other than 66840, 66850, 66852)

(66945 has been deleted. To report, see 66920-66940)

(For removal of intralenticular foreign body without lens extraction, see 65235)

(For repair of operative wound, see 66250)

(66980 has been deleted. To report, see 66983, 66984)

66983   Intracapsular cataract extraction with insertion of intraocular lens prosthesis (one stage procedure)

66984   Extracapsular cataract removal with insertion of intraocular lens prosthesis (one stage procedure), manual or mechanical technique (eg, irrigation and aspiration or phacoemulsification)

66985   Insertion of intraocular lens prosthesis (secondary implant), not associated with concurrent cataract removal

(To code implant at time of concurrent cataract surgery, use 66983 or 66984)

(For intraocular lens prosthesis supplied by physician, use 99070)

(For ultrasonic determination of intraocular lens power, use 76519)

(For removal of implanted material from anterior segment, use 65920)

(For secondary fixation (separate procedure), use 66682)

66986 Exchange of intraocular lens

Other Procedures

66999 Unlisted procedure, anterior segment of eye

Posterior Segment

Vitreous

67005 Removal of vitreous, anterior approach (open sky technique or limbal incision); partial removal

67010 subtotal removal with mechanical vitrectomy

(For removal of vitreous by paracentesis of anterior chamber, see 65810)

(For removal of corneovitreal adhesions, see 65880)

67015 Aspiration or release of vitreous, subretinal or choroidal fluid, pars plana approach (posterior sclerotomy)

67025 Injection of vitreous substitute, pars plana or limbal approach, (fluid-gas exchange), with or without aspiration (separate procedure)

67028 Intravitreal injection of a pharmacologic agent (separate procedure)

67030 Discission of vitreous strands (without removal), pars plana approach

67031 Severing of vitreous strands, vitreous face adhesions, sheets, membranes or opacities, laser surgery (one or more stages)

(67035 has been deleted. To report, use 67036)

67036 Vitrectomy, mechanical, pars plana approach;

67038 with epiretinal membrane stripping

67039 with focal endolaser photocoagulation

67040 with endolaser panretinal photocoagulation

(For associated lensectomy, see 66850)

(For use of vitrectomy in retinal detachment surgery, see 67108)

(For associated removal of foreign body, see 65260, 65265)

(For unlisted procedures on vitreous, see 67299)

Retina or Choroid

Repair

(If diathermy, cryotherapy and/or photocoagulation are combined, report under principal modality used)

67101 Repair of retinal detachment, one or more sessions; cryotherapy or diathermy, with or without drainage of subretinal fluid

(67102, 67103 have been deleted. To report, use 67101)

(67104 has been deleted. To report, use 67105)

▲**67105** photocoagulation, with or without drainage of subretinal fluid

(67106 has been deleted. To report, use 67105)

▲**67107** Repair of retinal detachment; scleral buckling (such as lamellar scleral dissection, imbrication or encircling procedure), with or without implant, with or without cryotherapy, photocoagulation, and drainage of subretinal fluid

▲**67108** with vitrectomy, any method, with or without air or gas tamponade, focal endolaser photocoagulation, cryotherapy, drainage of subretinal fluid, scleral buckling, and/or removal of lens by same technique

(67109 has been deleted. To report see 67299)

67110 by injection of air or other gas (eg, pneumatic retinopexy)

▲**67112** by scleral buckling or vitrectomy, on patient having previous ipsilateral retinal detachment repair(s) using scleral buckling or vitrectomy techniques

(For aspiration or drainage of subretinal or subchoroidal fluid, see 67015)

67115 Release of encircling material (posterior segment)

67120 Removal of implanted material, posterior segment; extraocular

67121 intraocular

(For removal from anterior segment, use 65920)

(For removal of foreign body, see 65260, 65265)

Prophylaxis

Repetitive services. The services listed below are often performed in multiple sessions or groups of sessions. The methods of reporting vary.

The following descriptors are intended to include all sessions in a defined treatment period.

67141 Prophylaxis of retinal detachment (eg, retinal break, lattice degeneration) without drainage, one or more sessions; cryotherapy, diathermy

(67142, 67143 have been deleted. To report, use 67141)

(67144 has been deleted. To report, use 67145)

67145 photocoagulation (laser or xenon arc)

(67146 has been deleted. To report, use 67145)

Destruction

67208 Destruction of localized lesion of retina (eg, maculopathy, choroidopathy, small tumors), one or more sessions; cryotherapy, diathermy

67210 photocoagulation (laser or xenon arc)

(67212, 67213 have been deleted. To report, use 67208)

(67214, 67216 have been deleted. To report, use 67210)

67218 radiation by implantation of source (includes removal of source)

(67222, 67223 have been deleted. To report, use 67227)

(67224, 67226 have been deleted. To report, use 67228)

67227 Destruction of extensive or progressive retinopathy (eg, diabetic retinopathy), one or more sessions; cryotherapy, diathermy

67228 photocoagulation (laser or xenon arc)

(For unlisted procedures on retina, see 67299)

Sclera

Repair

(For excision lesion sclera, see 66130)

67250 Scleral reinforcement (separate procedure); without graft

67255 with graft

(For repair scleral staphyloma, see 66220, 66225)

Other Procedures

67299 Unlisted procedure, posterior segment

Ocular Adnexa

Extraocular Muscles

67311 Strabismus surgery, recession or resection procedure (patient not previously operated on); one horizontal muscle

67312 two horizontal muscles

(67313 has been deleted)

67314 one vertical muscle (excluding superior oblique)

67316 two or more vertical muscles (excluding superior oblique)

(For adjustable sutures, use 67335 in addition to primary procedure reflecting number of muscles operated on)

67318 Strabismus surgery, any procedure (patient not previously operated on), superior oblique muscle

(Use 67320, 67331, 67332, 67335, 67340, 67343 in addition to code for primary strabismus surgery (67311-67318))

67320 Transposition procedure (eg, for paretic extraocular muscle), any extraocular muscle (specify)

67331 Strabismus surgery on patient with previous eye surgery or injury that did not involve the extraocular muscles

67332 Strabismus surgery on patient with scarring of extraocular muscles (eg, prior ocular injury, strabismus or retinal detachment surgery) or restrictive myopathy (eg, dysthyroid ophthalmopathy)

67334 Strabismus surgery by posterior fixation suture technique, with or without muscle recession

67335 Placement of adjustable suture(s) during strabismus surgery, including postoperative adjustment(s) of suture(s) (Report in addition to code for specific strabismus surgery)

(Use also code for conventional muscle surgery, 67311-67334, to identify number of muscles involved)

67340 Strabismus surgery involving exploration and/or repair of detached extraocular muscle(s)

67343 Release of extensive scar tissue without detaching extraocular muscle (separate procedure)

67345 Chemodenervation of extraocular muscle

(For chemodenervation for blepharospasm and other neurological disorders, see 64612 and 64613)

Other Procedures

67350 Biopsy of extraocular muscle

(For repair of wound, extraocular muscle, tendon or Tenon's capsule, see 65290)

67399 Unlisted procedure, ocular muscle

Orbit

Exploration, Excision, Decompression

67400 Orbitotomy without bone flap (frontal or transconjunctival approach); for exploration, with or without biopsy

67405 with drainage only

67412 with removal of lesion

67413 with removal of foreign body

67414 with removal of bone for decompression

67415 Fine needle aspiration of orbital contents

(For exenteration, enucleation, and repair, see 65101 et seq; for optic nerve decompression, see 67570)

67420 Orbitotomy with bone flap or window, lateral approach (eg, Kroenlein); with removal of lesion

67430 with removal of foreign body

67440 with drainage

67445 with removal of bone for decompression

(For optic nerve sheath decompression, see 67570)

67450 for exploration, with or without biopsy

(For orbitotomy, transcranial approach, see 61330-61334)

(For orbital implant, see 67550, 67560)

(For removal of eyeball or for repair after removal, see 65091-65175)

Other Procedures

67500* Retrobulbar injection; medication (separate procedure, does not include supply of medication)

67505 alcohol

(67510 has been deleted. To report, use 67599)

67515* Injection of therapeutic agent into Tenon's capsule

(For subconjunctival injection, see 68200)

67550 Orbital implant (implant outside muscle cone); insertion

67560 removal or revision

(For ocular implant (implant inside muscle cone), see 65093-65105, 65130-65175)

(For treatment of fractures of malar area, orbit, see 21355 et seq)

67570 Optic nerve decompression (eg, incision or fenestration of optic nerve sheath)

67599 Unlisted procedure, orbit

Eyelids

Incision

67700* Blepharotomy, drainage of abscess, eyelid

67710* Severing of tarsorrhaphy

67715* Canthotomy (separate procedure)

(For canthoplasty, see 67950)

(For division of symblepharon, see 68340)

Excision

Codes for removal of lesion include more than skin (ie, involving lid margin, tarsus, and/or palpebral conjunctiva).

(For removal of lesion, involving mainly skin of eyelid, see 11440-11446; 11640-11646; 17000-17010)

(For repair of wounds, blepharoplasty, grafts, reconstructive surgery, see 67930-67975)

67800 Excision of chalazion; single

67801 multiple, same lid

67805 multiple, different lids

67808 under general anesthesia and/or requiring hospitalization, single or multiple

67810* Biopsy of eyelid

67820* Correction of trichiasis; epilation, by forceps only

▲**67825*** epilation by other than forceps (eg, by electrosurgery, cryotherapy, laser surgery)

67830 incision of lid margin

67835 incision of lid margin, with free mucous membrane graft

67840* Excision of lesion of eyelid (except chalazion) without closure or with simple direct closure

(For excision and repair of eyelid by reconstructive surgery, see 67961, 67966)

67850* Destruction of lesion of lid margin (up to 1 cm)

(For Mohs' micrographic surgery, see 17304-17310)

(For initiation or follow-up care of topical chemotherapy (eg, 5-FU or similar agents), see appropriate office visits)

Tarsorrhaphy

67875 Temporary closure of eyelids by suture (eg, Frost suture)

67880 Construction of intermarginal adhesions, median tarsorrhaphy, or canthorrhaphy;

67882 with transposition of tarsal plate

(For severing of tarsorrhaphy, see 67710)

(For canthoplasty, reconstruction canthus, see 67950)

(For canthotomy, see 67715)

Repair (Brow Ptosis, Blepharoptosis, Lid Retraction, Ectropion, Entropion)

67900 Repair of brow ptosis (supraciliary, mid-forehead or coronal approach)

(For forehead rhytidectomy, see 15824)

67901 Repair of blepharoptosis; frontalis muscle technique with suture or other material

67902 frontalis muscle technique with fascial sling (includes obtaining fascia)

67903   (tarso)levator resection or advancement, internal approach

67904   (tarso)levator resection or advancement, external approach

67906   superior rectus technique with fascial sling (includes obtaining fascia)

(67907 has been deleted. To report, use 67999)

67908   conjunctivo-tarso-Muller's muscle-levator resection (eg, Fasanella-Servat type)

67909   Reduction of overcorrection of ptosis

67911   Correction of lid retraction

(For obtaining autogenous graft materials, see 20920, 20922 or 20926)

(For correction of trichiasis by mucous membrane graft, see 67835)

67914   Repair of ectropion; suture

67915   thermocauterization

67916   blepharoplasty, excision tarsal wedge

67917   blepharoplasty, extensive (eg, Kuhnt-Szymanowski or tarsal strip operations)

(For correction of everted punctum, see 68705)

67921   Repair of entropion; suture

67922   thermocauterization

67923   blepharoplasty, excision tarsal wedge

67924   blepharoplasty, extensive (eg, Wheeler operation)

(For repair of cicatricial ectropion or entropion requiring scar excision or skin graft, see also 67961 et seq)

Reconstruction

Codes for blepharoplasty involve more than skin (ie, involving lid margin, tarsus, and/or palpebral conjunctiva).

67930   Suture of recent wound, eyelid, involving lid margin, tarsus, and/or palpebral conjunctiva direct closure; partial thickness

67935   full thickness

67938   Removal of embedded foreign body, eyelid

(For repair of skin of eyelid, see 12011-12018; 12051-12057; 13150, 13152, 13300)

(For tarsorrhaphy, canthorrhaphy, see 67880, 67882)

(For repair of blepharoptosis and lid retraction, see 67901-67911)

(For blepharoplasty for entropion, ectropion, see 67916, 67917, 67923, 67924)

(For correction of blepharochalasis (blepharorhytidectomy), see 15820-15823)

(For repair of skin of eyelid, adjacent tissue transfer, see 14060, 14061; preparation for graft, see 15000; free graft, see 15120, 15121, 15260, 15261)

(For excision of lesion of eyelid, see 67800 et seq)

(For repair of lacrimal canaliculi, see 68700)

67950   Canthoplasty (reconstruction of canthus)

67961   Excision and repair of eyelid, involving lid margin, tarsus, conjunctiva, canthus, or full thickness, may include preparation for skin graft or pedicle flap with adjacent tissue transfer or rearrangement; up to one-fourth of lid margin

67966   over one-fourth of lid margin

(For canthoplasty, see 67950)

(For free skin grafts, see 15120, 15121, 15260, 15261)

(For tubed pedicle flap preparation, see 15576; for delay, see 15630; for attachment, see 15630)

67971   Reconstruction of eyelid, full thickness by transfer of tarsoconjunctival flap from opposing eyelid; up to two-thirds of eyelid, one stage or first stage

67973   total eyelid, lower, one stage or first stage

67974   total eyelid, upper, one stage or first stage

67975   second stage

Other Procedures

67999 Unlisted procedure, eyelids

Conjunctiva

(For removal of foreign body, see 65205 et seq)

Incision and Drainage

68020 Incision of conjunctiva, drainage of cyst

68040 Expression of conjunctival follicles (eg, for trachoma)

Excision and/or Destruction

68100 Biopsy of conjunctiva

68110 Excision of lesion, conjunctiva; up to 1 cm

68115   over 1 cm

68130   with adjacent sclera

68135* Destruction of lesion, conjunctiva

Injection

(For injection into Tenon's capsule or retrobulbar injection, see 67500-67515)

68200* Subconjunctival injection

Conjunctivoplasty

(For wound repair, see 65270-65273)

68320 Conjunctivoplasty; with conjunctival graft or extensive rearrangement

68325   with buccal mucous membrane graft (includes obtaining graft)

68326 Conjunctivoplasty, reconstruction cul-de-sac; with conjunctival graft or extensive rearrangement

68328   with buccal mucous membrane graft (includes obtaining graft)

68330 Repair of symblepharon; conjunctivoplasty, without graft

68335   with free graft conjunctiva or buccal mucous membrane (includes obtaining graft)

68340   division of symblepharon, with or without insertion of conformer or contact lens

Other Procedures

68360 Conjunctival flap; bridge or partial (separate procedure)

68362   total (such as Gunderson thin flap or purse string flap)

(For conjunctival flap for perforating injury, see 65280, 65285)

(For repair of operative wound, see 66250)

(For removal of conjunctival foreign body, see 65205, 65210)

68399 Unlisted procedure, conjunctiva

Lacrimal System

Incision

68400 Incision, drainage of lacrimal gland

68420 Incision, drainage of lacrimal sac (dacryocystotomy or dacryocystostomy)

68440* Snip incision of lacrimal punctum

Excision

68500 Excision of lacrimal gland (dacryoadenectomy), except for tumor; total

68505   partial

68510 Biopsy of lacrimal gland

68520 Excision of lacrimal sac (dacryocystectomy)

68525 Biopsy of lacrimal sac

68530 Removal of foreign body or dacryolith, lacrimal passages

68540 Excision of lacrimal gland tumor; frontal approach

68550   involving osteotomy

Repair

68700 Plastic repair of canaliculi

68705 Correction of everted punctum, cautery

68720 Dacryocystorhinostomy (fistulization of lacrimal sac to nasal cavity)

68745 Conjunctivorhinostomy (fistulization of conjunctiva to nasal cavity); without tube

68750   with insertion of tube or stent

68760 Closure of the lacrimal punctum; by thermocauterization, ligation, or laser surgery

68761   by plug, each

68770 Closure of lacrimal fistula (separate procedure)

Probing and/or Related Procedures

68800* Dilation of lacrimal punctum, with or without irrigation, unilateral or bilateral

68820* Probing of nasolacrimal duct, with or without irrigation, unilateral or bilateral;

68825   requiring general anesthesia

(See also 92018)

68830   with insertion of tube or stent

68840* Probing of lacrimal canaliculi, with or without irrigation

68850* Injection of contrast medium for dacryocystography

(For radiological supervision and interpretation, see 70170)

Other Procedures

68899 Unlisted procedure, lacrimal system

Auditory System

(For diagnostic services (eg, audiometry, vestibular tests), see 92502 et seq)

External Ear

Incision

69000* Drainage external ear, abscess or hematoma; simple

69005 complicated

69020* Drainage external auditory canal, abscess

69090 Ear piercing

Excision

69100 Biopsy external ear

69105 Biopsy external auditory canal

69110 Excision external ear; partial, simple repair

69120 complete amputation

(For reconstruction of ear, see 15120 et seq)

69140 Excision exostosis(es), external auditory canal

69145 Excision soft tissue lesion, external auditory canal

69150 Radical excision external auditory canal lesion; without neck dissection

69155 with neck dissection

(For resection of temporal bone, see 69535)

(For skin grafting, see 15000-15261)

Removal of Foreign Body

69200 Removal foreign body from external auditory canal; without general anesthesia

69205 with general anesthesia

69210 Removal impacted cerumen (separate procedure), one or both ears

69220 Debridement, mastoidectomy cavity, simple (eg, routine cleaning)

(69221 has been deleted. To report, use 69220 with modifier -50 or 09950)

69222 Debridement, mastoidectomy cavity, complex (eg, with anesthesia or more than routine cleaning)

(69223 has been deleted. To report, use 69222 with modifier -50 or 09950)

Repair

(For suture of wound or injury of external ear, see 12011-14300)

69300 Otoplasty, protruding ear, with or without size reduction

(69301 has been deleted. To report, use 69300 with modifier -50 or 09950)

69310 Reconstruction of external auditory canal (meatoplasty) (eg, for stenosis due to trauma, infection) (separate procedure)

69320 Reconstruction external auditory canal for congenital atresia, single stage

(For combination with middle ear reconstruction, see 69631, 69641)

(For other reconstructive procedures with grafts (eg, skin, cartilage, bone), see 13150-15760, 21230-21235)

Other Procedures

(For otoscopy under general anesthesia, see 92502)

69399 Unlisted procedure, external ear

Middle Ear

Introduction

69400 Eustachian tube inflation, transnasal; with catheterization

69401 without catheterization

69405 Eustachian tube catheterization, transtympanic

Ear 69000–69979

69410 Focal application of phase control substance, middle ear (baffle technique)

Incision

69420* Myringotomy including aspiration and/or eustachian tube inflation

69421* Myringotomy including aspiration and/or eustachian tube inflation requiring general anesthesia

69424 Ventilating tube removal when originally inserted by another physician

(69425 has been deleted. To report, use 69424 with modifier -50 or 09950)

(Tympanostomy 69431-69435 has been revised as 69433-69437)

69433* Tympanostomy (requiring insertion of ventilating tube), local or topical anesthesia

(69434 has been deleted. To report, use 69433 with modifier -50 or 09950)

69436 Tympanostomy (requiring insertion of ventilating tube), general anesthesia

(69437 has been deleted. To report, use 69436 with modifier -50 or 09950)

69440 Middle ear exploration through postauricular or ear canal incision

(For atticotomy, see 69601 et seq)

69450 Tympanolysis, transcanal

Excision

69501 Transmastoid antrotomy ("simple" mastoidectomy)

69502 Mastoidectomy; complete

69505 modified radical

69511 radical

(For skin graft, see 15000 et seq)

(For mastoidectomy cavity debridement, see 69220, 69222)

69530 Petrous apicectomy including radical mastoidectomy

69535 Resection temporal bone, external approach

(For middle fossa approach, see 69950-69970)

69540 Excision aural polyp

69550 Excision aural glomus tumor; transcanal

69552 transmastoid

69554 extended (extratemporal)

Repair

69601 Revision mastoidectomy; resulting in complete mastoidectomy

69602 resulting in modified radical mastoidectomy

69603 resulting in radical mastoidectomy

69604 resulting in tympanoplasty

(For planned secondary tympanoplasty after mastoidectomy, see 69631, 69632)

69605 with apicectomy

(For skin graft, see 15120, 15121, 15260, 15261)

69610 Tympanic membrane repair, with or without site preparation or perforation for closure, with or without patch

(69611 has been deleted. To report, see 69610)

69620 Myringoplasty (surgery confined to drumhead and donor area)

69631 Tympanoplasty without mastoidectomy (including canalplasty, atticotomy and/or middle ear surgery), initial or revision; without ossicular chain reconstruction

69632 with ossicular chain reconstruction (eg, postfenestration)

69633 with ossicular chain reconstruction and synthetic prosthesis (eg, partial ossicular replacement prosthesis, (PORP), total ossicular replacement prosthesis (TORP))

Ear 69000–69979

69635 Tympanoplasty with antrotomy or mastoidotomy (including canalplasty, atticotomy, middle ear surgery, and/or tympanic membrane repair); without ossicular chain reconstruction

69636 with ossicular chain reconstruction

69637 with ossicular chain reconstruction and synthetic prosthesis (eg, partial ossicular replacement prosthesis, (PORP), total ossicular replacement prosthesis (TORP))

69641 Tympanoplasty with mastoidectomy (including canalplasty, middle ear surgery, tympanic membrane repair); without ossicular chain reconstruction

69642 with ossicular chain reconstruction

69643 with intact or reconstructed wall, without ossicular chain reconstruction

69644 with intact or reconstructed canal wall, with ossicular chain reconstruction

69645 radical or complete, without ossicular chain reconstruction

69646 radical or complete, with ossicular chain reconstruction

69650 Stapes mobilization

69660 Stapedectomy or stapedotomy with reestablishment of ossicular continuity, with or without use of foreign material;

69661 with footplate drill out

69662 Revision of stapedectomy or stapedotomy

69666 Repair oval window fistula

69667 Repair round window fistula

69670 Mastoid obliteration (separate procedure)

(69675 Tympanic neurectomy has been revised as 69676)

69676 Tympanic neurectomy

(69677 has been deleted. To report, use 69676 with modifier -50 or 09950)

Other Procedures

69700 Closure postauricular fistula, mastoid (separate procedure)

69710 Implantation or replacement of electromagnetic bone conduction hearing device in temporal bone

(Replacement procedure includes removal of old device)

69711 Removal or repair of electromagnetic bone conduction hearing device in temporal bone

69720 Decompression facial nerve, intratemporal; lateral to geniculate ganglion

69725 including medial to geniculate ganglion

69740 Suture facial nerve, intratemporal, with or without graft or decompression; lateral to geniculate ganglion

69745 including medial to geniculate ganglion

(For extracranial suture of facial nerve, see 64864)

69799 Unlisted procedure, middle ear

Inner Ear

Incision and/or Destruction

69801 Labyrinthotomy, with or without cryosurgery or other nonexcisional destructive procedures or tack procedure; transcanal

69802 with mastoidectomy

69805 Endolymphatic sac operation; without shunt

69806 with shunt

69820 Fenestration semicircular canal

69840 Revision fenestration operation

Excision

69905 Labyrinthectomy; transcanal

69910 with mastoidectomy

69915 Vestibular nerve section, translabyrinthine approach

(For transcranial approach, see 69950)

Introduction

69930 Cochlear device implantation, with or without mastoidectomy

Other Procedures

69949 Unlisted procedure, inner ear

Temporal Bone, Middle Fossa Approach

(For external approach, see 69535)

69950 Vestibular nerve section, transcranial approach

69955 Total facial nerve decompression and/or repair (may include graft)

69960 Decompression internal auditory canal

(69965 has been deleted. To report, use 69979)

69970 Removal of tumor, temporal bone

Other Procedures

69979 Unlisted procedure, temporal bone, middle fossa approach

Notes

Notes

Radiology Guidelines (Including Nuclear Medicine and Diagnostic Ultrasound)

Items used by all physicians in reporting their services are presented in the **Introduction.** Some of the commonalities are repeated here for the convenience of those physicians referring to this section on **Radiology (Including Nuclear Medicine and Diagnostic Ultrasound).** Other definitions and items unique to Radiology are also listed.

Subject Listings

Subject listings apply when radiological services are performed by or under the responsible supervision of a physician.

Multiple Procedures

It is appropriate to designate multiple procedures that are rendered on the same date by separate entries. This can be reported by using the multiple procedure modifier ('-51' or 09951). See item "Modifiers" on page 250 for modifier definitions.

Separate Procedures

Some of the listed procedures are commonly carried out as an integral part of a total service, and as such, do not warrant a separate identification. When, however, such a procedure is performed independently of, and is not immediately related to, other services, it may be listed as a "separate procedure." Thus, when a procedure that is ordinarily a component of a larger procedure is performed alone for a specific purpose, it may be reported as a separate procedure.

Subsection Information

Several of the subheadings or subsections have special needs or instructions unique to that section. Where these are indicated (eg, "Radiation Oncology") special **"Notes"** will be presented preceding those procedural terminology listings, referring to that subsection specifically. If there is an "Unlisted Procedure" code number (see section below) for the individual subsection, it will be shown. Those subsections with **"Notes"** are as follows:

Diagnostic Radiology........... 70010-76499
Diagnostic Ultrasound.......... 76506-76999
Radiation Oncology............. 77261-77799
Nuclear Medicine 78000-79999

Unlisted Service or Procedure

A service or procedure may be provided that is not listed in this edition of *CPT*. When reporting such a service, the appropriate "Unlisted Procedure" code may be used to indicate the service, identifying it by "Special Report" as discussed on page 250. The "Unlisted Procedures" and accompanying codes for **Radiology (Including Nuclear Medicine and Diagnostic Ultrasound)** are as follows:

76499	Unlisted diagnostic radiologic procedure
76999	Unlisted diagnostic ultrasound procedure
77299	Unlisted procedure, therapeutic radiology, clinical treatment planning
77399	Unlisted procedure, medical radiation physics, dosimetry and treatment devices
77499	Unlisted procedure, therapeutic radiology clinical treatment management
77799	Unlisted procedure, clinical brachytherapy

**Radiology
70010–79999**

78099	Unlisted endocrine procedure, diagnostic nuclear medicine
78199	Unlisted hematopoietic, reticuloendothelial and lymphatic procedure, diagnostic nuclear medicine
78299	Unlisted gastrointestinal procedure, diagnostic nuclear medicine
78399	Unlisted musculoskeletal procedure, diagnostic nuclear medicine
78499	Unlisted cardiovascular procedure, diagnostic nuclear medicine
78599	Unlisted respiratory procedure, diagnostic nuclear medicine
78699	Unlisted nervous system procedure, diagnostic nuclear medicine
78799	Unlisted genitourinary procedure, diagnostic nuclear medicine
78999	Unlisted miscellaneous procedure, diagnostic nuclear medicine
79999	Unlisted radiopharmaceutical therapeutic procedure

Special Report

A service that is rarely provided, unusual, variable, or new may require a special report in determining medical appropriateness of the service. Pertinent information should include an adequate definition or description of the nature, extent, and need for the procedure; and the time, effort, and equipment necessary to provide the service. Additional items which may be included are:

- complexity of symptoms;
- final diagnosis;
- pertinent physical findings;
- diagnostic and therapeutic procedures;
- concurrent problems;
- follow-up care.

Supervision and Interpretation

When a procedure is performed by two physicians, the radiologic portion of the procedure is designated as "radiological supervision and interpretation." When a physician performs both the procedure and provides imaging supervision and interpretation, a combination of procedure codes outside the 70000 series and imaging supervision and interpretation codes are to be used.

(The Radiological Supervision and Interpretation codes are not applicable to the Radiation Oncology subsection.)

Modifiers

Listed services and procedures may be modified under certain circumstances. When applicable, the modifying circumstances should be identified by the addition of the appropriate modifier code, which may be reported in either of two ways. The modifier may be reported by a two digit number placed after the usual procedure number from which it is separated by a hyphen. Or the modifier may be reported by a separate five digit code that is used in addition to the procedure code. If more than one modifier is used, place the "Multiple Modifiers" code immediately after the procedure code. This indicates that one or more additional modifier codes will follow. Modifiers commonly used in **Radiology (Including Nuclear Medicine and Diagnostic Ultrasound)** are as follows:

-22 Unusual Procedural Services: When the service(s) provided is greater than that usually required for the listed procedure, it may be identified by adding modifier '-22' to the usual procedure number or by use of the separate five digit modifier code 09922. A report may also be appropriate. **Note:** Modifier '-22' or 09922 may be utilized with computerized tomography numbers when additional slices are required or a more detailed examination is necessary.

-26 Professional Component: Certain procedures are a combination of a physician component and a technical component. When the physician component is reported separately, the service may be identified by adding the modifier '-26' to the usual procedure number or the service may be reported by use of the five digit modifier code 09926.

-32 Mandated Services: Services related to *mandated* consultation and/or related services (eg, PRO, 3rd party payor) may be identified by adding the modifier '-32' to the basic procedure or the service may be reported by use of the five digit modifier 09932.

-51 Multiple Procedures: When multiple procedures are performed on the same day or at the same session, the major procedure or service may be reported as listed. The secondary, additional, or lesser procedure(s) or service(s) may be identified by adding the modifier '-51' to the secondary procedure or service code(s) or by use of the separate five digit modifier code 09951. This modifier may be used to report multiple medical procedures performed at the same session, as well as a combination of medical and surgical procedures, or several surgical procedures performed at the same operative session.

-52 Reduced Services: Under certain circumstances, a service or procedure is partially reduced or eliminated at the physician's election. Under these circumstances, the service provided can be identified by its usual procedure number and the addition of the modifier '-52,' signifying that the service is reduced. This provides a means of reporting reduced services without disturbing the identification of the basic service. Modifier code 09952 may be used as an alternative to modifier '-52.' **Note:** Modifier '-52' or 09952 may be utilized with computerized tomography numbers for a limited study or a follow-up study.

-58 Staged or Related Procedure or Service by the Same Physician During the Postoperative Period: The physician may need to indicate that the performance of a procedure or service during the postoperative period was: a) planned prospectively at the time of the original procedure (staged); b) more extensive than the original procedure; or c) for therapy following a diagnostic surgical procedure. This circumstance may be reported by adding the modifier '-58' to the staged or related procedure, or the separate five digit modifier 09958 may be used. **Note:** This modifier is not used to report the treatment of a problem that requires a return to the operating room. See modifier '-78.'

-62 Two Surgeons: Under certain circumstances, the skills of two surgeons (usually with different skills) may be required in the management of a specific surgical procedure. Under such circumstances, the separate services may be identified by adding the modifier '-62' to the procedure number used by each surgeon for reporting his services. Modifier code 09962 may be used as an alternative to modifier '-62.'

-66 Surgical Team: Under some circumstances, highly complex procedures (requiring the concomitant services of several physicians, often of different specialties, plus other highly skilled, specially trained personnel, and various types of complex equipment) are carried out under the "surgical team" concept. Such circumstances may be identified by each participating physician with the addition of the modifier '-66' to the basic procedure number used for reporting services. Modifier code 09966 may be used as an alternative to modifier '-66'.

-76 Repeat Procedure by Same Physician: The physician may need to indicate that a procedure or service was repeated subsequent to the original service. This circumstance may be reported by adding the modifier '-76' to the repeated service or the separate five digit modifier code 09976 may be used.

-77 Repeat Procedure by Another Physician: The physician may need to indicate that a basic procedure performed by another physician had to be repeated. This situation may be reported by adding modifier '-77' to the repeated service or the separate five digit modifier code 09977 may be used.

-78 Return to the Operating Room for a Related Procedure During the Postoperative Period: The physician may need to indicate that another procedure was performed during the postoperative period of the initial procedure. When this subsequent procedure is related to the first, and requires the use of the operating room, it may be reported by adding the modifier '-78' to the related procedure, or by using the separate five digit modifier 09978. (For repeat procedures on the same day, see '-76').

-79 Unrelated Procedure or Service by the Same Physician During the Postoperative Period: The physician may need to indicate that the performance of a procedure or service during the postoperative period was unrelated to the original procedure. This circumstance may be reported by using the modifier '-79' or by using the separate five digit modifier 09979. (For repeat procedures on the same day, see '-76').

-80 Assistant Surgeon: Surgical assistant services may be identified by adding the modifier '-80' to the usual procedure number(s) or by use of the separate five digit modifier code 09980.

-90 Reference (Outside) Laboratory: When laboratory procedures are performed by a party other than the treating or reporting physician, the procedure may be identified by adding the modifier '-90' to the usual procedure number or by using the separate five digit modifier code 09990.

-99 Multiple Modifiers: Under certain circumstances, two or more modifiers may be necessary to completely delineate a service. In such situations, modifier '-99' should be added to the basic procedure, and other applicable modifiers may be listed as part of the description of the service. Modifier code 09999 may be used as an alternative to modifier '-99.'

Written Report(s)

A written report, signed by the interpreting physician, should be considered an integral part of a radiologic procedure or interpretation.

Radiology

Diagnostic Radiology (Diagnostic Imaging)

Head and Neck

(70002, 70003 have been deleted. To report, use 76499)

70010 Myelography, posterior fossa, radiological supervision and interpretation

(70011 (complete procedure) has been deleted, see 61055, 62284, 70010)

70015 Cisternography, positive contrast, radiological supervision and interpretation

(70016 (complete procedure) has been deleted, see 61055, 62284, 70015)

(70020, 70021 have been deleted. To report, use 76499)

(70022 has been deleted. To report CT guidance for stereotactic localization, use 76355)

70030 Radiologic examination, eye, for detection of foreign body

(70040, 70050 have been deleted)

70100 Radiologic examination, mandible; partial, less than four views

70110 complete, minimum of four views

70120 Radiologic examination, mastoids; less than three views per side

70130 complete, minimum of three views per side

70134 Radiologic examination, internal auditory meati, complete

70140 Radiologic examination, facial bones; less than three views

70150 complete, minimum of three views

70160 Radiologic examination, nasal bones, complete, minimum of three views

70170 Dacryocystography, nasolacrimal duct, radiological supervision and interpretation

(70171 (complete procedure) has been deleted, see 68850, 70170)

70190 Radiologic examination; optic foramina

70200 orbits, complete, minimum of four views

70210 Radiologic examination, sinuses, paranasal, less than three views

70220 Radiologic examination, sinuses, paranasal, complete, minimum of three views

(70230, 70231 have been deleted. To report, use 76499)

70240 Radiologic examination, sella turcica

70250 Radiologic examination, skull; less than four views, with or without stereo

70260 complete, minimum of four views, with or without stereo

70300 Radiologic examination, teeth; single view

70310 partial examination, less than full mouth

70320 complete, full mouth

70328 Radiologic examination, temporomandibular joint, open and closed mouth; unilateral

70330 bilateral

70332 Temporomandibular joint arthrography, radiological supervision and interpretation

(70333 (complete procedure) has been deleted, see 21116, 70332)

70336 Magnetic resonance (eg, proton) imaging, temporomandibular joint

70350 Cephalogram, orthodontic

70355 Orthopantogram

70360 Radiologic examination; neck, soft tissue

70370 pharynx or larynx, including fluoroscopy and/or magnification technique

70371 Complex dynamic pharyngeal and speech evaluation by cine or video recording

70373 Laryngography, contrast, radiological supervision and interpretation

(70374 (complete procedure) has been deleted, see 31708, 70373)

70380 Radiologic examination, salivary gland for calculus

70390 Sialography, radiological supervision and interpretation

(70391 (complete procedure) has been deleted, see 42550, 70390)

(70400, 70401 have been deleted. To report, use 76499)

70450 Computerized axial tomography, head or brain; without contrast material

70460 with contrast material(s)

70470 without contrast material, followed by contrast material(s) and further sections

(For coronal, sagittal, and/or oblique sections, see 76375)

70480 Computerized axial tomography, orbit, sella, or posterior fossa or outer, middle, or inner ear; without contrast material

70481 with contrast material(s)

70482 without contrast material, followed by contrast material(s) and further sections

(For coronal, sagittal, and/or oblique sections, see 76375)

70486 Computerized axial tomography, maxillofacial area; without contrast material

70487 with contrast material(s)

70488 without contrast material, followed by contrast material(s) and further sections

(For coronal, sagittal, and/or oblique sections, see 76375)

70490 Computerized axial tomography, soft tissue neck; without contrast material

70491 with contrast material(s)

70492 without contrast material followed by contrast material(s) and further sections

(For coronal, sagittal, and/or oblique sections, see 76375)

(For cervical spine, see 72125, 72126)

70540 Magnetic resonance (eg, proton) imaging, orbit, face, and neck

70541 Magnetic resonance angiography, head and/or neck, with or without contrast material(s)

(70550 has been deleted. To report, use 70551)

70551 Magnetic resonance (eg, proton) imaging, brain (including brain stem); without contrast material

70552 with contrast material(s)

70553 without contrast material, followed by contrast material(s) and further sequences

Chest

(71000 has been deleted)

71010 Radiologic examination, chest; single view, frontal

71015 stereo, frontal

71020 Radiologic examination, chest, two views, frontal and lateral;

71021 with apical lordotic procedure

71022 with oblique projections

71023 with fluoroscopy

71030 Radiologic examination, chest, complete, minimum of four views;

71034 with fluoroscopy

(For separate chest fluoroscopy, see 76000)

71035 Radiologic examination, chest, special views (eg, lateral decubitus, Bucky studies)

71036   Needle biopsy of intrathoracic lesion, including follow-up films, fluoroscopic localization only, radiological supervision and interpretation

(71037 (complete procedure) has been deleted, see 32400, 32405, 71036)

71038   Fluoroscopic localization for transbronchial biopsy or brushing

71040   Bronchography, unilateral, radiological supervision and interpretation

(71041 (complete procedure) has been deleted, see 31656, 31708, 31710, 31715, 71040)

71060   Bronchography, bilateral, radiological supervision and interpretation

(71061 (complete procedure) has been deleted, see 31656, 31708, 31710, 31715, 71060)

71090   Insertion pacemaker, fluoroscopy and radiography, radiological supervision and interpretation

71100   Radiologic examination, ribs, unilateral; two views

71101   including posteroanterior chest, minimum of three views

71110   Radiologic examination, ribs, bilateral; three views

71111   including posteroanterior chest, minimum of four views

71120   Radiologic examination; sternum, minimum of two views

71130   sternoclavicular joint or joints, minimum of three views

71250   Computerized axial tomography, thorax; without contrast material

71260   with contrast material(s)

71270   without contrast material, followed by contrast material(s) and further sections

(For coronal, sagittal, and/or oblique sections, see 76375)

71550   Magnetic resonance (eg, proton) imaging, chest (eg, for evaluation of hilar and mediastinal lymphadenopathy)

(For breast MRI, see 76093 and 76094)

71555   Magnetic resonance angiography, chest (excluding myocardium), with or without contrast material(s)

Spine and Pelvis

72010   Radiologic examination, spine, entire, survey study, anteroposterior and lateral

72020   Radiologic examination, spine, single view, specify level

72040   Radiologic examination, spine, cervical; anteroposterior and lateral

72050   minimum of four views

72052   complete, including oblique and flexion and/or extension studies

72069   Radiologic examination, spine, thoracolumbar, standing (scoliosis)

72070   Radiologic examination, spine; thoracic, anteroposterior and lateral

72072   thoracic, anteroposterior and lateral, including swimmer's view of the cervicothoracic junction

72074   thoracic, complete, including obliques, minimum of four views

72080   thoracolumbar, anteroposterior and lateral

72090   scoliosis study, including supine and erect studies

72100   Radiologic examination, spine, lumbosacral; anteroposterior and lateral

72110   complete, with oblique views

72114   complete, including bending views

72120   Radiologic examination, spine, lumbosacral, bending views only, minimum of four views

Contrast material in CT of spine is either by intrathecal or intravenous injection. For intrathecal injection, use also 61055 or 62284. IV injection of contrast material is part of the CT procedure.

72125   Computerized axial tomography, cervical spine; without contrast material

72126   with contrast material

72127   without contrast material, followed by contrast material(s) and further sections

(For intrathecal injection procedure, see 61055, 62284)

72128 Computerized axial tomography, thoracic spine; without contrast material

72129   with contrast material

(For intrathecal injection procedure, see 61055, 62284)

72130   without contrast material, followed by contrast material(s) and further sections

(For intrathecal injection procedure, see 61055, 62284)

72131 Computerized axial tomography, lumbar spine; without contrast material

72132   with contrast material

72133   without contrast material, followed by contrast material(s) and further sections

(For intrathecal injection procedure, see 61055, 62284)

(For coronal, sagittal, and/or oblique sections, see 76375)

(72140 has been deleted. To report, see 72141-72149)

72141 Magnetic resonance (eg, proton) imaging, spinal canal and contents, cervical; without contrast material

72142   with contrast material(s)

(For cervical spinal canal imaging without contrast material followed by contrast material, use 72156)

(72143 has been deleted. To report, see 72146, 72147)

(72144 has been deleted. To report, see 72148, 72149)

(72145 has been deleted. To report, see 72125-72133)

72146 Magnetic resonance (eg, proton) imaging, spinal canal and contents, thoracic; without contrast material

72147   with contrast material(s)

(For thoracic spinal canal imaging without contrast material followed by contrast material, use 72157)

72148 Magnetic resonance (eg, proton) imaging, spinal canal and contents, lumbar; without contrast material

72149   with contrast material(s)

(For lumbar spinal canal imaging without contrast material followed by contrast material, use 72158)

72156 Magnetic resonance (eg, proton) imaging, spinal canal and contents, without contrast material, followed by contrast material(s) and further sequences; cervical

72157   thoracic

72158   lumbar

72159 Magnetic resonance angiography, spinal canal and contents, with or without contrast material(s)

72170 Radiologic examination, pelvis; anteroposterior only

(72180 has been deleted. To report, use 72170)

72190   complete, minimum of three views

(For pelvimetry, see 74710)

72192 Computerized axial tomography, pelvis; without contrast material

72193   with contrast material(s)

72194   without contrast material, followed by contrast material(s) and further sections

(For coronal, sagittal, and/or oblique sections, see 76375)

72196 Magnetic resonance (eg, proton) imaging, pelvis

72198 Magnetic resonance angiography, pelvis, with or without contrast material(s)

72200 Radiologic examination, sacroiliac joints; less than three views

72202   three or more views

72220 Radiologic examination, sacrum and coccyx, minimum of two views

72240 Myelography, cervical, radiological supervision and interpretation

(72241 (complete procedure) has been deleted, see 61055, 62284, 72240)

72255 Myelography, thoracic, radiological supervision and interpretation

(72256 (complete procedure) has been deleted, see 61055, 62284, 72255)

72265 Myelography, lumbosacral, radiological supervision and interpretation

(72266 (complete procedure) has been deleted, see 61055, 62284, 72265)

72270 Myelography, entire spinal canal, radiological supervision and interpretation

(72271 (complete procedure) has been deleted, see 61055, 62284, 72270)

72285 Diskography, cervical, radiological supervision and interpretation

(72286 (complete procedure) has been deleted, see 62291, 72285)

72295 Diskography, lumbar, radiological supervision and interpretation

(72296 (complete procedure) has been deleted, see 62290, 72295)

Upper Extremities

73000 Radiologic examination; clavicle, complete

73010   scapula, complete

73020 Radiologic examination, shoulder; one view

73030   complete, minimum of two views

73040 Radiologic examination, shoulder, arthrography, radiological supervision and interpretation

(73041 (complete procedure) has been deleted, see 23350, 73040)

73050 Radiologic examination; acromioclavicular joints, bilateral, with or without weighted distraction

73060   humerus, minimum of two views

73070 Radiologic examination, elbow; anteroposterior and lateral views

73080   complete, minimum of three views

73085 Radiologic examination, elbow, arthrography, radiological supervision and interpretation

(73086 (complete procedure) has been deleted, see 24220, 73085)

73090 Radiologic examination; forearm, anteroposterior and lateral views

73092   upper extremity, infant, minimum of two views

73100 Radiologic examination, wrist; anteroposterior and lateral views

73110   complete, minimum of three views

73115 Radiologic examination, wrist, arthrography, radiological supervision and interpretation

(73116 (complete procedure) has been deleted, see 25246, 73115)

73120 Radiologic examination, hand; two views

73130   minimum of three views

73140 Radiologic examination, finger(s), minimum of two views

73200 Computerized axial tomography, upper extremity; without contrast material

73201   with contrast material(s)

73202   without contrast material, followed by contrast material(s) and further sections

(For coronal, sagittal, and/or oblique sections, see 76375)

73220 Magnetic resonance (eg, proton) imaging, upper extremity, other than joint

73221 Magnetic resonance (eg, proton) imaging, any joint of upper extremity

▲=Revised Code   ●=New Code

73225 Magnetic resonance angiography, upper extremity, with or without contrast material(s)

Lower Extremities

73500 Radiologic examination, hip, unilateral; one view

73510 complete, minimum of two views

73520 Radiologic examination, hips, bilateral, minimum of two views of each hip, including anteroposterior view of pelvis

73525 Radiologic examination, hip, arthrography, radiological supervision and interpretation

(73526 (complete procedure) has been deleted, see 27093, 27095, 73525)

73530 Radiologic examination, hip, during operative procedure

(73531 has been deleted. To report, use 73530)

73540 Radiologic examination, pelvis and hips, infant or child, minimum of two views

73550 Radiologic examination, femur, anteroposterior and lateral views

73560 Radiologic examination, knee; anteroposterior and lateral views

73562 anteroposterior and lateral, with oblique(s), minimum of three views

73564 complete, including oblique(s), and tunnel, and/or patellar and/or standing views

73565 both knees, standing, anteroposterior

(73570 has been deleted. To report, see 73562, 73564)

73580 Radiologic examination, knee, arthrography, radiological supervision and interpretation

(73581 (complete procedure) has been deleted, see 27370, 73580)

73590 Radiologic examination; tibia and fibula, anteroposterior and lateral views

73592 lower extremity, infant, minimum of two views

73600 Radiologic examination, ankle; anteroposterior and lateral views

73610 complete, minimum of three views

73615 Radiologic examination, ankle, arthrography, radiological supervision and interpretation

(73616 (complete procedure) has been deleted, see 27648, 73615)

73620 Radiologic examination, foot; anteroposterior and lateral views

73630 complete, minimum of three views

73650 Radiologic examination; calcaneus, minimum of two views

73660 toe(s), minimum of two views

73700 Computerized axial tomography, lower extremity; without contrast material

73701 with contrast material(s)

73702 without contrast material, followed by contrast material(s) and further sections

(For coronal, sagittal, and/or oblique sections, see 76375)

73720 Magnetic resonance (eg, proton) imaging, lower extremity, other than joint

73721 Magnetic resonance (eg, proton) imaging, any joint of lower extremity

73725 Magnetic resonance angiography, lower extremity, with or without contrast material(s)

Abdomen

74000 Radiologic examination, abdomen; single anteroposterior view

74010 anteroposterior and additional oblique and cone views

74020 complete, including decubitus and/or erect views

74022 complete acute abdomen series, including supine, erect, and/or decubitus views, upright PA chest

74150 Computerized axial tomography, abdomen; without contrast material

74160 with contrast material(s)

74170 without contrast material, followed by contrast material(s) and further sections

(For coronal, sagittal, and/or oblique sections, see 76375)

74181 Magnetic resonance (eg, proton) imaging, abdomen

74185 Magnetic resonance angiography, abdomen, with or without contrast material(s)

74190 Peritoneogram (eg, after injection of air or contrast), radiological supervision and interpretation

(For procedure, see 49400)

(For computerized axial tomography, see 72192 or 74150)

Gastrointestinal Tract

(For percutaneous placement of gastrostomy tube, see 43750)

74210 Radiologic examination; pharynx and/or cervical esophagus

74220   esophagus

74230 Swallowing function, pharynx and/or esophagus, with cineradiography and/or video

74235 Removal of foreign body(s), esophageal, with use of balloon catheter, radiological supervision and interpretation

(For procedure, see 43215, 43247)

74240 Radiologic examination, gastrointestinal tract, upper; with or without delayed films, without KUB

74241   with or without delayed films, with KUB

74245   with small bowel, includes multiple serial films

74246 Radiological examination, gastrointestinal tract, upper, air contrast, with specific high density barium, effervescent agent, with or without glucagon; with or without delayed films, without KUB

74247   with or without delayed films, with KUB

74249   with small bowel follow-through

74250 Radiologic examination, small bowel, includes multiple serial films;

74251   via enteroclysis tube

74260 Duodenography, hypotonic

74270 Radiologic examination, colon; barium enema, with or without KUB

(74275 has been deleted. To report, use 76499)

74280   air contrast with specific high density barium, with or without glucagon

74283 Barium enema, therapeutic, for reduction of intussusception

(74285 has been deleted. To report, see 74270, 74280)

74290 Cholecystography, oral contrast;

74291   additional or repeat examination or multiple day examination

74300 Cholangiography and/or pancreatography; intraoperative, radiological supervision and interpretation

74301   additional set intraoperative, radiological supervision and interpretation

74305   postoperative, radiological supervision and interpretation

(For procedure, see 47605, 48400, 56341, 56362, 56363)

(For biliary duct stone extraction, percutaneous, see 47630, 74327)

(74310, 74315 have been deleted. To report, use 76499)

74320 Cholangiography, percutaneous, transhepatic, radiological supervision and interpretation

(74321 (complete procedure) has been deleted, see 47500, 74320)

(74325, 74326 have been deleted. To report, use 76499)

▲=Revised Code   ●=New Code

74327 Postoperative biliary duct stone removal, percutaneous via T-tube tract, basket, or snare (eg, Burhenne technique), radiological supervision and interpretation

(For procedure, see 47630)

74328 Endoscopic catheterization of the biliary ductal system, radiological supervision and interpretation

(For procedure, see 43260-43272 as appropriate)

74329 Endoscopic catheterization of the pancreatic ductal system, radiological supervision and interpretation

(For procedure, see 43260-43272 as appropriate)

74330 Combined endoscopic catheterization of the biliary and pancreatic ductal systems, radiological supervision and interpretation

(For procedure, see 43260-43272 as appropriate)

(74331 has been deleted. To report, use 43262)

74340 Introduction of long gastrointestinal tube (eg, Miller-Abbott), including multiple fluoroscopies and films, radiological supervision and interpretation

(For tube placement, see 44500)

74350 Percutaneous placement of gastrostomy tube, radiological supervision and interpretation

(74351 (complete procedure) has been deleted, see 43246, 43750, 74350)

74355 Percutaneous placement of enteroclysis tube, radiological supervision and interpretation

(74356 (complete procedure) has been deleted, see 44015, 74355)

74360 Intraluminal dilation of strictures and/or obstructions (eg, esophagus), radiological supervision and interpretation

(74361 (complete procedure) has been deleted, see 43220, 43458, 74360)

74363 Percutaneous transhepatic dilatation of biliary duct stricture with or without placement of stent, radiological supervision and interpretation

(For procedure, see 47510, 47511, 47555, 47556)

Urinary Tract

74400 Urography (pyelography), intravenous, with or without KUB, with or without tomography;

74405   with special hypertensive contrast concentration and/or clearance studies

74410 Urography, infusion, drip technique and/or bolus technique;

74415   with nephrotomography

74420 Urography, retrograde, with or without KUB

74425 Urography, antegrade, (pyelostogram, nephrostogram, loopogram), radiological supervision and interpretation

(74426 (complete procedure) has been deleted, see 50394, 50684, 50690, 74425)

74430 Cystography, minimum of three views, radiological supervision and interpretation

(74431 (complete procedure) has been deleted, see 51600, 51605, 74430)

74440 Vasography, vesiculography, or epididymography, radiological supervision and interpretation

(74441 (complete procedure) has been deleted, see 52010, 55300, 74440)

74445 Corpora cavernosography, radiological supervision and interpretation

(74446 (complete procedure) has been deleted, use 54230, 74445)

74450 Urethrocystography, retrograde, radiological supervision and interpretation

(74451 (complete procedure) has been deleted, see 51610, 74450)

74455 Urethrocystography, voiding, radiological supervision and interpretation

(74456 (complete procedure) has been deleted, see 51600, 74455)

(74460, 74461 have been deleted. To report, use 76499)

74470 Radiologic examination, renal cyst study, translumbar, contrast visualization, radiological supervision and interpretation

(74471 (complete procedure) has been deleted, see 50390, 74470)

74475 Introduction of intracatheter or catheter into renal pelvis for drainage and/or injection, percutaneous, radiological supervision and interpretation

(74476 (complete procedure) has been deleted, see 50392-50398, 74475)

74480 Introduction of ureteral catheter or stent into ureter through renal pelvis for drainage and/or injection, percutaneous, radiological supervision and interpretation

(74481 (complete procedure) has been deleted, see 50392-50398, 74480)

(For transurethral surgery (ureter and pelvis), see 52320-52338)

74485 Dilation of nephrostomy, ureters, or urethra, radiological supervision and interpretation

(74486 (complete procedure) has been deleted, see 50395, 53600-53621, 74485)

(For dilation of ureter without radiologic guidance, use 52335)

(For change of nephrostomy or pyelostomy tube, use 50398)

Gynecological and Obstetrical

(For abdomen and pelvis, see 72170-72190, 74000-74170)

74710 Pelvimetry, with or without placental localization

(74720, 74725 have been deleted. To report, see 74000)

(74730, 74731 have been deleted. To report, use 76499)

74740 Hysterosalpingography, radiological supervision and interpretation

(74741 (complete procedure) has been deleted, see 58340, 74740)

74742 Transcervical catheterization of fallopian tube, radiological supervision and interpretation

(For procedure, see 58345)

(74760, 74761, 74770, 74771 have been deleted. To report, use 76499)

74775 Perineogram (eg, vaginogram, for sex determination or extent of anomalies)

Heart

(For separate injection procedures for vascular radiology, see **Surgery** section, 36000-36299)

(For cardiac catheterization procedures, see 93501-93556)

(75500 has been deleted. To report, use 93555)

(75501 (complete procedure) has been deleted, see 93501-93536, 93542, 93543, 93555)

(75505 has been deleted. To report, use 93555)

(75506 (complete procedure) has been deleted, see 36400-36425 for intravenous procedure, 36100-36248 for intra-arterial procedure and 93501-93536, 93542, 93543, 93555)

(75507 has been deleted. To report, use 93555)

(75509 (complete procedure) has been deleted. To report, see 36400-36425 for intravenous procedure, 36100-36248 for intra-arterial procedure and 93501-93536, 93542, 93543)

(75510, 75511 have been deleted. To report, use 76499)

(75519 has been deleted. To report, use 93555)

(75520 (complete procedure) has been deleted, see 36400-36425 for intravenous procedure, 36100-36248 for intra-arterial procedure, and 93501, 93542)

(75523 has been deleted. To report, use 93555)

(75524 has been deleted, see 36400-36425 for intravenous procedure, 36100-36248 for intra-arterial procedure, and 93510-93514, 93524, 93543)

(75527 has been deleted. To report, use 93555)

(75528 has been deleted, see 36400-36425 for intravenous procedure, 36100-36248 for intra-arterial procedure, and 93526-93529, 93543, and 93555)

75552 Cardiac magnetic resonance imaging for morphology; without contrast material

75553 with contrast material

75554 Cardiac magnetic resonance imaging for function, with or without morphology; complete study (eg, multiple chambers)

75555 limited study (eg, single chamber)

75556 Cardiac magnetic resonance imaging for velocity flow mapping

Aorta and Arteries

Selective vascular catheterizations should be coded to include introduction and all lesser order selective catheterizations used in the approach (eg, the description for a selective right middle cerebral artery catheterization includes the introduction and placement catheterization of the right common and internal carotid arteries).

Additional second and/or third order arterial catheterizations within the same family of arteries supplied by a single first order artery should be expressed by 36218 or 36248. Additional first order or higher catheterizations in vascular families supplied by a first order vessel different from a previously selected and coded family should be separately coded using the conventions described above.

(For intravenous procedure, see 36000-36013, 36400-36425 and 36100-36248 for intra-arterial procedure)

(For radiological supervision and interpretation, see 75600-75978)

75600 Aortography, thoracic, without serialography, radiological supervision and interpretation

(75601 (complete procedure) has been deleted, see 36000-36013, 36400-36425 for intravenous procedure, and 36100-36200 for intra-arterial procedure and 75600)

(For injection procedure, see 93544)

75605 Aortography, thoracic, by serialography, radiological supervision and interpretation

(75606 (complete procedure) has been deleted, see 36000-36013, 36400-36425 for intravenous procedure, and 36100-36200 for intra-arterial procedure and 75605)

(For injection procedure, see 93544)

(75620, 75621, 75622, 75623 have been deleted. To report, use 76499)

75625 Aortography, abdominal, by serialography, radiological supervision and interpretation

(75626, 75627 and 75628 have been deleted, see 36000-36013, 36400-36425 for intravenous procedure, and 36100-36200 for intra-arterial procedure and 75625)

(For injection procedure, see 93544)

75630 Aortography, abdominal plus bilateral iliofemoral lower extremity, catheter, by serialography, radiological supervision and interpretation

(75631 (complete procedure) has been deleted, see 36000-36013, 36400-36425 for intravenous procedure, and 36100-36200 and 36245-36248 for intra-arterial procedure and 75630)

75650 Angiography, cervicocerebral, catheter, including vessel origin, radiological supervision and interpretation

(75651-75657 (complete procedure) have been deleted, see 36000-36013, 36400-36425 for intravenous procedure, and 36100-36218 for intra-arterial procedure and 75650, 75660-75685 as appropriate)

75658 Angiography, brachial, retrograde, radiological supervision and interpretation

(75659 (complete procedure) has been deleted, see 36000-36013, 36400-36425 for intravenous procedure, and 36100-36218 for intra-arterial procedure and 75658)

75660   Angiography, external carotid, unilateral, selective, radiological supervision and interpretation

(75661 (complete procedure) has been deleted, see 36000-36013, 36400-36425 for intravenous procedure, and 36100-36218 and 75660)

75662   Angiography, external carotid, bilateral, selective, radiological supervision and interpretation

(75663 (complete procedure) has been deleted, see 36000-36013, 36400-36425 for intravenous procedure, and 36100-36218 for intra-arterial procedure and 75662)

75665   Angiography, carotid, cerebral, unilateral, radiological supervision and interpretation

(75667, 75669 (complete procedure) have been deleted, see 36000-36013, 36400-36425 for intravenous procedure, and 36100-36218 for intra-arterial procedure and 75665)

75671   Angiography, carotid, cerebral, bilateral, radiological supervision and interpretation

(75672, 75673 (complete procedure) have been deleted, see 36000-36013, 36400-36425 for intravenous procedure, and 36100-36218 for intra-arterial procedure and 75671)

75676   Angiography, carotid, cervical, unilateral, radiological supervision and interpretation

(75677, 75678 (complete procedure) have been deleted, see 36000-36013, 36400-36425 for intravenous procedure, and 36100-36218 for intra-arterial procedure and 75676)

75680   Angiography, carotid, cervical, bilateral, radiological supervision and interpretation

(75681, 75682 (complete procedure) have been deleted, see 36000-36013, 36400-36425 for intravenous procedure, and 36100-36218 for intra-arterial procedure and 75680)

75685   Angiography, vertebral, cervical, and/or intracranial, radiological supervision and interpretation

(75686 has been deleted)

(75687 (complete procedure) has been deleted, see 36000-36013, 36400-36425 for intravenous procedure, and 36100-36218 for intra-arterial procedure and 75685)

(75690 (complete procedure) has been deleted, see 36000-36013, 36400-36425 for intravenous procedure, and 36100-36218 for intra-arterial procedure and 75685)

(75691 has been deleted)

(75692 (complete procedure) has been deleted, see 36000-36013, 36400-36425 for intravenous procedure, and 36100-36218 for intra-arterial procedure and 75685)

(75695 (complete procedure) has been deleted, see 36000-36013, 36400-36425 for intravenous procedure, and 36100-36218 for intra-arterial procedure and 75685)

(75696 has been deleted)

(75697 (complete procedure) has been deleted, see 36000-36013, 36400-36425 for intravenous procedure, and 36100-36218 for intra-arterial procedure and 75685)

75705   Angiography, spinal, selective, radiological supervision and interpretation

(75706 (complete procedure) has been deleted, see 36000-36013, 36400-36425 for intravenous procedure, and 36100-36248 for intra-arterial procedure and 75705)

75710   Angiography, extremity, unilateral, radiological supervision and interpretation

(75711, 75712 (complete procedure) have been deleted, see 36000-36013, 36400-36425 for intravenous procedure, and 36100-36248 for intra-arterial procedure and 75710)

75716   Angiography, extremity, bilateral, radiological supervision and interpretation

(75717, 75718 (complete procedure) have been deleted, see 36000-36013, 36400-36425 for intravenous procedure, and 36100-36248 for intra-arterial procedure and 75716)

75722   Angiography, renal, unilateral, selective (including flush aortogram), radiological supervision and interpretation

(75723 (complete procedure) has been deleted, see 36000-36013, 36400-36425 for intravenous procedure, and 36100-36200 and 36245-36248 for intra-arterial procedure and 75722)

75724 Angiography, renal, bilateral, selective (including flush aortogram), radiological supervision and interpretation

(75725 (complete procedure) has been deleted, see 36000-36013, 36400-36425 for intravenous procedure, and 36100-36200 and 36245-36248 for intra-arterial procedure and 75724)

75726 Angiography, visceral, selective or supra-selective, (with or without flush aortogram), radiological supervision and interpretation

(For selective angiography, each additional visceral vessel studied after basic examination, see 75774)

(75727, 75728 (complete procedure) have been deleted, see 36000-36013, 36400-36425 for intravenous procedure, and 36100-36248 for intra-arterial procedure and 75726)

75731 Angiography, adrenal, unilateral, selective, radiological supervision and interpretation

(75732 (complete procedure) has been deleted, see 36000-36013, 36400-36425 for intravenous procedure, and 36100-36200 and 36245-36248 for intra-arterial procedure and 75731)

75733 Angiography, adrenal, bilateral, selective, radiological supervision and interpretation

(75734 (complete procedure) has been deleted, see 36000-36013, 36400-36425 for intravenous procedure, and 36100-36200 and 36245-36248 for intra-arterial procedure and 75733)

75736 Angiography, pelvic, selective or supra-selective, radiological supervision and interpretation

(75737, 75738 (complete procedure) have been deleted, see 36000-36013, 36400-36425 for intravenous procedure, and 36100-36200 and 36245-36248 for intra-arterial procedure and 75736)

75741 Angiography, pulmonary, unilateral, selective, radiological supervision and interpretation

(75742 (complete procedure) has been deleted, see 36000-36015, 36400-36425 for intravenous procedure and 75741)

(For injection procedure, see 93541)

75743 Angiography, pulmonary, bilateral, selective, radiological supervision and interpretation

(75744 (complete procedure) has been deleted, see 36000-36015, 36400-36425 for intravenous procedure and 75743)

(For injection procedure, see 93541)

75746 Angiography, pulmonary, by nonselective catheter or venous injection, radiological supervision and interpretation

(75747, 75748 (complete procedure) have been deleted, see 36000-36013, 36400-36425 for intravenous procedure, and 36100-36200 for intra-arterial procedure and 75746)

(For injection procedure, see 93541)

(75750 has been deleted. To report, use 93556)

(75751 (complete procedure) has been deleted, see 36000-36013, 36400-36425 for intravenous procedure, and 36100-36200 for intra-arterial procedure and 93556)

(For introduction of catheter, injection procedure, see 93501-93536, 93539, 93540, 93545, 93556)

(75752 has been deleted. To report, use 93556)

(75753 (complete procedure) has been deleted, see 36100-36218 for intra-arterial procedure and 93556)

(For introduction of catheter, injection procedure, see 93501-93536, 93545, 93556)

(75754 has been deleted. To report, use 93556)

(75755 (complete procedure) has been deleted, see 36100-36218 for intra-arterial procedure and 93556)

(For introduction of catheter, injection procedure, see 93501-93536, 93539, 93540, 93545, 93556)

75756   Angiography, internal mammary, radiological
supervision and interpretation

(75757 (complete procedure) has been
deleted, see 36000-36013, 36400-36425 for
intravenous procedure, and 36100-36218 for
intra-arterial procedure and 93556)

(75762 has been deleted. To report, use
93556)

(75764 (complete procedure) has been
deleted, see 36000-36013, 36400-36425 for
intravenous procedure, and 36100-36218 for
intra-arterial procedure and 93556)

(For introduction of catheter, injection
procedure, see 93501-93536, 93545, 93556)

(75766 has been deleted. To report, use
93556)

(75767 has been deleted. To report, see
36000-36013, 36400-36425 for intravenous
procedure, and 36100-36218 for intra-arterial
procedure and 93556)

(For introduction of catheter, injection
procedure, see 93501-93536, 93545, 93556)

(75772, 75773 have been deleted. To report,
see 75774)

75774   Angiography, selective, each additional vessel
studied after basic examination, radiological
supervision and interpretation

(75775 (complete procedure) has been
deleted, see 36000-36015, 36400-36425 for
intravenous procedure, and 36100-36248 for
intra-arterial procedure and 75774)

(For introduction of catheter, injection procedure, see 93501-93536, 93545, 93555,
93556)

75790   Angiography, arteriovenous shunt (eg, dialysis
patient), radiological supervision and
interpretation

(For introduction of catheter, see 36140,
36215-36217, 36245-36247)

Veins and Lymphatics

(For injection procedure for venous system,
see 36000-36015, 36400-36510)

(For injection procedure for lymphatic system,
see 38790)

75801   Lymphangiography, extremity only, unilateral,
radiological supervision and interpretation

(75802 (complete procedure) has been
deleted, see 38790, 75801)

75803   Lymphangiography, extremity only, bilateral,
radiological supervision and interpretation

(75804 (complete procedure) has been
deleted, see 38790, 75803)

75805   Lymphangiography, pelvic/abdominal,
unilateral, radiological supervision and
interpretation

(75806 (complete procedure) has been
deleted, see 38790, 75805)

75807   Lymphangiography, pelvic/abdominal, bilateral,
radiological supervision and interpretation

(75808 (complete procedure) has been
deleted, see 38790, 75807)

75809   Shuntogram for investigation of previously
placed indwelling nonvascular shunt
(eg, LeVeen shunt, ventriculoperitoneal shunt),
radiological supervision and interpretation

(For procedure, see 49427 or 61070)

75810   Splenoportography, radiological supervision
and interpretation

(75811 (complete procedure) has been
deleted, see 38200, 75810)

75820   Venography, extremity, unilateral, radiological
supervision and interpretation

(75821 (complete procedure) has been
deleted, see 36000, 36406, 36410, 36420,
36425, 75820)

75822   Venography, extremity, bilateral, radiological
supervision and interpretation

(75823 (complete procedure) has been
deleted, see 36000, 36406, 36410, 36420,
36425, 75822)

75825   Venography, caval, inferior, with serialography,
radiological supervision and interpretation

(75826 (complete procedure) has been
deleted, see 36010, 75825)

75827 Venography, caval, superior, with serialography, radiological supervision and interpretation

(75828 (complete procedure) has been deleted, see 36010, 75827)

75831 Venography, renal, unilateral, selective, radiological supervision and interpretation

(75832 (complete procedure) has been deleted, see 36000-36012, 75831)

75833 Venography, renal, bilateral, selective, radiological supervision and interpretation

(75834 (complete procedure) has been deleted, see 36000-36012, 75833)

75840 Venography, adrenal, unilateral, selective, radiological supervision and interpretation

(75841 (complete procedure) has been deleted, see 36000-36012, 75840)

75842 Venography, adrenal, bilateral, selective, radiological supervision and interpretation

(75843 (complete procedure) has been deleted, see 36000-36012, 75842)

(75845, 75846, 75847, 75850, 75851 have been deleted)

75860 Venography, sinus or jugular, catheter, radiological supervision and interpretation

(75861 (complete procedure) has been deleted, see 36000-36012 for intravenous procedure and 36100-36218 for intra-arterial procedure, 75860)

75870 Venography, superior sagittal sinus, radiological supervision and interpretation

(75871 (complete procedure) has been deleted, see 36000-36012 for intravenous procedure and 36100-36218 for intra-arterial procedure, 75870)

75872 Venography, epidural, radiological supervision and interpretation

(75873 (complete procedure) has been deleted, see 36000-36012 for intravenous procedure and 36100-36218 for intra-arterial procedure, 75872)

75880 Venography, orbital, radiological supervision and interpretation

(75881 (complete procedure) has been deleted, see 36000-36012 for intravenous procedure and 36100-36218 for intra-arterial procedure, 75880)

75885 Percutaneous transhepatic portography with hemodynamic evaluation, radiological supervision and interpretation

(75886 (complete procedure) has been deleted, see 36011, 36012, 36481, 75885)

75887 Percutaneous transhepatic portography without hemodynamic evaluation, radiological supervision and interpretation

(75888 (complete procedure) has been deleted, see 36011, 36012, 36481, 75887)

75889 Hepatic venography, wedged or free, with hemodynamic evaluation, radiological supervision and interpretation

(75890 (complete procedure) has been deleted, see 36000-36012, 75889)

75891 Hepatic venography, wedged or free, without hemodynamic evaluation, radiological supervision and interpretation

(75892 (complete procedure) has been deleted, see 36000-36012, 75891)

75893 Venous sampling through catheter, with or without angiography (eg, for parathyroid hormone, renin), radiological supervision and interpretation

(For procedure, see 36500)

Transcatheter Therapy and Biopsy

75894 Transcatheter therapy, embolization, any method, radiological supervision and interpretation

(75895 (complete procedure) has been deleted, see 37204, 61624, 61626, 75894)

75896 Transcatheter therapy, infusion, any method (eg, thrombolysis other than coronary), radiological supervision and interpretation

(75897 (complete procedure) has been deleted, see 37201, 37202, 75896)

(Infusion for coronary disease, see 92975, 92977)

75898   Angiogram through existing catheter for follow-up study for transcatheter therapy, embolization or infusion

75900   Exchange of a previously placed arterial catheter during thrombolytic therapy with contrast monitoring, radiological supervision and interpretation

(For procedure, see 37209)

75940   Percutaneous placement of IVC filter, radiological supervision and interpretation

(75941 (complete procedure) has been deleted, see 37620, 75940)

(75950, 75951, 75955, 75956 (complete procedure) have been deleted, see 37204, 61624, 61626, 75894)

75960   Transcatheter introduction of intravascular stent(s), (non-coronary vessel), percutaneous and/or open, radiological supervision and interpretation, each vessel

(For procedure, see 37205-37208)

75961   Transcatheter retrieval, percutaneous, of intravascular foreign body (eg, fractured venous or arterial catheter), radiological supervision and interpretation

(For procedure, see 37203)

75962   Transluminal balloon angioplasty, peripheral artery, radiological supervision and interpretation

(75963 (complete procedure) has been deleted, see 35450-35460 or 35470-35476 and 75962)

75964   Transluminal balloon angioplasty, each additional peripheral artery, radiological supervision and interpretation

(75965 (complete procedure) has been deleted, see 35450-35460 or 35470-35476 and 75964)

75966   Transluminal balloon angioplasty, renal or other visceral artery, radiological supervision and interpretation

(75967 (complete procedure) has been deleted, see 35450-35460 or 35470-35476 and 75966)

75968   Transluminal balloon angioplasty, each additional visceral artery, radiological supervision and interpretation

(75969 (complete procedure) has been deleted, see 35450-35460 or 35470-35476 and 75968)

(For percutaneous transluminal coronary angioplasty, see 92982-92984)

75970   Transcatheter biopsy, radiological supervision and interpretation

(For injection procedure only for transcatheter therapy or biopsy, see 36100-36299)

(75971 (complete procedure) has been deleted, see 37200, 75970)

(For transcatheter renal and ureteral biopsy, see 52007)

(For percutaneous needle biopsy of pancreas, see 48102; of retroperitoneal lymph node or mass, see 49180)

(75972-75977 have been deleted. To report, see 75962-75968)

75978   Transluminal balloon angioplasty, venous (eg, subclavian stenosis), radiological supervision and interpretation

(75979 (complete procedure) has been deleted, see 35460, 35476, 75978)

75980   Percutaneous transhepatic biliary drainage with contrast monitoring, radiological supervision and interpretation

(75981 (complete procedure) has been deleted, see 47510, 47511, 75980)

75982   Percutaneous placement of drainage catheter for combined internal and external biliary drainage or of a drainage stent for internal biliary drainage in patients with an inoperable mechanical biliary obstruction, radiological supervision and interpretation

(75983 (complete procedure) has been deleted, see 47511, 75982)

75984   Change of percutaneous tube or drainage catheter with contrast monitoring (eg, gastrointestinal system, genitourinary system, abscess), radiological supervision and interpretation

(75985 (complete procedure) has been deleted, see 43760, 47525, 47530, 50398, 50688, 75984)

(For change of nephrostomy or pyelostomy tube only, use 50398)

(For introduction procedure only for percutaneous biliary drainage, see 47510, 47511)

(For percutaneous cholecystostomy, use 47490)

(For change of percutaneous biliary drainage catheter only, use 47525)

(For percutaneous nephrostolithotomy or pyelostolithotomy, see 50080, 50081)

75989   Radiological guidance for percutaneous drainage of abscess, or specimen collection (ie, fluoroscopy, ultrasound, or computed tomography), with or without placement of indwelling catheter, radiological supervision and interpretation

(75990 (complete procedure) has been deleted, see appropriate organ or site and 75989)

Transluminal Atherectomy

75992   Transluminal atherectomy, peripheral artery, radiological supervision and interpretation

(For procedure, see 35481-35485, 35491-35495)

75993   Transluminal atherectomy, each additional peripheral artery, radiological supervision and interpretation

(For procedure, see 35481-35485, 35491-35495)

75994   Transluminal atherectomy, renal, radiological supervision and interpretation

(For procedure, see 35480, 35490)

75995   Transluminal atherectomy, visceral, radiological supervision and interpretation

(For procedure, see 35480, 35490)

75996   Transluminal atherectomy, each additional visceral artery, radiological supervision and interpretation

(For procedure, see 35480, 35490)

Other Procedures

(For arthrography of shoulder, see 73040; elbow, see 73085; wrist, see 73115; hip, see 73525; knee, see 73580; ankle, see 73615)

76000   Fluoroscopy (separate procedure), up to one hour physician time, other than 71023 or 71034 (eg, cardiac fluoroscopy)

76001   Fluoroscopy, physician time more than one hour, assisting a non-radiologic physician (eg, nephrostolithotomy, ERCP, bronchoscopy, transbronchial biopsy)

76003   Fluoroscopic localization for needle biopsy or fine needle aspiration

(See appropriate surgical code for location, eg, 20220, 20225, 32400, 32405, 47000, 47001, 48102, 50200, 50390, 60100)

76010   Radiologic examination from nose to rectum for foreign body, single film, child

76020   Bone age studies

76040   Bone length studies (orthoroentgenogram, scanogram)

(76060 has been deleted. See 76061, 76062)

76061   Radiologic examination, osseous survey; limited (eg, for metastases)

76062   complete (axial and appendicular skeleton)

76065   Radiologic examination, osseous survey, infant

76066   Joint survey, single view, one or more joints (specify)

76070   Computerized tomography, bone density study

76075   Dual energy x-ray absorptiometry (DEXA), bone density study

76080   Radiologic examination, fistula or sinus tract study, radiological supervision and interpretation

(76081 (complete procedure) has been deleted, see 20501, 76080)

76086   Mammary ductogram or galactogram, single duct, radiological supervision and interpretation

(76087 (complete procedure) has been deleted, see 19030, 76086)

76088 Mammary ductogram or galactogram, multiple ducts, radiological supervision and interpretation

(76089 (complete procedure) has been deleted, see 19030, 76088)

76090 Mammography; unilateral

76091 bilateral

76092 Screening mammography, bilateral (two view film study of each breast)

76093 Magnetic resonance imaging, breast, without and/or with contrast material(s); unilateral

76094 bilateral

76095 Stereotactic localization for breast biopsy, each lesion, radiological supervision and interpretation

(For procedure, see 19100, 88170)

76096 Preoperative placement of needle localization wire, breast, radiological supervision and interpretation

(For placement, see 19290, 19291)

(76097 has been deleted. To report, see 19291, 76096)

76098 Radiological examination, surgical specimen

76100 Radiologic examination, single plane body section (eg, tomography), other than with urography

76101 Radiologic examination, complex motion (ie, hypercycloidal) body section (eg, mastoid polytomography), other than with urography; unilateral

76102 bilateral

(For nephrotomography, see 74415)

76120 Cineradiography, except where specifically included

76125 Cineradiography to complement routine examination

(76127 has been deleted. The use of photographic media is not reported separately but is considered to be a component of the basic procedure)

(76130-76137 have been deleted. To report, use code for specific radiologic examination)

76140 Consultation on x-ray examination made elsewhere, written report

76150 Xeroradiography

(76150 is to be used for non-mammographic studies only)

(76300 has been deleted. To report, use 76499)

76350 Subtraction in conjunction with contrast studies

76355 Computerized tomography guidance for stereotactic localization

76360 Computerized tomography guidance for needle biopsy, radiological supervision and interpretation

(76361 (complete procedure) has been deleted, see appropriate organ or site and 76360)

76365 Computerized tomography guidance for cyst aspiration, radiological supervision and interpretation

(76366 (complete procedure) has been deleted, see appropriate organ or site and 76365)

76370 Computerized tomography guidance for placement of radiation therapy fields

76375 Computerized tomography, coronal, sagittal, multiplanar, oblique and/or 3-dimensional reconstruction

76380 Computerized tomography, limited or localized follow-up study

76400 Magnetic resonance (eg, proton) imaging, bone marrow blood supply

76499 Unlisted diagnostic radiologic procedure

Diagnostic Ultrasound

Definitions

A-mode implies a one-dimensional ultrasonic measurement procedure.

M-mode implies a one-dimensional ultrasonic measurement procedure with movement of the trace to record amplitude and velocity of moving echo-producing structures.

B-scan implies a two-dimensional ultrasonic scanning procedure with a two-dimensional display.

Real-time scani implies a two-dimensional ultrasonic scanning procedure with display of both two-dimensional structure and motion with time.

Head and Neck

(76500, 76505 have been deleted. To report, use 76999)

76506 Echoencephalography, B-scan and/or real time with image documentation (gray scale) (for determination of ventricular size, delineation of cerebral contents and detection of fluid masses or other intracranial abnormalities), including A-mode encephalography as secondary component where indicated

76511 Ophthalmic ultrasound, echography, diagnostic; A-scan only, with amplitude quantification

76512 contact B-scan (with or without simultaneous A-scan)

76513 immersion (water bath) B-scan

(76515 has been deleted. To report, use 76999)

76516 Ophthalmic biometry by ultrasound echography, A-scan;

(76517 has been deleted. To report, use 76999)

76519 with intraocular lens power calculation

76529 Ophthalmic ultrasonic foreign body localization

(76530 has been deleted. To report, use 76999)

(76535 has been deleted. To report, use 76536)

76536 Echography, soft tissues of head and neck (eg, thyroid, parathyroid, parotid), B-scan and/or real time with image documentation

(76550 has been deleted. To report, see 93880-93888)

Chest

(76601 has been deleted. To report, use 76999)

76604 Echography, chest, B-scan (includes mediastinum) and/or real time with image documentation

(76620, 76625 have been deleted)

(76627, 76628 have been deleted. To report, see 93307, 93308)

(76629 has been deleted)

(76632 has been deleted. To report, see 93320, 93321)

(76640 has been deleted. To report, use 76999)

76645 Echography, breast(s) (unilateral or bilateral), B-scan and/or real time with image documentation

Abdomen and Retroperitoneum

76700 Echography, abdominal, B-scan and/or real time with image documentation; complete

76705 limited (eg, single organ, quadrant, follow-up)

76770 Echography, retroperitoneal (eg, renal, aorta, nodes), B-scan and/or real time with image documentation; complete

76775 limited

76778 Echography of transplanted kidney, B-scan and/or real time with image documentation, with or without duplex Doppler studies

Spinal Canal

76800   Echography, spinal canal and contents

Pelvis

76805   Echography, pregnant uterus, B-scan and/or real time with image documentation; complete (complete fetal and maternal evaluation)

76810   complete (complete fetal and maternal evaluation), multiple gestation, after the first trimester

76815   limited (gestational age, heart beat, placental location, fetal position, or emergency in the delivery room)

76816   follow-up or repeat

76818   Fetal biophysical profile

76825   Echocardiography, fetal, cardiovascular system, real time with image documentation (2D), with or without M-mode recording;

76826   follow-up or repeat study

76827   Doppler echocardiography, fetal, cardio-vascular system, pulsed wave and/or continuous wave with spectral display; complete

76828   follow-up or repeat study

   (To report the use of color mapping, see 93325)

76830   Echography, transvaginal

   (76855 has been deleted. To report, see 93975-93979)

76856   Echography, pelvic (nonobstetric), B-scan and/or real time with image documentation; complete

76857   limited or follow-up (eg, for follicles)

Genitalia

76870   Echography, scrotum and contents

76872   Echography, transrectal

Extremities

76880   Echography, extremity, non-vascular, B-scan and/or real time with image documentation

Vascular Studies

   (76900-76920 have been deleted. To report, see 93920-93971; for cerebro-vascular studies, see 93875-93888)

   (76925 has been deleted. To report, see 93920-93931 or 93965-93971)

   (76926 has been deleted. To report, see 93875-93888 or 93975-93979)

Ultrasonic Guidance Procedures

76930   Ultrasonic guidance for pericardiocentesis, radiological supervision and interpretation

   (76931 (complete procedure) has been deleted, see 33010, 33011, 76930)

76932   Ultrasonic guidance for endomyocardial biopsy, radiological supervision and interpretation

   (76933 (complete procedure) has been deleted, see 93505, 76932)

76934   Ultrasonic guidance for thoracentesis or abdominal paracentesis, radiological supervision and interpretation

   (76935 (complete procedure) has been deleted, see 32000, 76934)

76936   Ultrasound guided compression repair of arterial pseudo-aneurysm or arteriovenous fistulae (includes diagnostic ultrasound evaluation, compression of lesion and imaging)

76938   Ultrasonic guidance for cyst (any location), or renal pelvis aspiration, radiological supervision and interpretation

   (76939 (complete procedure) has been deleted, see appropriate organ or site and 76938)

76941   Ultrasonic guidance for intrauterine fetal transfusion or cordocentesis, radiological supervision and interpretation

(For procedure, see 36460, 59012)

76942 Ultrasonic guidance for needle biopsy, radiological supervision and interpretation

(76943 (complete procedure) has been deleted, see appropriate organ or site and 76942)

(76944 has been deleted. To report, use 75989)

76945 Ultrasonic guidance for chorionic villus sampling, radiological supervision and interpretation

(For procedure, see 59015)

76946 Ultrasonic guidance for amniocentesis, radiological supervision and interpretation

(76947 (complete procedure) has been deleted, see 59000, 76946)

76948 Ultrasonic guidance for aspiration of ova, radiological supervision and interpretation

(76949 (complete procedure) has been deleted, see 58970, 76948)

76950 Echography for placement of radiation therapy fields, B-scan

76960 Ultrasonic guidance for placement of radiation therapy fields, except for B-scan echography

● **76965** Ultrasonic guidance for interstitial radioelement application

---

Other Procedures

76970 Ultrasound study follow-up (specify)

76975 Gastrointestinal endoscopic ultrasound, radiological supervision and interpretation

(For procedure, see 43259)

(76980 has been deleted. To report, use code for specific ultrasound examination)

(76985 has been deleted. To report, use 76986)

76986 Echography, intraoperative

(76990 has been deleted. To report, use 76999)

(76991 has been deleted. To report, see 76830, 76872)

76999 Unlisted ultrasound procedure

Radiation Oncology

Listings for Radiation Oncology provide for teletherapy and brachytherapy to include initial consultation, clinical treatment planning, simulation, medical radiation physics, dosimetry, treatment devices, special services, and clinical treatment management procedures. They include normal follow-up care during course of treatment and for three months following its completion.

When a service or procedure is provided that is not listed in this edition of *CPT* it should be identified by a Special Report (see page 250) and one of the unlisted procedure codes listed below:

77299 Unlisted procedure, therapeutic radiology clinical treatment planning
77399 Unlisted procedure, medical radiation physics, dosimetry and treatment devices
77499 Unlisted procedure, therapeutic radiology clinical treatment management
77799 Unlisted procedure, clinical brachytherapy

For treatment by injectable or ingestible isotopes, see subsection Nuclear Medicine.

Consultation: Clinical Management

Preliminary consultation, evaluation of patient prior to decision to treat, or full medical care (in addition to treatment management) when provided by the therapeutic radiologist may be identified by the appropriate procedure codes from **Evaluation and Management, Medicine,** or **Surgery** sections.

Clinical Treatment Planning (External and Internal Sources)

The clinical treatment planning process is a complex service including interpretation of special testing, tumor localization, treatment volume determination, treatment time/dosage determination, choice of treatment modality, determination of number and size of treatment ports, selection of appropriate treatment devices, and other procedures.

Definitions

Simple planning requires a single treatment area of interest encompassed in a single port or simple parallel opposed ports with simple or no blocking.

Intermediate planning requires three or more converging ports, two separate treatment areas, multiple blocks, or special time dose constraints.

Complex planning requires highly complex blocking, custom shielding blocks, tangential ports, special wedges or compensators, three or more separate treatment areas, rotational or special beam considerations, combination of therapeutic modalities.

(77260, 77265, 77270, 77275 have been deleted. To report, see 77261-77263)

77261   Therapeutic radiology treatment planning; simple

77262   intermediate

77263   complex

Simple—simulation of a single treatment area with either a single port or parallel opposed ports. Simple or no blocking.

Intermediate—simulation of three or more converging ports, two separate treatment areas, multiple blocks.

Complex—simulation of tangential portals, three or more treatment areas, rotation or arc therapy, complex blocking, custom shielding blocks, brachytherapy source verification, hyperthermia probe verification, any use of contrast materials.

Simulation may be carried out on a dedicated simulator, a radiation therapy treatment unit, or diagnostic x-ray machine.

77280   Therapeutic radiology simulation-aided field setting; simple

77285   intermediate

77290   complex

▲77295   by three-dimensional reconstruction of tumor volume in preparation for treatment with non-coplanar therapy beams

77299   Unlisted procedure, therapeutic radiology clinical treatment planning

Medical Radiation Physics, Dosimetry, Treatment Devices, and Special Services

77300   Basic radiation dosimetry calculation, central axis depth dose, TDF, NSD, gap calculation, off axis factor, tissue inhomogeneity factors, as required during course of treatment, only when prescribed by the treating physician

77305   Teletherapy, isodose plan (whether hand or computer calculated); simple (one or two parallel opposed unmodified ports directed to a single area of interest)

77310   intermediate (three or more treatment ports directed to a single area of interest)

77315   complex (mantle or inverted Y, tangential ports, the use of wedges, compensators, complex blocking, rotational beam, or special beam considerations)

(Only one teletherapy isodose plan may be reported for a given course of therapy to a specific treatment area)

(77320 has been deleted. To report, see 77300-77399)

77321   Special teletherapy port plan, particles, hemibody, total body

(77325 has been deleted. To report, see 77300-77399)

77326   Brachytherapy isodose calculation; simple (calculation made from single plane, one to four sources/ribbon application, remote afterloading brachytherapy, 1 to 8 sources)

(For definition of source/ribbon, see page 275)

77327   intermediate (multiplane dosage calculations, application involving five to ten sources/ribbons, remote afterloading brachytherapy, 9 to 12 sources)

77328   complex (multiplane isodose plan, volume implant calculations, over ten sources/ribbons used, special spatial reconstruction, remote afterloading brachytherapy, over 12 sources)

(77330 has been deleted. To report, see 77300-77399)

▲=Revised Code   ●=New Code

77331   Special dosimetry (eg, TLD, microdosimetry) (specify), only when prescribed by the treating physician

77332   Treatment devices, design and construction; simple (simple block, simple bolus)

77333   intermediate (multiple blocks, stents, bite blocks, special bolus)

77334   complex (irregular blocks, special shields, compensators, wedges, molds or casts)

(77335 has been deleted. To report, see 77300-77399)

77336   Continuing medical radiation physics consultation in support of therapeutic radiologist including continuing quality assurance reported per week of therapy

(77340 has been deleted. To report, see 77300-77399)

(77345-77360 have been deleted. To report, see 77300-77399)

77370   Special medical radiation physics consultation

77399   Unlisted procedure, medical radiation physics, dosimetry and treatment devices

Radiation Treatment Delivery

(Radiation treatment delivery (77401-77416) recognizes the technical component and the various energy levels.)

(77400 has been deleted)

77401   Radiation treatment delivery, superficial and/or ortho voltage

77402   Radiation treatment delivery, single treatment area, single port or parallel opposed ports, simple blocks or no blocks; up to 5 MeV

77403   6-10 MeV

77404   11-19 MeV

(77405 has been deleted)

77406   20 MeV or greater

77407   Radiation treatment delivery, two separate treatment areas, three or more ports on a single treatment area, use of multiple blocks; up to 5 MeV

77408   6-10 MeV

77409   11-19 MeV

(77410 has been deleted)

77411   20 MeV or greater

77412   Radiation treatment delivery, three or more separate treatment areas, custom blocking, tangential ports, wedges, rotational beam, compensators, special particle beam (eg, electron or neutrons); up to 5 MeV

77413   6-10 MeV

77414   11-19 MeV

(77415 has been deleted. To report, use 77417)

77416   20 MeV or greater

77417   Therapeutic radiology port film(s)

Clinical Treatment Management

Weekly clinical management is based on five fractions delivered comprising one week regardless of the time interval separating the delivery of treatments.

Definitions

Simple management is a single treatment area, single port or parallel opposed ports or simple blocks.

Intermediate management is two separate treatment areas, three or more ports on a single treatment area, or use of special blocks.

Complex management is three or more separate treatment areas, highly complex blocking (mantle, inverted Y), tangential ports, wedges, rotational compensators or other special beam considerations.

Conformal management is multiple custom megavoltage treatment beams focused on a large 3-dimensional reconstructed target.

77419   Weekly radiation therapy management; conformal

(This code may be reported once per every five sessions of treatment management. This code excludes the use of 77420, 77425, 77430, and 77431)

77420   simple

77425   intermediate

77430   complex

77431   Radiation therapy management with complete course of therapy consisting of one or two fractions only

(77431 is not to be used to fill in the last week of a long course of therapy)

77432   Stereotactic radiation treatment management of cerebral lesion(s) (complete course of treatment consisting of one session)

(77435-77460 have been deleted. To report, see 77401-77499)

(77465 has been deleted)

77470   Special treatment procedure (eg, total body irradiation, hemibody irradiation, per oral, vaginal cone irradiation)

(77470 assumes that the procedure is performed one or more times during the course of therapy, in addition to daily or weekly patient management)

77499   Unlisted procedure, therapeutic radiology clinical treatment management

Hyperthermia

Hyperthermia treatments as listed in this section include external (superficial and deep), interstitial, and intracavitary. Radiation therapy when given concurrently is listed separately.

Hyperthermia is used only as an adjunct to radiation therapy or chemotherapy. It may be induced by a variety of sources (eg, microwave, ultrasound, low energy radio-frequency conduction, or by probes).

The listed treatments include management during the course of therapy and follow-up care for three months after completion. Preliminary consultation is not included (see **Medicine** 99241-99263). Physics planning and interstitial insertion of temperature sensors, and use of external or interstitial heat generating sources are included.

The following descriptors are included in the treatment schedule:

77600   Hyperthermia, externally generated; superficial (ie, heating to a depth of 4 cm or less)

77605   deep (ie, heating to depths greater than 4 cm)

77610   Hyperthermia generated by interstitial probe(s); 5 or fewer interstitial applicators

77615   more than 5 interstitial applicators

Clinical Intracavitary Hyperthermia

77620   Hyperthermia generated by intracavitary probe(s)

Clinical Brachytherapy

Clinical brachytherapy requires the use of either natural or man-made radioelements applied into or around a treatment field of interest. The supervision of radioelements and dose interpretation are performed solely by the therapeutic radiologist.

When a procedure requires the service of a surgeon(s) in addition, either modifier '-66' or 09966 or modifier '-62' or 09962 may be used (see Modifiers in **Radiology Guidelines,** pages 250-251).

Services 77750-77799 include admission to the hospital and daily visits.

Definitions

(Sources refer to intracavitary placement or permanent interstitial placement; ribbons refer to temporary interstitial placement)

A simple application has one to four sources/ribbons.

An intermediate application has five to ten sources/ribbons.

A complex application has greater than ten sources/ribbons.

(77700-77749 have been deleted. To report, see 77761-77799)

77750   Infusion or instillation of radioelement solution

(77755, 77760 have been deleted. To report, see 77761-77799)

77761   Intracavitary radioelement application; simple

77762   intermediate

77763   complex

(77765, 77770, 77775 have been deleted. To report, see 77761-77799)

77776 Interstitial radioelement application; simple

77777   intermediate

77778   complex

(77780 has been deleted. To report, see 77761-77799)

77781 Remote afterloading high intensity brachytherapy; 1-4 source positions or catheters

77782   5-8 source positions or catheters

77783   9-12 source positions or catheters

77784   over 12 source positions or catheters

(77785 has been deleted. To report, see 77761-77799)

77789 Surface application of radioelement

77790 Supervision, handling, loading of radioelement

77799 Unlisted procedure, clinical brachytherapy

(77800 has been deleted. To report, use 77331)

(77805-77810 have been deleted. To report, use 77305-77321 or 77326-77328)

(77850 has been deleted. To report, see 77300, 77336, 77370)

(77860 has been deleted. To report, use 77336)

(77999 has been deleted. To report, use 77399)

Nuclear Medicine

Listed procedures may be performed independently or in the course of overall medical care. If the physician providing these services is also responsible for diagnostic work-up and/or follow-up care of patient, see appropriate sections also.

Radioimmunoassay tests are found in the Clinical Pathology section (codes 82000-84999). These codes can be appropriately used by any specialist performing such tests in a laboratory licensed and/or certified for radioimmunoassays. The reporting of these tests is not confined to clinical pathology laboratories alone.

The services listed do not include the provision of radium or other radioelements. Those materials supplied by the physician should be listed separately and identified by the code 78990 for diagnostic radiopharmaceutical and 79900 for therapeutic radiopharmaceutical.

Diagnostic

Endocrine System

78000 Thyroid uptake; single determination

78001   multiple determinations

78003   stimulation, suppression or discharge (not including initial uptake studies)

78006 Thyroid imaging, with uptake; single determination

78007   multiple determinations

78010 Thyroid imaging; only

78011   with vascular flow

78015 Thyroid carcinoma metastases imaging; limited area (eg, neck and chest only)

78016   with additional studies (eg, urinary recovery)

78017   multiple areas

78018   whole body

(For triiodothyronine (true TT-3), RIA, see 84480)

(For calcitonin, RIA, see 82308)

(For triiodothyronine, free (FT-3), RIA (unbound T-3 only), see 84481)

(For TT-4 thyroxine, RIA, see 84436)

(For T-4 thyroxine, neonatal, see 84437)

(For FT-4 thyroxine, free, RIA (unbound T-4 only), see 84439)

78070 Parathyroid imaging

(For parathormone (parathyroid hormone), RIA, see 83970)

78075 Adrenal imaging, cortex and/or medulla

(For cortisol, RIA, plasma, see 82533)

(For cortisol, RIA, urine, see 82534)

(For aldosterone, double isotope technique, see 82087)

(For aldosterone, RIA, blood, see 82088)

(For aldosterone, RIA, urine, see 82088)

(For 17-ketosteroids, RIA, see 83586)

(For 17-OH ketosteroids, RIA, see 83586)

(For 17-hydroxycorticosteroids, RIA, see 83491)

(For insulin, RIA, see 83525)

(For insulin antibodies, RIA, see 86337)

(For proinsulin, RIA, see 84206)

(For glucagon, RIA, see 82943)

(For adrenocorticotropic hormone (ACTH), RIA, see 82024)

(For human growth hormone (HGH), (somatotropin), RIA, see 83003)

(For human growth antibody, RIA, see 86277)

(For thyroglobulin antibody, RIA, see 86800)

(For thyroid microsomal antibody, RIA, see 86376)

(For thyroid stimulating hormone (TSH), RIA, see 84443)

(For thyrotropin releasing factor, RIA, see 80438, 80439)

(For plus long-acting thyroid stimulator (LATS), see 84445)

(For follicle stimulating hormone (FSH component of pituitary gonadotropin), RIA, see 83001)

(For luteinizing hormone (LH component of pituitary gonadotropin), (ICSH), RIA, see 83002)

(For luteinizing releasing factor (LRH), RIA, see 83727)

(For prolactin level (mammotropin), RIA, see 84146)

(For vasopressin level (antidiuretic hormone), RIA, see 84588)

(For estradiol, RIA, see 82670)

(For progesterone, RIA, see 84144)

(For testosterone, blood, RIA, see 84403)

(For testosterone, urine, RIA, see 84403)

(For etiocholanolone, RIA, see 82696)

78099 Unlisted endocrine procedure, diagnostic nuclear medicine

(For chemical analysis, RIA tests, see Chemistry section)

Hematopoietic, Reticuloendothelial and Lymphatic System

78102 Bone marrow imaging; limited area

78103   multiple areas

78104   whole body

78110 Plasma volume, radiopharmaceutical volume-dilution technique (separate procedure); single sampling

78111   multiple samplings

78120 Red cell volume determination (separate procedure); single sampling

78121   multiple samplings

78122 Whole blood volume determination, including separate measurement of plasma volume and red cell volume (radiopharmaceutical volume-dilution technique)

78130 Red cell survival study;

78135   differential organ/tissue kinetics, (eg, splenic and/or hepatic sequestration)

78140 Labeled red cell sequestration, differential organ/tissue, (eg, splenic and/or hepatic)

78160 Plasma radioiron disappearance (turnover) rate

78162 Radioiron oral absorption

78170 Radioiron red cell utilization

78172 Chelatable iron for estimation of total body iron

(78180 has been deleted. To report, use 78199)

(For hemosiderin, RIA, see 83071)

(For intrinsic factor antibodies, RIA, see 82607)

(For cyanocobalamin (vitamin B-12), RIA, see 82607)

(For folic acid (folate) serum, RIA, see 82746)

(For human hepatitis antigen, hepatitis associated agent, (Australian antigen) (HAA), RIA, see 86287)

(For hepatitis A antibody (HAAb), RIA, see 86296)

(For hepatitis B core antibody (HBcAb), RIA, see 86289)

(For hepatitis B surface antigen (HBsAb), RIA, see 86287)

(For hepatitis B surface antibody (HBsAb), RIA, see 86291)

(For hepatitis Be antigen (HBeAg), RIA, see 86293)

(For hepatitis Be antibody (HBeAb), RIA, see 86295)

78185 Spleen imaging only, with or without vascular flow

(If combined with liver study, use procedures 78215 and 78216)

(78186 has been deleted)

78190 Kinetics, study of platelet survival, with or without differential organ/tissue localization

78191 Platelet survival study

(78192 has been deleted. To report, use 78805)

(78193 has been deleted. To report, use 78806)

78195 Lymphatics and lymph glands imaging

78199 Unlisted hematopoietic, reticuloendothelial and lymphatic procedure, diagnostic nuclear medicine

(For chemical analysis, RIA tests, see Chemistry section)

Gastrointestinal System

78201 Liver imaging; static only

78202 with vascular flow

(For spleen imaging only, use 78185)

78205 Liver imaging (SPECT)

78215 Liver and spleen imaging; static only

78216 with vascular flow

78220 Liver function study with hepatobiliary agents, with serial images

(78221 has been deleted. To report, use 78299)

78223 Hepatobiliary ductal system imaging, including gallbladder, with or without pharmacologic intervention, with or without quantitative measurement of gallbladder function

(78225 has been deleted)

78230 Salivary gland imaging;

78231 with serial images

78232 Salivary gland function study

(78240 has been deleted. To report pancreas imaging, use 78299)

78258 Esophageal motility

78261 Gastric mucosa imaging

78262 Gastroesophageal reflux study

78264 Gastric emptying study

78270　Vitamin B-12 absorption study (eg, Schilling test); without intrinsic factor

78271　　with intrinsic factor

78272　Vitamin B-12 absorption studies combined, with and without intrinsic factor

　　(78276 has been deleted)

78278　Acute gastrointestinal blood loss imaging

　　(78280 has been deleted)

78282　Gastrointestinal protein loss

　　(78285, 78286 have been deleted. To report, use 78299)

　　(For gastrin, RIA, see 82941)

　　(For intrinsic factor level, see 83528)

　　(For carcinoembryonic antigen level (CEA), RIA, see 82378)

78290　Bowel imaging (eg, ectopic gastric mucosa, Meckel's localization, volvulus)

78291　Peritoneal-venous shunt patency test (eg, for LeVeen, Denver shunt)

78299　Unlisted gastrointestinal procedure, diagnostic nuclear medicine

　　(For chemical analysis, RIA tests, see Chemistry section)

Musculoskeletal System

Bone and joint imaging can be used in the diagnosis of a variety of infectious inflammatory diseases (eg, osteomyelitis), as well as for localization of primary and/or metastatic neoplasms.

78300　Bone and/or joint imaging; limited area

78305　　multiple areas

78306　　whole body

　　(78310 has been deleted. To report, see 78445)

78315　　three phase study

78320　　tomographic (SPECT)

78350　Bone density (bone mineral content) study; single photon absorptiometry

78351　　dual photon absorptiometry

　　(78380, 78381 have been deleted. To report, see 78300, 78305)

78399　Unlisted musculoskeletal procedure, diagnostic nuclear medicine

Cardiovascular System

Myocardial perfusion and cardiac blood pool imaging studies may be performed at rest and/or during stress. When performed during exercise and/or pharmacologic stress, the appropriate stress testing code from the 93015-93018 series should be reported in addition to code(s) 78460-78465, 78472, 78473, 78481, and 78483.

　　(78401-78412 have been deleted. To report, see 78472-78483)

78414　Determination of central c-v hemodynamics (non-imaging) (eg, ejection fraction with probe technique) with or without pharmacologic intervention or exercise, single or multiple determinations

　　(78415 has been deleted. To report, see 78472)

　　(78418-78424 have been deleted. To report, see 78460-78469)

　　(78425 has been deleted. To report, see 78472)

78428　Cardiac shunt detection

　　(78435 has been deleted. To report, see 78481)

78445　Vascular flow imaging (ie, angiography, venography)

78455　Venous thrombosis study (eg, radioactive fibrinogen)

78457　Venous thrombosis imaging (eg, venogram); unilateral

78458　　bilateral

●**78459**　Myocardial imaging, positron emission tomography (PET), metabolic evaluation

78460 Myocardial perfusion imaging; single study, at rest or stress (exercise and/or pharmacologic), qualitative or quantitative

78461 multiple studies, at rest and/or stress (exercise and/or pharmacologic), and redistribution and/or rest injection, qualitative or quantitative

(78462, 78463 have been deleted. To report, see 78460, 78461)

78464 tomographic (SPECT), single study at rest or stress (exercise and/or pharmacologic), with or without quantitation

78465 tomographic (SPECT), multiple studies, at rest and/or stress (exercise and/or pharmacologic) and redistribution and/or rest injection, qualitative or quantitative

78466 Myocardial imaging, infarct avid, planar; qualitative or quantitative

(78467 has been deleted. To report, see 78466)

78468 with ejection fraction by first pass technique

78469 tomographic SPECT with or without quantitation

(78470 has been deleted. To report, see 78472, 78473 or 78481)

(78471 has been deleted. To report, see 78472)

78472 Cardiac blood pool imaging, gated equilibrium; single study at rest or stress (exercise and/or pharmacologic), wall motion study plus ejection fraction, with or without additional quantitative processing

78473 multiple studies, wall motion study plus ejection fraction, at rest and stress (exercise and/or pharmacologic), with or without additional quantification

(78474 has been deleted. To report, see 78472)

(78475-78477 have been deleted. To report, see 78473)

78478 Myocardial perfusion study with wall motion, qualitative or quantitative study (list separately in addition to code for primary procedure) (Use only for codes 78460, 78461, 78464, 78465)

(78479 has been deleted)

78480 Myocardial perfusion study with ejection fraction (list separately in addition to code for primary procedure) (Use only for codes 78460, 78461, 78464, 78465)

78481 Cardiac blood pool imaging, first pass technique; single study, at rest or during stress (exercise and/or pharmacologic), wall motion study plus ejection fraction, with or without quantitative processing

78483 multiple studies, at rest and during stress (exercise and/or pharmacologic), wall motion study plus ejection fraction, with or without additional quantitative processing

(78484 has been deleted. To report, see 78481)

(78485, 78486 have been deleted. To report, see 78483)

(78487 and 78489 have been deleted. To report, see 78483)

(78490 has been deleted. To report, use 78499)

(For digoxin, RIA, see 80162)

(For cerebral blood flow study, see 78615)

78499 Unlisted cardiovascular procedure, diagnostic nuclear medicine

(For chemical analysis, RIA tests, see Chemistry section)

Respiratory System

78580 Pulmonary perfusion imaging, particulate

(78581 and 78582 have been deleted)

78584 Pulmonary perfusion imaging, particulate, with ventilation; single breath

78585 rebreathing and washout, with or without single breath

78586 Pulmonary ventilation imaging, aerosol; single projection

78587   multiple projections (eg, anterior, posterior, lateral views)

78591 Pulmonary ventilation imaging, gaseous, single breath, single projection

78593 Pulmonary ventilation imaging, gaseous, with rebreathing and washout with or without single breath; single projection

78594   multiple projections (eg, anterior, posterior, lateral views)

78596 Pulmonary quantitative differential function (ventilation/perfusion) study

78599 Unlisted respiratory procedure, diagnostic nuclear medicine

Nervous System

78600 Brain imaging, limited procedure; static

78601   with vascular flow

78605 Brain imaging, complete study; static

78606   with vascular flow

78607   tomographic (SPECT)

78608 Brain imaging, positron emission tomography (PET); metabolic evaluation

78609   perfusion evaluation

78610 Brain imaging, vascular flow only

78615 Cerebral blood flow

78630 Cerebrospinal fluid flow, imaging (not including introduction of material); cisternography

(For injection procedure, see 61000-61070, 62270-62294)

78635   ventriculography

(For injection procedure, see 61000-61070, 62270-62294)

(78640 has been deleted. To report, use 78699)

78645   shunt evaluation

(For injection procedure, see 61000-61070, 62270-62294)

78647   tomographic (SPECT)

78650 CSF leakage detection and localization

(For injection procedure, see 61000-61070, 62270-62294)

(For myelin basic protein, CSF, RIA, see 83873)

(78652 has been deleted. To report, use 78647)

(78655 has been deleted. To report, see 78800)

78660 Radiopharmaceutical dacryocystography

78699 Unlisted nervous system procedure, diagnostic nuclear medicine

Genitourinary System

78700 Kidney imaging; static only

78701   with vascular flow

78704   with function study (ie, imaging renogram)

78707   with vascular flow and function study

(For introduction of radioactive substance in association with renal endoscopy, see 50559, 50578)

78710   tomographic (SPECT)

78715 Kidney vascular flow only

(78720 has been deleted. To report, use 78704)

78725 Kidney function study without pharmacologic intervention

78726 Kidney function study including pharmacologic intervention

(For renin (angiotensin I), RIA, see 84244)

(For angiotensin II, RIA, see 82163)

(For beta-2 microglobulin, RIA, see 82232)

78727 Kidney transplant evaluation

78730 Urinary bladder residual study

(For introduction of radioactive substance in association with cystotomy or cystostomy, see 51020; in association with cystourethroscopy, see 52250)

78740   Ureteral reflux study (radiopharmaceutical voiding cystogram)

(For estradiol, RIA, see 82670)

(For estriol, RIA, see 82677)

(For progesterone, RIA, see 84144)

(For prostatic acid phosphatase, RIA, see 84066)

78760   Testicular imaging;

78761   with vascular flow

(For testosterone, blood or urine, RIA, see 84403)

(For introduction of radioactive substance in association with ureteral endoscopy, see 50959, 50978)

(78770, 78775 have been deleted. To report, use 78799)

(For lactogen, human placental (HPL) chorionic somatomammotropin, RIA, see 83632)

(For chorionic gonadotropin, RIA or beta subunit, see 84702, 84703)

(For pregnanediol, RIA, see 84135)

(For pregnanetriol, RIA, see 84138)

78799   Unlisted genitourinary procedure, diagnostic nuclear medicine

(For chemical analysis, RIA tests, see **Chemistry** section)

Other Procedures

(For specific organ, see appropriate heading)

(For radiophosphorus tumor identification, ocular, see 78655)

78800   Radiopharmaceutical localization of tumor; limited area

(For specific organ, see appropriate heading)

78801   multiple areas

78802   whole body

78803   tomographic (SPECT)

78805   Radiopharmaceutical localization of abscess; limited area

78806   whole body

(For imaging bone infectious inflammatory disease, see 78300, 78305)

(For Rast, see 82785, 83518, 86003, 86005)

(For gamma-E immunoglobulin, RIA, see 82785)

(For gamma-G immunoglobulin, see 82784)

(For alpha-1 antitrypsin, RIA, see 82103, 82104)

(For alpha-1 fetoprotein, RIA, see 82105, 82106)

(For amikacin, see 80150)

(For aminophylline, see 80198)

(For amitriptyline, see 80152)

(For amphetamine, chemical quantitative, see 82145)

(For chlordiazepoxide, see code for specific method)

(For chlorpromazine, see phenothiazine, urine 84022)

(For clonazepam, see 80154)

(For cocaine, quantitative, see 82520)

(For diazepam, see 80154)

(For dihydromorphinone, quantitative, see 82649)

(For diphenylhydantoin, see 80185)

(For flucytosine, see code for specific method)

(For gentamicin, see 80170)

(For lactic dehydrogenase, RIA, see 83615)

(For lysergic acid diethylamide (LSD), RIA, see 80100-80103, 80299)

(For morphine (heroin), RIA, see 80100-80103, 83925)

(For phencyclidine (PCP), see 80100-80103, 83992)

(For phenobarbital, see barbiturates 82205, 82210)

(For phenytoin (diphenylthydantoin), see 80185)

(For tobramycin, see 80200)

78807   tomographic (SPECT)

●**78810**   Tumor imaging, positron emission tomography (PET), metabolic evaluation

78890   Generation of automated data: interactive process involving nuclear physician and/or allied health professional personnel; simple manipulations and interpretation, not to exceed 30 minutes

78891   complex manipulations and interpretation, exceeding 30 minutes

(Use 78890 or 78891 in addition to primary procedure)

(78895 has been deleted)

78990   Provision of diagnostic radiopharmaceutical(s)

78999   Unlisted miscellaneous procedure, diagnostic nuclear medicine

Therapeutic

79000   Radiopharmaceutical therapy, hyperthyroidism; initial, including evaluation of patient

79001   subsequent, each therapy

(For follow-up visit, see 99211-99215)

79020   Radiopharmaceutical therapy, thyroid suppression (euthyroid cardiac disease), including evaluation of patient

79030   Radiopharmaceutical ablation of gland for thyroid carcinoma

79035   Radiopharmaceutical therapy for metastases of thyroid carcinoma

79100   Radiopharmaceutical therapy, polycythemia vera, chronic leukemia, each treatment

79200   Intracavitary radioactive colloid therapy

79300   Interstitial radioactive colloid therapy

79400   Radiopharmaceutical therapy, nonthyroid, nonhematologic

79420   Intravascular radiopharmaceutical therapy, particulate

79440   Intra-articular radiopharmaceutical therapy

79900   Provision of therapeutic radiopharmaceutical(s)

79999   Unlisted radiopharmaceutical therapeutic procedure

Notes

Pathology and Laboratory Guidelines

Items used by all physicians in reporting their services are presented in the **Introduction.** Some of the commonalities are repeated here for the convenience of those physicians referring to this section on **Pathology and Laboratory.** Other definitions and items unique to Pathology and Laboratory are also listed.

Services in Pathology and Laboratory

Services in Pathology and Laboratory are provided by the pathologist or by technologists under responsible supervision of a physician.

Separate or Multiple Procedures

It is appropriate to designate multiple procedures that are rendered on the same date by separate entries.

Subsection Information

Several of the subheadings or subsections have special needs or instructions unique to that section. Where these are indicated, (eg, "Panel Tests"), special **"Notes"** will be presented preceding those procedural terminology listings referring to that subsection specifically. If there is an "Unlisted Procedure" code number (see section below) for the individual subsection, it will be shown. Those subsections with **"Notes"** are as follows:

Automated,
Multichannel Tests 80002-80019
Organ or Disease Panels 80050-80092
Drug Testing 80100-80103
Therapeutic Drug Assays 80150-80299

Evocative/Suppression Testing . 80400-80440
Consultations
(Clinical Pathology) 80500-80502
Urinalysis 81000-81099
Chemistry 82000-84999
Surgical Pathology 88300-88399

Unlisted Service or Procedure

A service or procedure may be provided that is not listed in this edition of *CPT.* When reporting such a service, the appropriate "Unlisted Procedure" code may be used to indicate the service, identifying it by "Special Report" as discussed below. The "Unlisted Procedures" and accompanying codes for **Pathology and Laboratory** are as follows:

80299 Unlisted quantitation of drug
81099 Unlisted urinalysis procedure
84999 Unlisted chemistry procedure
85999 Unlisted hematology procedure
86849 Unlisted immunology procedure
86999 Unlisted transfusion medicine procedure
87999 Unlisted microbiology procedure
88099 Unlisted necropsy (autopsy) procedure
88199 Unlisted cytopathology procedure
88299 Unlisted cytogenetic study
88399 Unlisted surgical pathology procedure
89399 Unlisted miscellaneous pathology test

Special Report

A service that is rarely provided, unusual, variable, or new may require a special report in determining medical appropriateness of the service. Pertinent information should include an adequate definition or description of the nature, extent, and need for the procedure; and the time, effort, and equipment necessary to provide the service. Additional items which may be included are:

- complexity of symptoms;
- final diagnosis;

- pertinent physical findings;
- diagnostic and therapeutic procedures;
- concurrent problems;
- follow-up care.

Modifiers

Listed services and procedures may be modified under certain circumstances. When applicable, the modifying circumstances should be identified by the addition of the appropriate modifier code, which may be reported in either of two ways. The modifier may be reported by a two digit number placed after the usual procedure number, from which it is separated by a hyphen. Or, the modifier may be reported by a separate five digit code that is used in addition to the procedure code. If more than one modifier is used, place the "Multiple Modifiers" code '-99' immediately after the procedure code. This indicates that one or more additional modifier codes will follow. Modifiers commonly used in **Pathology and Laboratory** are as follows:

-22 Unusual Procedural Services: When the service(s) provided is greater than that usually required for the listed procedure, it may be identified by adding modifier '-22' to the usual procedure number or by use of the separate five digit modifier code 09922. A report may also be appropriate.

-26 Professional Component: Certain procedures are a combination of a physician component and a technical component. When the physician component is reported separately, the service may be identified by adding the modifier '-26' to the usual procedure number or the service may be reported by use of the five digit modifier code 09926.

-32 Mandated Services: Services related to *mandated* consultation and/or related services (eg, PRO, 3rd party payor) may be identified by adding the modifier '-32' to the basic procedure or the service may be reported by use of the five digit modifier 09932.

-52 Reduced Services: Under certain circumstances, a service or procedure is partially reduced or eliminated at the physician's election. Under these circumstances, the service provided can be identified by its usual procedure number and the addition of the modifier '-52,' signifying that the service is reduced. This provides a means of reporting reduced services without disturbing the identification of the basic service. Modifier code 09952 may be used as an alternative to modifier '-52.'

-90 Reference (Outside) Laboratory: When laboratory procedures are performed by a party other than the treating or reporting physician, the procedure may be identified by adding the modifier '-90' to the usual procedure number or by using the separate five digit modifier code 09990.

80072 Arthritis panel

This panel must include the following:

Uric acid, blood, chemical (84550)

Sedimentation rate, erythrocyte, non-automated (85651)

Fluorescent antibody, screen, each antibody (86255)

Rheumatoid factor, qualitative (86430)

(80073 has been deleted. To report, see automated multichannel test codes (80002-80019))

(80075 has been deleted. To report, see codes for specific tests)

(80080 has been deleted. To report PSA, see 84153)

(80082 has been deleted. To report, see codes for specific tests)

(80084 has been deleted. To report, see codes for specific tests)

(80085 has been deleted. To report, see codes for specific tests)

(80086 has been deleted. To report, see codes for specific tests)

(80088 has been deleted. To report, see codes for specific tests)

(80089 has been deleted. To report, see codes for specific tests)

80090 TORCH antibody panel

This panel must include the following tests:

Antibody, cytomegalovirus (CMV) (86644)

Antibody, herpes simplex, non-specific type test (86694)

Antibody, rubella (86762)

Antibody, toxoplasma (86777)

80091 Thyroid panel

This panel must include the following tests:

Thyroxine, total (84436)

Triiodothyronine (T-3), resin uptake (84479);

80092 with thyroid stimulating hormone (TSH) (84443)

(80099 has been deleted. To report, use codes for specific tests)

Drug Testing

The following list contains examples of drugs or classes of drugs that are commonly assayed by qualitative screen, followed by confirmation with a second method.

Alcohols

Amphetamines

Barbiturates

Benzodiazepines

Cocaine and Metabolites

Methadones

Methaqualones

Opiates

Phencyclidines

Phenothiazines

Propoxyphenes

Tetrahydrocannabinoids

Tricyclic Antidepressants

Confirmed drugs may also be quantitated. Qualitative screening tests are coded by procedure, not method or analyte. For example, if chromatography is being used, code each combination of stationary and mobile phases separately using 80100 if the analysis is designed to detect multiple drug classes or 80101 if the procedure is capable of detecting a single class of drugs.

Use 80102 for each procedure necessary for confirmation, eg, if confirmation of three drugs by chromatography requires three stationary or mobile phases, use 80102 three (3) times. However, if multiple drugs can be confirmed using a single analysis, use 80102 only once.

For quantitation of drugs screened, use appropriate code in Chemistry section (82000-84999) or Therapeutic Drug Assay section (80150-80299).

The following codes (80100-80103) should be used for testing of other drugs which may not be listed above.

80100 Drug, screen; multiple drug classes, each procedure

80101 single drug class, each drug class

80102 Drug, confirmation, each procedure

80103 Tissue preparation for drug analysis

Therapeutic Drug Assays

The material for examination may be from any source. Examination is quantitative. For nonquantitative testing, see Drug Testing (80100-80103).

80150 Amikacin

80152 Amitriptyline

80154 Benzodiazepines

80156 Carbamazepine

80158 Cyclosporine

80160 Desipramine

80162 Digoxin

80164 Dipropylacetic acid (valproic acid)

80166 Doxepin

80168 Ethosuximide

80170 Gentamicin

80172 Gold

80174 Imipramine

80176 Lidocaine

80178 Lithium

80182 Nortriptyline

80184 Phenobarbital

80185 Phenytoin; total

80186 free

80188 Primidone

80190 Procainamide;

80192 with metabolites (eg, n-acetyl procainamide)

80194 Quinidine

80196 Salicylate

80198 Theophylline

80200 Tobramycin

80202 Vancomycin

80299 Quantitation of drug, not elsewhere specified

Evocative/Suppression Testing

The following test panels involve the administration of evocative or suppressive agents, and the baseline and subsequent measurement of their effects on chemical constituents. These codes are to be used for the reporting of the laboratory component of the overall testing protocol. For the physician's administration of the evocative or suppressive agents, see 90780-90784; for the supplies and drugs, see 99070. To report physician attendance and monitoring during the testing, use the appropriate evaluation and management code, including the prolonged physician care codes if required. Prolonged physician care codes are not separately reported when evocative/suppression testing involves prolonged infusions reported with 90780 and 90781. In the code descriptors where reference is made to a particular analyte (eg, Cortisol (82533 x 2)) the "x 2" refers to the number of times the test for that particular analyte is performed.

80400 ACTH stimulation panel; for adrenal insufficiency

This panel must include the following:

Cortisol (82533 x 2)

80402   for 21 hydroxylase deficiency

This panel must include the following:

Cortisol (82533 x 2)

17 hydroxyprogesterone (83498 x 2)

80406   for 3 beta-hydroxydehydrogenase deficiency

This panel must include the following:

Cortisol (82533 x 2)

17 hydroxypregnenolone (84143 x 2)

80408 Aldosterone suppression evaluation panel
(eg, saline infusion)

This panel must include the following:

Aldosterone (82088 x 2)

Renin (84244 x 2)

▲**80410** Calcitonin stimulation panel (eg, calcium,
pentagastrin)

This panel must include the following:

Calcitonin (82308 x 3)

80412 Corticotropic releasing hormone (CRH)
stimulation panel

This panel must include the following:

Cortisol (82533 x 6)

Adrenocorticotropic hormone (ACTH)
(82024 x 6)

80414 Chorionic gonadotropin stimulation panel;
testosterone response

This panel must include the following:

Testosterone (84403 x 2 on three pooled
blood samples)

80415   estradiol response

This panel must include the following:

Estradiol (82670 x 2 on three pooled blood
samples)

●**80416** Renal vein renin stimulation panel
(eg, captopril)

This panel must include the following:

Renin (84244 x 6)

●**80417** Peripheral vein renin stimulation panel
(eg, captopril)

This panel must include the following:

Renin (84244 x 2)

80418 Combined rapid anterior pituitary evaluation
panel

This panel must include the following:

Adrenocorticotropic hormone (ACTH)
(82024 x 4)

Luteinizing hormone (LH) (83002 x 4)

Follicle stimulating hormone (FSH)
(83001 x 4)

Prolactin (84146 x 4)

Human growth hormone (HGH) (83003 x 4)

Cortisol (82533 x 4)

Thyroid stimulating hormone (TSH)
(84443 x 4)

80420 Dexamethasone suppression panel, 48 hour

This panel must include the following:

Free cortisol, urine (82530 x 2)

Cortisol (82533 x 2)

Volume measurement for timed collection
(81050 x 2)

(For single dose dexamethasone, use 82533)

80422 Glucagon tolerance panel; for insulinoma

This panel must include the following:

Glucose (82947 x 3)

Insulin (83525 x 3)

80424   for pheochromocytoma

This panel must include the following:

Catecholamines, fractionated (82384 x 2)

80426 Gonadotropin releasing hormone stimulation panel

This panel must include the following:

Follicle stimulating hormone (FSH) (83001 x 4)

Luteinizing hormone (LH) (83002 x 4)

80428 Growth hormone stimulation panel (eg, arginine infusion, l-dopa administration)

This panel must include the following:

Human growth hormone (HGH) (83003 x 4)

80430 Growth hormone suppression panel (glucose administration)

This panel must include the following:

Glucose (82947 x 3)

Human growth hormone (HGH) (83003 x 4)

80432 Insulin-induced C-peptide suppression panel

This panel must include the following:

Insulin (83525)

C-peptide (84681 x 5)

Glucose (82947 x 5)

80434 Insulin tolerance panel; for ACTH insufficiency

This panel must include the following:

Cortisol (82533 x 5)

Glucose (82947 x 5)

80435 for growth hormone deficiency

This panel must include the following:

Glucose (82947 x 5)

Human growth hormone (HGH) (83003 x 5)

80436 Metyrapone panel

This panel must include the following:

Cortisol (82533 x 2)

11 deoxycortisol (82634 x 2)

80438 Thyrotropin releasing hormone (TRH) stimulation panel; one hour

This panel must include the following:

Thyroid stimulating hormone (TSH) (84443 x 3)

80439 two hour

This panel must include the following:

Thyroid stimulating hormone (TSH) (84443 x 4)

80440 for hyperprolactinemia

This panel must include the following:

Prolactin (84146 x 3)

Consultations (Clinical Pathology)

A clinical pathology consultation is a service, including a written report, rendered by the pathologist in response to a request from an attending physician in relation to a test result(s) requiring additional medical interpretive judgment. Reporting of a test result(s) without medical interpretive judgment is not considered a clinical pathology consultation.

80500 Clinical pathology consultation; limited, without review of patient's history and medical records

80502 comprehensive, for a complex diagnostic problem, with review of patient's history and medical records

(These codes may also be used for pharmacokinetic consultations)

(For consultations involving the examination and evaluation of the patient, see 99241-99275)

Urinalysis

For specific analyses, see appropriate section.

▲**81000**   Urinalysis, by dip stick or tablet reagent for bilirubin, glucose, hemoglobin, ketones, leukocytes, nitrite, pH, protein, specific gravity, urobilinogen, any number of these constituents; non-automated, with microscopy

●**81001**   automated, with microscopy

81002   non-automated, without microscopy

81003   automated, without microscopy

(81004 has been deleted. To report, see 81000)

81005   Urinalysis; qualitative or semiquantitative, except immunoassays

(For non-immunoassay reagent strip urinalysis, see 81000, 81002)

(For immunoassay, qualitative or semiquantitative, see 83518)

(81006 has been deleted. To report, use 81099)

(For microalbumin, see 82043, 82044)

81007   bacteriuria screen, by non-culture technique, commercial kit (specify type)

(81010, 81011, and 81012 have been deleted)

81015   microscopic only

81020   two or three glass test

81025   Urine pregnancy test, by visual color comparison methods

(81030 has been deleted)

81050   Volume measurement for timed collection, each

81099   Unlisted urinalysis procedure

Chemistry

The material for examination may be from any source. Examination is quantitative unless specified. (For list of automated, multichannel tests, see 80002-80019).

Clinical information derived from the results of laboratory data that is mathematically calculated (eg, free thyroxine index (T7)) is considered part of the test procedure and therefore is not a separately reportable service.

82000   Acetaldehyde, blood

82003   Acetaminophen

(82005 has been deleted)

82009   Acetone or other ketone bodies, serum; qualitative

82010   quantitative

(82011 has been deleted. To report, use 80196)

(82012 has been deleted)

82013   Acetylcholinesterase

(Acid, gastric, see gastric acid, 82926, 82928)

(Acid phosphatase, see 84060-84066)

(82015 has been deleted)

82024   Adrenocorticotropic hormone (ACTH)

82030   Adenosine, 5'-monophosphate, cyclic (cyclic AMP)

(82035 has been deleted)

82040   Albumin; serum

82042   urine, quantitative

82043   urine, microalbumin, quantitative

82044   urine, microalbumin, semiquantitative (eg, reagent strip assay)

(For prealbumin, see 84134)

82055   Alcohol (ethanol); any specimen except breath

(For other volatiles, alcohol, see 84600)

(82060, 82065, 82070 have been deleted. To report, use 82055)

(82072 has been deleted)

82075   breath

(82076, 82078 have been deleted. For ethanol, see 82055; for volatiles, see 84600)

82085 Aldolase

(82086 has been deleted. To report, use 82085)

(82087 has been deleted. To report, use 82088)

82088 Aldosterone

(82089 has been deleted. To report, use 82088)

(82091 has been deleted. To report, use 80408)

(82095 has been deleted. To report, see 80100, 80101 and 80103)

(82096 has been deleted. To report, use code for specific drug and 80103)

(82100 has been deleted. To report, use 80100 and 80101)

(Alkaline phosphatase, see 84075, 84080)

82101 Alkaloids, urine, quantitative

(Alphaketoglutarate, see 82009, 82010)

(Alpha tocopherol (Vitamin E), see 84446)

82103 Alpha-1-antitrypsin; total

82104 phenotype

82105 Alpha-fetoprotein; serum

82106 amniotic fluid

82108 Aluminum

(82112 has been deleted. To report, use 80150)

(82126 has been deleted)

82128 Amino acids, qualitative

82130 Amino acids, urine or plasma, chromatographic fractionation

82131 Amino acids, quantitation, each

(82134 has been deleted)

82135 Aminolevulinic acid, delta (ALA)

(82137 has been deleted. To report, use 80198)

(82138 has been deleted. To report, use 80152)

82140 Ammonia

(82141 has been deleted. To report, use 82140)

(82142 has been deleted)

82143 Amniotic fluid scan (spectrophotometric)

(For L/S ratio, see 83661)

(Amobarbital, see 80100-80103 for qualitative analysis, 82205 for quantitative analysis)

82145 Amphetamine or methamphetamine

(For qualitative analysis, see 80100-80103)

82150 Amylase

82154 Androstanediol glucuronide

(82155 has been deleted)

(82156 has been deleted. To report, use 82150)

82157 Androstenedione

(82159 has been deleted. To report, use 82160)

82160 Androsterone

82163 Angiotensin II

82164 Angiotensin I - converting enzyme (ACE)

(82165 has been deleted)

(Antidiuretic hormone (ADH), see 84588)

(82168 has been deleted. For antihistamines, see code for specific method)

(82170 has been deleted. To report, see 83015, 83018)

(Antimony, see 83015)

(Antitrypsin, alpha-1-, see 82103, 82104)

82172   Apolipoprotein, each

(82173 has been deleted. To report, see 80428)

82175   Arsenic

(For heavy metal screening, see 83015)

82180   Ascorbic acid (Vitamin C), blood

(Aspirin, see acetylsalicylic acid, 80196)

(Atherogenic index, blood, ultracentrifugation, quantitative, see 83717)

82190   Atomic absorption spectroscopy, each analyte

82205   Barbiturates, not elsewhere specified

(For qualitative analysis, see 80100-80103)

(82210 has been deleted. To report, see 80100-80103, 82205)

(82225, 82230 have been deleted. To report, see 83015, 83018)

(82231 has been deleted. To report, use 82232)

82232   Beta-2 microglobulin

(82235, 82236 have been deleted)

(Bicarbonate, use 82374)

82239   Bile acids; total

82240   cholylglycine

(For bile pigments, urine, see 81000-81005)

(82245 has been deleted. To report, see 81000, 81002, 81005)

82250   Bilirubin; total OR direct

82251   total AND direct

82252   feces, qualitative

(82260 has been deleted. To report, use 82250)

(82265 has been deleted. To report spectrophotometric scan, see 82143)

(82268 has been deleted. To report, see 83015, 83018)

82270   Blood, occult; feces screening, 1-3 simultaneous determinations

82273   other sources, qualitative

(Blood urea nitrogen (BUN), see 84520, 84525)

(82280, 82285 have been deleted. To report, see code for specific method)

82286   Bradykinin

(82290, 82291 have been deleted. To report, use 84311)

82300   Cadmium

(82305 has been deleted. To report, see 82486, 82491)

82306   Calcifediol (25-OH Vitamin D-3)

82307   Calciferol (Vitamin D)

(For 1,25-Dihydroxyvitamin D, use 82652)

82308   Calcitonin

82310   Calcium; total

(82315, 82320, 82325 have been deleted. To report, use 82310)

82330   ionized

82331   after calcium infusion test

(82335 has been deleted)

82340   urine quantitative, timed specimen

(82345 has been deleted)

82355   Calculus (stone); qualitative analysis

82360   quantitative analysis, chemical

82365   infrared spectroscopy

82370   x-ray diffraction

(82372 has been deleted. To report, use 80156)

(Carbamates, see individual listings)

82374   Carbon dioxide (bicarbonate)

(See also 82802, 82803)

82375 Carbon monoxide, (carboxyhemoglobin); quantitative

82376   qualitative

82378 Carcinoembryonic antigen (CEA)

82380 Carotene

82382 Catecholamines; total urine

82383   blood

82384   fractionated

(For urine metabolites, see 83835, 84585)

82387 Cathepsin-D

82390 Ceruloplasmin

82397 Chemiluminescent assay

(82400 has been deleted. To report, use code for specific method)

(82405 has been deleted)

82415 Chloramphenicol

(82418, 82420, 82425 have been deleted. To report, use code for specific method)

82435 Chloride; blood

82436   urine

(82437 has been deleted)

82438   other source

(For sweat collection by iontophoresis, see 89360)

82441 Chlorinated hydrocarbons, screen

(82443 has been deleted. To report, use code for specific method)

(Chlorpromazine, see 84022)

(Cholecalciferol (Vitamin D), see 82307)

82465 Cholesterol, serum, total

(For high density lipoprotein (HDL), see 83718)

(82470 has been deleted)

82480 Cholinesterase; serum

82482   RBC

(82484 has been deleted. To report, use 82480 and 82482)

82485 Chondroitin B sulfate, quantitative

(Chorionic gonadotropin, see gonadotropin, 84702, 84703)

82486 Chromatography, qualitative; column (eg, gas liquid or high performance liquid chromatography), analyte not elsewhere specified

82487   paper, 1-dimensional, analyte not elsewhere specified

82488   paper, 2-dimensional, analyte not elsewhere specified

82489   thin layer, analyte not elsewhere specified

(82490 has been deleted)

82491 Chromatography, quantitative, column (eg, gas liquid or high performance liquid chromatography), analyte not elsewhere specified

82495 Chromium

(82505 has been deleted)

82507 Citrate

(82512 has been deleted. To report, use 80154)

82520 Cocaine or metabolite

(Cocaine, qualitative analysis, see 80100-80103)

(Codeine, qualitative analysis, see 80100-80103)

(Codeine, quantitative analysis, see 82101)

(Complement, see 86160-86162)

82525 Copper

(82526 has been deleted. To report, use 82525)

(Coproporphyrin, see 84119, 84120)

(Corticosteroids, see 83491)

82528   Corticosterone

(82529 has been deleted. To report, use 82533)

82530   Cortisol; free

(82531, 82532 have been deleted)

82533   total

(82534 has been deleted. To report, use 82533)

(82536 has been deleted. To report, see 80400-80406)

(82537 has been deleted. To report, see 80400-80406)

(82538 has been deleted. To report, see 80436)

(82539 has been deleted. To report, see 80420)

(C-peptide, use 84681)

82540   Creatine

(82545 has been deleted. To report, use 82540)

(82546 has been deleted. To report, use 82540 and 82565)

82550   Creatine kinase (CK), (CPK); total

82552   isoenzymes

82553   MB fraction only

82554   isoforms

(82555 has been deleted)

82565   Creatinine; blood

82570   other source

82575   clearance

82585   Cryofibrinogen

82595   Cryoglobulin

(Crystals, pyrophosphate vs. urate, see 89060)

82600   Cyanide

(82601 has been deleted. To report, use 80103, 82600)

(82606 has been deleted)

82607   Cyanocobalamin (Vitamin B-12);

82608   unsaturated binding capacity

(Cyclic AMP, see 82030)

(Cyclic GMP, see 83008)

(Cyclosporine, use 80158)

(82610, 82614 have been deleted)

82615   Cystine and homocystine, urine, qualitative

(82620 has been deleted. For cystine and homocystine, quantitative, see 82130)

(82624 has been deleted)

82626   Dehydroepiandrosterone (DHEA)

82627   Dehydroepiandrosterone-sulfate (DHEA-S)

(82628 has been deleted. To report, see 80100-80103 for qualitative analysis; see 80160 for quantitative analysis)

(Delta-aminolevulinic acid (ALA), see 82135)

82633   Desoxycorticosterone, 11-

82634   Deoxycortisol, 11-

(Dexamethasone suppression test, see 80420)

(82635 has been deleted)

(Diastase, urine, see 82150)

(82636 has been deleted. To report, see 80100-80103, 80154)

82638   Dibucaine number

(82639 has been deleted. To report, use code for specific method)

(Dichloroethane, see 84600)

(Dichloromethane, see 84600)

(Diethylether, see 84600)

(82640, 82641 have been deleted)

(82643 has been deleted. To report, use 80162)

82646 Dihydrocodeinone

(For qualitative analysis, see 80100-80103)

82649 Dihydromorphinone

(For qualitative analysis, see 80100-80103)

82651 Dihydrotestosterone (DHT)

82652 Dihydroxyvitamin D, 1,25-

82654 Dimethadione

(For qualitative analysis, see 80100-80103)

(Diphenylhydantoin, see 80185)

(Dipropylacetic acid, see 80164)

(Dopamine, see 82382-82384)

(82656 has been deleted. To report, use 80166)

(Duodenal contents, see individual enzymes; for intubation and collection, see 89100)

(82660 has been deleted. To report, see 80100, 80101)

(82662 has been deleted. To report, see 80100-80103)

82664 Electrophoretic technique, not elsewhere specified

(Endocrine receptor assays, see 84233-84235)

82666 Epiandrosterone

(Epinephrine, see 82382-82384)

82668 Erythropoietin

82670 Estradiol

82671 Estrogens; fractionated

82672   total

(82673, 82674, 82676 have been deleted. To report, use 82677)

(Estrogen receptor assay, see 84233)

82677 Estriol

(82678 has been deleted. To report, use 82679)

82679 Estrone

(Ethanol, see 82055 and 82075)

82690 Ethchlorvynol

(82691 has been deleted. To report, see 82690)

(82692 has been deleted. To report, use 80168)

(Ethyl alcohol, see 82055 and 82075)

82693 Ethylene glycol

(82694 has been deleted. To report, use 82696)

82696 Etiocholanolone

(For fractionation of ketosteroids, see 83593)

82705 Fat or lipids, feces; qualitative

82710   quantitative

82715 Fat differential, feces, quantitative

(82720 has been deleted)

82725 Fatty acids, nonesterified

(82727 has been deleted. To report ferric chloride test, urine, use 81005)

82728 Ferritin

(Fetal hemoglobin, see hemoglobin 83030, 83033, and 85460)

(Fetoprotein, alpha-1, see 82105, 82106)

(82730 has been deleted. To report fibrinogen, see 85384, 85385)

82735 Fluoride

(82740 has been deleted. To report, use 82735)

(82741 has been deleted. To report, see code for specific method)

82742 Flurazepam

(For qualitative analysis, see 80100-80103)

(Foam stability test, see 83662)

(82745 has been deleted)

82746 Folic acid; serum

82747   RBC

(Follicle stimulating hormone (FSH), see 83001)

(82750 has been deleted. To report, use code for specific method)

(82755, 82756 have been deleted)

82757 Fructose, semen

(Fructosamine, see 82985)

(Fructose, TLC screen, see 84375)

82759 Galactokinase, RBC

82760 Galactose

(82763 has been deleted. To report, use 82760 and codes for administration)

(82765 has been deleted. To report, use 82760)

82775 Galactose-1-phosphate uridyl transferase; quantitative

82776   screen

(82780 has been deleted. To report gallium, use code for specific method)

82784 Gammaglobulin; IgA, IgD, IgG, IgM, each

82785   IgE

(For allergen specific IgE, see 86003, 86005)

(82786 has been deleted)

82787   immunoglobulin subclasses, (IgG1, 2, 3, and 4)

(Gamma-glutamyltransferase (GGT), see 82977)

(82790, 82791 have been deleted)

(82792 has been deleted. To report, see 82805, 82810)

(82793, 82795 have been deleted)

82800 Gases, blood, pH only

(82801, 82802 have been deleted. To report, see 82803)

82803 Gases, blood, any combination of pH, pCO_2, pO_2, CO_2, HCO_3 (including calculated O_2 saturation);

(Use 82803 for two or more of the above listed analytes)

(82804 has been deleted. To report, see 82803)

82805   with O_2 saturation, by direct measurement, except pulse oximetry

82810 Gases, blood, O_2 saturation only, by direct measurement, except pulse oximetry

(For pulse oximetry, use 94760)

(82812 has been deleted. To report, use 82803)

(82817 has been deleted. To report, use 82803)

82820 Hemoglobin-oxygen affinity (pO_2 for 50% hemoglobin saturation with oxygen)

82926 Gastric acid, free and total, each specimen

(82927 has been deleted. To report, use 82926)

82928 Gastric acid, free or total; each specimen

(82929, 82931, and 82932 have been deleted. To report, use 82928)

82938 Gastrin after secretin stimulation

82941 Gastrin

(Gentamicin, see 80170)

(GGT, see 82977)

(GLC, gas liquid chromatography, see 82486)

(82942 has been deleted)

82943 Glucagon

(82944 has been deleted)

82946 Glucagon tolerance test

82947 Glucose; quantitative

82948   blood, reagent strip

(82949 has been deleted)

82950   post glucose dose (includes glucose)

82951   tolerance test (GTT), three specimens (includes glucose)

82952   tolerance test, each additional beyond three specimens

82953   tolbutamide tolerance test

(For insulin tolerance test, see 80434, 80435)

(For leucine tolerance test, see 80428)

(82954 has been deleted. To report, use 82947)

(For semiquantitative urine glucose, see 81000, 81002, 81005, 81099)

82955 Glucose-6-phosphate dehydrogenase (G6PD); quantitative

82960   screen

(82961 has been deleted)

(For glucose tolerance test with medication, use 90784 in addition)

82962 Glucose, blood by glucose monitoring device(s) cleared by the FDA specifically for home use

82963 Glucosidase, beta

82965 Glutamate dehydrogenase

82975 Glutamine (glutamic acid amide)

82977 Glutamyltransferase, gamma (GGT)

82978 Glutathione

82979 Glutathione reductase, RBC

82980 Glutethimide

(Glycohemoglobin, see 83036)

82985 Glycated protein

(82995 has been deleted. To report, use 80172)

(82996-82998 have been deleted. To report, see 84702, 84703)

(Gonadotropin, chorionic, see 84702, 84703)

(83000 has been deleted)

83001 Gonadotropin; follicle stimulating hormone (FSH)

83002   luteinizing hormone (LH)

(For luteinizing releasing factor (LRH), see 83727)

83003 Growth hormone, human (HGH) (somatotropin)

(83004 has been deleted. To report, use 80430)

(For antibody to human growth hormone, see 86277)

(83005 has been deleted)

83008 Guanosine monophosphate (GMP), cyclic

83010 Haptoglobin; quantitative

(83011 has been deleted. To report, use 83010)

83012   phenotypes

83015 Heavy metal (arsenic, barium, beryllium, bismuth, antimony, mercury); screen

83018   quantitative, each

83020 Hemoglobin, electrophoresis (eg, A2, S, C)

83026 Hemoglobin; by copper sulfate method, non-automated

83030   F(fetal), chemical

83033   F(fetal), qualitative (APT) test, fecal

83036   glycated

(83040 has been deleted. To report, see 83050)

83045   methemoglobin, qualitative

83050   methemoglobin, quantitative

83051   plasma

(83052, 83053 have been deleted. To report, use 85660)

83055   sulfhemoglobin, qualitative

83060   sulfhemoglobin, quantitative

83065   thermolabile

83068   unstable, screen

83069   urine

83070 Hemosiderin; qualitative

83071   quantitative

(Heroin, see 80100-80103)

(HIAA, see 83497)

(High performance liquid chromatography (HPLC), see 82486)

(83086, 83087 have been deleted. To report, use 82128)

83088 Histamine

(Hollander test, see 91052)

(Homocystine, see 82128, 82130)

(83093, 83095 have been deleted. For homogentisic acid, qualitative urine screen, see 81005. For quantitative assay, see code for specific method)

83150 Homovanillic acid (HVA)

(Hormones, see individual alphabetic listings in Chemistry section)

(Hydrogen breath test, see 91065)

(83485, 83486 have been deleted)

83491 Hydroxycorticosteroids, 17- (17-OHCS)

(83492 has been deleted. To report, use 83491)

(83493 has been deleted)

(83494-83496 have been deleted. To report, use 83491)

(For cortisol, see 82530, 82533. For deoxycortisol, see 82634)

83497 Hydroxyindolacetic acid, 5-(HIAA)

(For urine qualitative test, see 81005)

(5-Hydroxytryptamine, see 84260)

83498 Hydroxyprogesterone, 17-d

83499 Hydroxyprogesterone, 20-

83500 Hydroxyproline; free

83505   total

(83510 has been deleted. To report, use 83500 and 83505)

83516 Immunoassay for analyte other than antibody or infectious agent antigen, qualitative or semiquantitative; multiple step method

83518   single step method (eg, reagent strip)

83519 Immunoassay, analyte, quantitative; by radiopharmaceutical technique (eg, RIA)

83520   not otherwise specified

(83523 has been deleted. To report, use 80174)

(For immunoassays for antibodies to infectious agent antibodies, see analyte and method specific codes in the Immunology section)

(For immunoassay of tumor antigen not elsewhere specified, see 86316)

(Immunoglobulins, see 82784, 82785)

(83524 has been deleted)

83525 Insulin; total

(For proinsulin, see 84206)

(83526 has been deleted. To report, see 80434, 80435)

83527   free

83528 Intrinsic factor

(For intrinsic factor antibodies, see 86340)

(83530 has been deleted)

(83533, 83534 have been deleted. To report, use 84999)

83540 Iron

(83545, 83546 have been deleted. To report, use 83540)

83550 Iron binding capacity

(83555, 83565 have been deleted. To report, use 83550)

83570 Isocitric dehydrogenase (IDH)

(83571 has been deleted. To report, use 83570)

(Isopropyl alcohol, see 84600)

(83576 has been deleted. To report, see code for specific method)

(Isonicotinic acid hydrazide, INH, see code for specific method)

(83578 has been deleted)

83582 Ketogenic steroids, fractionation

(83583, 83584 have been deleted)

(Ketone bodies, for serum, see 82009, 82010; for urine, see 81000-81003)

83586 Ketosteroids, 17- (17-KS); total

(83587 has been deleted. To report, use 83593)

(83588, 83589 have been deleted. To report, use 83586)

(83590 has been deleted)

83593   fractionation

(83596 has been deleted)

(83597 has been deleted)

(83599 has been deleted. To report, use 83586)

(83600 has been deleted. To report, use code for specific method)

83605 Lactate (lactic acid)

(83610 has been deleted. To report, use 83615)

83615 Lactate dehydrogenase (LD), (LDH);

(83620 has been deleted. To report, use 83615)

(83624 has been deleted)

83625   isoenzymes, separation and quantitation

(83626 has been deleted)

(83628 has been deleted. To report, use 83625)

(83629, 83631 have been deleted. To report, use 83615)

83632 Lactogen, human placental (HPL) human chorionic somatomammotropin

83633 Lactose, urine; qualitative

83634   quantitative

(For tolerance, see 82951, 82952)

(For breath hydrogen test for lactase deficiency, see 91065)

(83645 has been deleted. To report, see quantitative code or screening for toxicity)

(83650 has been deleted)

83655 Lead

(83660 has been deleted. To report, use 83655)

83661 Lecithin-sphingomyelin ratio (L/S ratio); quantitative

83662   foam stability test

83670 Leucine aminopeptidase (LAP)

(83675, 83680 have been deleted. To report, see 83670)

(83681 has been deleted. To report, see 80428)

(83685 has been deleted. To report, use 80176)

83690 Lipase

(83700, 83705 have been deleted. For cholesterol, see 82465, 83718-83721. For triglycerides, see 84478)

83715 Lipoprotein, blood; electrophoretic separation and quantitation

83717 ultracentrifugation and quantitation

83718 Lipoprotein, direct measurement; high density cholesterol (HDL cholesterol)

83719 VLDL cholesterol

(83720 has been deleted)

83721 LDL cholesterol

(Luteinizing hormone (LH), see 83002)

(83725 has been deleted. To report, use 80178)

83727 Luteinizing releasing factor (LRH)

(83728 has been deleted. To report, see 80100-80103, 80299)

(83730 has been deleted)

(For qualitative analysis, see 80100-80103)

(Macroglobulins, alpha-2, see 86329)

83735 Magnesium

(83740, 83750, 83755, 83760, 83765 have been deleted. To report, use 83735)

83775 Malate dehydrogenase

(Maltose tolerance, see 82951, 82952)

(Mammotropin, see 84146)

83785 Manganese

(83790 has been deleted)

(Marijuana, see 80100-80103)

(83795 has been deleted)

(83799 has been deleted. To report, use 83925)

83805 Meprobamate

(For qualitative analysis, see 80100-80103)

83825 Mercury, quantitative

(83830 has been deleted. To report, use 83825)

(Mercury screen, see 83015)

83835 Metanephrines

(For catecholamines, see 82382-82384)

83840 Methadone

(For methadone qualitative analysis, see 80100-80103)

(Methamphetamine, see 80100-80103, 82145)

(Methanol, see 84600)

(83842 has been deleted. To report, see code for specific method)

(83845 has been deleted. To report, see 80101-80103)

83857 Methemalbumin

(Methemoglobin, see hemoglobin 83045, 83050)

83858 Methsuximide

(Methyl alcohol, see 84600)

(Microalbumin, see 82043 for quantitative, see 82044 for semiquantitative)

(Microglobulin, beta-2, see 82232)

(83859 has been deleted)

(83860-83862 have been deleted. To report, see 80100-80103 for qualitative analysis, 83925 for quantitative analysis)

83864 Mucopolysaccharides, acid; quantitative

(83865 has been deleted. To report, use 83864)

83866 screen

(83870 has been deleted. To report, use 84999)

83872 Mucin, synovial fluid (Ropes test)

83873 Myelin basic protein, CSF

(For oligoclonal bands, see 83916)

83874 Myoglobin

(83875 has been deleted)

(83880 has been deleted. To report, see 83925)

83883 Nephelometry, each analyte not elsewhere specified

83885 Nickel

83887 Nicotine

Molecular Diagnostics

This series of codes 83890-83912 is intended for use with molecular diagnostic techniques for analysis of nucleic acids. These services are coded by procedure rather than analyte. Code separately for each procedure used in an analysis. For example, a procedure requiring isolation of DNA, restriction endonuclease digestion, electrophoresis, and nucleic acid probe amplification would be coded 83890, 83892, 83894, and 83898.

(For microbial identification, see 87178, 87179)

83890 Nuclear molecular diagnostics; molecular isolation or extraction

83892 enzymatic digestion

83894 separation (eg, dot blot, electrophoresis)

(83895 has been deleted)

83896 nucleic acid probe, each

83898 nucleic acid probe with amplification, eg, polymerase chain reaction (PCR), each

(83900 has been deleted)

(83910 has been deleted)

83912 interpretation and report

(83913 has been deleted. To report, see 83898)

83915 Nucleotidase 5'-

83916 Oligoclonal immunoglobulin (oligoclonal bands)

(83917 has been deleted)

83918 Organic acids, quantitative

(83920 has been deleted. To report, use code for specific method)

83925 Opiates, (eg, morphine, meperidine)

83930 Osmolality; blood

83935 urine

83937 Osteocalcin (bone g1a protein)

(83938 has been deleted)

83945 Oxalate

(83946 has been deleted. To report, use 80154)

(83947 has been deleted. To report, see 82009, 82010)

(83948 has been deleted. To report, see 80100-80103, 83925)

(83949 has been deleted)

(83965 has been deleted. To report, use code for specific method)

83970 Parathormone (parathyroid hormone)

(83971, 83972 have been deleted. To report, use code for specific method)

(83973 has been deleted. To report, use 84375)

(83974 has been deleted)

(83975, 83985 have been deleted. To report, use code for specific method)

(Pesticide, quantitative, see code for specific method. For screen for chlorinated hydrocarbons, see 82441)

83986 pH, body fluid, except blood

(For blood pH, see 82800, 82803)

83992 Phencyclidine (PCP)

(For qualitative analysis, see 80100-80103)

(Phenobarbital, see 80184)

(83995 has been deleted. To report, use code for specific method)

(84005 has been deleted)

(84021 has been deleted. To report, see 80100, 80101, 84022)

84022   Phenothiazine

(For qualitative analysis, see 80100, 80101)

84030   Phenylalanine (PKU), blood

(Phenylalanine-tyrosine ratio, see 84030, 84510)

(84031 has been deleted)

(84033 has been deleted. To report, use code for specific method)

84035   Phenylketones, qualitative

(84037 has been deleted. To report, use 84035)

(84038 has been deleted. To report, use code for specific method)

(84039, 84040 have been deleted)

(84045 has been deleted. To report, see 80185, 80186)

84060   Phosphatase, acid; total

84061   forensic examination

(84065 has been deleted. To report, use 84066)

84066   prostatic

84075   Phosphatase, alkaline;

84078   heat stable (total not included)

84080   isoenzymes

84081   Phosphatidylglycerol

(84082 has been deleted)

(Phosphates inorganic, see 84100)

(Phosphates, organic, see code for specific method. For cholinesterase, see 82480, 82482)

(84083 has been deleted)

84085   Phosphogluconate, 6-, dehydrogenase, RBC

84087   Phosphohexose isomerase

(84090 has been deleted)

84100   Phosphorus inorganic (phosphate);

84105   urine

(Pituitary gonadotropins, see 83001-83002)

(PKU, see 84030, 84035)

84106   Porphobilinogen, urine; qualitative

84110   quantitative

(84118 has been deleted. To report, use 84120)

84119   Porphyrins, urine; qualitative

84120   quantitation and fractionation

(84121 has been deleted. To report, use 84120)

84126   Porphyrins, feces; quantitative

84127   qualitative

(84128 has been deleted)

(Porphyrin precursors, see 82135, 84106, 84110)

(For protoporphyrin, RBC, see 84202, 84203)

84132   Potassium; serum

84133   urine

84134   Prealbumin

(For microalbumin, see 82043, 82044)

84135   Pregnanediol

(84136 has been deleted. To report, use 84135)

84138   Pregnanetriol

(84139 has been deleted. To report, use 84138)

84140 Pregnenolone

(84141 has been deleted. To report, use 80188)

(84142 has been deleted. To report, see 80190, 80192)

84143 17-hydroxypregnenolone

84144 Progesterone

(Progesterone receptor assay, see 84234)

(For proinsulin, see 84206)

84146 Prolactin

(84147 has been deleted. To report, see 80100-80103)

(84149 has been deleted)

84150 Prostaglandin, each

84153 Prostate specific antigen (PSA)

84155 Protein; total, except refractometry

84160 refractometric

84165 electrophoretic fractionation and quantitation

(84170 has been deleted)

(84175 has been deleted. To report, use 84165)

(84176 has been deleted)

(84180 has been deleted. To report, use 81050 and 84155)

84181 Western Blot, with interpretation and report, blood or other body fluid

84182 Western Blot, with interpretation and report, blood or other body fluid, immunological probe for band identification, each

(For Western Blot tissue analysis, see 88371)

(84185 has been deleted)

(84190 has been deleted. To report, use 84165)

(84195 has been deleted)

(84200 has been deleted. To report, use 84165)

(84201 has been deleted. To report, see 80438, 80439)

84202 Protoporphyrin, RBC; quantitative

84203 screen

(84205 has been deleted. To report, use code for specific method)

84206 Proinsulin

(Pseudocholinesterase, see 82480)

84207 Pyridoxal phosphate (Vitamin B-6)

(84208 has been deleted. To report, use 89060)

84210 Pyruvate

84220 Pyruvate kinase

84228 Quinine

(84230 has been deleted. To report, use 80194)

(84231 has been deleted. To report radioimmunoassay not elsewhere specified, see 83519)

(84232 has been deleted)

84233 Receptor assay; estrogen

84234 progesterone

84235 endocrine, other than estrogen or progesterone (specify hormone)

(84236 has been deleted. To report, use 84233 and 84234)

84238 non-endocrine (eg, acetylcholine) (specify receptor)

84244 Renin

(84246 has been deleted)

(84250, 84251 have been deleted. To report, use 84479)

84252 Riboflavin (Vitamin B-2)

(Salicylates, see 80196)

(Secretin test, see 99070, 89100 and appropriate analyses)

84255 Selenium

84260 Serotonin

(For urine metabolites (HIAA), see 83497)

84270 Sex hormone binding globulin (SHBG)

84275 Sialic acid

(Sickle hemoglobin, see 85660)

84285 Silica

84295 Sodium; serum

84300 urine

(Somatomammotropin, see 83632)

(Somatotropin, see 83003)

84305 Somatomedin

84307 Somatostatin

(84310 has been deleted)

84311 Spectrophotometry, analyte not elsewhere specified

84315 Specific gravity (except urine)

(For specific gravity, urine, see 81000-81003)

(84317 has been deleted)

(84318 has been deleted)

(Stone analysis, see 82355-82370)

(84324 has been deleted. To report, use code for specific method)

84375 Sugars, chromatographic, TLC or paper chromatography

(Sulfhemoglobin, see hemoglobin, 83055, 83060)

(84382 has been deleted)

84392 Sulfate, urine

(84395 has been deleted)

(84397 has been deleted)

(T-3, see 84479-84481)

(T-4, see 84435-84439)

(84401 has been deleted)

84402 Testosterone; free

84403 total

(84404 has been deleted)

(84405 has been deleted. To report, use 84403)

(84406 has been deleted. For testosterone binding protein, see sex hormone binding globulin, 84270)

(84407 has been deleted. To report, use code for specific method)

(84408 has been deleted. To report, see 80100-80103, 80299)

(84409, 84410 have been deleted. To report, use code for specific method)

(84420 has been deleted. To report, use 80198)

84425 Thiamine (Vitamin B-1)

84430 Thiocyanate

84432 Thyroglobulin

(Thyroglobulin, antibody, see 86800)

(84434 has been deleted. To report, use 84022)

(Thyrotropin releasing hormone (TRH) test, see 84201)

(84435 has been deleted)

84436 Thyroxine; total

84437 requiring elution (eg, neonatal)

84439 free

(84441 has been deleted. To report, use 84436-84439)

84442 Thyroxine binding globulin (TBG)

84443 Thyroid stimulating hormone (TSH)

(84444 has been deleted. To report, see 80438, 80439)

84445 Thyroid stimulating immunoglobulins (TSI)

(Tobramycin, use 80200)

84446 Tocopherol alpha (Vitamin E)

(Tolbutamide tolerance, use 82953)

(84447, 84448 have been deleted. To report, see 80100-80103)

84449 Transcortin (cortisol binding globulin)

84450 Transferase; aspartate amino (AST) (SGOT)

(84455 has been deleted. To report, use 84450)

84460   alanine amino (ALT) (SGPT)

(84465 has been deleted. To report, use 84460)

84466 Transferrin

(Iron binding capacity, see 83550)

(84472 has been deleted. To report, use code for specific method)

(84474 has been deleted. To report, use code for specific method)

(84476 has been deleted. To report, see 84022)

84478 Triglycerides

84479 Triiodothyronine (T-3); resin uptake

84480   total (TT-3)

84481   free

84482   reverse

(84483 has been deleted. To report, see 80100-80103, 80299)

84485 Trypsin; duodenal fluid

84488   feces, qualitative

84490   feces, quantitative, 24-hour collection

84510 Tyrosine

(Urate crystal identification, see 89060)

84520 Urea nitrogen; quantitative

84525   semiquantitative (eg, reagent strip test)

84540 Urea nitrogen, urine

84545 Urea nitrogen, clearance

84550 Uric acid; blood

(84555 has been deleted. To report, use 84550)

84560   other source

(84565, 84570, 84575 have been deleted)

84577 Urobilinogen, feces, quantitative

84578 Urobilinogen, urine; qualitative

84580   quantitative, timed specimen

84583   semiquantitative

(84584 has been deleted)

(Uroporphyrins, see 84120)

(Valproic acid (dipropylacetic acid), see 80164)

84585 Vanillylmandelic acid (VMA), urine

84586 Vasoactive intestinal peptide (VIP)

84588 Vasopressin (antidiuretic hormone, ADH)

(84589 has been deleted. To report, use 85810)

84590 Vitamin A

(84595 has been deleted. To report, use 82380 and 84590)

(Vitamin B-1, see 84425)

(Vitamin B-2, see 84252)

(Vitamin B-6, see 84207)

(Vitamin B-12, see 82607)

(Vitamin B-12, absorption (Schilling), see 78270, 78271)

(Vitamin C, see 82180)

(Vitamin D, see 82306, 82307, 82652)

(Vitamin E, see 84446)

84597   Vitamin K

(VMA, see 84585)

84600   Volatiles (eg, acetic anhydride, carbon tetrachloride, dichloroethane, dichloromethane, diethylether, isopropyl alcohol, methanol)

(For acetaldehyde, see 82000)

(84605 has been deleted)

(84610 has been deleted)

(Volume, blood, RISA or Cr-51, see 78110, 78111)

(84613 has been deleted)

(84615 has been deleted. To report, use code for specific method)

84620   Xylose absorption test, blood and/or urine

(For administration, see 99070)

84630   Zinc

(84635 has been deleted. To report, use 84630)

(84645 has been deleted)

(84680 has been deleted. To report, use 82677)

84681   C-peptide

(84695 has been deleted. To report, use 80170)

(84701 has been deleted. To report, see 84702-84703)

84702   Gonadotropin, chorionic (hCG); quantitative

84703   qualitative

(For urine pregnancy test by visual color comparison, see 81025)

(84800 has been deleted. To report, see 84443)

(84810 has been deleted. To report, use 80200)

84830   Ovulation tests, by visual color comparison methods for human luteinizing hormone

84999   Unlisted chemistry procedure

Hematology and Coagulation

(For blood banking procedures, see Transfusion Medicine)

(Agglutinins, see Immunology)

(Antiplasmin, see 85410)

(Antithrombin III, see 85300, 85301)

(85000 has been deleted. To report, use 85002)

85002   Bleeding time

(85003 has been deleted. To report, use 85999)

(85005 has been deleted)

85007   Blood count; manual differential WBC count (includes RBC morphology and platelet estimation)

85008   manual blood smear examination without differential parameters

(See also 85585)

(For other fluids (eg, CSF), see 89050, 89051)

85009   differential WBC count, buffy coat

(85012 has been deleted)

(Eosinophils, nasal smear, see 89190)

85013   spun microhematocrit

85014   other than spun hematocrit

85018   hemoglobin

(For other hemoglobin determination, see 83020-83069)

85021   hemogram, automated (RBC, WBC, Hgb, Hct and indices only)

85022   hemogram, automated, and manual differential WBC count (CBC)

85023   hemogram and platelet count, automated, and manual differential WBC count (CBC)

85024   hemogram and platelet count, automated, and automated partial differential WBC count (CBC)

85025   hemogram and platelet count, automated, and automated complete differential WBC count (CBC)

85027   hemogram and platelet count, automated

(85028 has been deleted. To report, use 85023-85025)

85029 Additional automated hemogram indices (eg, red cell distribution width (RDW), mean platelet volume (MPV), red blood cell histogram, platelet histogram, white blood cell histogram); one to three indices

85030   four or more indices

85031 Blood count; hemogram, manual, complete CBC (RBC, WBC, Hgb, Hct, differential and indices)

85041   red blood cell (RBC) only

(See also 85021-85031, 89050)

85044   reticulocyte count, manual

85045   reticulocyte count, flow cytometry

85048   white blood cell (WBC)

(See also 85021-85031)

85060 Blood smear, peripheral, interpretation by physician with written report

85095 Bone marrow; aspiration only

(85096 has been deleted. For interpretation of smear, use 85097; for cell block interpretation, see 88305)

85097   smear interpretation only, with or without differential cell count

(85100 has been deleted. To report, use 85095 and 85097)

(85101 has been deleted. For aspiration, see 85095)

(For special stains, see 85540, 88312, 88313)

85102 Bone marrow biopsy, needle or trocar

(For bone biopsy, use 20220)

(85103, 85105 have been deleted. For bone marrow biopsy interpretation, see 88305)

(85109 has been deleted)

(85120 has been deleted. To report, see 38230-38240)

85130 Chromogenic substrate assay

(85150, 85160, 85165 have been deleted)

(Circulating anti-coagulant screen (mixing studies), see 85611, 85732)

85170 Clot retraction

(85171, 85172 have been deleted)

85175 Clot lysis time, whole blood dilution

(Clotting factor I (fibrinogen), see 85384, 85385)

85210 Clotting; factor II, prothrombin, specific

(See also 85610-85613)

85220   factor V (AcG or proaccelerin), labile factor

85230   factor VII (proconvertin, stable factor)

85240   factor VIII (AHG), one stage

(85242 has been deleted)

85244   factor VIII related antigen

85245   factor VIII, VW factor, ristocetin cofactor

85246   factor VIII, VW factor antigen

85247   factor VIII, Von Willebrand's factor, multimetric analysis

85250   factor IX (PTC or Christmas)

85260   factor X (Stuart-Prower)

85270   factor XI (PTA)

85280   factor XII (Hageman)

85290   factor XIII (fibrin stabilizing)

85291   factor XIII (fibrin stabilizing), screen solubility

85292   prekallikrein assay (Fletcher factor assay)

85293   high molecular weight kininogen assay (Fitzgerald factor assay)

85300   Clotting inhibitors or anticoagulants; antithrombin III, activity

85301   antithrombin III, antigen assay

85302   protein C, antigen

85303   protein C, activity

85305   protein S, total

85306   protein S, free

(85310, 85311 have been deleted)

(85320 has been deleted)

(85330 has been deleted. To report, see 85335)

85335   Factor inhibitor test

85337   Thrombomodulin

(For mixing studies for inhibitors, use 85732)

(85340, 85341 have been deleted)

85345   Coagulation time; Lee and White

85347   activated

85348   other methods

(Differential count, see 85007 et seq)

(Duke bleeding time, see 85002)

(Eosinophils, nasal smear, see 89190)

85360   Euglobulin lysis

(Fetal hemoglobin, see 83030, 83033, 85460)

85362   Fibrin(ogen) degradation (split) products (FDP)(FSP); agglutination slide, semiquantitative

(85363, 85364 have been deleted)

(85365 has been deleted. To report, use 86320)

(Immunoelectrophoresis, see 86320)

85366   paracoagulation

(85367 has been deleted)

(85368 has been deleted. To report, use 85366)

(85369 has been deleted)

85370   quantitative

(85371 has been deleted. To report, see 85384, 85385)

(85372 has been deleted)

(85376, 85377 have been deleted. To report, use 85384, 85385)

85378   Fibrin degradation products, D-dimer; semiquantitative

85379   quantitative

85384   Fibrinogen; activity

85385   antigen

85390   Fibrinolysins or coagulopathy screen, interpretation and report

(85392 has been deleted)

(85395 has been deleted)

(85398 has been deleted)

85400   Fibrinolytic factors and inhibitors; plasmin

85410   alpha-2 antiplasmin

85415   plasminogen activator

85420   plasminogen, except antigenic assay

85421   plasminogen, antigenic assay

▲=Revised Code   ●=New Code

(85426 has been deleted. For von Willebrand factor assay, see 85245-85247)

(Fragility, red blood cell, see 85547, 85555-85557)

85441 Heinz bodies; direct

85445   induced, acetyl phenylhydrazine

(Hematocrit (PCV), see 85014, 85021-85031)

(Hemoglobin, see 83020-83068, 85018-85031)

85460 Hemoglobin or RBCs, fetal, for fetomaternal hemorrhage; differential lysis (Kleihauer-Betke)

(See also 83030, 83033)

(Hemogram, see 85021-85031)

(Hemolysins, see 86940, 86941)

85461   rosette

85475 Hemolysin, acid

(See also 86940, 86941)

85520 Heparin assay

85525 Heparin neutralization

85530 Heparin-protamine tolerance test

85535 Iron stain (RBC or bone marrow smears)

(85538 has been deleted. For leder stain, esterase, blood or bone marrow, see 88319)

85540 Leukocyte alkaline phosphatase with count

(85544 has been deleted)

85547 Mechanical fragility, RBC

(85548 has been deleted. To report, see 85008)

85549 Muramidase

(Nitroblue tetrazolium dye test, see 86384)

85555 Osmotic fragility, RBC; unincubated

(85556 has been deleted)

85557   incubated

(Packed cell volume, see 85013)

(Partial thromboplastin time, see 85730, 85732)

(Parasites, blood (eg, malaria smears), see 87207)

(Plasmin, see 85400)

(Plasminogen, see 85420)

(Plasminogen activator, see 85415)

(85560 has been deleted. For peroxidase stain, WBC, see 88319)

(85575 has been deleted)

85576 Platelet; aggregation (in vitro), each agent

(85577 has been deleted)

(85580 has been deleted. To report, use 85590)

85585   estimation on smear, only

(See also 85008)

85590   manual count

85595   automated count

85597 Platelet neutralization

85610 Prothrombin time;

85611   substitution, plasma fractions, each

85612 Russell viper venom time (includes venom); undiluted

85613   diluted

(85614 has been deleted)

(85615 has been deleted)

(85618 has been deleted)

(Red blood cell count, see 85021, 85031, 85041)

(85630 has been deleted. To report, use 85029, 85030)

(85632 has been deleted)

85635 Reptilase test

(Reticulocyte count, see 85044, 85045)

(85650 has been deleted)

85651 Sedimentation rate, erythrocyte;
non-automated

●**85652** automated

85660 Sickling of RBC, reduction

(Hemoglobin electrophoresis, see 83020)

(Smears (eg, for parasites, malaria), see
87207)

(85665 has been deleted. For plasminogen
activator, see 85415)

(85667 has been deleted)

85670 Thrombin time; plasma

85675 titer

(85700 has been deleted)

85705 Thromboplastin inhibition; tissue

(85710, 85711 have been deleted)

(85720 has been deleted)

(For individual clotting factors, see 85245-
85247)

85730 Thromboplastin time, partial (PTT); plasma or
whole blood

85732 substitution, plasma fractions, each

85810 Viscosity

(85820 has been deleted. To report, use
85810)

(von Willebrand factor assay, see 85245-
85247)

(WBC count, see 85021-85031, 85048,
89050)

85999 Unlisted hematology and coagulation
procedure

Immunology

(Acetylcholine receptor antibody, see 86255,
86256)

(Actinomyces, antibodies to, see 86602)

(Adrenal cortex antibodies, see 86255,
86256)

86000 Agglutinins, febrile (eg, Brucella, Francisella,
Murine typhus, Q fever, Rocky Mountain
spotted fever, scrub typhus), each antigen

(For antibodies to infectious agents, see
86602-86793)

(86002 has been deleted)

(Agglutinins and autohemolysins, see 86940,
86941)

▲**86003** Allergen specific IgE; quantitative or
semiquantitative, each allergen

(For total quantitative IgE, use 82785)

(86004 has been deleted. To report, see
86940, 86941)

▲**86005** qualitative, multiallergen screen (dipstick,
paddle or disk)

(For MAST, see 86005)

(For total qualitative IgE, use 83518)

(Alpha-1 antitrypsin, see 82103, 82104)

(Alpha-1 feto-protein, see 82105, 82106)

(Anti-AChR (acetylcholine receptor) antibody
titer, see 86255, 86256)

(86006 has been deleted. To report, see
83519, 86318, 86403)

(86007, 86008, 86009 have been deleted)

(86011 has been deleted. To report, see
86021)

(86012 has been deleted. To report, see
86978)

(86013 has been deleted)

(86014 has been deleted. To report, see 86022)

(86016 has been deleted. To report, see 86850)

(86017 has been deleted. To report, see 86850 and 86901)

(86018 has been deleted)

(86019 has been deleted. To report, see 86860)

(Anticardiolipin antibody, see 86147)

(Anti-DNA, see 86225)

(Anti-deoxyribonuclease titer, see 86215)

86021 Antibody identification; leukocyte antibodies

86022 platelet antibodies

86023 platelet associated immunoglobulin assay

(86024 has been deleted. For RBC antibodies, see 86870)

(86026, 86028 have been deleted)

(86031 has been deleted. To report, see 86880)

(86032 has been deleted. To report, see 86885)

(86033 has been deleted. To report, see 86886)

(86034 has been deleted. To report, see 86880-86886 and 86971)

(86035 has been deleted. To report, use 86970)

86038 Antinuclear antibodies (ANA);

86039 titer

(86045 has been deleted)

(Antistreptococcal antibody, ie, anti-DNAse, see 86215)

(Antistreptokinase titer, see 86590)

86060 Antistreptolysin O; titer

(For antibodies to infectious agents, see 86602-86793)

86063 screen

(For antibodies to infectious agents, see 86602-86793)

(86064 has been deleted. For antitrypsin, alpha-1 see 82103, for phenotyping see 82104)

(86066 has been deleted. To report, see 82104)

(86067 has been deleted. To report, see 82103)

(86068 has been deleted. For blood compatibility test, see 86920-86922)

(Blastomyces, antibodies to, see 86612)

(86069 has been deleted)

(86070 has been deleted. To report, see 86920)

(86072 has been deleted)

(86073 has been deleted. To report, see 86156, 86157, 86904)

(86074 has been deleted)

(86075, 86076 have been deleted)

86077 Blood bank physician services; difficult cross match and/or evaluation of irregular antibody(s), interpretation and written report

86078 investigation of transfusion reaction including suspicion of transmissible disease, interpretation and written report

86079 authorization for deviation from standard blood banking procedures (eg, use of outdated blood, transfusion of Rh incompatible units), with written report

(86080 has been deleted. For blood typing, see 86900-86910)

(86082 has been deleted. To report, see 86900, 86901)

(86083 has been deleted. To report, use 86850 and 86900 or 86901)

(86084 has been deleted. To report, use 86903)

(86085 has been deleted. To report, see 86904)

(86090 has been deleted)

(86095 has been deleted. To report, see 86905)

(86096 has been deleted)

(86100 has been deleted. To report, see 86901)

(86105 has been deleted. To report, see 86906)

(86115 has been deleted)

(86120 has been deleted. To report, use 86905)

(86128 has been deleted. To report, see 86890)

(86129 has been deleted)

(86130 has been deleted. To report, see 86891)

(86131, 86134, 86138 and 86139 have been deleted)

(Brucella, antibodies to, see 86622)

(Candida, antibodies to, see 86628. For skin testing, see 86485)

86140 C-reactive protein

(Candidiasis, see 86628)

86147 Cardiolipin (phospholipid) antibody

(86149 has been deleted. To report, see 82378)

(86151 has been deleted. To report, see 82378)

86155 Chemotaxis assay, specify method

(Clostridium difficile toxin, see 87230)

(Coccidioides, antibodies to, see 86635. For skin testing, see 86490)

86156 Cold agglutinin; screen

86157   titer

(86158 has been deleted)

(86159 has been deleted. To report, see 86160 and 86161)

86160 Complement; antigen, each component

86161   functional activity, each component

86162   total hemolytic (CH50)

(86163, 86164 have been deleted. To report, see 86160 and 86161)

86171 Complement fixation tests, each antigen

(Coombs test, see 86880-86886)

86185 Counterimmunoelectrophoresis, each antigen

(86201, 86202 have been deleted)

(Cryptococcus, antibodies to, see 86641)

(86209 has been deleted. To report, use 86999)

86215 Deoxyribonuclease, antibody

86225 Deoxyribonucleic acid (DNA) antibody; native or double stranded

(Echinococcus, antibodies to, see code for specific method)

(For HIV antibody tests, see 86701-86703)

86226   single stranded

(Anti D.S., DNA, IFA, eg, using C.Lucilae, see 86255 and 86256)

(86227, 86228 have been deleted. To report, use 86317)

(86229 has been deleted)

86235 Extractable nuclear antigen, antibody to, any method (eg, nRNP, SS-A, SS-B, Sm, RNP, Sc170, J01), each antibody

(86240, 86241 have been deleted)

86243 Fc receptor

(86244 has been deleted. To report fetoprotein, alpha-1, see 82105, 82106)

(86245 has been deleted)

(Filaria, antibodies to, see code for specific method)

86255   Fluorescent antibody; screen, each antibody

86256   titer, each antibody

(Fluorescent technique for antigen identification in tissue, see 88346; for indirect fluorescence, see 88347)

(86265 has been deleted. To report, see 86930)

(86266 has been deleted. To report, see 86931)

(FTA, see 86781)

(86267 has been deleted. To report, see 86932)

(Gel (agar) diffusion tests, see 86331)

(86272, 86273 have been deleted)

(86274 has been deleted. To report, see 90742)

86277   Growth hormone, human (HGH), antibody

86280   Hemagglutination inhibition test (HAI)

(For rubella, see 86762)

(86281 has been deleted. To report, see 85475)

(86282 has been deleted. To report, see 86940)

(86283 has been deleted. To report, see 86941)

(86285, 86286 have been deleted)

86287   Hepatitis B surface antigen (HBsAg)

(86288 has been deleted)

86289   Hepatitis B core antibody (HBcAb); IgG and IgM

(For antibodies to infectious agents, see 86602-86793)

86290   IgM antibody

(For antibodies to infectious agents, see 86602-86793)

86291   Hepatitis B surface antibody (HBsAb)

(For antibodies to infectious agents, see 86602-86793)

86293   Hepatitis Be antigen (HBeAg)

(For antibodies to infectious agents, see 86602-86793)

86295   Hepatitis Be antibody (HBeAb)

(For antibodies to infectious agents, see 86602-86793)

86296   Hepatitis A antibody (HAAb); IgG and IgM

(For antibodies to infectious agents, see 86602-86793)

(86297 has been deleted. To report, use 86296)

(86298 has been deleted)

86299   IgM antibody

(For antibodies to infectious agents, see 86602-86793)

(86300 has been deleted. To report, see 86308)

86302   Hepatitis C antibody;

(For antibodies to infectious agents, see 86602-86793)

(86305 has been deleted. To report, use 86309)

86303   confirmatory test (eg, immunoblot)

86306   Hepatitis, delta agent

(For hepatitis delta agent, antibody, see 86692)

86308   Heterophile antibodies; screening

(For antibodies to infectious agents, see 86602-86793)

86309 titer

(For antibodies to infectious agents, see 86602-86793)

86310 titers after absorption with beef cells and guinea pig kidney

(Histoplasma, antibodies to, see 86698. For skin testing, see 86510)

(For antibodies to infectious agents, see 86602-86793)

86311 HIV, antigen

(86312 has been deleted. To report, see 86701-86703)

(Human growth hormone antibody, see 86277)

86313 Immunoassay for infectious agent antigen, qualitative or semiquantitative; multiple step method

(86314 has been deleted. To report, use 86689)

86315 single step method (eg, reagent strip)

86316 Immunoassay for tumor antigen (eg, cancer antigen 125), each

86317 Immunoassay for infectious agent antibody, quantitative, not elsewhere specified

(For immunoassay techniques for antigens, see 83516, 83518, 83519, 83520, 86313, 86315)

(For particle agglutination procedures, see 86403)

86318 Immunoassay for infectious agent antibody, qualitative or semiquantitative, single step method (eg, reagent strip)

(86319 has been deleted. To report immunoassays for drugs, see 80100-80103)

86320 Immunoelectrophoresis; serum

86325 other fluids (eg, urine, CSF) with concentration

86327 crossed (2-dimensional assay)

86329 Immunodiffusion; not elsewhere specified

86331 gel diffusion, qualitative (Ouchterlony), each antigen or antibody

86332 Immune complex assay

(86333 has been deleted. To report, see 86332)

86334 Immunofixation electrophoresis

(86335 has been deleted)

86337 Insulin antibodies

(86338 has been deleted. To report, see 86337)

86340 Intrinsic factor antibodies

(Leptospira, antibodies to, see 86720)

(Leukoagglutinins, see 86021)

86341 Islet cell antibody

(86342 has been deleted. To report, see 86945)

86343 Leukocyte histamine release test (LHR)

86344 Leukocyte phagocytosis

(86345, 86346, 86347 have been deleted)

(86349 has been deleted. To report, see 86950)

(86351 has been deleted)

86353 Lymphocyte transformation, mitogen (phytomitogen) or antigen induced blastogenesis

(86357 has been deleted. To report, see 88180, 88342, 88346)

(Lymphocytes immunophenotyping, see 88180 for cytometry; see 88342, 88346 for microscopic techniques)

(86358 has been deleted. To report, see 88180, 88342, 88346)

(Malaria antibodies, see 86750)

86359 T cells; total count

86360 T4 and T8, including ratio

(86365 has been deleted)

86376 Microsomal antibodies (eg, thyroid or liver-kidney), each

(86377 has been deleted. To report, see 86376)

86378 Migration inhibitory factor test (MIF)

(Mitochondrial antibody, liver, see 86255, 86256)

(Mononucleosis, see 86308-86310)

86382 Neutralization test, viral

86384 Nitroblue tetrazolium dye test (NTD)

(Ouchterlony diffusion, see 86331)

(86385, 86386 have been deleted. To report, see 86910, 86911)

(86388, 86389, 86391 have been deleted)

(Platelet antibodies, see 86022, 86023)

(86392, 86393, 86398 have been deleted)

(86402 has been deleted)

86403 Particle agglutination; screen, each antibody

(86404 has been deleted. To report, see 86965)

(86405 has been deleted)

86406 titer, each antibody

(Pregnancy test, see 84702, 84703)

(86410 has been deleted. To report, see 86970)

(86411 has been deleted. To report, see 86971)

(86412 has been deleted. To report, see 86972)

(86415, 86416 have been deleted)

(86417 has been deleted. To report, see 86975)

(86418 has been deleted. To report, see 86976)

(86419 has been deleted. To report, see 86977)

(86420 has been deleted. To report, see 86978)

(86421-86423 have been deleted. To report, see 82785, 83518, 86003, 86005)

(Rapid plasma reagin test (RPR), see 86592, 86593)

(86424, 86425, 86427 have been deleted)

86430 Rheumatoid factor; qualitative

86431 quantitative

(Serologic test for syphilis, see 86592, 86593)

(86450 has been deleted)

(86455 has been deleted. To report, use 86586)

(86460, 86470, 86480 have been deleted)

86485 Skin test; candida

(For antibody, candida, see 86628)

86490 coccidioidomycosis

(86495, 86500 have been deleted)

86510 histoplasmosis

(For histoplasma, antibody, see 86698)

(86520, 86530 have been deleted)

(86540 has been deleted. For mumps antibody, see 86735)

(86550, 86565, 86570 have been deleted)

86580 tuberculosis, intradermal

86585 tuberculosis, tine test

(For skin tests for allergy, see 95010-95199)

(Smooth muscle antibody, see 86255, 86256)

(Sporothrix, antibodies to, see code for specific method)

86586 unlisted antigen, each

(86587 has been deleted. To report, see 86985)

86588   Streptococcus, screen, direct

86590   Streptokinase, antibody

(For antibodies to infectious agents, see 86602-86793)

(Streptolysin O antibody, see antistreptolysin O, 86060, 86063)

86592   Syphilis test; qualitative (eg, VDRL, RPR, ART)

(For antibodies to infectious agents, see 86602-86793)

86593   quantitative

(For antibodies to infectious agents, see 86602-86793)

(Tetanus antibody, see 86774)

(Thyroglobulin antibody, see 86800)

(Thyroglobulin, see 84432)

(86594 has been deleted. To report, see 86376 and 86800)

(Thyroid microsomal antibody, see 86376)

(86595 has been deleted)

(86597 has been deleted. To report use 86812-86822)

(86600 has been deleted)

(For toxoplasma antibody, see 86777-86778)

The following codes (86602-86793) are qualitative or semiquantitative immunoassays performed by multiple step methods. For immunoassays by single step method (eg, reagent strips), use code 86318. Procedures for the identification of antibodies should be coded as precisely as possible. For example, an antibody to a virus could be coded with increasing specificity for virus, family, genus, species, or type. In some cases, further precision may be added to codes by specifying the class of immunoglobulin being detected. When multiple tests are done to detect antibodies to organisms classified more precisely than the specificity allowed by available codes, it is appropriate to code each as a separate service. For example, a test for antibody to an enterovirus is coded as 86658.

Coxsackie viruses are enteroviruses, but there are no codes for the individual species of enterovirus. If assays are performed for antibodies to Coxsackie A and B species, each assay should be separately coded. Similarly, if multiple assays are performed for antibodies of different immunoglobulin classes, each assay should be coded separately.

86602   Antibody; actinomyces

86603   adenovirus

86606   Aspergillus

86609   bacterium, not elsewhere specified

86612   Blastomyces

86615   Bordetella

86617   Borrelia burgdorferi (Lyme disease) confirmatory test (eg, Western blot or immunoblot)

86618   Borrelia burgdorferi (Lyme disease)

86619   Borrelia (relapsing fever)

86622   Brucella

86625   Campylobacter

86628   Candida

(For skin test, candida, see 86485)

(86630 has been deleted)

86631   Chlamydia

86632   Chlamydia, IgM

(For chlamydia antigen, see 83518. For fluorescent technique, see 86255, 86256)

86635   Coccidioides

86638   Coxiella Brunetii (Q fever)

86641   Cryptococcus

86644   cytomegalovirus (CMV)

(For TORCH panel, see 80090)

86645   cytomegalovirus (CMV), IgM

86648   Diphtheria

(86650 has been deleted. To report, use 86781)

86651   encephalitis, California (La Crosse)

86652   encephalitis, Eastern equine

86653   encephalitis, St. Louis

86654   encephalitis, Western equine

86658   enterovirus (eg, coxsackie, echo, polio)

(86662 has been deleted. To report, use 86781)

(Trichinella, antibodies to, see 86784)

(Trypanosoma, antibodies to, see code for specific method)

(Tuberculosis, see 86580 for skin testing)

(Viral antibodies, see code for specific method)

86663   Epstein-Barr (EB) virus, early antigen (EA)

86664   Epstein-Barr (EB) virus, nuclear antigen (EBNA)

86665   Epstein-Barr (EB) virus, viral capsid (VCA)

86668   Francisella Tularensis

86671   fungus, not elsewhere specified

86674   Giardia Lamblia

86677   Helicobacter Pylori

(86681 has been deleted. To report, see 86255, 86256)

86682   helminth, not elsewhere specified

86684   Hemophilus influenza

(86685 has been deleted. To report, see 86255, 86256)

86687   HTLV I

86688   HTLV-II

86689   HTLV or HIV antibody, confirmatory test (eg, Western Blot)

86692   hepatitis, delta agent

(For hepatitis delta agent, antigen, see 86306)

86694   herpes simplex, non-specific type test

(For TORCH panel, see 80090)

86695   herpes simplex, type I

86698   histoplasma

86701   HIV-1

86702   HIV-2

86703   HIV-1 and HIV-2, single assay

(For HIV antigen, see 86311)

(For confirmatory test for HIV antibody (eg, Western Blot), see 86689)

86710   influenza virus

86713   Legionella

86717   Leishmania

86720   Leptospira

86723   Listeria monocytogenes

86727   lymphocytic choriomeningitis

86729   Lymphogranuloma Venereum

86732   mucormycosis

86735   mumps

86738   Mycoplasma

86741   Neisseria meningitidis

86744   Nocardia

86747   parvovirus

86750   Plasmodium (malaria)

86753   protozoa, not elsewhere specified

86756   respiratory syncytial virus

86759   rotavirus

86762   rubella

86765   rubeola

86768   Salmonella

86771 Shigella

86774 tetanus

86777 Toxoplasma

86778 Toxoplasma, IgM

86781 Treponema Pallidum, confirmatory test (eg, FTA-abs)

86784 trichinella

86787 varicella-zoster

86790 virus, not elsewhere specified

86793 Yersinia

86800 Thyroglobulin antibody

(For thyroglobulin, see 84432)

Tissue Typing

(For pretransplant cross-match, use appropriate code or codes)

86805 Lymphocytotoxicity assay, visual crossmatch; with titration

86806 without titration

86807 Serum screening for cytotoxic percent reactive antibody (PRA); standard method

86808 quick method

(86810 has been deleted)

86812 HLA typing; A, B, or C (eg, A10, B7, B27), single antigen

86813 A, B, or C, multiple antigens

86816 DR/DQ, single antigen

86817 DR/DQ, multiple antigens

86821 lymphocyte culture, mixed (MLC)

86822 lymphocyte culture, primed (PLC)

86849 Unlisted immunology procedure

Transfusion Medicine

(For apheresis, see 36520)

(For therapeutic phlebotomy, see 99195)

86850 Antibody screen, RBC, each serum technique

86860 Antibody elution (RBC), each elution

86870 Antibody identification, RBC antibodies, each panel for each serum technique

86880 Antihuman globulin test (Coombs test); direct, each antiserum

86885 indirect, qualitative, each antiserum

86886 indirect, titer, each antiserum

86890 Autologous blood or component, collection processing and storage; predeposited

86891 intra- or postoperative salvage

(For physician services to autologous donors, see 99201-99204)

86900 Blood typing; ABO

86901 Rh (D)

86903 antigen screening for compatible blood unit using reagent serum, per unit screened

86904 antigen screening for compatible unit using patient serum, per unit screened

86905 RBC antigens, other than ABO or Rh (D), each

86906 Rh phenotyping, complete

86910 Blood typing, for paternity testing, per individual, ABO, Rh and MN;

86911 each additional antigen system

86915 Bone marrow, modification or treatment to eliminate cell (eg, T-cells, metastatic carcinoma)

86920 Compatibility test each unit; immediate spin technique

86921 incubation technique

86922 antiglobulin technique

86927 Fresh frozen plasma, thawing, each unit

86930 Frozen blood, preparation for freezing, each unit;

▲=Revised Code ●=New Code

86931   with thawing

86932   with freezing and thawing

86940 Hemolysins and agglutinins, auto, screen, each;

86941   incubated

86945 Irradiation of blood product, each unit

86950 Leukocyte transfusion

(For leukapheresis, see 36520)

86965 Pooling of platelets or other blood products

86970 Pretreatment of RBC's for use in RBC antibody detection, identification, and/or compatibility testing; incubation with chemical agents or drugs, each

86971   incubation with enzymes, each

86972   by density gradient separation

86975 Pretreatment of serum for use in RBC antibody identification; incubation with drugs, each

86976   by dilution

86977   incubation with inhibitors, each

86978   by differential red cell absorption using patient RBC's or RBC's of known phenotype, each absorption

86985 Splitting of blood or blood products, each unit

86999 Unlisted transfusion medicine procedure

Microbiology

Includes bacteriology, mycology, parasitology, and virology.

87001 Animal inoculation, small animal; with observation

87003   with observation and dissection

87015 Concentration (any type), for parasites, ova, or tubercle bacillus (TB, AFB)

87040 Culture, bacterial, definitive; blood (includes anaerobic screen)

87045   stool

87060   throat or nose

87070   any other source

(For urine, see 87086-87088)

87072 Culture or direct bacterial identification method, each organism, by commercial kit, any source except urine

(For urine, see 87087)

87075 Culture, bacterial, any source; anaerobic (isolation)

87076   definitive identification, each anaerobic organism, including gas chromatography

(For anaerobe without GC, see 87072)

87081 Culture, bacterial, screening only, for single organisms

87082 Culture, presumptive, pathogenic organisms, screening only, by commercial kit (specify type); for single organisms

87083   multiple organisms

87084   with colony estimation from density chart

87085   with colony count

(For urine colony count, see 87086)

87086 Culture, bacterial, urine; quantitative, colony count

87087   commercial kit

87088   identification, in addition to quantitative or commercial kit

87101 Culture, fungi, isolation (with or without presumptive identification); skin

87102   other source (except blood)

87103   blood

87106 Culture, fungi, definitive identification of each fungus (use in addition to codes 87101, 87102, or 87103 when appropriate)

87109 Culture, mycoplasma, any source

87110 Culture, chlamydia

87116 Culture, tubercle or other acid-fast bacilli (eg, TB, AFB, mycobacteria); any source, isolation only

87117 concentration plus isolation

87118 Culture, mycobacteria, definitive identification of each organism

87140 Culture, typing; fluorescent method, each antiserum

87143 gas liquid chromatography (GLC) method

87145 phage method

87147 serologic method, agglutination grouping, per antiserum

87151 serologic method, speciation

87155 precipitin method, grouping, per antiserum

87158 other methods

87163 Culture, any source, additional identification methods required (use in addition to primary culture code)

87164 Dark field examination, any source (eg, penile, vaginal, oral, skin); includes specimen collection

87166 without collection

(87173 has been deleted)

87174 Endotoxin, bacterial (pyrogens); chemical

87175 biological assay (eg, Limulus lysate)

87176 homogenization, tissue, for culture

87177 Ova and parasites, direct smears, concentration and identification

(Individual smears and procedures, see 87015, 87208-87211)

(Trichrome, iron hemotoxylin and other special stains, see 88312)

87178 Microbial identification, nucleic acid probes, each probe used;

(For nucleic acid probes in cytologic material, use 88365)

87179 with amplification, eg, polymerase chain reaction (PCR)

(For molecular diagnostics, see 83890-83898)

87181 Sensitivity studies, antibiotic; agar diffusion method, per antibiotic

87184 disk method, per plate (12 or less disks)

87186 microtiter, minimum inhibitory concentration (MIC), any number of antibiotics

87187 minimum bactericidal concentration (MBC) (use in addition to 87186 or 87188)

87188 macrotube dilution method, each antibiotic

87190 tubercle bacillus (TB, AFB), each drug

87192 fungi, each drug

87197 Serum bactericidal titer (Schlicter test)

87205 Smear, primary source, with interpretation; routine stain for bacteria, fungi, or cell types

87206 fluorescent and/or acid fast stain for bacteria, fungi, or cell types

87207 special stain for inclusion bodies or intracellular parasites (eg, malaria, kala azar, herpes)

87208 direct or concentrated, dry, for ova and parasites

(For concentration, see 87015; complete examination, see 87177)

(For complex special stains, see 88312, 88313)

(For fat, meat, fibers, nasal eosinophils, and starch, see miscellaneous section)

87210 wet mount with simple stain, for bacteria, fungi, ova, and/or parasites

87211 wet and dry mount, for ova and parasites

87220 Tissue examination for fungi (eg, KOH slide)

87230 Toxin or antitoxin assay, tissue culture (eg, Clostridium difficile toxin)

87250 Virus identification; inoculation of embryonated eggs, or small animal, includes observation and dissection

87252 tissue culture inoculation and observation

87253 tissue culture, additional studies (eg, hemabsorption, neutralization) each isolate

(Electron microscopy, see 88348)

(Inclusion bodies in tissue sections, see 88304-88309; in smears, see 87207-87210; in fluids, see 88106)

(87300 has been deleted. To report, use 87999)

87999 Unlisted microbiology procedure

Anatomic Pathology

Postmortem Examination

Procedures 88000 through 88099 represent physician services only. Use modifier '-90' or 09990 for outside laboratory services.

88000 Necropsy (autopsy), gross examination only; without CNS

88005 with brain

88007 with brain and spinal cord

88012 infant with brain

88014 stillborn or newborn with brain

88016 macerated stillborn

88020 Necropsy (autopsy), gross and microscopic; without CNS

88025 with brain

88027 with brain and spinal cord

88028 infant with brain

88029 stillborn or newborn with brain

88036 Necropsy (autopsy), limited, gross and/or microscopic; regional

88037 single organ

88040 Necropsy (autopsy); forensic examination

88045 coroner's call

88099 Unlisted necropsy (autopsy) procedure

Cytopathology

88104 Cytopathology, fluids, washings or brushings, except cervical or vaginal; smears with interpretation

88106 filter method only with interpretation

88107 smears and filter preparation with interpretation

88108 concentration technique, smears and interpretation (eg, Saccomanno technique)

(88109 has been deleted. For interpretation of smear, use 88104; for cell block interpretation, see 88305)

(For cervical or vaginal smears, see 88150-88156)

(For gastric intubation with lavage, see 89130-89141, 91055)

(For x-ray localization, see 74340)

88125 Cytopathology, forensic (eg, sperm)

88130 Sex chromatin identification; Barr bodies

88140 peripheral blood smear, polymorphonuclear "drumsticks"

(For Guard stain, see 88313)

88150 Cytopathology, smears, cervical or vaginal, up to three smears; screening by technician under physician supervision

88151 requiring interpretation by physician

88155 with definitive hormonal evaluation (eg, maturation index, karyopyknotic index, estrogenic index)

88156 Cytopathology, smears, cervical or vaginal, (the Bethesda System (TBS)), up to three smears; screening by technician under physician supervision

88157 requiring interpretation by physician

88160 Cytopathology, smears, any other source; screening and interpretation

88161 preparation, screening and interpretation

88162 extended study involving over 5 slides and/or multiple stains

(For obtaining specimen, see percutaneous needle biopsy under individual organ in **Surgery**)

(For aerosol collection of sputum, see 89350)

(For special stains, see 88312-88314)

88170 Fine needle aspiration with or without preparation of smears; superficial tissue (eg, thyroid, breast, prostate)

(For percutaneous needle biopsy, see 60100 for thyroid, 19100 for breast, 55700 for prostate)

88171 deep tissue under radiologic guidance

(For radiological supervision and interpretation, see 76003, 76360, 76942)

(For percutaneous needle biopsy, see 32405 for lung, 47000, 47001 for liver, 48102 for pancreas, 49180 for abdominal or retroperitoneal mass)

88172 Evaluation of fine needle aspirate with or without preparation of smears; immediate cytohistologic study to determine adequacy of specimen(s)

88173 interpretation and report

88180 Flow cytometry; each cell surface marker

88182 cell cycle or DNA analysis

(For tumor morphometry and DNA and ploidy analysis by imaging techniques, use 88358)

88199 Unlisted cytopathology procedure

(For electron microscopy, see 88348, 88349)

Cytogenetic Studies

(For acetylcholinesterase, see 82013)

(For alpha-fetoprotein, serum or amniotic fluid, see 82105, 82106)

88230 Tissue culture for chromosome analysis; lymphocyte

88233 skin or other solid tissue biopsy

88235 amniotic fluid or chorionic villus cells

88237 bone marrow (myeloid) cells

88239 other tissue

88245 Chromosome analysis for breakage syndromes; score 25 cells (SCE study), count 5 cells, 1 karyotype, with banding (eg, Bloom syndrome)

88248 score 100 cells, count 20 cells, 2 karyotypes, with banding (eg, ataxia telangiectasia, Fanconi anemia)

88250 Chromosome analysis for fragile X associated with fragile X-linked mental retardation, score 100 cells, count 20 cells, 2 karyotypes, with banding

88260 Chromosome analysis; count 5 cells, screening, with banding

88261 count 5 cells, 1 karyotype, with banding

88262 count 15-20 cells, 2 karyotypes, with banding

88263 count 45 cells for mosaicism, 2 karyotypes, with banding

(88265 has been deleted. To report, use 88262)

88267 Chromosome analysis, amniotic fluid or chorionic villus, count 15 cells, 1 karyotype, with banding

(88268 has been deleted. To report, see 88261)

88269 Chromosome analysis, in situ for amniotic fluid cells, count cells from 6-12 colonies, 1 karyotype, with banding

(88270 has been deleted. To report, see 88261)

88280 Chromosome analysis; additional karyotypes, each study

88283 additional specialized banding technique (eg, NOR, C-banding)

88285 additional cells counted, each study

88289 additional high resolution study

88299 Unlisted cytogenetic study

Surgical Pathology

Services 88300 through 88309 include accession, examination, and reporting. They do not include the services designated in codes 88311 through 88365 and 88399, which are coded in addition when provided.

The unit of service for codes 88300 through 88309 is the specimen. A specimen is defined as tissue or tissues that is (are) submitted for individual and separate attention, requiring individual examination and pathologic diagnosis. Two or more such specimens from the same patient (eg, separately identified endoscopic biopsies, skin lesions, etc.) are each appropriately assigned an individual code reflective of its proper level of service.

Service code 88300 is used for any specimen that in the opinion of the examining pathologist can be accurately diagnosed without microscopic examination. Service code 88302 is used when gross and microscopic examination is performed on a specimen to confirm identification and the absence of disease. Service codes 88304 through 88309 describe all other specimens requiring gross and microscopic examination, and represent additional ascending levels of physician work. Levels 88302 through 88309 are specifically defined by the assigned specimens.

Any unlisted specimen should be assigned to the code which most closely reflects the physician work involved when compared to other specimens assigned to that code.

88300 **Level I -** Surgical pathology, gross examination only

88302 **Level II -** Surgical pathology, gross and microscopic examination

Appendix, Incidental
Fallopian Tube, Sterilization
Fingers/Toes, Amputation, Traumatic
Foreskin, Newborn
Hernia Sac, Any Location
Hydrocele Sac
Nerve
Skin, Plastic Repair
Sympathetic Ganglion
Testis, Castration
Vaginal Mucosa, Incidental
Vas Deferens, Sterilization

88304 **Level III -** Surgical pathology, gross and microscopic examination

Abortion, Induced
Abscess
Aneurysm - Arterial/Ventricular
Anus, Tag
Appendix, Other than Incidental
Artery, Atheromatous Plaque
Bartholin's Gland Cyst
Bone Fragment(s), Other than Pathologic Fracture
Bursa/Synovial Cyst
Carpal Tunnel Tissue
Cartilage, Shavings
Cholesteatoma
Colon, Colostomy Stoma
Conjunctiva - Biopsy/Pterygium
Cornea
Diverticulum - Esophagus/Small Bowel
Dupuytren's Contracture Tissue
Femoral Head, Other than Fracture
Fissure/Fistula
Foreskin, Other than Newborn
Gallbladder
Ganglion Cyst
Hematoma
Hemorrhoids
Hydatid of Morgagni
Intervertebral Disc
Joint, Loose Body
Meniscus
Mucocele, Salivary
Neuroma - Morton's/Traumatic
Pilonidal Cyst/Sinus
Polyps, Inflammatory - Nasal/Sinusoidal
Skin - Cyst/Tag/Debridement
Soft Tissue, Debridement
Soft Tissue, Lipoma
Spermatocele
Tendon/Tendon Sheath
Testicular Appendage
Thrombus or Embolus
Tonsil and/or Adenoids
Varicocele
Vas Deferens, Other than Sterilization
Vein, Varicosity

88305 **Level IV -** Surgical pathology, gross and microscopic examination

Abortion - Spontaneous/Missed
Artery, Biopsy
Bone Marrow, Biopsy
Bone Exostosis
Brain/Meninges, Other than for Tumor Resection
Breast, Biopsy
Breast, Reduction Mammoplasty

Bronchus, Biopsy
Cell Block, Any Source
Cervix, Biopsy
Colon, Biopsy
Duodenum, Biopsy
Endocervix, Curettings/Biopsy
Endometrium, Curettings/Biopsy
Esophagus, Biopsy
Extremity, Amputation, Traumatic
Fallopian Tube, Biopsy
Fallopian Tube, Ectopic Pregnancy
Femoral Head, Fracture
Fingers/Toes, Amputation, Non-traumatic
Gingiva/Oral Mucosa, Biopsy
Heart Valve
Joint, Resection
Kidney, Biopsy
Larynx, Biopsy
Leiomyoma(s), Uterine Myomectomy - without
    Uterus
Lip, Biopsy/Wedge Resection
Lung, Transbronchial Biopsy
Lymph Node, Biopsy
Muscle, Biopsy
Nasal Mucosa, Biopsy
Nasopharynx/Oropharynx, Biopsy
Nerve, Biopsy
Odontogenic/Dental Cyst
Omentum, Biopsy
Ovary with or without Tube, Non-neoplastic
Ovary, Biopsy/Wedge Resection
Parathyroid Gland
Peritoneum, Biopsy
Pituitary Tumor
Placenta, Other than Third Trimester
Pleura/Pericardium - Biopsy/Tissue
Polyp, Cervical/Endometrial
Polyp, Colorectal
Polyp, Stomach/Small Bowel
Prostate, Needle Biopsy
Prostate, TUR
Salivary Gland, Biopsy
Sinus, Paranasal Biopsy
Skin, Other than Cyst/Tag/Debridement/
    Plastic Repair
Small Intestine, Biopsy
Soft Tissue, Other than Tumor/Mass/Lipoma/
    Debridement
Spleen
Stomach, Biopsy
Synovium
Testis, Other than Tumor/Biopsy/Castration
Thyroglossal Duct/Brachial Cleft Cyst
Tongue, Biopsy
Tonsil, Biopsy
Trachea, Biopsy
Ureter, Biopsy
Urethra, Biopsy
Urinary Bladder, Biopsy

Uterus, with or without Tubes & Ovaries, for
    Prolapse
Vagina, Biopsy
Vulva/Labia, Biopsy

88307 **Level V -** Surgical pathology, gross and
microscopic examination

Adrenal, Resection
Bone - Biopsy/Curettings
Bone Fragment(s), Pathologic Fracture
Brain, Biopsy
Brain/Meninges, Tumor Resection
Breast, Mastectomy - Partial/Simple
Cervix, Conization
Colon, Segmental Resection, Other than for
    Tumor
Extremity, Amputation, Non-traumatic
Eye, Enucleation
Kidney, Partial/Total Nephrectomy
Larynx, Partial/Total Resection
Liver, Biopsy - Needle/Wedge
Liver, Partial Resection
Lung, Wedge Biopsy
Lymph Nodes, Regional Resection
Mediastinum, Mass
Myocardium, Biopsy
Odontogenic Tumor
Ovary with or without Tube, Neoplastic
Pancreas, Biopsy
Placenta, Third Trimester
Prostate, Except Radical Resection
Salivary Gland
Small Intestine, Resection, Other than for
    Tumor
Soft Tissue Mass (except Lipoma) - Biopsy/
    Simple Excision
Stomach - Subtotal/Total Resection, Other
    than for Tumor
Testis, Biopsy
Thymus, Tumor
Thyroid, Total/Lobe
Ureter, Resection
Urinary Bladder, TUR
Uterus, with or without Tubes & Ovaries,
    Other than Neoplastic/Prolapse

88309 **Level VI -** Surgical pathology, gross and
microscopic examination

Bone Resection
Breast, Mastectomy - with Regional Lymph
    Nodes
Colon, Segmental Resection for Tumor
Colon, Total Resection
Esophagus, Partial/Total Resection
Extremity, Disarticulation
Fetus, with Dissection
Larynx, Partial/Total Resection - with Regional
    Lymph Nodes

Lung - Total/Lobe/Segment Resection
Pancreas, Total/Subtotal Resection
Prostate, Radical Resection
Small Intestine, Resection for Tumor
Soft Tissue Tumor, Extensive Resection
Stomach - Subtotal/Total Resection for Tumor
Testis, Tumor
Tongue/Tonsil - Resection for Tumor
Urinary Bladder, Partial/Total Resection
Uterus, with or without Tubes & Ovaries,
  Neoplastic
Vulva, Total/Subtotal Resection

(For fine needle aspiration, preparation, and interpretation of smears, see 88170-88173)

88311 Decalcification procedure (List separately in addition to code for surgical pathology examination)

88312 Special stains (List separately in addition to code for surgical pathology examination); Group I for microorganisms (eg, Gridley, acid fast, methenamine silver), each

88313 Group II, all other, (eg, iron, trichrome), except immunocytochemistry and immunoperoxidase stains, each

(For immunocytochemistry and immunoperoxidase tissue studies, use 88342)

88314 histochemical staining with frozen section(s)

(88316 has been deleted. To report, use 99070)

(88317 has been deleted)

88318 Determinative histochemistry to identify chemical components (eg, copper, zinc)

88319 Determinative histochemistry or cytochemistry to identify enzyme constituents, each

88321 Consultation and report on referred slides prepared elsewhere

88323 Consultation and report on referred material requiring preparation of slides

88325 Consultation, comprehensive, with review of records and specimens, with report on referred material

88329 Pathology consultation during surgery;

88331 with frozen section(s), single specimen

88332 each additional tissue block with frozen section(s)

88342 Immunocytochemistry (including tissue immunoperoxidase), each antibody

(88345 has been deleted. To report, use 88346)

88346 Immunofluorescent study, each antibody; direct method

88347 indirect method

88348 Electron microscopy; diagnostic

88349 scanning

88355 Morphometric analysis; skeletal muscle

88356 nerve

88358 tumor

When semi-thin plastic-embedded sections are performed in conjunction with morphometric analysis, only the morphometric analysis should be coded; if performed as an independent procedure, see codes 88300-88309 for surgical pathology.

(88360 has been deleted. To report, use 88399)

88362 Nerve teasing preparations

(For physician interpretation of peripheral blood smear, use 85060)

88365 Tissue in situ hybridization, interpretation and report

(88370 has been deleted. To report, use 88342)

88371 Protein analysis of tissue by Western Blot, with interpretation and report;

88372 immunological probe for band identification, each

88399 Unlisted surgical pathology procedure

Other Procedures

(Basal metabolic rate has been deleted. If necessary to report, use 89399)

(89005-89007 have been deleted)

89050   Cell count, miscellaneous body fluids (eg, CSF, joint fluid), except blood;

89051   with differential count

89060   Crystal identification by light microscopy with or without polarizing lens analysis, any body fluid (except urine)

(89070, 89080 have been deleted)

89100   Duodenal intubation and aspiration; single specimen (eg, simple bile study or afferent loop culture) plus appropriate test procedure

89105   collection of multiple fractional specimens with pancreatic or gallbladder stimulation, single or double lumen tube

(For radiological localization, see 74340)

(For chemical analyses, see Chemistry)

(Electrocardiogram, see 93000-93268)

(Esophagus acid perfusion test (Bernstein), see 91030)

89125   Fat stain, feces, urine, or sputum

89130   Gastric intubation and aspiration, diagnostic, each specimen, for chemical analyses or cytopathology;

89132   after stimulation

89135   Gastric intubation, aspiration, and fractional collections (eg, gastric secretory study); one hour

89136   two hours

89140   two hours including gastric stimulation (eg, histalog, pentagastrin)

89141   three hours, including gastric stimulation

(For gastric lavage, therapeutic, see 91105)

(For radiologic localization of gastric tube, see 74340)

(For chemical analyses, see 82926, 82928)

(Joint fluid chemistry, see Chemistry, this section)

89160   Meat fibers, feces

(89180 has been deleted. To report, use 89190)

89190   Nasal smear for eosinophils

(89205 has been deleted. To report, use 82273)

(Occult blood, feces, see 82270)

(Paternity tests, see 86910)

(89210 has been deleted)

● **89250**   Culture and fertilization of oocyte(s)

89300   Semen analysis; presence and/or motility of sperm including Huhner test

89310   motility and count

89320   complete (volume, count, motility and differential)

(Skin tests, see 86485-86585 and 95010-95199)

(89323 has been deleted. To report, use 89325)

89325   Sperm antibodies

(For medicolegal identification of sperm, see 88125)

89329   Sperm evaluation; hamster penetration test

89330   cervical mucus penetration test, with or without spinnbarkeit test

(89345 has been deleted)

89350   Sputum, obtaining specimen, aerosol induced technique (separate procedure)

89355   Starch granules, feces

89360   Sweat collection by iontophoresis

(For chloride and sodium analysis, see 84295)

89365   Water load test

89399   Unlisted miscellaneous pathology test

Notes

Medicine Guidelines

In addition to the definitions and commonly used terms presented in the **Introduction,** several other items unique to this section on **Medicine** are defined or identified here.

Multiple Procedures

It is appropriate to designate multiple procedures that are rendered on the same date by separate entries. For example: If individual medical psycho-therapy (90841) is rendered in addition to sub-sequent hospital care (eg, 99231), the psycho-therapy would be reported separately from the hospital visit. In this instance, both 99231 and 90841 would be reported.

Separate Procedures

Some of the listed procedures are commonly car-ried out as an integral part of a total service, and as such, do not warrant a separate identification. When, however, such a procedure is performed independently of, and is not immediately related to, other services, it may be listed as a "separate procedure." Thus, when a procedure that is ordi-narily a component of a larger procedure is per-formed alone for a specific purpose, it may be reported as a separate procedure.

Subsection Information

Several of the subheadings or subsections have special instructions unique to that section. These special instructions will be presented preceding those procedural terminology listings, referring to that subsection specifically. If there is an "Unlisted Procedure" code number (see section below) for the individual subsection, it will also be shown. Those subsections within the **Medicine** section that have special instructions are as follows:

Immunization Injections 90700-90749
Therapeutic or
    Diagnostic Infusions 90780-90781

Psychiatry 90801-90899
Dialysis......................... 90918-90999
Ophthalmology 92002-92499
Otorhinolaryngology 92502-92599
Non-Invasive Vascular
    Diagnostic Studies........... 93875-93990
Pulmonary 94010-94799
Allergy and
    Clinical Immunology........ 95004-95199
Neurology and Neuromuscular . 95805-95999
Central Nervous System
    Assessments/Tests 96100-96117
Chemotherapy Administration . 96400-96549
Dermatological Procedures..... 96900-96999
Special Services & Reports 99000-99199

Unlisted Service or Procedure

A service or procedure may be provided that is not listed in this edition of *CPT.* When reporting such a service, the appropriate "Unlisted Procedure" code may be used to indicate the service, identify-ing it by "Special Report" as discussed on page 332. The "Unlisted Procedures" and accompany-ing codes for **Medicine** are as follows:

90749 Unlisted immunization procedure
90799 Unlisted therapeutic or diagnostic injection
90899 Unlisted psychiatric service or procedure
90915 Unlisted biofeedback procedure
90999 Unlisted dialysis procedure, inpatient or outpatient
91299 Unlisted diagnostic gastroenterology procedure
92499 Unlisted ophthalmological service or procedure
92599 Unlisted otorhinolaryngological service or procedure
93799 Unlisted cardiovascular service or procedure
94799 Unlisted pulmonary service or procedure
95199 Unlisted allergy/clinical immunologic service or procedure
95999 Unlisted neurological or neuromuscular diagnostic procedure
96549 Unlisted chemotherapy procedure
96999 Unlisted special dermatological service or procedure
97039 Unlisted physical medicine modality

97139   Unlisted physical medicine therapeutic
procedure
97799   Unlisted physical medicine service or
procedure
99199   Unlisted special service or report

Special Report

A service that is rarely provided, unusual, variable, or new may require a special report in determining medical appropriateness of the service. Pertinent information should include an adequate definition or description of the nature, extent, and need for the procedure; and the time, effort, and equipment necessary to provide the service. Additional items which may be included are:

- complexity of symptoms;
- final diagnosis;
- pertinent physical findings;
- diagnostic and therapeutic procedures;
- concurrent problems;
- follow-up care.

Modifiers

Listed services and procedures may be modified under certain circumstances. When applicable, the modifying circumstance should be identified by the addition of the appropriate modifier code, which may be reported in either of two ways. The modifier may be reported by a two digit number placed *after* the usual procedure number, from which it is separated by a hyphen. Or, the modifier may be reported by a separate five digit code that is used *in addition* to the procedure code. If more than one modifier is used, place the "Multiple Modifiers" code immediately after the procedure code. This indicates that one or more additional modifier codes will follow. Modifiers commonly used in **Medicine** are as follows:

-22 Unusual Procedural Services: When the service(s) provided is greater than that usually required for the listed procedure, it may be identified by adding modifier '-22' to the usual procedure number or by use of the separate five digit modifier code 09922. A report may also be appropriate.

-26 Professional Component: Certain procedures are a combination of a physician component

and a technical component. When the physician component is reported separately, the service may be identified by adding the modifier '-26' to the usual procedure number or the service may be reported by use of the five digit modifier code 09926.

-32 Mandated Services: Services related to *mandated* consultation and/or related services (eg, PRO, 3rd party payor) may be identified by adding the modifier '-32' to the basic procedure or the service may be reported by use of the five digit modifier 09932.

-51 Multiple Procedures: When multiple procedures are performed on the same day or at the same session, the major procedure or service may be reported as listed. The secondary, additional, or lesser procedure(s) or service(s) may be identified by adding the modifier '-51' to the secondary procedure or service code(s) or by use of the separate five digit modifier code 09951. This modifier may be used to report multiple medical procedures performed at the same session, as well as a combination of medical and surgical procedures, or several surgical procedures performed at the same operative session.

-52 Reduced Services: Under certain circumstances, a service or procedure is partially reduced or eliminated at the physician's election. Under these circumstances, the service provided can be identified by its usual procedure number and the addition of the modifier '-52,' signifying that the service is reduced. This provides a means of reporting reduced services without disturbing the identification of the basic service. Modifier code 09952 may be used as an alternative to modifier '-52.'

-55 Postoperative Management Only: When one physician performs the postoperative management and another physician has performed the surgical procedure, the postoperative component may be identified by adding the modifier '-55' to the usual procedure number or by use of the separate five digit modifier code 09955.

-56 Preoperative Management Only: When one physician performs the preoperative care and evaluation and another physician performs the surgical procedure, the preoperative component may be identified by adding the modifier '-56' to the usual procedure number or by use of the separate five digit modifier code 09956.

-57 Decision for Surgery. An evaluation and management service that resulted in the initial decision to perform the surgery may be identified by adding the modifier '-57' to the appropriate level of E/M service or the separate five digit modifier 09957 may be used.

-58 Staged or Related Procedure or Service by the Same Physician During the Postoperative Period: The physician may need to indicate that the performance of a procedure or service during the postoperative period was: a) planned prospectively at the time of the original procedure (staged); b) more extensive than the original procedure; or c) for therapy following a diagnostic surgical procedure. This circumstance may be reported by adding the modifier '-58' to the staged or related procedure, or the separate five digit modifier 09958 may be used. **Note:** This modifier is not used to report the treatment of a problem that requires a return to the operating room. See modifier '-78'.

-76 Repeat Procedure by Same Physician: The physician may need to indicate that a procedure or service was repeated subsequent to the original service. This circumstance may be reported by adding the modifier '-76' to the repeated service or the separate five digit modifier code 09976 may be used.

-77 Repeat Procedure by Another Physician: The physician may need to indicate that a basic procedure performed by another physician had to be repeated. This situation may be reported by adding modifier '-77' to the repeated service or the separate five digit modifier code 09977 may be used.

-78 Return to the Operating Room for a Related Procedure During the Postoperative Period: The physician may need to indicate that another procedure was performed during the postoperative period of the initial procedure. When this subsequent procedure is related to the first, and requires the use of the operating room, it may be reported by adding the modifier '-78' to the related procedure, or by using the separate five digit modifier 09978. (For repeat procedures on the same day, see '-76').

-79 Unrelated Procedure or Service by the Same Physician During the Postoperative Period: The physician may need to indicate that the performance of a procedure or service during the postoperative period was unrelated to the original procedure. This circumstance may be reported by using the modifier '-79' or by using the separate five digit modifier 09979. (For repeat procedures on the same day, see '-76').

-90 Reference (Outside) Laboratory: When laboratory procedures are performed by a party other than the treating or reporting physician, the procedure may be identified by adding the modifier '-90' to the usual procedure number or by using the separate five digit modifier code 09990.

-99 Multiple Modifiers: Under certain circumstances, two or more modifiers may be necessary to completely delineate a service. In such situations, modifier '-99' should be added to the basic procedure, and other applicable modifiers may be listed as part of the description of the service. Modifier code 09999 may be used as an alternative to modifier '-99.'

Materials Supplied by Physician

Supplies and materials provided by the physician (eg, sterile trays/drugs), over and above those usually included with the office visit or other services rendered may be listed separately. List drugs, trays, supplies, and materials provided. Identify as 99070.

(90000-90080 have been deleted. To report, see 99201-99215)

(90100-90170 have been deleted. To report, see 99341-99353)

(90200-90220 have been deleted. To report, see 99221-99223)

(90225 has been deleted. To report, use 99431)

(90240-90280 have been deleted. To report, see 99231-99233)

(90282 has been deleted. To report, see 99433)

(90292 has been deleted. To report, see 99238)

(90300-90370 have been deleted. To report, see 99301-99313)

(90400-90470 have been deleted. To report, see 99321-99333)

(90500-90580 have been deleted. To report, see 99281-99288)

(90590 has been deleted. To report, see 99288)

(90600-90630 have been deleted. To report, see 99241-99255)

(90640-90643 have been deleted. To report, see 99241-99245 or 99261-99263)

(90650-90654 have been deleted. To report, see 99271-99275)

(90699 has been deleted. To report, use 99499)

Immunization Injections

Immunizations are usually given in conjunction with a medical service.

When an immunization is the only service performed, a minimal service may be listed in addition to the injection. Immunization procedures include the supply of materials.

(For allergy testing, see 95004 et seq)

(For skin testing of bacterial, viral, fungal extracts, see 86485-86586)

(For therapeutic or diagnostic injections, see 90782-90799)

90700 Immunization, active; diphtheria, tetanus toxoids, and acellular pertussis vaccine (DTaP)

90701 diphtheria and tetanus toxoids and pertussis vaccine (DTP)

90702 diphtheria and tetanus toxoids (DT)

90703 tetanus toxoid

90704 mumps virus vaccine, live

90705 measles virus vaccine, live, attenuated

90706 rubella virus vaccine, live

90707 measles, mumps and rubella virus vaccine, live

90708 measles and rubella virus vaccine, live

90709 rubella and mumps virus vaccine, live

90710 measles, mumps, rubella, and varicella vaccine

90711 diphtheria, tetanus toxoids, and pertussis (DTP) and injectable poliomyelitis vaccine

90712 poliovirus vaccine, live, oral (any type(s))

90713 poliomyelitis vaccine

90714 typhoid vaccine

90716 varicella (chicken pox) vaccine

90717 yellow fever vaccine

90718 tetanus and diphtheria toxoids absorbed, for adult use (Td)

90719 diphtheria toxoid

90720 diphtheria, tetanus toxoids, and pertussis (DTP) and Hemophilus influenza B (HIB) vaccine

●**90721** diphtheria, tetanus toxoids, and acellular pertussis vaccine (DTaP) and Hemophilus influenza B (HIB) vaccine

90724 influenza virus vaccine

90725 cholera vaccine

90726 rabies vaccine

90727 plague vaccine

90728 BCG vaccine

90730 hepatitis A vaccine

(90731 has been deleted. To report, see 90744-90747)

90732 pneumococcal vaccine, polyvalent

90733 meningococcal polysaccharide vaccine (any group(s))

90735 encephalitis virus vaccine

90737 Hemophilus influenza B

90741 Immunization, passive; immune serum globulin, human (ISG)

90742 specific hyperimmune serum globulin (eg, hepatitis B, measles, pertussis, rabies, Rho(D), tetanus, vaccinia, varicella-zoster)

●**90744** Immunization, active, hepatitis B vaccine; newborn to 11 years

●**90745** 11-19 years

●**90746** 20 years and above

●**90747** dialysis or immunosuppressed patient, any age

90749 Unlisted immunization procedure

(90750-90754 have been deleted. To report, see 99381-99387)

(90755 has been deleted)

(90757 has been deleted. To report, use 99432)

(90760-90764 have been deleted. To report, see 99391-99397)

(90774 has been deleted. To report, use 99178)

(90778 has been deleted. To report, use 94772)

Therapeutic or Diagnostic Infusions (Excludes Chemotherapy)

These procedures encompass prolonged intravenous injections. These codes require the presence of the physician during the infusion. These codes are not to be used for intradermal, subcutaneous or intramuscular or routine IV drug injections. For these services, see 90782-90788.

These codes may not be used in addition to prolonged services codes.

90780 IV infusion for therapy/diagnosis, administered by physician or under direct supervision of physician; up to one hour

90781 each additional hour, up to eight (8) hours

Therapeutic or Diagnostic Injections

90782 Therapeutic or diagnostic injection (specify material injected); subcutaneous or intramuscular

90783 intra-arterial

90784 intravenous

(90782-90784 do not include injections for allergen immunotherapy. For allergen immunotherapy injections, see 95115-95117)

90788 Intramuscular injection of antibiotic (specify)

▲=Revised Code ●=New Code

(90790-90796 have been deleted. To report, see 96408-96414, 96420-96425, 96440, 96450, 96530, 96545, 96549)

(90798 has been deleted. To report, see 90780, 90781, 90784)

90799 Unlisted therapeutic or diagnostic injection

(For allergy immunizations, see 95004 et seq)

Psychiatry

Hospital care by the attending physician in treating a psychiatric inpatient or partial hospitalization may be initial or subsequent in nature (see 99221-99233) and may include exchanges with nursing and ancillary personnel. Hospital care services involve a variety of responsibilities unique to the medical management of inpatients, such as physician hospital orders, interpretation of laboratory or other medical diagnostic studies and observations, review of activity therapy reports, supervision of nursing and ancillary personnel, and the programming of all hospital resources for diagnosis and treatment.

When services include not only a visit to the patient, but also activity in leadership or direction of a treatment team as related to that patient, a code may be selected based upon the services provided that day.

Some patients receive hospital evaluation and management services only and others receive evaluation and management services and other procedures. If other procedures such as electroconvulsive therapy or medical psychotherapy are rendered in addition to hospital evaluation and management services, these should be listed separately (ie, hospital care service plus electroconvulsive therapy or plus medical psychotherapy if rendered).

Psychiatric care may be reported without time dimensions according to the procedure or service as are other medical or surgical procedures.

In reporting medical psychotherapy procedures, time is only one aspect and may be expressed as is customary in the local area. For example, the usual appointment length of an individual medical psychotherapy procedure may be signified by the procedure code alone. The modifier '-52' or 09952 may be used to signify a service that is reduced or less extensive than the usual procedure. The modifier '-22' or 09922 may be used to indicate a more extensive service. Thus, medical psychotherapy procedures may be reported by the procedure code alone or by the procedure code with a modifier. If appropriate and customary in the local area, codes 90841, 90842, 90843 or 90844 may be used.

Other evaluation and management services, such as office medical service or other patient encounters, may be described as listed in the section on **Evaluation and Management,** if appropriate.

General Clinical Psychiatric Diagnostic or Evaluative Interview Procedures

90801 Psychiatric diagnostic interview examination including history, mental status, or disposition (may include communication with family or other sources, ordering and medical interpretation of laboratory or other medical diagnostic studies. In certain circumstances other informants will be seen in lieu of the patient).

Consultation for psychiatric evaluation of a patient includes examination of a patient and exchange of information with primary physician and other informants such as nurses or family members, and preparation of report. These consultation services (99241-99263) are limited to initial or follow-up evaluation and do not involve psychiatric treatment. For treatment, see 99221 et seq or 90841 et seq.

Special Clinical Psychiatric Diagnostic or Evaluative Procedures

Interactive procedures (90820) are distinct forms of diagnostic procedures which predominately use physical aids and non-verbal communication to overcome barriers to therapeutic interaction between the physician and a patient who has lost, or has not yet developed either the expressive language communication skills to explain his/her symptoms and response to treatment or the receptive communication skills to understand the physician if he/she were to use ordinary adult language for communication.

90820 Interactive medical psychiatric diagnostic interview examination

90825 Psychiatric evaluation of hospital records, other psychiatric reports, psychometric and/or projective tests, and other accumulated data for medical diagnostic purposes

(90830 has been deleted. To report, use 96100)

(90831 has been deleted. To report, see 99371-99373)

Psychiatric Therapeutic Procedures

Interactive procedures (90855, 90857) are distinct medical psychotherapeutic procedures which predominantly use physical aids and non-verbal communication to overcome barriers to therapeutic interaction between the physician and a patient who has lost, or has not yet developed either the expressive language communication skills to explain his/her symptoms and response to treatment, or the receptive communication skills to understand the physician if he/she were to use ordinary adult language for communication.

90835 Narcosynthesis for psychiatric diagnostic and therapeutic purposes (eg, sodium amobarbital (Amytal) interview)

▲**90841** Individual medical psychotherapy by a physician, with continuing medical diagnostic evaluation, and drug management when indicated, including insight oriented, behavior modifying or supportive psychotherapy (face-to-face with the patient); time unspecified

90842   approximately 75 to 80 minutes

90843   approximately 20 to 30 minutes

90844   approximately 45 to 50 minutes

90845 Medical psychoanalysis

90846 Family medical psychotherapy (without the patient present)

90847 Family medical psychotherapy (conjoint psychotherapy) by a physician, with continuing medical diagnostic evaluation, and drug management when indicated

(90848 has been deleted. To report, use 90847)

90849 Multiple-family group medical psychotherapy by a physician, with continuing medical diagnostic evaluation, and drug management when indicated

90853 Group medical psychotherapy (other than of a multiple-family group) by a physician, with continuing medical diagnostic evaluation and drug management when indicated

90855 Interactive individual medical psychotherapy

90857 Interactive group medical psychotherapy

Psychiatric Somatotherapy

90862 Pharmacologic management, including prescription, use, and review of medication with no more than minimal medical psychotherapy

90870 Electroconvulsive therapy (includes necessary monitoring); single seizure

90871   multiple seizures, per day

(90872 has been deleted. To report, use 90899)

Other Psychiatric Therapy

90880 Medical hypnotherapy

90882 Environmental intervention for medical management purposes on a psychiatric patient's behalf with agencies, employers, or institutions

90887 Interpretation or explanation of results of psychiatric, other medical examinations and procedures, or other accumulated data to family or other responsible persons, or advising them how to assist patient

90889 Preparation of report of patient's psychiatric status, history, treatment, or progress (other than for legal or consultative purposes) for other physicians, agencies, or insurance carriers

Other Procedures

90899 Unlisted psychiatric service or procedure

Biofeedback

90900   Biofeedback training; by electromyogram application (eg, in tension headache, muscle spasm)

90902   in conduction disorder (eg, arrhythmia)

90904   regulation of blood pressure (eg, in essential hypertension)

90906   regulation of skin temperature or peripheral blood flow

90908   by electroencephalogram application (eg, in anxiety, insomnia)

90910   by electro-oculogram application (eg, in blepharospasm)

90911   anorectal, including EMG and/or manometry

90915   other

Dialysis

Evaluation and management services unrelated to the dialysis procedure that cannot be rendered during the dialysis session may be reported in addition to the dialysis procedure. All evaluation and management services related to the patient's end stage renal disease that are rendered on a day when dialysis is performed and all other patient care services that are rendered during the dialysis procedure are included in the dialysis procedure, 90935-90947.

End Stage Renal Disease Services

90918   End stage renal disease (ESRD) related services per full month; for patients under two years of age to include monitoring for the adequacy of nutrition, assessment of growth and development, and counseling of parents

▲**90919**   for patients between two and eleven years of age to include monitoring for the adequacy of nutrition, assessment of growth and development, and counseling of parents

▲**90920**   for patients between twelve and nineteen years of age to include monitoring for the adequacy of nutrition, assessment of growth and development, and counseling of parents

90921   for patients twenty years of age and over

▲**90922**   End stage renal disease (ESRD) related services (less than full month), per day; for patients under two years of age

●**90923**   for patients between two and eleven years of age

●**90924**   for patients between twelve and nineteen years of age

●**90925**   for patients twenty years of age and over

Hemodialysis

(For cannula declotting, see 36860, 36861)

(For prolonged physician attendance, see 99354-99360)

90935   Hemodialysis procedure with single physician evaluation

90937   Hemodialysis procedure requiring repeated evaluation(s) with or without substantial revision of dialysis prescription

(90941-90944 have been deleted. To report, see 90935-90937)

Peritoneal Dialysis

(For insertion of cannula or catheter, see 49420, 49421)

(For prolonged physician attendance, see 99354-99360)

90945   Dialysis procedure other than hemodialysis (eg, peritoneal, hemofiltration), with single physician evaluation

90947   Dialysis procedure other than hemodialysis (eg, peritoneal, hemofiltration) requiring repeated evaluations, with or without substantial revision of dialysis prescription

(90951-90958 have been deleted. To report, see 90935, 90937)

(90966-90985 have been deleted. To report, see 90945, 90947)

Miscellaneous Dialysis Procedures

(90988, 90991 and 90994 have been deleted. To report, see 90995 and 90998)

90989 Dialysis training, patient, including helper where applicable, any mode, completed course

(90990, 90992 have been deleted. To report, see 90989 and 90993)

90993 Dialysis training, patient, including helper where applicable, any mode, course not completed, per training session

(90995 has been deleted. To report, see 90918-90921)

90997 Hemoperfusion (eg, with activated charcoal or resin)

(90998 has been deleted. To report, see 90922)

90999 Unlisted dialysis procedure, inpatient or outpatient

Gastroenterology

(For duodenal intubation and aspiration, see 89100-89105)

(For gastrointestinal radiologic procedures, see 74210-74363)

(For esophagoscopy procedures, see 43200-43228; upper GI endoscopy 43234-43259; endoscopy, small bowel and stomal 44360-44393; proctosigmoidoscopy 45300-45321; sigmoidoscopy 45330-45339; colonoscopy 45355-45385; anoscopy 46600-46615)

91000 Esophageal intubation and collection of washings for cytology, including preparation of specimens (separate procedure)

91010 Esophageal motility study;

91011   with mecholyl or similar stimulant

91012   with acid perfusion studies

91020 Esophagogastric manometric studies

91030 Esophagus, acid perfusion (Bernstein) test for esophagitis

91032 Esophagus, acid reflux test, with intraluminal pH electrode for detection of gastroesophageal reflux;

91033   prolonged recording

91052 Gastric analysis test with injection of stimulant of gastric secretion (eg, histamine, insulin, pentagastrin, calcium and secretin)

(For gastric biopsy by capsule, peroral, via tube, one or more specimens, see 43600)

(For gastric laboratory procedures, see also 89130-89141)

91055 Gastric intubation, washings, and preparing slides for cytology (separate procedure)

(For gastric lavage, therapeutic, see 91105)

91060 Gastric saline load test

(For biopsy by capsule, small intestine, per oral, via tube (one or more specimens), see 44100)

91065 Breath hydrogen test (eg, for detection of lactase deficiency)

(91090 has been deleted)

91100 Intestinal bleeding tube, passage, positioning and monitoring

91105 Gastric intubation, and aspiration or lavage for treatment (eg, for ingested poisons)

(For cholangiography, see 47500, 74320)

(For abdominal paracentesis, see 49080, 49081; with instillation of medication, see 96535)

(For peritoneoscopy, see 56360; with biopsy, see 56361)

(For peritoneoscopy and guided transhepatic cholangiography, see 56362; with biopsy, see 56363)

(For splenoportography, see 38200, 75810)

91122 Anorectal manometry

91299 Unlisted diagnostic gastroenterology procedure

Ophthalmology

(For surgical procedures, see **Surgery,** Eye and Ocular Adnexa, 65091 et seq)

Definitions

Intermediate ophthalmological services describes a level of service pertaining to the evaluation of a new or existing condition complicated with a new diagnostic or management problem not necessarily relating to the primary diagnosis, including history, general medical observation, external ocular and adnexal examination and other diagnostic procedures as indicated; may include the use of mydriasis.

For example:

a. Review of history, external examination, ophthalmoscopy, biomicroscopy for an acute complicated condition (eg, iritis) not requiring comprehensive ophthalmological services.

b. Review of interval history, external examination, ophthalmoscopy, biomicroscopy and tonometry in established patient with known cataract not requiring comprehensive ophthalmological services.

Comprehensive ophthalmological services describes a level of service in which a general evaluation of the complete visual system is made. The comprehensive services constitute a single service entity but need not be performed at one session. The service includes history, general medical observation, external and ophthalmoscopic examination, gross visual fields and basic sensorimotor examination. It often includes, as indicated, biomicroscopy, examination with cycloplegia or mydriasis and tonometry. It always includes initiation of diagnostic and treatment programs as indicated.

For example:

The comprehensive services required for diagnosis and treatment of a patient with symptoms indicating possible disease of the visual system, such as glaucoma, cataract or retinal disease, or to rule out disease of the visual system, new or established patient.

Initiation of diagnostic and treatment program includes the prescription of medication, lenses and other therapy and arranging for special ophthalmological diagnostic or treatment services, consultations, laboratory procedures and radiological services as may be indicated.

Prescription of lenses may be deferred to a subsequent visit, but in any circumstance is not reported separately. ("Prescription of lenses" does not include anatomical facial measurements for or writing of laboratory specifications for spectacles. For Spectacle Services, see 92340 et seq.)

Special ophthalmological services describes services in which a special evaluation of part of the visual system is made, which goes beyond the services included under general ophthalmological services, or in which special treatment is given. Special ophthalmological services may be reported in addition to the general ophthalmological services or evaluation and management services.

For example:

Fluorescein angioscopy, quantitative visual field examination, or extended color vision examination (such as Nagel's anomaloscope) should be specifically reported as special ophthalmological services.

Medical diagnostic evaluation by the physician is an integral part of all ophthalmological services. Technical procedures (which may or may not be performed by the physician personally) are often part of the service, but should not be mistaken to constitute the service itself.

Intermediate and comprehensive ophthalmological services constitute integrated services in which medical diagnostic evaluation cannot be separated from the examining techniques used. Itemization of service components, such as slit lamp examination, keratometry, ophthalmoscopy, retinoscopy, tonometry, motor evaluation is not applicable.

General Ophthalmological Services

New Patient

A new patient is one who has not received any professional services from the physician or another physician of the same specialty who belongs to the same group practice within the past three years.

92002 Ophthalmological services: medical examination and evaluation with initiation of diagnostic and treatment program; intermediate, new patient

92004 comprehensive, new patient, one or more visits

Established Patient

An established patient is one who has received professional services from the physician or another physician of the same specialty who belongs to the same group practice within the past three years.

92012 Ophthalmological services: medical examination and evaluation, with initiation or continuation of diagnostic and treatment program; intermediate, established patient

92014 comprehensive, established patient, one or more visits

(For surgical procedures, see **Surgery,** Eye and Ocular Adnexa, 65091 et seq)

Special Ophthalmological Services

92015 Determination of refractive state

92018 Ophthalmological examination and evaluation, under general anesthesia, with or without manipulation of globe for passive range of motion or other manipulation to facilitate diagnostic examination; complete

92019 limited

▲**92020** Gonioscopy (separate procedure)

(For gonioscopy under general anesthesia, see 92018)

▲**92060** Sensorimotor examination with multiple measurements of ocular deviation (eg, restrictive or paretic muscle with diplopia) with interpretation and report (separate procedure)

92065 Orthoptic and/or pleoptic training, with continuing medical direction and evaluation

92070 Fitting of contact lens for treatment of disease, including supply of lens

▲**92081** Visual field examination, unilateral or bilateral, with interpretation and report; limited examination (eg, tangent screen, Autoplot, arc perimeter, or single stimulus level automated test, such as Octopus 3 or 7 equivalent)

92082 intermediate examination (eg, at least 2 isopters on Goldmann perimeter, or semi-quantitative, automated suprathreshold screening program, Humphrey suprathreshold automatic diagnostic test, Octopus program 33)

92083 extended examination (eg, Goldmann visual fields with at least 3 isopters plotted and static determination within the central 30°, or quantitative, automated threshold perimetry, Octopus program G-1, 32 or 42, Humphrey visual field analyzer full threshold programs 30-2, 24-2, or 30/60-2)

(Gross visual field testing (eg, confrontation testing) is a part of general ophthalmological services and is not reported separately)

▲**92100** Serial tonometry (separate procedure) with multiple measurements of intraocular pressure over an extended time period with interpretation and report, same day (eg, diurnal curve or medical treatment of acute elevation of intraocular pressure)

▲**92120** Tonography with interpretation and report, recording indentation tonometer method or perilimbal suction method

92130 Tonography with water provocation

▲**92140** Provocative tests for glaucoma, with interpretation and report, without tonography

Ophthalmoscopy

Routine ophthalmoscopy is part of general and special ophthalmologic services whenever indicated. It is a non-itemized service and is not reported separately.

▲**92225** Ophthalmoscopy, extended, with retinal drawing (eg, for retinal detachment, melanoma), with interpretation and report; initial

92226 subsequent

▲**92230** Fluorescein angioscopy with interpretation and report

▲**92235**   Fluorescein angiography (includes multiframe imaging) with interpretation and report

▲**92250**   Fundus photography with interpretation and report

92260   Ophthalmodynamometry

(For ophthalmoscopy under general anesthesia, see 92018)

Other Specialized Services

▲**92265**   Needle oculoelectromyography, one or more extraocular muscles, one or both eyes, with interpretation and report

▲**92270**   Electro-oculography with interpretation and report

▲**92275**   Electroretinography with interpretation and report

(92280 has been deleted. To report visual evoked potential testing of the central nervous system, see 95930)

(For electronystagmography for vestibular function studies, see 92541 et seq)

(For ophthalmic echography (diagnostic ultrasound), see 76511-76529)

92283   Color vision examination, extended, eg, anomaloscope or equivalent

(Color vision testing with pseudoisochromatic plates (such as HRR or Ishihara) is not reported separately. It is included in the appropriate general or ophthalmological service.)

▲**92284**   Dark adaptation examination, with interpretation and report

▲**92285**   External ocular photography with interpretation and report for documentation of medical progress (eg, close-up photography, slit lamp photography, goniophotography, stereophotography)

▲**92286**   Special anterior segment photography with interpretation and report; with specular endothelial microscopy and cell count

92287   with fluorescein angiography

Contact Lens Services

The prescription of contact lens includes specification of optical and physical characteristics (such as power, size, curvature, flexibility, gaspermeability). It is NOT a part of the general ophthalmological services.

The fitting of contact lens includes instruction and training of the wearer and incidental revision of the lens during the training period.

Follow-up of successfully fitted extended wear lenses is reported as part of a general ophthalmological service (92012 et seq).

The supply of contact lenses may be reported as part of the service of fitting. It may also be reported separately by using 92391 or 92396 and modifier '-26' or 09926 for the service of fitting without supply.

(For therapeutic or surgical use of contact lens, see 68340, 92070)

92310   Prescription of optical and physical characteristics of and fitting of contact lens, with medical supervision of adaptation; corneal lens, both eyes, except for aphakia

(For prescription and fitting of one eye, add modifier -52 or 09952)

92311   corneal lens for aphakia, one eye

92312   corneal lens for aphakia, both eyes

92313   corneoscleral lens

92314   Prescription of optical and physical characteristics of contact lens, with medical supervision of adaptation and direction of fitting by independent technician; corneal lens, both eyes except for aphakia

(For prescription and fitting of one eye, add modifier -52 or 09952)

92315   corneal lens for aphakia, one eye

92316   corneal lens for aphakia, both eyes

92317   corneoscleral lens

92325   Modification of contact lens (separate procedure), with medical supervision of adaptation

92326   Replacement of contact lens

Ocular Prosthetics, Artificial Eye

92330   Prescription, fitting, and supply of ocular prosthesis (artificial eye), with medical supervision of adaptation

(If supply is not included, use modifier -26 or 09926; to report supply separately, see 92393)

92335   Prescription of ocular prosthesis (artificial eye) and direction of fitting and supply by independent technician, with medical supervision of adaptation

Spectacle Services (Including Prosthesis for Aphakia)

Prescription of spectacles, when required, is an integral part of general ophthalmological services and is not reported separately. It includes specification of lens type (monofocal, bifocal, other), lens power, axis, prism, absorptive factor, impact resistance, and other factors.

Fitting of spectacles is a separate service; when provided by the physician, it is reported as indicated by 92340-92371. Fitting includes measurement of anatomical facial characteristics, the writing of laboratory specifications, and the final adjustment of the spectacles to the visual axes and anatomical topography. Presence of physician is not required.

Supply of materials is a separate service component; it is not part of the service of fitting spectacles.

92340   Fitting of spectacles, except for aphakia; monofocal

92341   bifocal

92342   multifocal, other than bifocal

92352   Fitting of spectacle prosthesis for aphakia; monofocal

92353   multifocal

92354   Fitting of spectacle mounted low vision aid; single element system

92355   telescopic or other compound lens system

92358   Prosthesis service for aphakia, temporary (disposable or loan, including materials)

92370   Repair and refitting spectacles; except for aphakia

92371   spectacle prosthesis for aphakia

Supply of Materials

92390   Supply of spectacles, except prosthesis for aphakia and low vision aids

92391   Supply of contact lenses, except prosthesis for aphakia

(For supply of contact lenses reported as part of the service of fitting, see 92310-92313)

(For replacement of contact lens, see 92326)

92392   Supply of low vision aids (A low vision aid is any lens or device used to aid or improve visual function in a person whose vision cannot be normalized by conventional spectacle correction. Includes reading additions up to 4D.)

92393   Supply of ocular prosthesis (artificial eye)

(For supply reported as part of the service of fitting, see 92330)

92395   Supply of permanent prosthesis for aphakia; spectacles

(For temporary spectacle correction, see 92358)

92396   contact lenses

(For supply reported as part of the service of fitting, see 92311, 92312)

(See 99070 for the supply of other materials, drugs, trays, etc.)

Other Procedures

92499   Unlisted ophthalmological service or procedure

Special Otorhinolaryngologic Services

Diagnostic or treatment procedures usually included in a comprehensive otorhinolaryngologic evaluation or office visit, are reported as an integrated medical service, using appropriate descriptors from the 99201 series. Itemization of component procedures (eg, otoscopy, rhinoscopy, tuning fork test) does not apply.

Special otorhinolaryngologic services are those diagnostic and treatment services not usually included in a comprehensive otorhinolaryngologic evaluation or office visit. These services are reported separately, using descriptors from the 92500 series.

All services include medical diagnostic evaluation. Technical procedures (which may or may not be performed by the physician personally) are often part of the service, but should not be mistaken to constitute the service itself.

(For laryngoscopy with stroboscopy, use 31579)

92502 Otolaryngologic examination under general anesthesia

92504 Binocular microscopy (separate diagnostic procedure)

▲**92506** Evaluation of speech, language, voice, communication, auditory processing, and/or aural rehabilitation status

▲**92507** Treatment of speech, language, voice, communication, and/or auditory processing disorder (includes aural rehabilitation); individual

▲**92508**   group, two or more individuals

●**92510** Aural rehabilitation following cochlear implant (includes evaluation of aural rehabilitation status and hearing, therapeutic services) with or without speech processor programming

92511 Nasopharyngoscopy with endoscope (separate procedure)

92512 Nasal function studies (eg, rhinomanometry)

▲**92516** Facial nerve function studies (eg, electroneuronography)

92520 Laryngeal function studies

●**92525** Evaluation of swallowing and oral function for feeding

●**92526** Treatment of swallowing dysfunction and/or oral function for feeding

Vestibular Function Tests, With Observation and Evaluation by Physician, Without Electrical Recording

92531 Spontaneous nystagmus, including gaze

92532 Positional nystagmus

92533 Caloric vestibular test, each irrigation (binaural, bithermal stimulation constitutes four tests)

92534 Optokinetic nystagmus

Vestibular Function Tests, With Recording (eg, ENG, PENG), and Medical Diagnostic Evaluation

92541 Spontaneous nystagmus test, including gaze and fixation nystagmus, with recording

92542 Positional nystagmus test, minimum of 4 positions, with recording

92543 Caloric vestibular test, each irrigation (binaural, bithermal stimulation constitutes four tests), with recording

92544 Optokinetic nystagmus test, bidirectional, foveal or peripheral stimulation, with recording

92545 Oscillating tracking test, with recording

▲**92546** Sinusoidal vertical axis rotational testing

92547 Use of vertical electrodes in any or all of above tests counts as one additional test

(For unlisted vestibular tests, see 92599)

Audiologic Function Tests With Medical Diagnostic Evaluation

The audiometric tests listed below imply the use of calibrated electronic equipment. Other hearing tests (such as whispered voice, tuning fork) are considered part of the general otorhinolaryngologic services and are not reported separately. All descriptors refer to testing both ears. Use the modifier '-52' or 09952, if a test is applied to one ear instead of to two ears. All descriptors (except 92559) apply to testing of individuals; for testing of groups, use 92559 and specify test(s) used.

(For evaluation of speech, language and/or hearing problems through observation and assessment of performance, see 92506)

92551 Screening test, pure tone, air only

92552 Pure tone audiometry (threshold); air only

92553   air and bone

▲**92555** Speech audiometry threshold;

▲**92556**   with speech recognition

▲**92557** Comprehensive audiometry threshold evaluation and speech recognition (92553 and 92556 combined)

(For hearing aid evaluation and selection, see 92590-92595)

92559 Audiometric testing of groups

92560 Bekesy audiometry; screening

92561   diagnostic

92562 Loudness balance test, alternate binaural or monaural

92563 Tone decay test

92564 Short increment sensitivity index (SISI)

92565 Stenger test, pure tone

(92566 has been deleted. To report, use 92567)

92567 Tympanometry (impedance testing)

92568 Acoustic reflex testing

92569 Acoustic reflex decay test

92571 Filtered speech test

92572 Staggered spondaic word test

92573 Lombard test

(92574 has been deleted)

92575 Sensorineural acuity level test

92576 Synthetic sentence identification test

92577 Stenger test, speech

(92578 has been deleted)

●**92579** Visual reinforcement audiometry (VRA)

(92580 has been deleted)

(92581 has been deleted. To report, use 92585)

92582 Conditioning play audiometry

92583 Select picture audiometry

92584 Electrocochleography

▲**92585** Auditory evoked potentials for evoked response audiometry and/or testing of the central nervous system

92587 Evoked otoacoustic emissions; limited (single stimulus level, either transient or distortion products)

▲**92588**   comprehensive or diagnostic evaluation (comparison of transient and/or distortion product otoacoustic emissions at multiple levels and frequencies)

92589 Central auditory function test(s) (specify)

92590 Hearing aid examination and selection; monaural

92591   binaural

92592 Hearing aid check; monaural

92593   binaural

92594 Electroacoustic evaluation for hearing aid; monaural

92595   binaural

92596 Ear protector attenuation measurements

▲=Revised Code ●=New Code

●**92597** Evaluation for use and/or fitting of voice prosthetic or augmentative/alternative communication device to supplement oral speech

●**92598** Modification of voice prosthetic or augmentative/alternative communication device to supplement oral speech

Other Procedures

92599 Unlisted otorhinolaryngological service or procedure

Cardiovascular

Therapeutic Services

92950 Cardiopulmonary resuscitation (eg, in cardiac arrest)

(See also critical care services, 99291, 99292)

92953 Temporary transcutaneous pacing

(For physician direction of ambulance or rescue personnel outside the hospital, see 99288)

92960 Cardioversion, elective, electrical conversion of arrhythmia, external

92970 Cardioassist-method of circulatory assist; internal

92971 external

(For balloon atrial-septostomy, see 92992)

(For placement of catheters for use in circulatory assist devices such as intra-aortic balloon pump, see 33970)

92975 Thrombolysis, coronary; by intracoronary infusion, including selective coronary angiography

92977 by intravenous infusion

(For thrombolysis of vessels other than coronary, see 37201, 75896)

92980 Transcatheter placement of an intracoronary stent(s), percutaneous, with or without other therapeutic intervention, any method; single vessel

92981 each additional vessel

(To report additional vessels treated by angioplasty or atherectomy only during the same session, see 92984, 92996)

92982 Percutaneous transluminal coronary balloon angioplasty; single vessel

92984 each additional vessel

(For stent placement following completion of angioplasty or atherectomy, see 92980, 92981)

92986 Percutaneous balloon valvuloplasty; aortic valve

●**92987** mitral valve

92990 pulmonary valve

92992 Atrial septectomy or septostomy; transvenous method, balloon, Rashkind type (includes cardiac catheterization)

92993 blade method (Park septostomy) (includes cardiac catheterization)

92995 Percutaneous transluminal coronary atherectomy, with or without balloon angioplasty; single vessel

92996 each additional vessel

(For stent placement following completion of angioplasty or atherectomy, see 92980, 92981)

(To report additional vessels treated by angioplasty only during the same session, see 92984)

Cardiography

(For echocardiography, see 93307-93350)

93000 Electrocardiogram, routine ECG with at least 12 leads; with interpretation and report

93005 tracing only, without interpretation and report

93010 interpretation and report only

(For ECG monitoring, see 99354-99360)

93012 Telephonic transmission of post-symptom electrocardiogram rhythm strip(s), per 30 day period of time; tracing only

93014 physician review with interpretation and report only

93015 Cardiovascular stress test using maximal or submaximal treadmill or bicycle exercise, continous electrocardiographic monitoring, and/or pharmacological stress; with physician supervision, with interpretation and report

93016 physician supervision only, without interpretation and report

93017 tracing only, without interpretation and report

93018 interpretation and report only

93024 Ergonovine provocation test

93040 Rhythm ECG, one to three leads; with interpretation and report

93041 tracing only without interpretation and report

93042 interpretation and report only

(93045 has been deleted. To report, use 93615)

93201 Phonocardiogram with or without ECG lead; with supervision during recording with interpretation and report (when equipment is supplied by the physician)

93202 tracing only, without interpretation and report (eg, when equipment is supplied by the hospital, clinic)

93204 interpretation and report

93205 Phonocardiogram with ECG lead, with indirect carotid artery and/or jugular vein tracing, and/or apex cardiogram; with interpretation and report

93208 tracing only, without interpretation and report

93209 interpretation and report only

93210 Phonocardiogram, intracardiac

93220 Vectorcardiogram (VCG), with or without ECG; with interpretation and report

93221 tracing only, without interpretation and report

93222 interpretation and report only

93224 Electrocardiographic monitoring for 24 hours by continuous original ECG waveform recording and storage, with visual superimposition scanning; includes recording, scanning analysis with report, physician review and interpretation

93225 recording (includes hook-up, recording, and disconnection)

93226 scanning analysis with report

93227 physician review and interpretation

93230 Electrocardiographic monitoring for 24 hours by continuous original ECG waveform recording and storage without superimposition scanning utilizing a device capable of producing a full miniaturized printout; includes recording, microprocessor-based analysis with report, physician review and interpretation

93231 recording (includes hook-up, recording, and disconnection)

93232 microprocessor-based analysis with report

93233 physician review and interpretation

93235 Electrocardiographic monitoring for 24 hours by continuous computerized monitoring and non-continuous recording, and real-time data analysis utilizing a device capable of producing intermittent full-sized waveform tracings, possibly patient activated; includes monitoring and real-time data analysis with report, physician review and interpretation

93236 monitoring and real-time data analysis with report

93237 physician review and interpretation

(93255 has been deleted)

(93258, 93259, 93262, 93263, 93266 have been deleted. To report, see 93224-93237)

93268 Patient demand single or multiple event recording with presymptom memory loop, per 30 day period of time; includes transmission, physician review and interpretation

(93269 has been deleted. To report, see 93268)

93270 recording (includes hook-up, recording, and disconnection)

93271 monitoring, receipt of transmissions, and analysis

93272 physician review and interpretation only

(For postsymptom recording, see 93012, 93014)

(93273-93277 have been deleted. To report, see 93224-93237)

93278 Signal-averaged electrocardiography (SAECG), with or without ECG

(For interpretation and report only, use 93278 with modifier -26)

(For unlisted cardiographic procedure, see 93799)

(93280 has been deleted. To report, see 76000)

Echocardiography

Echocardiography includes obtaining ultrasonic signals from the heart and great arteries, with two-dimensional image and/or Doppler ultrasonic signal documentation, and interpretation and report. When interpretation is performed separately use modifier '-26' or 09926.

(For fetal echocardiography, see 76825-76828)

(93300, 93305 have been deleted)

93307 Echocardiography, real-time with image documentation (2D) with or without M-mode recording; complete

93308 follow-up or limited study

(93309 has been deleted. To report, see 93307, 93308)

93312 Echocardiography, real time with image documentation (2D) (with or without M-mode recording), transesophageal; including probe placement, image acquisition, interpretation and report

93313 placement of transesophageal probe only

93314 image acquisition, interpretation and report only

93320 Doppler echocardiography, pulsed wave and/or continuous wave with spectral display; complete

93321 follow-up or limited study

93325 Doppler color flow velocity mapping (list separately in addition to code for echo-cardiography 76825, 76826, 76827, 76828, 93307, 93308, 93312, 93314, 93320, 93321)

93350 Echocardiography, real-time with image documentation (2D), with or without M-mode recording, during rest and cardiovascular stress test using maximal or submaximal treadmill, bicycle exercise and/or pharmacologically induced stress, including electrocardiographic monitoring, with interpretation and report

(When performed during exercise and/or pharmacologic stress, the appropriate stress testing code from the 93015-93018 series should be reported in addition to 93350)

Cardiac Catheterization

Cardiac catheterization is a diagnostic medical procedure which includes introduction, positioning and repositioning of catheter(s), when necessary, recording of intracardiac and intravascular pressure, obtaining blood samples for measurement of blood gases or dilution curves and cardiac output measurements (Fick or other method, with or without rest and exercise and/or studies) with or without electrode catheter placement, final evaluation and report of procedure. When selective injection procedures are performed without a preceding cardiac catheterization, these services should be reported using codes in the Vascular Injection Procedures section, 36011-36015 and 36215-36218. Modifier '-51' should not be appended to codes 93501-93556.

93501 Right heart catheterization

(For bundle of His recording, see 93600)

93503 Insertion and placement of flow directed catheter (eg, Swan-Ganz) for monitoring purposes

(For subsequent monitoring, see 99354-99360)

93505   Endomyocardial biopsy

93510   Left heart catheterization, retrograde, from the brachial artery, axillary artery or femoral artery; percutaneous

93511   by cutdown

93514   Left heart catheterization by left ventricular puncture

(93515 has been deleted. To report, use 93524)

93524   Combined transseptal and retrograde left heart catheterization

93526   Combined right heart catheterization and retrograde left heart catheterization

93527   Combined right heart catheterization and transseptal left heart catheterization through intact septum (with or without retrograde left heart catheterization)

93528   Combined right heart catheterization with left ventricular puncture (with or without retrograde left heart catheterization)

93529   Combined right heart catheterization and left heart catheterization through existing septal opening (with or without retrograde left heart catheterization)

(93535 has been deleted. To report, see 33971, 93536)

93536   Percutaneous insertion of intra-aortic balloon catheter

When injection procedures are performed in conjunction with cardiac catheterization, these services do not include introduction of catheters but do include repositioning of catheters when necessary and use of automatic power injectors. Injection procedures 93539-93545 represent separate identifiable services and may be coded in conjunction with one another when appropriate. The technical details of angiography, supervision of filming and processing, interpretation and report are not included. To report imaging supervision, interpretation and report, use code 93555 and/or 93556. Modifier -51 should not be appended to codes 93539-93556.

93539   Injection procedure during cardiac catheterization; for selective opacification of arterial conduits (eg, internal mammary), whether native or used for bypass

93540   for selective opacification of aortocoronary venous bypass grafts, one or more coronary arteries

93541   for pulmonary angiography

93542   for selective right ventricular or right atrial angiography

93543   for selective left ventricular or left atrial angiography

93544   for aortography

93545   for selective coronary angiography (injection of radiopaque material may be by hand)

(93546 has been deleted. To report, use 93510 and 93543)

(To report imaging supervision and interpretation, use 93555)

(93547 has been deleted. To report, use 93510, 93543, and 93545)

(To report imaging supervision and interpretation, use 93555 and 93556)

(93548 has been deleted. To report, see 93510, 93543, 93544, 93545)

(To report imaging supervision and interpretation, use 93555 and 93556)

(93549 has been deleted. To report, use 93526, 93527 or 93528; 93543, 93545)

(To report imaging supervision and interpretation, use 93555 and 93556)

(93550 has been deleted. To report, use 93526 or 93527 or 93528; 93540, 93543; and 93545)

(To report imaging supervision and interpretation, use 93555 and 93556)

(93551 has been deleted. To report, use 93539 or 93540)

(93552 has been deleted. To report, use 93510; 93539 or 93540; 93543 and 93545)

▲=Revised Code   ●=New Code

(To report imaging supervision and interpretation, use 93555 and 93556)

(93553 has been deleted. To report, use 93510; 93539 or 93540; 93543, 93544, 93545)

(To report imaging supervision and interpretation, use 93555 and 93556)

93555   Imaging supervision, interpretation and report for injection procedure(s) during cardiac catheterization; ventricular and/or atrial angiography

93556   pulmonary angiography, aortography, and/or selective coronary angiography including venous bypass grafts and arterial conduits (whether native or used in bypass)

Codes 93561 and 93562 are not to be used with cardiac catheterization codes.

93561   Indicator dilution studies such as dye or thermal dilution, including arterial and/or venous catheterization; with cardiac output measurement (separate procedure)

93562   subsequent measurement of cardiac output

(For radioisotope method of cardiac output, see 78472, 78473, or 78481)

(93570 has been deleted. To report, use 92982)

(For unlisted cardiac catheterization procedure, see 93799)

Intracardiac Electrophysiological Procedures

93600   Bundle of His recording

93602   Intra-atrial recording

93603   Right ventricular recording

(93604, 93606 have been deleted. To report, see 93603, 93607, and 93609 as appropriate)

(93605 has been deleted. To report, use 93609)

93607   Left ventricular recording

(93608 has been deleted. To report, use 93609)

93609   Intraventricular and/or intra-atrial mapping of tachycardia site(s) with catheter manipulation to record from multiple sites to identify origin of tachycardia

93610   Intra-atrial pacing

93612   Intraventricular pacing

(93614 has been deleted)

93615   Esophageal recording of atrial electrogram with or without ventricular electrogram(s);

93616   with pacing

93618   Induction of arrhythmia by electrical pacing

(For intracardiac phonocardiogram, see 93210)

93619   Comprehensive electrophysiologic evaluation with right atrial pacing and recording, right ventricular pacing and recording, His bundle recording, including insertion and repositioning of multiple electrode catheters; without induction of arrhythmia (This code is to be used when 93600 is combined with 93602, 93603, 93610, 93612)

93620   with induction of arrhythmia (This code is to be used when 93618 is combined with 93619)

93621   with left atrial recordings from coronary sinus or left atrium, with or without pacing

93622   with left ventricular recordings, with or without pacing

93623   Programmed stimulation and pacing after intravenous drug infusion (Use this code with 93620, 93621, 93622)

93624   Electrophysiologic follow-up study with pacing and recording to test effectiveness of therapy, including induction or attempted induction of arrhythmia

(93630 has been deleted. To report, use 93631 and 33261)

93631   Intra-operative epicardial and endocardial pacing and mapping to localize the site of tachycardia or zone of slow conduction for surgical correction

93640 Electrophysiologic evaluation of cardioverter-defibrillator leads (includes defibrillation threshold testing and sensing function) at time of initial implantation or replacement;

93641 with testing of cardioverter-defibrillator pulse generator

93642 Electrophysiologic evaluation of cardioverter-defibrillator (includes defibrillation threshold evaluation, induction of arrhythmia, evaluation of sensing and pacing for arrhythmia termination, and programming or reprogramming of sensing or therapeutic parameters)

93650 Intracardiac catheter ablation of atrioventricular node function, atrioventricular conduction for creation of complete heart block, with or without temporary pacemaker placement

93651 Intracardiac catheter ablation of arrhythmogenic focus; for treatment of supraventricular tachycardia by ablation of fast or slow atrioventricular pathways, accessory atrioventricular connections or other atrial foci, singly or in combination

93652 for treatment of ventricular tachycardia

▲**93660** Evaluation of cardiovascular function with tilt table evaluation, with continuous ECG monitoring and intermittent blood pressure monitoring, with or without pharmacological intervention

Other Vascular Studies

(For arterial cannulization and recording of direct arterial pressure, see 36620)

(For radiographic injection procedures, see 36000-36299)

(For vascular cannulization for hemodialysis, see 36800-36821)

(For chemotherapy for malignant disease, see 96500-96549)

(For penile plethysmography, see 54240)

(93700 has been deleted)

(93710 has been deleted)

93720 Plethysmography, total body; with interpretation and report

93721 tracing only, without interpretation and report

93722 interpretation and report only

(For regional plethysmography, see 93875-93910)

93724 Electronic analysis of antitachycardia pacemaker system (includes electrocardiographic recording, programming of device, induction and termination of tachycardia via implanted pacemaker, and interpretation of recordings)

(93725-93730 have been deleted. To report, see 93875-93971)

93731 Electronic analysis of dual-chamber pacemaker system (includes evaluation of programmable parameters at rest and during activity where applicable, using electrocardiographic recording and interpretation of recordings at rest and during exercise, analysis of event markers and device response); without reprogramming

93732 with reprogramming

93733 Electronic analysis of dual chamber internal pacemaker system (may include rate, pulse amplitude and duration, configuration of wave form, and/or testing of sensory function of pacemaker), telephonic analysis

93734 Electronic analysis of single chamber pacemaker system (includes evaluation of programmable parameters at rest and during activity where applicable, using electrocardiographic recording and interpretation of recordings at rest and during exercise, analysis of event markers and device response); without reprogramming

93735 with reprogramming

93736 Electronic analysis of single chamber internal pacemaker system (may include rate, pulse amplitude and duration, configuration of wave form, and/or testing of sensory function of pacemaker), telephonic analysis

93737 Electronic analysis of cardioverter/defibrillator only (interrogation, evaluation of pulse generator status); without reprogramming

93738 with reprogramming

93740 Temperature gradient studies

(93750 has been deleted. To report, see 93875-93971)

93760 Thermogram; cephalic

93762   peripheral

93770 Determination of venous pressure

(For central venous cannulization and pressure measurements, see 36488-36491, 36500)

(93780, 93781 have been deleted)

93784 Ambulatory blood pressure monitoring, utilizing a system such as magnetic tape and/or computer disk, for 24 hours or longer; including recording, scanning analysis, interpretation and report

93786   recording only

93788   scanning analysis with report

93790   physician review with interpretation and report

(93791-93796 have been deleted. To report, see 93731-93736)

Other Procedures

93797 Physician services for outpatient cardiac rehabilitation; without continuous ECG monitoring (per session)

93798   with continuous ECG monitoring (per session)

93799 Unlisted cardiovascular service or procedure

Non-Invasive Vascular Diagnostic Studies

Vascular studies include patient care required to perform the studies, supervision of the studies and interpretation of study results with copies for patient records of hard copy output with analysis of all data, including bidirectional vascular flow or imaging when provided.

The use of a simple hand-held or other Doppler device that does not produce hard copy output, or that produces a record that does not permit analysis of bidirectional vascular flow, is considered to be part of the physical examination of the vascular system and is not separately reported.

Duplex scan describes an ultrasonic scanning procedure with display of both two-dimensional structure and motion with time and Doppler ultrasonic signal documentation with spectral analysis and/or color flow velocity mapping or imaging.

Cerebrovascular Arterial Studies

(93850, 93860 have been deleted. To report, see 93875-93882)

(93870 has been deleted. To report, see 93880 and 93882)

93875 Non-invasive physiologic studies of extra-cranial arteries, complete bilateral study (eg, periorbital flow direction with arterial compression, ocular pneumoplethysmography, Doppler ultrasound spectral analysis)

93880 Duplex scan of extracranial arteries; complete bilateral study

93882   unilateral or limited study

93886 Transcranial Doppler study of the intracranial arteries; complete study

93888   limited study

Extremity Arterial Studies (Including Digits)

(93890, 93910 have been deleted. To report, see 93922-93931)

(93920, 93921 have been deleted. To report, see 93922-93924)

93922 Non-invasive physiologic studies of upper or lower extremity arteries, single level, bilateral (eg, ankle/brachial indices, Doppler waveform analysis, volume plethysmography, transcutaneous oxygen tension measurement)

93923 Non-invasive physiologic studies of upper or lower extremity arteries, multiple levels or with provocative functional maneuvers, complete bilateral study (eg, segmental blood pressure measurements, segmental Doppler waveform analysis, segmental volume plethysmography, segmental transcutaneous oxygen tension measurements, measurements with postural provocative tests, measurements with reactive hyperemia)

93924 Non-invasive physiologic studies of lower extremity arteries, at rest and following treadmill stress testing, complete bilateral study

93925 Duplex scan of lower extremity arteries or arterial bypass grafts; complete bilateral study

93926 unilateral or limited study

93930 Duplex scan of upper extremity arteries or arterial bypass grafts; complete bilateral study

93931 unilateral or limited study

Extremity Venous Studies (Including Digits)

(93950, 93960 have been deleted. To report, see 93965-93971)

93965 Non-invasive physiologic studies of extremity veins, complete bilateral study (eg, Doppler waveform analysis with responses to compression and other maneuvers, phlebo-rheography, impedance plethysmography)

93970 Duplex scan of extremity veins including responses to compression and other maneuvers; complete bilateral study

93971 unilateral or limited study

Visceral and Penile Vascular Studies

93975 Duplex scan of arterial inflow and venous outflow of abdominal, pelvic, and/or retroperitoneal organs; complete study

93976 limited study

93978 Duplex scan of aorta, inferior vena cava, iliac vasculature, or bypass grafts; complete study

93979 unilateral or limited study

93980 Duplex scan of arterial inflow and venous outflow of penile vessels; complete study

93981 follow-up or limited study

Extremity Arterial-Venous Studies

93990 Duplex scan of hemodialysis access (including arterial inflow, body of access and venous outflow)

Pulmonary

Items 94010-94799 include laboratory procedure(s) and interpretation of test results. If a separate identifiable Evaluation and Management service is performed, the appropriate E/M service code should be reported in addition to 94010-94799.

94010 Spirometry, including graphic record, total and timed vital capacity, expiratory flow rate measurement(s), and/or maximal voluntary ventilation

94060 Bronchospasm evaluation: spirometry as in 94010, before and after bronchodilator (aerosol or parenteral) or exercise

94070 Prolonged postexposure evaluation of bronchospasm with multiple spirometric determinations after test dose of bronchodilator (aerosol only) antigen, exercise, cold air, methocholine or other chemical agent, with spirometry as in 94010

94150 Vital capacity, total (separate procedure)

94160 Vital capacity screening tests: total capacity, with timed forced expiratory volume (state duration), and peak flow rate

94200 Maximum breathing capacity, maximal voluntary ventilation

94240 Functional residual capacity or residual volume: helium method, nitrogen open circuit method, or other method

94250 Expired gas collection, quantitative, single procedure (separate procedure)

94260 Thoracic gas volume

(For plethysmography, see 93720-93722)

94350 Determination of maldistribution of inspired gas: multiple breath nitrogen washout curve including alveolar nitrogen or helium equilibration time

94360 Determination of resistance to airflow, oscillatory or plethysmographic methods

94370 Determination of airway closing volume, single breath tests

94375 Respiratory flow volume loop

94400 Breathing response to CO_2 (CO_2 response curve)

94450 Breathing response to hypoxia (hypoxia response curve)

94620 Pulmonary stress testing, simple or complex

94640 Nonpressurized inhalation treatment for acute airway obstruction

94642 Aerosol inhalation of pentamidine for pneumocystis carinii pneumonia treatment or prophylaxis

94650 Intermittent positive pressure breathing (IPPB) treatment, air or oxygen, with or without nebulized medication; initial demonstration and/or evaluation

94651 subsequent

94652 newborn infants

94656 Ventilation assist and management, initiation of pressure or volume preset ventilators for assisted or controlled breathing; first day

94657 subsequent days

94660 Continuous positive airway pressure ventilation (CPAP), initiation and management

94662 Continuous negative pressure ventilation (CNP), initiation and management

94664 Aerosol or vapor inhalations for sputum mobilization, bronchodilation, or sputum induction for diagnostic purposes; initial demonstration and/or evaluation

94665 subsequent

94667 Manipulation chest wall, such as cupping, percussing, and vibration to facilitate lung function; initial demonstration and/or evaluation

94668 subsequent

94680 Oxygen uptake, expired gas analysis; rest and exercise, direct, simple

94681 including CO_2 output, percentage oxygen extracted

94690 rest, indirect (separate procedure)

(94700, 94705, 94710 have been deleted. For analysis of arterial blood gas results, see appropriate Evaluation and Management code. For test procedure, see 82800-82817)

(For single arterial puncture, see 36600)

(94715 has been deleted. To report, use 82820)

94720 Carbon monoxide diffusing capacity, any method

94725 Membrane diffusion capacity

94750 Pulmonary compliance study, any method

94760 Noninvasive ear or pulse oximetry for oxygen saturation; single determination

(For blood gases, see 82803-82810)

94761 multiple determinations (eg, during exercise)

94762 by continuous overnight monitoring (separate procedure)

94770 Carbon dioxide, expired gas determination by infrared analyzer

(For bronchoscopy, see 31622-31659)

(For placement of flow directed catheter, see 93503)

(For venipuncture, see 36410)

(For central venous catheter placement, see 36488-36491)

(For arterial puncture, see 36600)

(For arterial catheterization, see 36620)

(For thoracentesis, see 32000)

(For phlebotomy, therapeutic, see 99195)

(For lung biopsy, needle, see 32405)

(For intubation, orotracheal or nasotracheal, see 31500)

94772 Circadian respiratory pattern recording (pediatric pneumogram), 12 to 24 hour continuous recording, infant

(Separate procedure codes for electro-myograms, EEG, ECG, and recordings of respiration are excluded when 94772 is reported.)

94799 Unlisted pulmonary service or procedure

Allergy and Clinical Immunology

Definitions

Allergy sensitivity tests describe the performance and evaluation of selective cutaneous and mucous membrane tests in correlation with the history, physical examination, and other observations of the patient. The number of tests performed should be judicious and dependent upon the history, physical findings, and clinical judgment. All patients should not necessarily receive the same tests nor the same number of sensitivity tests.

Immunotherapy (desensitization, hyposensitization) is the parenteral administration of allergenic extracts as antigens at periodic intervals, usually on an increasing dosage scale to a dosage which is maintained as maintenance therapy. Indications for immunotherapy are determined by appropriate diagnostic procedures coordinated with clinical judgment and knowledge of the natural history of allergic diseases.

Other therapy: for medical conferences on the use of mechanical and electronic devices (precipitators, air conditioners, air filters, humidifiers, dehumidifiers), climatotherapy, physical therapy, occupational and recreational therapy, see **Evaluation and Management** section.

Allergy Testing

(95000-95003 have been deleted. To report, use 95004)

95004 Percutaneous tests (scratch, puncture, prick) with allergenic extracts, immediate type reaction, specify number of tests

(95005-95007 have been deleted. To report, use 95010)

95010 Percutaneous tests (scratch, puncture, prick) sequential and incremental, with drugs, biologicals or venoms, immediate type reaction, specify number of tests

(95011 has been deleted. To report, use 95010)

(95014 has been deleted. To report, use 95015)

95015 Intracutaneous (intradermal) tests, sequential and incremental, with drugs, biologicals, or venoms, immediate type reaction, specify number of tests

(95016-95018 have been deleted. To report, use 95015)

(95020-95023 have been deleted. To report, use 95024)

95024 Intracutaneous (intradermal) tests with allergenic extracts, immediate type reaction, specify number of tests

95027 Skin end point titration

95028 Intracutaneous (intradermal) tests with allergenic extracts, delayed type reaction, including reading, specify number of tests

(95030-95034 have been deleted. To report, use 95028)

(95040-95043 have been deleted. To report, use 95044)

95044 Patch or application test(s) (specify number of tests)

(95050, 95051 have been deleted. To report, use 95052)

95052 Photo patch test(s) (specify number of tests)

95056 Photo tests

95060 Ophthalmic mucous membrane tests

95065 Direct nasal mucous membrane test

95070 Inhalation bronchial challenge testing (not including necessary pulmonary function tests); with histamine, methacholine, or similar compounds

95071   with antigens or gases, specify

(For pulmonary function tests, see 94060, 94070)

95075   Ingestion challenge test (sequential and incremental ingestion of test items, eg, food, drug or other substance such as metabisulfite)

(95077 has been deleted)

95078   Provocative testing (eg, Rinkel test)

(95080-95082 have been deleted)

(For allergy laboratory tests, see 86000-86999)

(For intravenous therapy for severe or intractable allergic disease, see 90780, 90781, 90784)

(95105 has been deleted. To report, see appropriate E/M codes(s))

Allergen Immunotherapy

Codes 95115-95199 include the professional services necessary for allergen immunotherapy. Office visit codes may be used in addition to allergen immunotherapy if, and only if, other identifiable services are provided at that time.

95115   Professional services for allergen immunotherapy not including provision of allergenic extracts; single injection

▲**95117**   two or more injections

95120   Professional services for allergen immunotherapy in prescribing physician's office or institution, including provision of allergenic extract; single injection

▲**95125**   two or more injections

95130   single stinging insect venom

95131   two stinging insect venoms

95132   three stinging insect venoms

95133   four stinging insect venoms

95134   five stinging insect venoms

(95135 has been deleted. To report, use 95144)

(95140 has been deleted. To report, use 95144)

95144   Professional services for the supervision and provision of antigens for allergen immunotherapy, single or multiple antigens, single dose vials (specify number of vials)

▲**95145**   Professional services for the supervision and provision of antigens for allergen immunotherapy (specify number of doses); single stinging insect venom

▲**95146**   two single stinging insect venoms

▲**95147**   three single stinging insect venoms

▲**95148**   four single stinging insect venoms

▲**95149**   five single stinging insect venoms

(95150, 95155 have been deleted. To report, use 95165)

(95160 has been deleted. To report, see 95145-95149)

▲**95165**   Professional services for the supervision and provision of antigens for allergen immunotherapy; single or multiple antigens (specify number of doses)

95170   whole body extract of biting insect or other arthropod (specify number of doses)

95180   Rapid desensitization procedure, each hour (eg, insulin, penicillin, horse serum)

95199   Unlisted allergy/clinical immunologic service or procedure

(For skin testing of bacterial, viral, fungal extracts, see 95030-95034, 86485-86586)

(For special reports on allergy patients, see 99080)

(For testing procedures such as radio-allergosorbent testing (RAST), rat mast cell technique (RMCT), mast cell degranulation test (MCDT), lymphocytic transformation test (LTT), leukocyte histamine release (LHR), migration inhibitory factor test (MIF), transfer factor test (TFT), nitroblue tetrazolium dye test (NTD), see Immunology section in **Pathology** or use 95199)

Neurology and Neuromuscular Procedures

Neurologic services are typically consultative, and any of the levels of consultation (99241-99263) may be appropriate.

In addition, services and skills outlined under **Evaluation and Management** levels of service appropriate to neurologic illnesses should be coded similarly.

The EEG, evoked potential and sleep services (95805-95829, 95920-95925 and 95950-95962) include tracing, interpretation and report. For interpretation only, use modifier '-26' or 09926.

Sleep Testing

Sleep studies and polysomnography refer to the continuous and simultaneous monitoring and recording of various physiological and pathophysiological parameters of sleep for 6 or more hours with physician review, interpretation and report. The studies are performed to diagnose a variety of sleep disorders and to evaluate a patient's response to therapies such as nasal continuous positive airway pressure (NCPAP). Polysomnography is distinguished from sleep studies by the inclusion of sleep staging which is defined to include a 1-4 lead electroencephalogram (EEG), and electro-oculogram (EOG), and a submental electro-myogram (EMG). Additional parameters of sleep include: 1) ECG; 2) airflow; 3) ventilation and respiratory effort; 4) gas exchange by oximetry, transcutaneous monitoring, or end tidal gas analysis; 5) extremity muscle activity, motor activity-movement; 6) extended EEG monitoring; 7) penile tumescence; 8) gastroesophageal reflux; 9) continuous blood pressure monitoring; 10) snoring; 11) body positions; etc.

For a study to be reported as polysomnography, sleep must be recorded and staged.

(Report with a -52 modifier if less than 6 hours of recording or in other cases of reduced services as appropriate)

(For unattended sleep study/polysomnography, use 94799)

95805 Multiple sleep latency testing (MSLT), recording, analysis and interpretation of physiological measurements of sleep during multiple nap opportunities

95807 Sleep study, 3 or more parameters of sleep other than sleep staging, attended by a technologist

95808 Polysomnography; sleep staging with 1-3 additional parameters of sleep, attended by a technologist

95810 sleep staging with 4 or more additional parameters of sleep, attended by a technologist

95812 Electroencephalogram (EEG) extended monitoring; up to one hour

95813 greater than one hour

95816 Electroencephalogram (EEG) including recording awake and drowsy, with hyperventilation and/or photic stimulation

(For extended EEG monitoring, see 95812, 95813)

(95817 has been deleted. To report, use 95816)

95819 Electroencephalogram (EEG) including recording awake and asleep, with hyperventilation and/or photic stimulation

(For extended EEG monitoring, see 95812, 95813)

(For digital analysis of EEG, see 95957)

(95821 has been deleted. To report, use 95819)

95822 Electroencephalogram (EEG); sleep only

(For extended EEG monitoring, see 95812, 95813)

(95823 has been deleted. To report, use 95954)

95824 cerebral death evaluation only

(95826 has been deleted. To report, use 95829, 95951 or 95956)

95827 all night sleep only

(For ambulatory 24 hour EEG monitoring, see 95950)

(For EEG during nonintracranial surgery, use 95955)

(For Wada activation test, use 95958)

(95828 has been deleted. To report, see 95807-95810)

(For recording of circadian respiratory patterns of infants, see 94772)

95829 Electrocorticogram at surgery (separate procedure)

95830 Insertion by physician of sphenoidal electrodes for electroencephalographic (EEG) recording

95831 Muscle testing, manual (separate procedure); extremity (excluding hand) or trunk, with report

95832 hand (with or without comparison with normal side)

95833 total evaluation of body, excluding hands

95834 total evaluation of body, including hands

(95842 has been deleted. To report, use 95999)

95851 Range of motion measurements and report (separate procedure); each extremity (excluding hand) or each trunk section (spine)

95852 hand, with or without comparison with normal side

95857 Tensilon test for myasthenia gravis;

95858 with electromyographic recording

95860 Needle electromyography, one extremity and related paraspinal areas

95861 Needle electromyography, two extremities and related paraspinal areas

95863 Needle electromyography, three extremities and related paraspinal areas

95864 Needle electromyography, four extremities and related paraspinal areas

95867 Needle electromyography, cranial nerve supplied muscles, unilateral

95868 Needle electromyography, cranial nerve supplied muscles, bilateral

95869 Needle electromyography, limited study of specific muscles (eg, thoracic spinal muscles)

(For anal or urethral sphincter, detrusor, urethra, perineum or abdominal musculature, see 51785-51792)

(For eye muscles, see 92265)

▲**95872** Needle electromyography using single fiber electrode, with quantitative measurement of jitter, blocking and/or fiber density, any/all sites of each muscle studied

95875 Ischemic limb exercise with needle electromyography, with lactic acid determination

(95880 has been deleted. To report, see 96105)

(95881 has been deleted. To report, see 96111)

(95882 has been deleted. To report, see 96115)

(95883 has been deleted. To report, use 96117)

▲**95900** Nerve conduction, amplitude and latency/velocity study, each nerve, any/all site(s) along the nerve; motor, without F-wave study

●**95903** motor, with F-wave study

▲**95904** sensory

95920 Intraoperative neurophysiology testing, per hour

(Use code 95920 in addition to the evoked potential study performed, 92280, 92585, 95925)

▲**95925** Short-latency somatosensory evoked potential study, stimulation of any/all peripheral nerves or skin sites, recording from the central nervous system; in upper limbs

●**95926** in lower limbs

●**95927** in the trunk or head

(To report a unilateral study, use modifier -52 or 09952)

(For visual evoked potentials, see 95930)

(For brainstem evoked response recording, see 92585)

(For auditory evoked potentials, see 92585)

●**95930** Visual evoked potential (VEP) testing central nervous system, checkerboard or flash

95933 Orbicularis oculi (blink) reflex, by electrodiagnostic testing

●**95934** H-reflex, amplitude and latency study; record gastrocnemius/soleus muscle

(95935 has been deleted. To report, see 95903, 95934, 95936)

●**95936** record muscle other than gastrocnemius/ soleus muscle

(To report a bilateral study, use modifier -50 or 09950)

95937 Neuromuscular junction testing (repetitive stimulation, paired stimuli), each nerve, any one method

95950 Monitoring for identification and lateralization of cerebral seizure focus by attached electrodes; electroencephalographic (eg, 8 channel EEG) recording and interpretation, each 24 hours

95951 combined electroencephalographic (EEG) and video recording and interpretation, each 24 hours

(95952 has been deleted. To report, see 95950)

95953 Monitoring for localization of cerebral seizure focus by computerized portable 16 or more channel EEG; electroencephalographic (EEG) recording and interpretation, each 24 hours

95954 Pharmacological or physical activation requiring physician attendance during EEG recording of activation phase (eg, thiopental activation test)

(For digital analysis of EEG, see 95957)

95955 Electroencephalogram (EEG) during nonintracranial surgery (eg, carotid surgery)

95956 Monitoring for localization of cerebral seizure focus by cable or radio, 16 or more channel telemetry, electroencephalographic (EEG) recording and interpretation, each 24 hours

95957 Digital analysis of electroencephalogram (EEG) (eg, for epileptic spike analysis) (list separately in addition to code for primary procedure)

(Use 95957 only for codes 95816, 95819, or 95954)

95958 Wada activation test for hemispheric function, including electroencephalographic (EEG) monitoring

95961 Functional cortical mapping by stimulation of electrodes on brain surface, or of depth electrodes, to provoke seizures or identify vital cortex; initial hour of physician attendance

95962 each additional hour of physician attendance

95999 Unlisted neurological or neuromuscular diagnostic procedure

Central Nervous System Assessments/Tests (eg, Neuro-Cognitive, Mental Status, Speech Testing)

The following codes are used to report the services provided during testing of the cognitive function of the central nervous system. The testing of cognitive processes, visual motor responses, and abstractive abilities is accomplished by the combination of several types of testing procedures. It is expected that the administration of these tests will generate material that will be formulated into a report.

(For development of cognitive skills, see 97770)

●**96100** Psychological testing (includes psycho-diagnostic assessment of personality, psychopathology, emotionality, intellectual abilities, eg, WAIS-R, Rorschach, MMPI) with interpretation and report, per hour

---

▲=Revised Code ●=New Code

●**96105** Assessment of aphasia (includes assessment of expressive and receptive speech and language function, language comprehension, speech production ability, reading, spelling, writing, eg, by Boston Diagnostic Aphasia Examination) with interpretation and report, per hour

●**96110** Developmental testing; limited (eg, Developmental Screening Test II, Early Language Milestone Screen), with interpretation and report

●**96111** extended (includes assessment of motor, language, social, adaptive and/or cognitive functioning by standardized developmental instruments, eg, Bayley Scales of Infant Development) with interpretation and report, per hour

●**96115** Neurobehavorial status exam (clinical assessment of thinking, reasoning and judgment, eg, acquired knowledge, attention, memory, visual spatial abilities, language functions, planning) with interpretation and report, per hour

●**96117** Neuropsychological testing battery (eg, Halstead-Reitan, Luria, WAIS-R) with interpretation and report, per hour

Chemotherapy Administration

Procedures 96400-96549 are independent of the patient's visit. Either may occur independently on any date of service, or they may occur sequentially on the same day.

Preparation of chemotherapy agent(s) is included in the service for administration of the agent.

Regional (isolation) chemotherapy perfusion should be reported using the codes for arterial infusion. Placement of the intra-arterial catheter should be reported using the appropriate code from the Cardiovascular Surgery section.

Report separate codes for each parenteral method of administration employed when chemotherapy is administered by different techniques.

96400 Chemotherapy administration, subcutaneous or intramuscular, with or without local anesthesia

96405 Chemotherapy administration, intralesional; up to and including 7 lesions

96406 more than 7 lesions

96408 Chemotherapy administration, intravenous; push technique

96410 infusion technique, up to one hour

96412 infusion technique, one to 8 hours, each additional hour

96414 infusion technique, initiation of prolonged infusion (more than 8 hours), requiring the use of a portable or implantable pump

(For pump or reservoir refilling, see 96520, 96530)

96420 Chemotherapy administration, intra-arterial; push technique

96422 infusion technique, up to one hour

96423 infusion technique, one to 8 hours, each additional hour

96425 infusion technique, initiation of prolonged infusion (more than 8 hours), requiring the use of a portable or implantable pump

(For pump or reservoir refilling, see 96520, 96530)

96440 Chemotherapy administration into pleural cavity, requiring and including thoracentesis

96445 Chemotherapy administration into peritoneal cavity, requiring and including peritoneocentesis

96450 Chemotherapy administration, into CNS (eg, intrathecal), requiring and including lumbar puncture

(For intravesical (bladder) chemotherapy administration, see 51720)

(For insertion of subarachnoid catheter and reservoir for infusion of drug, see 63750, 63780; for insertion of intraventricular catheter and reservoir, see 61210, 61215)

(96500-96512 have been deleted. To report, see 96408-96414)

96520 Refilling and maintenance of portable pump

(96524, 96526 have been deleted. To report, see 96420-96425)

96530 Refilling and maintenance of implantable pump or reservoir

(Access of pump port is included in filling of implantable pump)

(96535 has been deleted. To report, see 96440, 96445)

(96540 has been deleted. To report, see 96542)

96542 Chemotherapy injection, subarachnoid or intraventricular via subcutaneous reservoir, single or multiple agents

96545 Provision of chemotherapy agent

(For radioactive isotope therapy, see 79000-79999)

96549 Unlisted chemotherapy procedure

Special Dermatological Procedures

Dermatologic services are typically consultative, and any of the five levels of consultation (99241-99263) may be appropriate.

In addition, services and skills outlined under **Evaluation and Management** levels of service appropriate to dermatologic illnesses should be coded similarly.

(For intralesional injections, see 11900, 11901)

(For Tzanck smear, use 87207)

96900 Actinotherapy (ultraviolet light)

96910 Photochemotherapy; tar and ultraviolet B (Goeckerman treatment) or petrolatum and ultraviolet B

96912 psoralens and ultraviolet A (PUVA)

96913 Photochemotherapy (Goeckerman and/or PUVA) for severe photoresponsive dermatoses requiring at least four to eight hours of care under direct supervision of the physician (includes application of medication and dressings)

96999 Unlisted special dermatological service or procedure

Physical Medicine and Rehabilitation

(97000 has been deleted. To report, use 97010-97039)

(For muscle testing, range of joint motion, electromyography, see 95831 et seq)

(For biofeedback training by EMG, see 90900)

(For transcutaneous nerve stimulation (TNS), see 64550)

Modalities

Any physical agent applied to produce therapeutic changes to biologic tissue; includes but not limited to thermal, acoustic, light, mechanical, or electric energy.

Supervised

The application of a modality that does not require direct (one on one) patient contact by the provider.

97010 Application of a modality to one or more areas; hot or cold packs

97012 traction, mechanical

97014 electrical stimulation (unattended)

97016 vasopneumatic devices

97018 paraffin bath

97020 microwave

97022 whirlpool

97024 diathermy

97026 infrared

97028   ultraviolet

Constant Attendance

The application of a modality that requires direct (one on one) patient contact by the provider.

97032   Application of a modality to one or more areas; electrical stimulation (manual), each 15 minutes

97033   iontophoresis, each 15 minutes

97034   contrast baths, each 15 minutes

97035   ultrasound, each 15 minutes

97036   Hubbard tank, each 15 minutes

97039   Unlisted modality (specify type and time if constant attendance)

Therapeutic Procedures

A manner of effecting change through the application of clinical skills and/or services that attempt to improve function.

Physician or therapist required to have direct (one on one) patient contact.

(97100 has been deleted. To report, see 97110-97139)

(97101 has been deleted. To report, see 97110-97139)

97110   Therapeutic procedure, one or more areas, each 15 minutes; therapeutic exercises to develop strength and endurance, range of motion and flexibility

97112   neuromuscular reeducation of movement, balance, coordination, kinesthetic sense, posture, and proprioception

97113   aquatic therapy with therapeutic exercises

(97114 has been deleted. To report, see 97530)

▲**97116**   gait training (includes stair climbing)

(97118 has been deleted. To report, see 97032)

(97120 has been deleted. To report, see 97033)

97122   traction, manual

97124   massage, including effleurage, petrissage and/or tapotement (stroking, compression, percussion)

(For myofascial release, see 97250)

(97126 has been deleted. To report, see 97034)

(97128 has been deleted. To report, see 97035)

97139   unlisted therapeutic procedure (specify)

(97145 has been deleted. To report, see 97110-97139)

97150   Therapeutic procedure(s), group (2 or more individuals)

(97200, 97201 have been deleted. To report, see 97010-97039, 97110-97139)

(97220, 97221 have been deleted. To report, see 97036)

(97240, 97241 have been deleted. To report, see 97036, 97113)

97250   Myofascial release/soft tissue mobilization, one or more regions

97260   Manipulation (cervical, thoracic, lumbosacral, sacroiliac, hand, wrist) (separate procedure), performed by physician; one area

97261   each additional area

(For manipulation under general anesthesia, see appropriate anatomic section in Musculoskeletal System)

(For osteopathic manipulative treatment (OMT), see 98925-98929)

97265   Joint mobilization, one or more areas (peripheral or spinal)

97500   Orthotics training (dynamic bracing, splinting), upper and/or lower extremities; initial 30 minutes, each visit

97501   each additional 15 minutes

(Codes 97500, 97501 should not be reported with 97116)

97520   Prosthetic training; initial 30 minutes, each visit

97521   each additional 15 minutes

97530   Therapeutic activities, direct (one on one) patient contact by the provider (use of dynamic activities to improve functional performance), each 15 minutes

(97531 has been deleted. To report, use 97530)

●**97535**   Self care/home management training (eg, activities of daily living (ADL) and compensatory training, meal preparation, safety procedures, and instructions in use of adaptive equipment) direct one on one contact by provider, each 15 minutes

●**97537**   Community/work reintegration training (eg, shopping, transportation, money management, avocational activities and/or work environment/modification analysis, work task analysis), direct one on one contact by provider, each 15 minutes

(97540 has been deleted. To report, see 97535, 97537)

(97541 has been deleted. To report, see 97535, 97537)

(For wheelchair management/propulsion training, use 97542)

●**97542**   Wheelchair management/propulsion training, each 15 minutes

97545   Work hardening/conditioning; initial 2 hours

97546   each additional hour

Tests and Measurements

(For muscle testing, manual or electrical, joint range of motion, electromyography or nerve velocity determination, see 95831-95904)

(97700, 97701 have been deleted. To report, use 97703)

●**97703**   Checkout for orthotic/prosthetic use, established patient, each 15 minutes

(97720, 97721 have been deleted. To report, see 97750)

(97740, 97741 have been deleted. To report, use 97530)

97750   Physical performance test or measurement (eg, musculoskeletal, functional capacity), with written report, each 15 minutes

(97752 has been deleted. To report, see 97750)

Other Procedures

97770   Development of cognitive skills to improve attention, memory, problem solving, includes compensatory training and/or sensory integrative activities, direct (one on one) patient contact by the provider, each 15 minutes

97799   Unlisted physical medicine/rehabilitation service or procedure

(98900-98902 have been deleted. To report, use appropriate category and level of Evaluation and Management codes)

(98910-98912 have been deleted. To report, see 99361-99362)

(98920-98922 have been deleted. To report, see 99371-99373)

Osteopathic Manipulative Treatment

Osteopathic manipulative treatment is a form of manual treatment applied by a physician to eliminate or alleviate somatic dysfunction and related disorders. This treatment may be accomplished by a variety of techniques.

Evaluation and management services may be reported separately if, and only if, the patient's condition requires a significant separately identifiable E/M service, above and beyond the usual preservice and postservice work associated with the procedure.

Body regions referred to are: head region; cervical region; thoracic region; lumbar region; sacral region; pelvic region; lower extremities; upper extremities; rib cage region; abdomen and viscera region.

▲=Revised Code   ●=New Code

98925 Osteopathic manipulative treatment (OMT);
one to two body regions involved

98926 three to four body regions involved

98927 five to six body regions involved

98928 seven to eight body regions involved

98929 nine to ten body regions involved

Special Services and Reports

The procedures with code numbers 99000 through 99090 provide the reporting physician with the means of identifying the completion of special reports and services that are an adjunct to the basic services rendered. The specific number assigned indicates the special circumstances under which a basic procedure is performed.

Miscellaneous Services

99000 Handling and/or conveyance of specimen for transfer from the physician's office to a laboratory

99001 Handling and/or conveyance of specimen for transfer from the patient in other than a physician's office to a laboratory (distance may be indicated)

99002 Handling, conveyance, and/or any other service in connection with the implementation of an order involving devices (eg, designing, fitting, packaging, handling, delivery or mailing) when devices such as orthotics, protectives, prosthetics are fabricated by an outside laboratory or shop but which items have been designed, and are to be fitted and adjusted by the attending physician

(For routine collection of venous blood, use 36415)

(99012, 99013, 99014, 99015 have been deleted. To report, see 99371-99373)

99024 Postoperative follow-up visit, included in global service

(As a component of a surgical "package", see **Surgery** guidelines)

99025 Initial (new patient) visit when starred (*) surgical procedure constitutes major service at that visit

99050 Services requested after office hours in addition to basic service

99052 Services requested between 10:00 PM and 8:00 AM in addition to basic service

99054 Services requested on Sundays and holidays in addition to basic service

99056 Services provided at request of patient in a location other than physician's office which are normally provided in the office

99058 Office services provided on an emergency basis

(99062, 99064, 99065 have been deleted. To report, see 99281-99285)

99070 Supplies and materials (except spectacles), provided by the physician over and above those usually included with the office visit or other services rendered (list drugs, trays, supplies, or materials provided)

(For spectacles, see 92390-92395)

99071 Educational supplies, such as books, tapes, and pamphlets, provided by the physician for the patient's education at cost to physician

99075 Medical testimony

99078 Physician educational services rendered to patients in a group setting (eg, prenatal, obesity, or diabetic instructions)

99080 Special reports such as insurance forms, more than the information conveyed in the usual medical communications or standard reporting form

99082 Unusual travel (eg, transportation and escort of patient)

99090 Analysis of information data stored in computers (eg, ECGs, blood pressures, hematologic data)

Qualifying Circumstances for Anesthesia

(For explanation of these services, see **Anesthesia** guidelines)

99100   Anesthesia for patient of extreme age, under one year and over seventy

99116   Anesthesia complicated by utilization of total body hypothermia

99135   Anesthesia complicated by utilization of controlled hypotension

99140   Anesthesia complicated by emergency conditions (specify)

    (An emergency is defined as existing when delay in treatment of the patient would lead to a significant increase in the threat to life or body part.)

    (99150, 99151 have been deleted. To report, see 99354-99360)

Other Services

99175   Ipecac or similar administration for individual emesis and continued observation until stomach adequately emptied of poison

    (For diagnostic intubation, see 82926-82928, 89130-89141)

    (For gastric lavage for diagnostic purposes, see 91055)

    (99178 has been deleted. To report, see 96110)

    (99180 has been deleted. To report, use 99183)

    (99182 has been deleted. To report, use 99183)

99183   Physician attendance and supervision of hyperbaric oxygen therapy, per session

    (Evaluation and Management services and/or procedures (eg, wound debridement) provided in a hyperbaric oxygen treatment facility in conjunction with a hyperbaric oxygen therapy session should be reported separately)

99185   Hypothermia; regional

99186   total body

99190   Assembly and operation of pump with oxygenator or heat exchanger (with or without ECG and/or pressure monitoring); each hour

99191   3/4 hour

99192   1/2 hour

99195   Phlebotomy, therapeutic (separate procedure)

99199   Unlisted special service or report

Notes

Appendix A

Modifiers

This list includes all of the modifiers applicable to *CPT 1996* codes.

-20 Microsurgery: When the surgical services are performed using the techniques of micro-surgery, requiring the use of an operating microscope, modifier '-20' may be added to the surgical procedure or the separate five digit modifier code 09920 may be used. Modifier '-20' is not to be used when a magnifying surgical loupe is used, whether attached to the eyeglasses or on a headband. A special report may be appropriate to document the necessity of the microsurgical approach.

-21 Prolonged Evaluation and Management Services: When the face-to-face or floor/unit service(s) provided is prolonged or otherwise greater than that usually required for the high-est level of evaluation and management service within a given category, it may be identified by adding modifier '-21' to the evaluation and management code number or by use of the separate five digit modifier code 09921. A report may also be appropriate.

-22 Unusual Procedural Services: When the ser-vice(s) provided is greater than that usually required for the listed procedure, it may be identified by adding modifier '-22' to the usual procedure number or by use of the separate five digit modifier code 09922. A report may also be appropriate.

-23 Unusual Anesthesia: Occasionally, a proce-dure, which usually requires either no anesthe-sia or local anesthesia, because of unusual circumstances must be done under general anesthesia. This circumstance may be reported by adding the modifier '-23' to the procedure code of the basic service or by use of the separate five digit modifier code 09923.

-24 Unrelated Evaluation and Management Service by the Same Physician During a Post-operative Period: The physician may need to indicate that an evaluation and management service was performed during a postoperative period for a reason(s) unrelated to the original procedure. This circumstance may be reported by adding the modifier '-24' to the appropriate level of E/M service, or the separate five digit modifier 09924 may be used.

-25 Significant, Separately Identifiable Evaluation and Management Service by the Same Physi-cian on the Same Day of the Procedure or Other Service: The physician may need to indicate that on the day a procedure or service identified by a CPT code was performed, the patient's condition required a significant, sepa-rately identifiable E/M service above and be-yond the other service provided or beyond the usual preoperative and postoperative care asso-ciated with the procedure that was performed. This circumstance may be reported by adding the modifier '-25' to the appropriate level of E/M service, or the separate five digit modifier 09925 may be used. **Note:** This modifier is not used to report an E/M service that resulted in a decision to perform surgery. See modifier '-57'.

-26 Professional Component: Certain procedures are a combination of a physician component and a technical component. When the physi-cian component is reported separately, the service may be identified by adding the modifi-er '-26' to the usual procedure number or the service may be reported by use of the five digit modifier code 09926.

-32 Mandated Services: Services related to *man-dated* consultation and/or related services (eg, PRO, 3rd party payor) may be identified by adding the modifier '-32' to the basic proce-dure or the service may be reported by use of the five digit modifier 09932.

-47 Anesthesia by Surgeon: Regional or general anesthesia provided by the surgeon may be reported by adding the modifier '-47' to the basic service or by use of the separate five digit modifier code 09947. (This does not include local anesthesia.) **Note:** Modifier '-47' or 09947 would not be used as a modifier for the anesthesia procedures 00100-01999.

-50 Bilateral Procedure: Unless otherwise identi-fied in the listings, bilateral procedures that are performed at the same operative session, should be identified by the appropriate five digit code describing the first procedure. The second (bilateral) procedure is identified either by adding modifier '-50' to the procedure number or by use of the separate five digit modifier code 09950.

-51 Multiple Procedures: When multiple procedures are performed on the same day or at the same session, the major procedure or service may be reported as listed. The secondary additional, or lesser procedure(s) or service(s) may be identified by adding the modifier '-51' to the secondary procedure or service code(s) or by use of the separate five digit modifier code 09951. This modifier may be used to report multiple medical procedures performed at the same session, as well as a combination of medical and surgical procedures, or several surgical procedures performed at the same operative session.

-52 Reduced Services: Under certain circumstances a service or procedure is partially reduced or eliminated at the physician's election. Under these circumstances the service provided can be identified by its usual procedure number and the addition of the modifier '-52', signifying that the service is reduced. This provides a means of reporting reduced services without disturbing the identification of the basic service. Modifier code 09952 may be used as an alternative to modifier '-52'.

-54 Surgical Care Only: When one physician performs a surgical procedure and another provides preoperative and/or postoperative management, surgical services may be identified by adding the modifier '-54' to the usual procedure number or by use of the separate five digit modifier code 09954.

-55 Postoperative Management Only: When one physician performs the postoperative management and another physician has performed the surgical procedure, the postoperative component may be identified by adding the modifier '-55' to the usual procedure number or by use of the separate five digit modifier code 09955.

-56 Preoperative Management Only: When one physician performs the preoperative care and evaluation and another physician performs the surgical procedure, the preoperative component may be identified by adding the modifier '-56' to the usual procedure number or by use of the separate five digit modifier code 09956.

-57 Decision for Surgery: An evaluation and management service that resulted in the initial decision to perform the surgery, may be identified by adding the modifier '-57' to the appropriate level of E/M service, or the separate five digit modifier 09957 may be used.

-58 Staged or Related Procedure or Service by the Same Physician During the Postoperative Period: The physician may need to indicate that the performance of a procedure or service during the postoperative period was: a) planned prospectively at the time of the original procedure (staged); b) more extensive than the original procedure; or c) for therapy following a diagnostic surgical procedure. This circumstance may be reported by adding the modifier '-58' to the staged or related procedure, or the separate five digit modifier 09958 may be used. **Note:** This modifier is not used to report the treatment of a problem that requires a return to the operating room. See modifier '-78'.

-62 Two Surgeons: Under certain circumstances the skills of two surgeons (usually with different skills) may be required in the management of a specific surgical procedure. Under such circumstances the separate services may be identified by adding the modifier '-62' to the procedure number used by each surgeon for reporting his services. Modifier code 09962 may be used as an alternative to modifier '-62'.

-66 Surgical Team: Under some circumstances, highly complex procedures (requiring the concomitant services of several physicians, often of different specialties, plus other highly skilled, specially trained personnel, various types of complex equipment) are carried out under the "surgical team" concept. Such circumstances may be identified by each participating physician with the addition of the modifier '-66' to the basic procedure number used for reporting services. Modifier code 09966 may be used as an alternative to modifier '-66'.

-76 Repeat Procedure by Same Physician: The physician may need to indicate that a procedure or service was repeated subsequent to the original service. This circumstance may be reported by adding the modifier '-76' to the repeated service or the separate five digit modifier code 09976 may be used.

-77 Repeat Procedure by Another Physician: The physician may need to indicate that a basic procedure performed by another physician had to be repeated. This situation may be reported by adding modifier '-77' to the repeated service or the separate five digit modifier code 09977 may be used.

-78 Return to the Operating Room for a Related Procedure During the Postoperative Period: The physician may need to indicate that another procedure was performed during the postoperative period of the initial procedure. When this subsequent procedure is related to the first, and requires the use of the operating room, it may be reported by adding the modifier '-78' to the related procedure, or by using the separate five digit modifier 09978. (For repeat procedures on the same day, see '-76').

-79 Unrelated Procedure or Service by the Same Physician During the Postoperative Period: The physician may need to indicate that the performance of a procedure or service during the postoperative period was unrelated to the original procedure. This circumstance may be reported by using the modifier '-79' or by using the separate five digit modifier 09979. (For repeat procedures on the same day, see '-76').

-80 Assistant Surgeon: Surgical assistant services may be identified by adding the modifier '-80' to the usual procedure number(s) or by use of the separate five digit modifier code 09980.

-81 Minimum Assistant Surgeon: Minimum surgical assistant services are identified by adding the modifier '-81' to the usual procedure number or by use of the separate five digit modifier code 09981.

-82 Assistant Surgeon (when qualified resident surgeon not available): The unavailability of a qualified resident surgeon is a prerequisite for use of modifier '-82' appended to the usual procedure code number(s) or by use of the separate five digit modifier code 09982.

-90 Reference (Outside) Laboratory: When laboratory procedures are performed by a party other than the treating or reporting physician, the procedure may be identified by adding the modifier '-90' to the usual procedure number or by use of the separate five digit modifier code 09990.

-99 Multiple Modifiers: Under certain circumstances two or more modifiers may be necessary to completely delineate a service. In such situations modifier '-99' should be added to the basic procedure, and other applicable modifiers may be listed as part of the description of the service. Modifier code 09999 may be used as an alternative to modifier '-99'.

Appendix B

Summary of Additions, Deletions and Revisions

This listing is a summary of additions, deletions and revisions applicable to *CPT 1996* codes.

Please refer to the notes, introductory paragraphs and cross-references in the main text of *CPT* for additional changes. The descriptors of the codes listed with an asterisk have not been substantially altered, but contain minor grammatical changes. These codes will not be identified in *CPT* with a ▲ symbol.

00520 Terminology revised

00540 Terminology revised

00865 Anesthesia for radical prostatectomy code added

17110 Terminology revised

20100 Wound exploration trauma code added

20101 Wound exploration trauma code added

20102 Wound exploration trauma code added

20103 Wound exploration trauma code added

*20802 Terminology revised

20804 Code deleted. To report, see specific repair codes and use modifier -52

*20805 Terminology revised

20806 Code deleted. To report, see specific repair codes and use modifier -52

*20808 Terminology revised

20812 Code deleted. To report, see specific repair codes and use modifier -52

*20816 Terminology revised

20820 Code deleted. To report, see specific repair codes and use modifier -52

*20822 Terminology revised

20823 Code deleted. To report, see specific repair codes and use modifier -52

*20824 Terminology revised

20826 Code deleted. To report, see specific repair codes and use modifier -52

*20827 Terminology revised

20828 Code deleted. To report, see specific repair codes and use modifier -52

20832 Code deleted. To report, see specific repair codes and use modifier -52

20834 Code deleted. To report, see specific repair codes and use modifier -52

*20838 Terminology revised

20840 Code deleted. To report, see specific repair codes and use modifier -52

20930 Spinal bone allograft code added

20931 Spinal bone allograft code added

20936 Spinal bone autograft code added

20937 Spinal bone autograft code added

20938 Spinal bone autograft code added

21076 Surgical obturator prosthesis code added

21077 Orbital prosthesis code added

*21079 Terminology revised

21141 Midface reconstruction without bone graft code added

21142 Midface reconstruction without bone graft code added

21143 Midface reconstruction without bone graft code added

21144 Code deleted. To report, see 21141

21145 Terminology revised

21146 Terminology revised

21147 Terminology revised

21193 Terminology revised

21195 Terminology revised

22100 Terminology revised

22103 Partial excision of vertebra, extra segment code added

22105 Code deleted. To report, see 22100

22106 Code deleted. To report, see 22101

22107 Code deleted. To report, see 22102

22110 Terminology revised

22116 Partial excision of vertebra, extra segment code added

22140 Code deleted. To report, use 63081 and 22554 and 20931 or 20938

22141 Code deleted. To report, use 63085 or 63087 and 22556 and 20931 or 20938

22142 Code deleted. To report, use 63087 or 63090 and 22558 and 20931 or 20938

22145 Code deleted. To report, use 63082 or 63086 or 63088 or 63091, and 22585

22148 Code deleted. To report, see 20931 or 20938

22150 Code deleted. To report, use 63081 and 22554 and 20931 or 20938 and 22851

22151 Code deleted. To report, use 63085 or 63087 and 22556 and 20931 or 20938 and 22851

22152 Code deleted. To report, use 63087 or 63090 and 22558, and 20931 or 20938 and 22851

22210 Terminology revised

22216 Osteotomy of spine, extra segment code added

22220 Terminology revised

22226 Osteotomy of spine, extra segment code added

22230 Code deleted. To report, use 22216 or 22226

22310 Terminology revised

22315 Terminology revised

22325 Terminology revised

22326 Terminology revised

22327 Terminology revised

22328 Vertebral fracture add-on code added

22548 Terminology revised

22554 Terminology revised

22556 Terminology revised

22558 Terminology revised

22585 Terminology revised

22590 Terminology revised

22595 Terminology revised

22600 Terminology revised

22610 Terminology revised

22612 Terminology revised

22614 Spinal arthrodesis, extra segment code added

22625 Code deleted. To report, use 22612 and 22840-22855, and 20930-20938

22630 Terminology revised

22632 Spinal arthrodesis, additional interspace code added

22650 Code deleted. To report, see 22614

22800 Terminology revised

22802 Terminology revised

22804 Posterior spinal arthrodesis code added

22808 Anterior spinal arthrodesis code added

22810 Terminology revised

22812 Terminology revised

22820 Code deleted. To report, see 20930-20938

22840 Terminology revised

22841 Internal spinal fixation code added

22842 Terminology revised

22843 Spinal instrumentation code added

22844 Spinal instrumentation code added

22845 Terminology revised

22846 Spinal instrumentation code added

22847 Spinal instrumentation code added

22848 Pelvic fixation code added

22851 Application of prosthetic device code added

27691 Terminology revised

28236 Code deleted. To report, see 27690, 27691

31579 Terminology revised

32485 Code deleted. To report, use 32501

32501 Bronchoplasty add-on code added

33253 Reconstruction of atria code added

33260 Code deleted. To report, use 33261

33261 Terminology revised

33350 Code deleted

33696 Code deleted. To report, see 33924

*33697 Terminology revised

33698 Code deleted. To report, see 33924

33924 Removal of pulmonary artery shunt with congenital heart procedure code added

38231 Stem cell collection code added

38240 Terminology revised

47350 Terminology revised

47355 Code deleted

47360 Terminology revised

47361 Hepatic wound exploration/suture code added

47362 Hepatic wound reexploration code added

55859 Insertion of needles into prostate for radiotherapy code added

56343 Laparoscopic salpingostomy code added

56344 Laparoscopic fimbrioplasty code added

57284 Paravaginal defect repair code added

58100 Terminology revised

58972 Code deleted. To report, see 89250

58974 Terminology revised

58976	Terminology revised
59610	VBAC code added
59612	VBAC code added
59614	VBAC code added
59618	VBAC code added
59620	VBAC code added
59622	VBAC code added
62274	Terminology revised
62288	Terminology revised
62350	Implant of spinal catheter for drug infusion code added
62351	Implant of spinal catheter for drug infusion code added
62355	Removal of implanted spinal catheter code added
62360	Implant of device for spinal drug infusion code added
62361	Implant of pump for spinal drug infusion code added
62362	Implant of pump for spinal drug infusion code added
62365	Removal of implanted spinal device for drug infusion code added
62367	Analysis of implanted spinal infusion pump code added
62368	Analysis of implanted spinal infusion pump code added
63750	Code deleted. To report, see 62351 and 62360, 62361 or 62362
63780	Code deleted. To report, see 62350 and 62360, 62361 or 62362
67105	Terminology revised
67107	Terminology revised
67108	Terminology revised
67109	Code deleted. To report, see 67299
67112	Terminology revised
67825	Terminology revised
76965	Ultrasonic guidance for radiotherapy code added
77295	Terminology revised
78459	Myocardial imaging, PET code added
78655	Code deleted. To report, see 78800
78810	Tumor imaging, PET code added
80019	Terminology revised
80410	Terminology revised

80416	Renin stimulation panel code added
80417	Renin stimulation panel code added
81000	Terminology revised
81001	Urinalysis code added
*81002	Terminology revised
*81003	Terminology revised
*85651	Terminology revised
85652	Erythrocyte sedimentation rate code added
86003	Terminology revised
86005	Terminology revised
89250	Culture & fertilization of oocyte(s) code added
*90711	Terminology revised
*90720	Terminology revised
90721	DTaP & HIB vaccine code added
90731	Code deleted. To report, see 90765-90768
90744	Hepatitis B vaccine code added
90745	Hepatitis B vaccine code added
90746	Hepatitis B vaccine code added
90747	Hepatitis B vaccine code added
90830	Code deleted. To report, use 96100
90841	Terminology revised
90919	Terminology revised
90920	Terminology revised
90922	Terminology revised
90923	ESRD service code added
90924	ESRD service code added
90925	ESRD service code added
92020	Terminology revised
92060	Terminology revised
92081	Terminology revised
92100	Terminology revised
92120	Terminology revised
92140	Terminology revised
92225	Terminology revised
92230	Terminology revised
92235	Terminology revised
92250	Terminology revised
92265	Terminology revised
92270	Terminology revised
92275	Terminology revised

92280 Code deleted. To report, see 95930

92284 Terminology revised

92285 Terminology revised

92286 Terminology revised

92506 Terminology revised

92507 Terminology revised

92508 Terminology revised

92510 Rehabilitation following cochlear implant code added

92516 Terminology revised

92525 Evaluation of swallowing & oral function code added

92526 Treatment of swallowing dysfunction code added

92546 Terminology revised

92555 Terminology revised

92556 Terminology revised

92557 Terminology revised

92574 Code deleted

92578 Code deleted

92579 Visual reinforcement audiometry code added

92580 Code deleted

92585 Terminology revised

92588 Terminology revised

92597 Evaluation/fitting of prosthetic communication device code added

92598 Modification of prosthetic communication device code added

92987 Percutaneous balloon mitral valvuloplasty code added

93660 Terminology revised

95117 Terminology revised

95125 Terminology revised

95145 Terminology revised

95146 Terminology revised

95147 Terminology revised

95148 Terminology revised

95149 Terminology revised

95165 Terminology revised

95872 Terminology revised

95880 Code deleted. To report, see 96105

95881 Code deleted. To report, see 96111

95882 Code deleted. To report, see 96115

95883 Code deleted. To report, use 96117

95900 Terminology revised

95903 Nerve conduction of motor function code added

95904 Terminology revised

95925 Terminology revised

95926 Somatosensory evoked potential study code added

95927 Somatosensory evoked potential study code added

95930 Visual evoked potential code added

95934 H-reflex code added

95935 Code deleted. To report, see 95903, 95934, 95936

95936 H-reflex code added

96100 Psychological testing code added

96105 Assessment of aphasia code added

96110 Developmental testing code added

96111 Developmental testing code added

96115 Neurobehavorial status exam code added

96117 Neuropsychological testing battery code added

97116 Terminology revised

97535 Self care management training code added

97537 Community reintegration training code added

97540 Code deleted. To report, see 97535, 97537

97541 Code deleted. To report, see 97535, 97537

97542 Wheelchair management training code added

97700 Code deleted. To report, use 97703

97701 Code deleted. To report, use 97703

97703 Orthotic/prosthetic checkout code added

99178 Code deleted. To report, see 96110

99238 Terminology revised

99239 Hospital discharge day management code added

99291 Terminology revised

99295 Terminology revised

99296 Terminology revised

99297 Terminology revised

99435 Newborn hospital discharge day code added

99440 Terminology revised

Appendix C

Update to Short Descriptors

This listing includes changes necessary to update the short descriptors on the *CPT 1996* data file.

The descriptors have been changed to reflect additions, revisions or deletions to the *CPT 1996* codes, or to enhance or correct the data file. The descriptors which have been enhanced, but do not necessarily reflect a change to the *CPT 1996* codes, are indicated with a asterisk.

00865	Add:	Anesth, removal of prostate
20100	Add:	Explore wound, neck
20101	Add:	Explore wound, chest
20102	Add:	Explore wound, abdomen
20103	Add:	Explore wound, extremity
20804	Delete	
20806	Delete	
20812	Delete	
20820	Delete	
20823	Delete	
20826	Delete	
20828	Delete	
20832	Delete	
20834	Delete	
20840	Delete	
20930	Add:	Spinal bone allograft
20931	Add:	Spinal bone allograft
20936	Add:	Spinal bone autograft
20937	Add:	Spinal bone autograft
20938	Add:	Spinal bone autograft
21076	Add:	Prepare face/oral prosthesis
21077	Add:	Prepare face/oral prosthesis
21141	Add:	Reconstruct midface, LeFort
21142	Add:	Reconstruct midface, LeFort
21143	Add:	Reconstruct midface, LeFort
21144	Delete	

22103	Add:	Remove extra spine segment
22105	Delete	
22106	Delete	
22107	Delete	
22116	Add:	Remove extra spine segment
22140	Delete	
22141	Delete	
22142	Delete	
22145	Delete	
22148	Delete	
22150	Delete	
22151	Delete	
22152	Delete	
22216	Add:	Revise, extra spine segment
22226	Add:	Revise, extra spine segment
22230	Delete	
22328	Add:	Repair each add spine fx
22614	Add:	Spine fusion, extra segment
22625	Delete	
22632	Add:	Spine fusion, extra segment
22650	Delete	
22804	Add:	Fusion of spine
22808	Add:	Fusion of spine
22820	Delete	
22841	Add:	Insert spine fixation device
22843	Add:	Insert spine fixation device
22844	Add:	Insert spine fixation device
22846	Add:	Insert spine fixation device
22847	Add:	Insert spine fixation device
22848	Add:	Insert pelvic fixation device
22851	Add:	Apply spine prosth device
28236	Delete	
32485	Delete	
32501	Add:	Repair bronchus (add-on)
33253	Add:	Reconstruct atria
33260	Delete	
33350	Delete	
33696	Delete	
33698	Delete	
33924	Add:	Remove pulmonary shunt

38231	Add:	Stem cell collection	85652	Add:	RBC sed rate, auto
38240	Revise:	Bone marrow/stem transplant	89250	Add:	Fertilization of oocyte
*38241	Revise:	Bone marrow/stem transplant	90721	Add:	DTaP/HIB vaccine
47355	Delete		90731	Delete	
47361	Add:	Repair liver wound	90744	Add:	Hepatitis B vaccine,under 11
47362	Add:	Repair liver wound	90745	Add:	Hepatitis B vaccine, 11-19
55859	Add:	Percut/needle insert, pros	90746	Add:	Hepatitis B vaccine, over 20
56343	Add:	Laparoscopic salpingostomy	90747	Add:	Hepatitis B vaccine, ill pat
56344	Add:	Laparoscopic fimbrioplasty	90830	Delete	
57284	Add:	Repair paravaginal defect	90923	Add:	ESRD related services, day
58972	Delete		90924	Add:	ESRD related services, day
59610	Add:	VBAC delivery	90925	Add:	ESRD related services, day
59612	Add:	VBAC delivery only	92280	Delete	
59614	Add:	VBAC care after delivery	92510	Add:	Rehab for ear implant
59618	Add:	Attempted VBAC delivery	92525	Add:	Oral function evaluation
59620	Add:	Attempted VBAC delivery only	92526	Add:	Oral function therapy
59622	Add:	Attempted VBAC after care	92546	Revise:	Sinusoidal rotational test
62350	Add:	Implant spinal canal catheter	92574	Delete	
62351	Add:	Implant spinal canal catheter	92578	Delete	
62355	Add:	Remove spinal canal catheter	92579	Add:	Visual audiometry (VRA)
62360	Add:	Insert spine infusion device	92580	Delete	
62361	Add:	Implant spine infusion pump	92585	Revise:	Auditory evoked potential
62362	Add:	Implant spine infusion pump	92597	Add:	Oral speech device eval
62365	Add:	Remove spine infusion device	92598	Add:	Modify oral speech device
62367	Add:	Analyze spine infusion pump	92987	Add:	Revision of mitral valve
62368	Add:	Analyze spine infusion pump	95880	Delete	
63750	Delete		95881	Delete	
63780	Delete		95882	Delete	
67109	Delete		95883	Delete	
76965	Add:	Echo guidance radiotherapy	95903	Add:	Motor nerve conduction test
78459	Add:	Heart muscle imaging (PET)	95926	Add:	Somatosensory testing
78655	Delete		95927	Add:	Somatosensory testing
78810	Add:	Tumor imaging (PET)	95930	Add:	Visual evoked potential test
80019	Revise:	19 blood/urine tests	95934	Add:	"H" reflex test
80410	Revise:	Calcitonin stimul panel	95935	Delete	
80416	Add:	Renin stimulation panel	95936	Add:	"H" reflex test
80417	Add:	Renin stimulation panel	96100	Add:	Psychological testing
81000	Revise:	Urinalysis, nonauto, w/scope	96105	Add:	Assessment of aphasia
81001	Add:	Urinalysis, auto, w/scope	96110	Add:	Developmental test, lim
*85651	Revise:	RBC sed rate, nonauto	96111	Add:	Developmental test, extend

96115 Add: Neurobehavior status exam

96117 Add: Neuropsych test battery

97535 Add: Self care mngment training

97537 Add: Community/work reintegration

97540 Delete

97541 Delete

97542 Add: Wheelchair mngement training

97700 Delete

97701 Delete

97703 Add: Prosthetic checkout

99178 Delete

99239 Add: Hospital discharge day

99435 Add: Hospital NB discharge day

Appendix D

Clinical Examples Supplement

As described in *CPT 1996,* clinical examples of the CPT codes for evaluation and management (E/M) services are intended to be an important element of the coding system. The clinical examples, when used with the E/M descriptors contained in the full text of *CPT,* provide a comprehensive and powerful new tool for physicians to report the services provided to their patients.

The American Medical Association is pleased to provide you with this clinical examples supplement to *CPT 1996.* The clinical examples that are provided in this supplement are limited to Office or Other Outpatient Services, Hospital Inpatient Services, Consultations, Critical Care, Prolonged Services and Care Plan Oversight.

It is important to note that these clinical examples do not encompass the entire scope of medical practice. Inclusion or exclusion of any particular specialty group does not infer any judgement of importance or lack thereof, nor does it limit the applicability of the example to any particular specialty.

Of utmost importance is the fact that these clinical examples are just that; examples. A particular patient encounter, depending on the specific circumstances must be judged by the services provided by the physician for that particular patient. Simply because the patient's complaints, symptoms or diagnoses match those of a particular clinical example, does not automatically assign that patient encounter to that particular level of service. It is important that the three key components (history, examination and medical decision making) be met and documented in the medical record to report a particular level of service.

New Patient

99201 Initial office visit for a 50-year-old male from out-of-town who needs a prescription refill for a nonsteroidal anti-inflammatory drug. (Anesthesiology)

Initial office visit for a 40-year-old female, new patient, requesting information about local pain clinics. (Anesthesiology/Pain Medicine)

Initial office visit for a 10-year-old girl for determination of visual acuity as part of a summer camp physical (does not include determination of refractive error). (Ophthalmology)

Initial office visit for an out-of-town patient requiring topical refill. (Dermatology)

Initial office visit for a 65-year-old male for reassurance about an isolated seborrheic keratosis on upper back. (Plastic Surgery)

Initial office visit for an out-of-state visitor who needs refill of topical steroid to treat lichen planus. (Dermatology)

Initial office visit for 86-year-old male, out-of-town visitor, who needs prescription refilled for an anal skin preparation that he forgot. (General Surgery/Colon & Rectal Surgery)

Initial office visit for a transient patient with alveolar osteitis for repacking. (Oral & Maxillofacial Surgery)

Initial office visit for a patient with a pedunculated lesion of the neck which is unsightly. (Dermatology)

Initial office visit for a 10-year-old male, for limited subungual hematoma not requiring drainage. (Internal Medicine)

99202 Initial office visit for a 13-year-old patient with comedopapular acne of the face unresponsive to over-the-counter medications. (Family Medicine)

Initial office visit for a patient with a clinically benign lesion or nodule of the lower leg which has been present for many years. (Dermatology)

Initial office visit for a patient with a circumscribed patch of dermatitis of the leg. (Dermatology)

Initial office visit for a patient with papulosquamous eruption of elbows. (Dermatology)

Initial office visit for a 9-year-old patient with erythematous, grouped, vesicular eruption of the lip of three days duration. (Pediatrics)

Initial office visit for an 18-year-old male referred by an orthodontist for advice regarding removal of four wisdom teeth. (Oral & Maxillofacial Surgery)

Initial office visit for a 14-year-old male, who was referred by his orthodontist, for advice on the exposure of impacted maxillary cuspids. (Oral & Maxillofacial Surgery)

Initial office visit for a patient presenting with itching patches on the wrists and ankles. (Dermatology)

Initial office visit for a 30-year-old male for evaluation and discussion of treatment of rhinophyma. (Plastic Surgery)

99203 Initial office visit for a 76-year-old male with a stasis ulcer of three months duration. (Dermatology)

Initial office visit for a 30-year-old female with pain in the lateral aspect of the forearm. (Physical Medicine & Rehabilitation)

Initial office visit for a 15-year-old patient with a four year history of moderate comedopapular acne of the face, chest and back with early scarring. Discussion of use of systemic medication. (Dermatology)

Initial office visit for a patient with papulosquamous eruption of the elbow with pitting of nails and itchy scalp. (Dermatology)

Initial office visit for a 57-year-old female who complains of painful parotid swelling for one week's duration. (Oral & Maxillofacial Surgery)

Initial office visit for a patient with an ulcerated non-healing lesion or nodule on the tip of the nose. (Dermatology)

Initial office visit for a patient with dermatitis of the antecubital and popliteal fossae. (Dermatology)

Initial office visit for a 22-year-old female with irregular menses. (Family Medicine)

Initial office visit for a 50-year-old female with dyspepsia and nausea. (Family Medicine)

Initial office visit for a 53-year-old laborer with degenerative joint disease of the knee with no prior treatment. (Orthopaedic Surgery)

Initial office visit for 60-year-old male with Dupuytren's contracture of one hand with multiple digit involvement. (Orthopaedic Surgery)

Initial office visit for a 33-year-old male with painless gross hematuria without cystoscopy. (Internal Medicine)

Initial office visit for a 55-year-old female with chronic blepharitis. There is a history of use of many medications. (Ophthalmology)

Initial office visit for an 18-year-old female with a two day history of acute conjunctivitis. Extensive history of possible exposures, prior normal ocular history, and medication use is obtained. (Ophthalmology)

Initial office visit for a 14-year-old male with unilateral anterior knee pain. (Physical Medicine & Rehabilitation)

An initial office visit of an adult who presents with symptoms of an upper-respiratory infection that has progressed to unilateral purulent nasal discharge and discomfort in the right maxillary teeth. (Otolaryngology, Head & Neck Surgery)

Initial office visit of a 40-year-old female with symptoms of atopic allergies including eye and sinus congestion, often associated with infections. She would like to be tested for allergies. (Otolaryngology, Head & Neck Surgery)

Initial office visit of a 65-year-old with nasal stuffiness. (Otolaryngology, Head & Neck Surgery)

99204 Initial office visit for a 13-year-old female with progressive scoliosis. (Orthopaedic Surgery)

Initial office visit for a 34-year-old female with primary infertility for evaluation and counseling. (Obstetrics & Gynecology)

Initial office visit for a 6-year-old male with multiple upper respiratory infections. (Allergy & Immunology)

Initial office visit for a patient with generalized dermatitis of 80% of the body surface area. (Dermatology)

Initial office visit for adolescent who was referred by school counselor because of repeated skipping school. (Psychiatry)

Initial office visit for a 50-year-old machinist with a generalized eruption. (Dermatology)

Initial office visit for a 45-year-old female, who has been abstinent from alcohol and benzodiazepines for three months, but complains of headaches, insomnia, and anxiety. (Psychiatry)

Initial office visit for a 60-year-old male with recent change in bowel habits, weight loss and abdominal pain. (Abdominal Surgery/General Surgery)

Initial office visit for 50-year-old male with an aortic aneurysm who is considering surgery. (General Surgery)

Initial office visit for a 17-year-old female with depression. (Internal Medicine)

Initial office visit of a 40-year-old with chronic draining ear, imbalance and probablecholesteatoma. (Otolaryngology, Head & Neck Surgery)

99205 Initial office visit for a patient with disseminated lupus erythematosus with kidney disease, edema, purpura and scarring lesions on the extremities plus cardiac symptoms. (Dermatology/General Surgery/Internal Medicine)

Initial office visit for a 25-year-old female with systemic lupus erythematosus, fever, seizures and profound thrombocytopenia. (Rheumatology/Allergy & Immunology)

Initial office visit for an adult with multiple cutaneous blisters, denuded secondarily infected ulcerations, oral lesions, weight loss and increasing weakness refractory to high dose corticosteroid. Initiation of new immunosuppressive therapy. (Dermatology)

Initial office visit for a 28-year-old male with systemic vasculitis and compromised circulation to the limbs. (Rheumatology)

Initial office visit for a 41-year-old female, new to the area requesting rheumatologic care, on disability due to scleroderma and recent hospitalization for malignant hypertension. (Rheumatology)

Initial office visit for a 52-year-old female with acute four extremity weakness and shortness of breath one week post-flu vaccination. (Physical Medicine & Rehabilitation)

Initial office visit for a 60-year-old male with previous back surgery; now presents with back and pelvic pain, two month history of bilateral progressive calf and thigh tightness and weakness when walking, causing several falls. (Orthopaedic Surgery)

Initial office visit for adolescent referred from ER after making suicide gesture. (Psychiatry)

Initial office visit for a 49-year-old female with a history of headaches and dependence on opioids. She reports weight loss, progressive headache, and depression. (Psychiatry)

Initial office visit for a 50-year-old female with symptoms of rash, swellings, recurrent arthritic complaints, and diarrhea and lymphadenopathy. Patient has had a 25 lb. weight loss and was recently camping in the Amazon. (Allergy & Immunology)

Initial office visit for a 34-year-old uremic type I diabetic patient referred for ESRD modality assessment and planning. (Nephrology)

Initial office visit for a 75-year-old female with neck and bilateral shoulder pain, brisk deep tendon reflexes and stress incontinence. (Physical Medicine & Rehabilitation)

Initial office visit for an 8-year-old male with cerebral palsy and spastic quadriparesis. (Physical Medicine & Rehabilitation)

Initial office visit for a 73-year-old male with known prostate malignancy, who presents with severe back pain and a recent onset of lower extremity weakness. (Physical Medicine & Rehabilitation)

Initial office visit for a 38-year-old male with paranoid delusions and a history of alcohol abuse. (Psychiatry)

Initial office visit for 12-week-old infant with bilateral hip dislocations and bilateral club feet. (Orthopaedic Surgery)

Initial office visit for a 29-year-old female with acute orbital congestion, eyelid retraction, and bilateral visual loss from optic neuropathy. (Ophthalmology)

Initial office visit for a 70-year-old diabetic patient with progressive visual field loss, advanced optic disc cupping and neovascularization of retina. (Ophthalmology)

Initial office visit for a newly diagnosed Type I diabetic patient. (Endocrinology)

Established Patient

99211 Office visit for an 82-year-old female, established patient, for a monthly B12 injection with documented Vitamin B12 deficiency. (Geriatrics/Internal Medicine/Family Medicine)

Office visit for a 50-year-old male, established patient, for removal of uncomplicated facial sutures. (Plastic Surgery)

Office visit for an established patient who lost prescription for lichen planus. Returned for new copy. (Dermatology)

Office visit for an established patient undergoing ortho-dontics who complains of a wire which is irritating his/her cheek and asks you to check it. (Oral & Maxillofacial Surgery)

Office visit for a 50-year-old female, established patient, seen for her gold injection by the nurse. (Rheumatology)

Office visit for a 73-year-old female, established patient, with pernicious anemia for weekly B12 injection. (Gastroenterology)

Office visit for an established patient for dressing change on a skin biopsy. (Dermatology)

Office visit for a 19-year-old established patient, for removal of sutures from a two cm. laceration of forehead, which you placed four days ago in ER. (Plastic Surgery)

Office visit of a 20-year-old female established patient who receives an allergy vaccine injection and is observed for a reaction by the nurse. (Otolaryngology, Head & Neck Surgery)

Office visit for a 45-year-old male, established patient, with chronic renal failure for the administration of erythropoietin. (Nephrology)

Office visit for an established patient, a Peace Corps enlistee, who requests documentation that third molars have been removed. (Oral & Maxillofacial Surgery)

Office visit for a 69-year-old female, established patient, for partial removal of antibiotic gauze from an infected wound site. (Plastic Surgery)

Office visit for a 9-year-old established patient, successfully treated for impetigo, requiring release to return to school. (Dermatology/Pediatrics)

Office visit for an established patient requesting a return-to-work certificate for resolving contact dermatitis. (Dermatology)

Office visit for an established patient who is performing glucose monitoring and wants to check accuracy of machine with lab blood glucose by technician who checks accuracy and function of patient machine. (Endocrinology)

Follow-up office visit for a 65-year-old female with a chronic indwelling percutaneous nephrostomy catheter who is seen for routine pericatheter skin care and dressing change. (Interventional Radiology)

99212 Office visit for an 11-year-old established patient seen in follow-up for mild comedonal acne of the cheeks on topical desquamating agents. (Dermatology/Family Medicine/Pediatrics)

Office visit for a 10-year-old female, established patient, who has been swimming in a lake, now presents with a one day history of left ear pain with purulent drainage. (Family Medicine)

Office visit of a child established patient with chronic secretory otitis media. (Otolaryngology, Head & Neck Surgery)

Office visit for an established patient seen in follow-up of clearing patch of localized contact dermatitis. (Family Medicine/Dermatology)

Office visit for an established patient returning for evaluation of response to treatment of lichen planus on wrists and ankles. (Dermatology)

Office visit for an established patient with tinea pedis being treated with topical therapy. (Dermatology)

Office visit for an established patient with localized erythematous plaque of psoriasis with topical hydration. (Dermatology)

Office visit for 50-year-old male, established patient, recently seen for acute neck pain, diagnosis of spondylosis, responding to physical therapy and intermittent cervical traction. Returns for evaluation for return to work. (Neurology)

Office visit for an established patient with recurring episodes of herpes simplex who has developed a clustering of vesicles on the upper lip. (Oral & Maxillofacial Surgery)

Evaluation for a 50-year-old male, established patient, who has experienced a recurrence of knee pain after he discontinued NSAID. (Anesthesiology/Pain Medicine)

Office visit for an established patient with an irritated skin tag for reassurance. (Dermatology)

Office visit for a 40-year-old established patient who has experienced a systemic allergic reaction following administration of immunotherapy. The dose must be readjusted. (Allergy & Immunology)

Office visit for a 6-year-old child, established patient, with sore throat and headache. (Family Medicine)

Office visit for 33-year-old established patient for contusion and abrasion of lower extremity. (Orthopaedic Surgery)

Office visit for 22-year-old male, established patient, one month after I & D of "wrestler's ear." (Plastic Surgery)

Office visit for a 21 year old established patient who is seen in follow-up after antibiotic therapy for acute bacterial tonsillitis. (Otolaryngology, Head & Neck Surgery)

Office visit for a 4-year old child established patient with tympanostomy tubes, check-up. (Otolaryngology, Head & Neck Surgery)

Office visit for an established patient who has had needle aspiration of a peritonsillar abscess. (Otolaryngology, Head & Neck Surgery)

Follow-up office examination for evaluation and treatment of acute draining ear in a 5-year-old child with tympanotomy tubes. (Otolaryngology, Head & Neck Surgery)

99213 Office visit for an established patient with new lesions of lichen planus in spite of topical therapies. (Dermatology)

Office visit for the quarterly follow-up of 45-year-old male with stable chronic asthma requiring regular drug therapy. (Allergy & Immunology)

Office visit for 13-year-old established patient with comedopapular acne of the face which has shown poor response to topical medication. Discussion of use of systemic medication. (Dermatology)

Office visit for a 62-year-old female, established patient, for follow-up for stable cirrhosis of the liver. (Internal Medicine/Family Medicine)

Office visit for a 3-year-old established patient with atopic dermatitis and food hypersensitivity for quarterly follow-up evaluation. The patient is on topical lotions and steroid creams, as well as oral antihistamines. (Allergy & Immunology)

Office visit for a 80-year-old female, established patient, to evaluate medical management of osteoarthritis of the temporomandibular joint. (Rheumatology)

Office visit for a 70-year-old female, established patient, one year post excision of basal cell carcinoma of nose with nasolabial flap. Now presents with new suspicious recurrent lesion and suspicious lesion of the back. (Plastic Surgery)

Office visit for a 68-year-old female, established patient, with polymyalgia rheumatic, maintained on chronic low-dose corticosteroid, with no new complaints. (Rheumatology)

Office visit for a 3-year-old female, established patient, for earache and dyshidrosis of feet. (Pediatrics/Family Medicine)

Office visit for an established patient for 18 months post-operative follow-up of TMJ repair. (Oral & Maxillofacial Surgery)

Office visit for a 45-year-old male, established patient, being re-evaluated for recurrent acute prostatitis. (Urology)

Office visit for a 43-year-old male, established patient, with known reflex sympathetic dystrophy. (Anesthesiology)

Office visit for an established patient with an evenly pigmented superficial nodule of leg which is symptomatic. (Dermatology)

Office visit for an established patient with psoriasis involvement of the elbows, pitting of the nails, and itchy scalp. (Dermatology)

Office visit for a 27-year-old male, established patient, with deep follicular and perifollicular inflammation unable to tolerate systemic antibiotics due to GI upset, requires change of systemic medication. (Dermatology)

Office visit for a 16-year-old male, established patient, who is on medication for exercise-induced bronchospasm. (Allergy & Immunology)

Office visit for a 60-year-old established patient, with chronic essential hypertension on multiple drug regimen, for blood pressure check. (Family Medicine)

Office visit for a 20-year-old male, established patient, for removal of sutures in hand. (Family Medicine)

Office visit for 58-year-old female, established patient, with unilateral painful bunion. (Orthopaedic Surgery)

Office visit for a 45-year-old female, established patient, with known osteoarthritis and painful swollen knees. (Rheumatology)

Office visit for 25-year-old female, established patient, complaining of bleeding and heavy menses. (Obstetrics & Gynecology)

Office visit for a 55-year-old male, established patient, with hypertension managed by a beta blocker/thiazide regime; now experiencing mild fatigue. (Nephrology)

Office visit for a 65-year-old female, established patient, with primary glaucoma for interval determination of intraocular pressure and possible adjustment of medication. (Ophthalmology)

Office visit for a 56-year-old man, established patient, with stable exertional angina who complains of new onset of calf pain while walking. (Cardiology)

Office visit for a 63-year-old female, established patient, with rheumatoid arthritis on auranofin and ibuprofin, seen for routine follow-up visit. (Rheumatology)

Office visit for an established patient with Graves' disease, three months post I-131 therapy, who presents with lassitude and malaise. (Endocrinology)

Office visit for the quarterly follow-up of a 63-year-old male, established patient, with chronic myofascial pain syndrome, effectively managed by doxepin, who presents with new onset urinary hesitancy. (Pain Medicine)

Office visit for the biannual follow-up of an established patient with migraine variant having infrequent, intermittent, moderate to severe headaches with nausea and vomiting, which are sometimes effectively managed by ergotamine tartrate and an antiemetic, but occasionally requiring visits to an emergency department. (Pain Medicine)

Office visit for an established patient after discharge from a pain rehabilitation program to review and adjust medication dosage. (Pain Medicine)

99214 Office visit for an established patient now presenting with generalized dermatitis of 80% of the body surface area. (Dermatology)

Office visit for a 32-year-old female, established patient, with new onset RLQ pain. (Family Medicine)

Office visit for reassessment and reassurance/counseling of a 40-year-old female, established patient, who is experiencing increased symptoms while on a pain management treatment program. (Pain Medicine)

Office visit for a 30-year-old established patient under management for intractable low back pain, who now presents with new onset right posterior thigh pain. (Pain Medicine)

Office visit for an established patient with frequent intermittent, moderate to severe headaches requiring beta blocker or tricyclic antidepressant prophylaxis, as well as four symptomatic treatments, but who is still experiencing headaches at a frequency of several times a month that are unresponsive to treatment. (Pain Medicine)

Office visit for an established patient with psoriasis with extensive involvement of scalp, trunk, palms and soles with joint pain. Combinations of topical and systemic treatments discussed and instituted. (Dermatology)

Office visit for 55-year-old male, established patient, with increasing night pain, limp and progressive varus of both knees. (Orthopaedic Surgery)

Follow-up visit for a 15-year-old withdrawn patient with four year history of papulocystic acne of the face, chest and back with early scarring and poor response to past treatment. Discussion of use of systemic medication. (Dermatology)

Office visit for a 28-year-old male, established patient, with regional enteritis, diarrhea and low-grade fever. (Internal Medicine)

Office visit for a 25-year-old female, established patient, following recent arthrogram and MR imaging for TMJ pain. (Oral & Maxillofacial Surgery)

Office visit for a 32-year-old female, established patient, with large obstructing stone in left mid-ureter, to discuss management options including urethroscopy with extraction or ESWL. (Urology)

Evaluation for a 28-year-old male, established patient, with new onset of low back pain. (Anesthesiology/Pain Medicine)

Office visit for a 28-year-old female, established patient, with right lower quadrant abdominal pain, fever and anorexia. (Internal Medicine/Family Medicine)

Office visit for a 45-year-old male, established patient, four months follow-up of L4-5 diskectomy, with persistent incapacitating low back and leg pain. (Orthopaedic Surgery)

Outpatient visit for a 77-year-old male, established patient, with hypertension, presenting with a three month history of episodic substernal chest pain on exertion. (Cardiology)

Office visit for a 25-year-old female, established patient, for evaluation of progressive saddle nose deformity of unknown etiology. (Plastic Surgery)

Office visit for a 65-year-old male, established patient, with BPH and severe bladder outlet obstruction, to discuss management options such as TURP. (Urology)

Office visit for an adult diabetic established patient with a past history of recurrent sinusitis who presents with a one week history of double vision. (Otolaryngology, Head & Neck Surgery)

Office visit for an established patient with lichen planus and 60% of the cutaneous surface involved, not responsive to systemic steroids, as well as developing symptoms of progressive heartburn and paranoid ideation. (Dermatology)

Office visit for a 52-year-old male, established patient, with a 12 year history of bipolar disorder responding to lithium carbonate and brief psychotherapy. Psychotherapy and prescription provided. (Psychiatry)

Office visit for a 63-year-old female, established patient, with a history of familial polyposis, status post-colectomy with sphincter sparing procedure, who now presents with rectal bleeding and increase in stooling frequency. (General Surgery)

Office visit for a 68-year-old male, established patient, with the sudden onset of multiple flashes and floaters in the right eye due to a posterior vitreous detachment. (Ophthalmology)

Office visit for a 55-year-old female, established patient, on cyclosporin for treatment of resistant, small vessel vasculitis. (Rheumatology)

Follow-up office visit for a 55-year-old male, two months after iliac angioplasty with new onset of contralateral extremity claudication. (Interventional Radiology)

99215 Office visit for an established patient who developed persistent cough, rectal bleeding, weakness and diarrhea plus pustular infection on skin. Patient on immunosuppressive therapy. (Dermatology)

Office visit for an established patient with disseminated lupus erythematosus, extensive edema of extremities kidney disease, and weakness requiring monitored course on azathioprene, corticosteroid and complicated by acute depression. (Dermatology/Internal Medicine/Rheumatology)

Office visit for an established patient with progressive dermatomyositis and recent onset of fever, nasal speech and regurgitation of fluids through the nose. (Dermatology)

Office visit for a 28-year-old female, established patient, who is abstinent from previous cocaine dependence, but reports progressive panic attacks and chest pains. (Psychiatry)

Office visit for an established adolescent patient with history of bipolar disorder treated with lithium; seen on urgent basis at family's request because of severe depressive symptoms. (Psychiatry)

Office visit for an established patient having acute migraine with new onset neurological symptoms and whose headaches are unresponsive to previous attempts at management with a combination of preventive and abortive medication. (Pain Medicine)

Office visit for an established patient with exfoliative lichen planus with daily fever spikes, disorientation and shortness of breath. (Dermatology)

Office visit for a 25-year-old established patient, two years post-burn with bilateral ectropion, hypertrophic facial burn scars, near absence of left breast, and burn syndactyly of both hands. Discussion of treatment options following examination. (Plastic Surgery)

Office visit for a 6-year-old child, established patient, to review newly diagnosed immune deficiency with recommendations for therapy including IV immuno-globulin and chronic antibiotics. (Allergy & Immunology)

Office visit for a 36-year-old established patient, three months status post-transplant, with new onset of

peripheral edema, increased blood pressure and progressive fatigue. (Nephrology)

Office visit for an established patient with Kaposi's sarcoma who presents with fever and widespread vesicles. (Dermatology)

Office visit for a 27-year-old female, established patient, with bipolar disorder who was stable on lithium carbonate and monthly supportive psychotherapy but now has developed symptoms of hypomania. (Psychiatry)

Office visit for a 25-year-old male, established patient with a history of schizophrenia who has been seen bi-monthly but is complaining of auditory hallucinations. (Psychiatry)

Office visit for 62-year-old male, established patient, three years post-op abdominal perineal resection, now with a rising CEA, weight loss and pelvic pain. (Abdominal Surgery)

Office visit for 42-year-old male, established patient, nine months post-op emergency vena cava shunt for variceal bleeding, now presents with complaints of one episode of "dark" bowel movement, weight gain, tightness in abdomen, whites of eyes seem "yellow" and occasional drowsiness after eating hamburgers. (Abdominal Surgery)

Office visit for 68-year-old male, established patient, with biopsy-proven rectal carcinoma, for evaluation and discussion of treatment options. (General Surgery)

Office visit for a 60-year-old established patient with diabetic nephropathy with increasing edema and dyspnea. (Endocrinology)

Hospital Inpatient Services

Initial Hospital Care

New or Established Patient

99221 Initial hospital visit following admission for a 42-year-old male for observation following an uncomplicated mandible fracture. (Plastic Surgery/Oral & Maxillofacial Surgery)

Initial hospital visit for a 40-year-old patient with a thrombosed synthetic AV conduit. (Nephrology)

Initial hospital visit for a healthy 24-year-old male with an acute onset of low back pain following a lifting injury. (Internal Medicine/Anesthesiology/Pain Medicine)

Initial hospital visit for a 69-year-old female with controlled hypertension, scheduled for surgery. (Internal Medicine/Cardiology)

Initial hospital visit for a 24-year-old healthy female with benign tumor of palate. (Oral & Maxillofacial Surgery)

Initial hospital visit for a 14-year-old female with infectious mononucleosis and dehydration. (Internal Medicine)

Initial hospital visit for a 62-year-old female with stable rheumatoid arthritis, admitted for total joint replacement. (Rheumatology)

Initial hospital visit for a 12-year-old patient with a laceration of the upper eyelid, involving the lid margin and superior canaliculus, admitted prior to surgery for IV antibiotic therapy. (Plastic Surgery)

Initial hospital visit for a 69-year-old female with controlled hypertension, scheduled for surgery. (Cardiology)

99222 Initial hospital visit for 50-year-old patient with lower quadrant abdominal pain and increased temperature, but without septic picture. (General Surgery/Abdominal Surgery/Colon & Rectal Surgery)

Initial hospital visit for airway management, due to a benign laryngeal mass. (Otolaryngology, Head & Neck Surgery)

Initial hospital visit for 66-year-old female with an L-2 vertebral compression fracture with acute onset of paralytic ileus; seen in the office two days previously. (Orthopaedic Surgery)

Initial hospital visit and evaluation of a 15-year-old male admitted with peritonsillar abscess or cellulitis requiring intravenous antibiotic therapy. (Otolaryngology, Head & Neck Surgery)

Initial hospital visit for 42-year-old male with vertebral compression fracture following a motor vehicle accident. (Orthopaedic Surgery)

Initial hospital visit for a patient with generalized atopic dermatitis and secondary infection. (Dermatology)

Initial hospital visit for a 3-year-old patient with high temperature, limp and painful hip motion of 18 hours duration. (Pediatrics/Orthopaedic Surgery)

Initial hospital visit for a young adult, presenting with an acute asthma attack unresponsive to outpatient therapy. (Allergy & Immunology)

Initial hospital visit for an 18-year-old male who has suppurative sialoadenitis and dehydration. (Oral & Maxillofacial Surgery)

Initial hospital visit for 65-year-old female for acute onset of thrombotic cerebrovascular accident with contralateral paralysis and aphasia. (Neurology)

Initial hospital visit for a 50-year-old male chronic paraplegic patient with pain and spasm below the lesion. (Anesthesiology)

Partial hospital admission for an adolescent patient from chaotic blended family, transferred from inpatient setting, for continued treatment to control symptomatic expressions of hostility and depression. (Psychiatry)

Initial hospital visit for a 15-year-old male with acute status asthmaticus, unresponsive to outpatient therapy. (Internal Medicine)

Initial hospital visit for a 61-year-old male with history of previous myocardial infarction, who now complains of chest pain. (Internal Medicine)

Initial hospital visit of a 15-year-old on medications for a sore throat over the last two weeks. The sore throat has worsened and now has dysphagia. The exam shows large necrotic tonsils with an adequate airway and small palpable nodes. The initial mono test was negative. (Otolaryngology, Head & Neck Surgery)

Initial hospital evaluation of a 23-year-old allergy patient admitted with eyelid edema and pain on 5th day of oral antibiotic therapy. (Otolaryngology, Head & Neck Surgery)

99223 Initial hospital visit for a 45-year-old female, who has a history of rheumatic fever as a child and now has anemia, fever, and congestive heart failure. (Cardiology)

Initial hospital visit for a 50-year-old male with acute chest pain and diagnostic electrocardiographic changes of an acute anterior myocardial infarction. (Cardiology/Family Medicine/Internal Medicine)

Initial hospital visit of a 75-year-old with progressive stridor and dysphagia with history of cancer of the larynx treated by radiation therapy in the past. Exam shows a large recurrent tumor of the glottis with a mass in the neck. (Otolaryngology, Head & Neck Surgery)

Initial hospital visit for a 70-year-old male admitted with chest pain, complete heart block and congestive heart failure. (Cardiology)

Initial hospital visit for an 82-year-old male who presents with syncope, chest pain, and ventricular arrhythmias. (Cardiology)

Initial hospital visit for a 75-year-old male with history of ASCVD, who is severely dehydrated, disoriented and experiencing auditory hallucinations. (Psychiatry)

Initial hospital visit for a 70-year-old male with alcohol and sedative-hypnotic dependence, admitted by family for severe withdrawal, hypertension and diabetes mellitus. (Psychiatry)

Initial hospital visit for a persistently suicidal latency-aged child whose parents have requested admission to provide safety during evaluation, but are anxious about separation from her. (Psychiatry)

Initial psychiatric visit for an adolescent patient without previous psychiatric history, who was transferred from the medical ICU after a significant overdose. (Psychiatry)

Initial hospital visit for a 35-year-old female with severe systemic lupus erythematosus on corticosteroid and cyclophosphamide, with new onset of fever, chills, rash and chest pain. (Rheumatology)

Initial hospital visit for a 52-year-old male with known rheumatic heart disease who presents with anasarca, hypertension, and history of alcohol abuse. (Cardiology)

Initial hospital visit for a 55-year-old female with a history of congenital heart disease; now presents with cyanosis. (Cardiology)

Initial hospital visit for psychotic, hostile, violently combative adolescent, involuntarily committed, for seclusion and restraint in order to provide for safety on unit. (Psychiatry)

Initial hospital visit for now subdued and sullen teen-age male with six month history of declining school performance, increasing self-endangerment and resistance of parental expectations including running away last weekend after physical fight with father. (Psychiatry)

Initial partial hospital admission for 17-year-old female with history of borderline mental retardation who has developed auditory hallucinations. Parents are known to abuse alcohol, and protective services is investigating allegations of sexual abuse of a younger sibling. (Psychiatry)

Initial hospital visit of a 67-year old male admitted with a large neck mass, dysphagia and history of myocardial infarction three months before. (Otolaryngology, Head & Neck Surgery)

Initial hospital visit for a patient with suspected cerebrospinal fluid rhinorrhea which developed two weeks after head injury. (Otolaryngology, Head & Neck Surgery)

Initial hospital visit for a 25-year-old female with history of poly-substance abuse and psychiatric disorder. The patient appears to be psychotic with markedly elevated vital signs. (Psychiatry)

Initial hospital visit for a 70-year-old male with cutaneous T-cell lymphoma who has developed fever and lymphadenopathy. (Internal Medicine)

Initial hospital visit for 62-year-old female with known coronary artery disease, for evaluation of increasing edema, dyspnea on exertion, confusion and sudden onset of fever with productive cough. (Internal Medicine)

Initial hospital visit for a 3-year-old female with 36 hour history of sore throat and high fever; now with sudden onset of lethargy, irritability, photophobia and nuchal rigidity. (Pediatrics)

Initial hospital visit for a 26-year-old female for evaluation of severe facial fractures (LeFort's II/III). (Plastic Surgery)

Initial hospital visit for a 55-year-old female for bilateral mandibular fractures resulting in flail mandible and airway obstruction. (Plastic Surgery)

Initial hospital visit for a 71-year-old patient with a red painful eye four days following uncomplicated cataract surgery due to endophthalmitis. (Ophthalmology)

Initial hospital visit for a 45-year-old patient involved in a motor vehicle accident who suffered a perforating corneoscleral laceration with loss of vision. (Ophthalmology)

Initial hospital visit for a 58-year-old male who has Ludwig's angina and progressive airway compromise. (Oral & Maxillofacial Surgery)

Initial hospital visit for a patient with generalized systemic sclerosis, receiving immunosuppressive therapy because of recent onset of cough, fever and inability to swallow. (Dermatology)

Initial hospital visit for an 82-year-old male who presents with syncope, chest pain and ventricular arrhythmias. (Cardiology)

Initial hospital visit for a 62-year-old male with history of previous myocardial infarction, comes in with recurrent, sustained ventricular tachycardia. (Cardiology)

Initial hospital visit for a chronic dialysis patient with infected PTFE fistula, septicemia and shock. (Nephrology)

Initial hospital visit for 1-year-old male, victim of child abuse, with central nervous system depression, skull fracture and retinal hemorrhage. (Family Medicine/Neurology)

Initial hospital visit for a 25-year-old female with recent C4-5 quadriplegia, admitted for rehabilitation. (Physical Medicine & Rehabilitation)

Initial hospital visit for an 18-year-old male, post-traumatic brain injury with multiple impairment. (Physical Medicine & Rehabilitation)

Initial partial hospital admission for 16-year-old male, sullen and subdued, with 6 month history of declining school performance, increasing self-endangerment, and resistance to parental expectations. (Psychiatry)

Initial hospital visit for a 16-year-old primigravida at 32 weeks gestation with severe hypertension (200/110), thrombocytopenia and headache. (Obstetrics & Gynecology)

Initial hospital visit for 49-year-old male with cirrhosis of liver with hematemesis, hepatic encephalopathy and fever. (Gastroenterology)

Initial hospital visit for a 55-year-old female in chronic pain who has attempted suicide. (Psychiatry)

Initial hospital visit for a 70-year-old male, with multiple organ system disease, admitted with history of being aneuric and septic for 24 hours prior to admission. (Urology)

Initial hospital visit for a 3-year-old female with 36 hour history of sore throat and high fever, now with sudden onset of lethargy, irritability, photophobia and nuchal ridigity. (Internal Medicine)

Initial hospital visit for a 78-year-old male, transfers from nursing home with dysuria and pyuria, increasing confusion and high fever. (Internal Medicine)

Initial hospital visit for a one-day-old male infant with cyanosis, respiratory distress and tachypnea. (Cardiology)

Initial hospital visit for a 3-year-old female child with recurrent tachycardia and syncope. (Cardiology)

Initial hospital visit for a thyrotoxic patient who presents with fever, atrial fibrillation and delirium. (Endocrinology)

Initial hospital visit for a 50-year-old Type I diabetic who presents with diabetic ketoacidosis with fever and obtundation. (Endocrinology)

Initial hospital visit for a 40-year-old female with anatomical stage 3, ARA functional class 3 rheumatoid arthritis on methotrexate, corticosteroid and nonsteroidal anti-inflammatory drugs. Patient presents with severe arthritis flare, new oral ulcers, abdominal pain and leukopenia. (Rheumatology)

Initial hospital exam of a pediatric patient with high fever and proptosis. (Otolaryngology, Head & Neck Surgery)

Initial hospital visit for a 25-year-old patient admitted for the first time to the rehab unit, with recent C-4-5 quadriplegia. (Physical Medicine & Rehabilitation)

Subsequent Hospital Care

99231 Subsequent hospital visit for a 65-year-old female, post-open reduction and internal fixation of a fracture. (Physical Medicine & Rehabilitation)

Subsequent hospital visit for a 33-year-old patient with pelvic pain that is responding to pain medication and observation. (Obstetrics & Gynecology)

Subsequent hospital visit for a 21-year-old female with hyperemesis that has responded well to intravenous fluids. (Obstetrics & Gynecology)

Subsequent hospital visit to re-evaluate post-op pain and titrate patient controlled analgesia for a 27-year-old female. (Anesthesiology)

Follow-up hospital visit for a 35-year-old female, status post-epidural analgesia. (Anesthesiology/Pain Medicine)

Subsequent hospital visit for a 56-year-old male, post-gastrectomy, for maintenance of analgesia using an intravenous dilaudid infusion. (Anesthesiology)

Subsequent hospital visit for a 4-year-old child on day three receiving medication for uncomplicated pneumonia. (Allergy & Immunology)

Subsequent hospital visit for a 30-year-old female with urticaria which has stabilized with medication. (Allergy & Immunology)

Subsequent hospital visit for a 76-year-old male with venous stasis ulcers. (Dermatology)

Subsequent hospital visit for a 24 year old female with otitis externa, seen two days before in consultation, now to have otic wick removal. (Otolaryngology, Head & Neck Surgery)

Subsequent hospital visit for a 27 year old with acute labyrinthitis. (Otolaryngology, Head & Neck Surgery)

Subsequent hospital visit for a 10-year-old male admitted for lobar pneumonia with vomiting and dehydration; is becoming afebrile and tolerating oral fluids. (Family Medicine/Pediatrics)

Subsequent hospital visit for a 62-year-old patient with resolving cellulitis of the foot. (Orthopaedic Surgery)

Subsequent hospital visit for a 25-year-old male admitted for supra-ventricular tachycardia and converted on medical therapy. (Cardiology)

Subsequent hospital visit for a 27-year-old male two days after open reduction and internal fixation for malar complex fracture. (Plastic Surgery)

Subsequent hospital visit for a 76-year-old male with venous stasis ulcers. (Geriatrics)

Subsequent hospital visit for a 67-year-old female admitted three days ago with bleeding gastric ulcer; now stable. (Gastroenterology)

Subsequent hospital visit for stable 33-year-old male, status post-lower gastrointestinal bleeding. (General Surgery/Gastroenterology)

Subsequent hospital visit for a 29-year-old auto mechanic with effort thrombosis of left upper extremity. (General Surgery)

Subsequent hospital visit for a 14-year-old female in middle phase of inpatient treatment, who is now behaviorally stable and making satisfactory progress in treatment. (Psychiatry)

Subsequent hospital visit for an 18-year-old male with uncomplicated asthma who is clinically stable. (Allergy & Immunology)

Subsequent hospital visit for a 55-year-old male with rheumatoid arthritis, two days following an uncomplicated total joint replacement. (Rheumatology)

Subsequent hospital visit for a 60-year-old dialysis patient with an access infection, now afebrile on antibiotic. (Nephrology)

Subsequent hospital visit for a 36-year-old female with stable post-rhinoplasty epistaxis. (Plastic Surgery)

Subsequent hospital visit for a 66-year-old female with L-2 vertebral compression fracture with resolving ileus. (Orthopaedic Surgery)

Subsequent hospital visit for a 3-year-old patient in traction for congenital (developmental) dislocation of the hip. (Orthopaedic Surgery)

Subsequent hospital visit for a patient with peritonsillar abscess. (Otolaryngology, Head & Neck Surgery)

Subsequent hospital visit for an 18-year old female responding to intravenous antibiotic therapy for ear or sinus infection. (Otolaryngology, Head & Neck Surgery)

Subsequent hospital visit for a 70-year-old male admitted with congestive heart failure who has responded to therapy. (Cardiology)

Follow-up hospital visit for a 32-year-old female with left ureteral calculus; being followed in anticipation of spontaneous passage. (Urology)

Subsequent hospital visit for a 4-year-old female, admitted for acute gastroenteritis and dehydration, requiring IV hydration; now stable. (Family Medicine)

Subsequent hospital visit for a 50-year-old Type II diabetic who is clinically stable and without complications requiring regulation of a single dose of insulin daily. (Endocrinology)

Subsequent hospital visit to reassesses the status of a 65-year-old patient post open reduction and internal fixation of hip fracture, on the rehab unit. (Physical Medicine & Rehabilitation)

Subsequent hospital visit for a 78-year-old male with cholangiocarcinoma managed by biliary drainage. (Interventional Radiology)

99232 Subsequent hospital visit for a patient with venous stasis ulcers who developed fever and red streaks adjacent to the ulcer. (Dermatology/Internal Medicine/Family Medicine)

Subsequent hospital visit for a 66-year-old male for dressing changes and observation. Patient has had a myocutaneous flap to close a pharyngeal fistula and now has a low-grade fever. (Plastic Surgery)

Subsequent hospital visit for a 54-year-old female admitted for myocardial infarction, but who is now having frequent premature ventricular contractions. (Internal Medicine)

Subsequent hospital visit for 80-year-old patient with a pelvic rim fracture, inability to walk and severe pain; now 36 hours post-injury, experiencing urinary retention. (Orthopaedic Surgery)

Subsequent hospital visit for a 17-year-old female with fever, pharyngitis and airway obstruction, who after 48 hours, develops a maculopapular rash. (Pediatrics/Family Medicine)

Follow-up hospital visit for a 32-year-old patient admitted the previous day for corneal ulcer. (Dermatology)

Follow-up visit for a 67-year-old male with congestive heart failure who has responded to antibiotics and diuretics, and has now developed a monoarthropathy. (Internal Medicine)

Follow-up hospital visit for a 58-year-old male receiving continuous opioids who is experiencing severe nausea and vomiting. (Pain Medicine)

Subsequent hospital visit for a patient after an auto accident who is slow to respond to ambulation training. (Physical Medicine & Rehabilitation)

Subsequent hospital visit for a 14-year-old child with unstable bronchial asthma complicated by pneumonia. (Allergy & Immunology)

Subsequent hospital visit for a 50-year-old diabetic, hypertensive male with back pain not responding to conservative inpatient management with continued radiation of pain to the lower left extremity. (Orthopaedic Surgery)

Subsequent hospital visit for a 37-year-old female on day five of antibiotics for bacterial endocarditis, who still has low grade fever. (Cardiology)

99233 Subsequent hospital visit for a 38-year-old male, quadriplegic with acute autonomic hyperreflexia, who is not responsive to initial care. (Physical Medicine & Rehabilitation)

Follow-up hospital visit for a teen-aged female who continues to experience severely disruptive, violent and

life-threatening symptoms in a complicated multi-system illness. Family/social circumstances also a contributing factor. (Psychiatry)

Subsequent hospital visit for a 42-year-old female with progressive systemic sclerosis (scleroderma), renal failure on dialysis, congestive heart failure, cardiac arrhythmias and digital ulcers. (Allergy & Immunology)

Subsequent hospital visit for a 50-year-old diabetic, hypertensive male with nonresponding back pain and radiating pain to the lower left extremity, who develops chest pain, cough and bloody sputum. (Orthopaedic Surgery)

Subsequent hospital visit for a 64-year-old female, status post-abdominal aortic aneurysm resection, with non-responsive coagulopathy and has now developed lower GI bleeding. (Abdominal Surgery/Colon & Rectal Surgery/General Surgery)

Follow-up hospital care of a patient with pansinusitis infection complicated by a brain abscess and asthma; no response to current treatment. (Otolaryngology, Head & Neck Surgery)

Subsequent hospital visit for a patient with a laryngeal neoplasm who develops airway compromise, suspected metastasis. (Otolaryngology, Head & Neck Surgery)

Subsequent hospital visit for a 49-year-old male with significant rectal bleeding, etiology undetermined, not responding to treatment. (Abdominal Surgery/General Surgery/Colon & Rectal Surgery)

Subsequent hospital visit for a 50-year-old male, post-aortocoronary bypass surgery; now develops hypotension and oliguria. (Cardiology)

Subsequent hospital visit for an adolescent patient who is violent, unsafe and noncompliant, with multiple expectations for participation in treatment plan and behavior on the treatment unit. (Psychiatry)

Subsequent hospital visit for an 18-year-old male being treated for presumed PCP psychosis. Patient is still moderately symptomatic with auditory hallucinations and is insisting on signing out against medical advice. (Psychiatry)

Subsequent hospital visit for an 8-year-old female with caustic ingestion, who now has fever, dyspnea and dropping hemoglobin. (Gastroenterology)

Follow-up hospital visit for a chronic renal failure patient on dialysis who develops chest pain and shortness of breath and a new onset pericardial friction rub. (Nephrology)

Subsequent hospital visit for a 44-year-old patient with electrical burns to the left arm with ascending infection. (Orthopaedic Surgery)

Subsequent hospital visit for a patient with systemic sclerosis who has aspirated and is short of breath. (Dermatology)

Subsequent hospital visit for a 65-year-old female, status post-op resection of abdominal aortic aneurysm, with suspected ischemic bowel. (General Surgery)

Subsequent hospital visit for a 50-year-old male, post-aortocoronary bypass surgery, now develops hypotension and oliguria. (Cardiology)

Subsequent hospital visit for a 65-year-old male, following an acute myocardial infarction who complains of shortness of breath and new chest pain. (Cardiology)

Subsequent hospital visit for a 65-year-old female with rheumatoid arthritis (stage 3, class 3) admitted for urosepsis. On the third hospital day, chest pain, dyspnea and fever develop. (Rheumatology)

Follow-up hospital care of a pediatric case with stridor, laryngomalcia, established tracheostomy, complicated by multiple medical problems in PICU. (Otolaryngology, Head & Neck Surgery)

Consultations

Office or Other Outpatient Consultations

New or Established Patient

99241 Initial office consultation for a 40-year-old female in pain from blister on lip following a cold. (Oral & Maxillofacial Surgery)

Initial office consultation for a 62-year-old construction worker with olecranon bursitis. (Orthopaedic Surgery)

99242 Initial office consultation for a 20-year-old male with acute upper respiratory tract symptoms. (Allergy & Immunology)

Initial office consultation for a 29-year-old soccer player with painful proximal thigh/groin injury. (Orthopaedic Surgery)

Initial office consultation for a 66-year-old female with wrist and hand pain, numbness of finger tips, suspected median nerve compression by carpal tunnel syndrome. (Plastic Surgery)

Initial office consultation for a patient with a solitary lesion of discoid lupus erythematosus on left cheek to rule out malignancy of self-induced lesion. (Dermatology)

99243 Initial office consultation for a 60-year-old male with avascular necrosis of the left femoral head with increasing pain. (Orthopaedic Surgery)

Office consultation for a 31-year-old woman complaining of palpitations and chest pains. Her internist had described a mild systolic click. (Cardiology)

99244 Initial office consultation for a 28-year-old male, HIV positive, with a recent change in visual acuity. (Ophthalmology)

Initial office consultation for a 15-year-old male with failing grades, suspected drug abuse. (Pediatrics)

Initial office consultation for a 36-year-old factory worker, who is four months status post occupational low back injury and requires management of intractable low back pain. (Pain Medicine)

Initial office consultation for a 45-year-old female with a history of chronic arthralgia of TMJ and associated myalgia and sudden progressive symptomatology over last two to three months. (Oral & Maxillofacial Surgery)

Initial office consultation for evaluation of a 70-year-old male with appetite loss and diminished energy. (Psychiatry)

Initial office consultation for an elementary school-aged patient, referred by pediatrician, with multiple systematic complaints and recent onset of behavioral discontrol. (Psychiatry)

Initial office consultation for a 23-year-old female with developmental facial skeletal anomaly and subsequent abnormal relationship of jaw(s) to cranial base. (Oral & Maxillofacial Surgery)

Initial office consultation for a 45-year-old myopic patient with a one week history of floaters and a partial retinal detachment. (Ophthalmology)

Initial office consultation for a 65-year-old female with moderate dementia, mild unsteadiness, back pain fatigue on ambulation, intermittent urinary incontinence. (Neurosurgery)

Initial office consultation for a 33-year-old female referred by endocrinologist with amenorrhea and galactorrhea, for evaluation of pituitary tumor. (Neurosurgery)

Initial office consultation for a 34-year-old male with new onset nephrotic syndrome. (Nephrology)

Initial office consultation for a 39-year-old female with intractable chest wall pain secondary to metastatic breast cancer. (Anesthesiology/Pain Medicine)

Initial office consultation for a patient with multiple giant tumors of jaws. (Oral & Maxillofacial Surgery)

Initial office consultation for a patient with a failed total hip replacement with loosening and pain upon walking. (Orthopaedic Surgery)

Initial office consultation for a 60-year-old female with three year history of intermittent tic-like unilateral facial pain; now constant pain for six weeks without relief by adequate carbamazepine dosage. (Neurosurgery)

Initial office consultation for a 45-year-old male heavy construction worker with prior lumbar disk surgery two years earlier; now gradually recurring low back and unilateral leg pain for three months, unable to work for two weeks. (Neurosurgery)

Initial office consultation of a patient who presents with a 30 year history of smoking and right neck mass. (Otolaryngology, Head & Neck Surgery)

99245 Initial office consultation for a 35-year-old multiple-trauma male patient with complex pelvic fractures, for evaluation and formulation of management plan. (Orthopaedic Surgery)

Initial emergency room consultation for 10-year-old male in status epilepticus, recent closed head injury, information about medication not available. (Neurosurgery)

Initial emergency room consultation for a 23-year-old patient with severe abdominal pain, guarding, febrile and unstable vital signs. (Obstetrics & Gynecology)

Office consultation for a 67-year-old female longstanding uncontrolled diabetic who presents with retinopathy, nephropathy, and a foot ulcer. (Endocrinology)

Office consultation for a 37-year-old male for initial evaluation and management of Cushing's disease. (Endocrinology)

Office consultation for a 60-year-old male who presents with thyrotoxicosis, exophthalmos, frequent premature ventricular contractions and congestive heart failure. (Endocrinology)

Initial office consultation for a 36-year-old patient, one year status post occupational herniated cervical disk treated by laminectomy, requiring management of multiple sites of intractable pain, depression, and narcotic dependence. (Pain Medicine)

Office consultation for a 58-year-old man with a history of MI and CHF who complains of the recent onset of rest angina and shortness of breath. The patient has a systolic blood pressure of 90mmHG and is in Class IV heart failure. (Cardiology)

Emergency room consultation for a 1-year-old infant with a three-day history of fever with increasing respiratory distress who is thought to have cardiac tamponade by the ER physician. (Cardiology)

Initial Inpatient Consultations

New or Established Patient

99251 Initial hospital consultation for a 27-year-old female with fractured incisor post-intubation. (Oral & Maxillofacial Surgery)

Initial hospital consultation for an orthopaedic patient on IV antibiotics that has developed an apparent candida infection of the oral cavity. (Oral & Maxillofacial Surgery)

99252 Initial hospital consultation for a 45-year-old male, previously abstinent alcoholic, who relapsed and was admitted for management of gastritis. The patient readily accepts the need for further treatment. (Addiction Medicine)

Initial hospital consultation for a 35-year-old dialysis patient with episodic oral ulcerations. (Oral & Maxillofacial Surgery)

Initial inpatient preoperative consultation for a 43-year-old woman with cholecystitis and well-controlled hypertension. (Cardiology)

99253 Initial hospital consultation for 50-year-old female with incapacitating knee pain due to generalized rheumatoid arthritis. (Orthopaedic Surgery)

Initial hospital consultation for 60-year-old male with avascular necrosis of the left femoral heal with increasing pain. (Orthopaedic Surgery)

Initial hospital consultation for a 45-year-old female with compound mandibular fracture and concurrent head, abdominal and/or orthopaedic injuries. (Oral & Maxillofacial Surgery)

Initial hospital consultation for 22-year-old female, paraplegic, to evaluate wrist and hand pain. (Orthopaedic Surgery)

Initial hospital consultation for 40-year-old male with 10 day history of incapacitating unilateral sciatica, unable to walk now, not improved by bed rest. (Neurosurgery)

Initial hospital consultation, requested by pediatrician, for treatment recommendations for a patient admitted with persistent inability to walk following soft tissue injury to ankle. (Psychiatry)

Initial hospital consultation for a 27-year-old previously healthy male who vomited during IV sedation and may have aspirated gastric contents. (Anesthesiology)

Initial hospital consultation for a 33-year-old female, post-abdominal surgery, who now has a fever. (Internal Medicine)

99254 Initial hospital consultation for 15-year-old patient with painless swelling of proximal humerus with lytic lesion by x-ray. (Orthopaedic Surgery)

Initial hospital consultation for evaluation of a 29-year-old female with a diffusely positive medical review of systems and history of multiple surgeries. (Psychiatry)

Initial hospital consultation for 70-year-old diabetic female with gangrene of the foot. (Orthopaedic Surgery)

Initial inpatient consultation for a 47-year-old female with progressive pulmonary infiltrate, hypoxemia, and diminished urine output. (Anesthesiology)

Initial hospital consultation for a 13-month-old child with spasmodic cough, respiratory distress and fever. (Allergy & Immunology)

Initial hospital consultation for patient with failed total hip replacement with loosening and pain upon walking. (Orthopaedic Surgery)

Initial hospital consultation for 62-year-old female with metastatic breast cancer to the femoral neck and thoracic vertebra. (Orthopaedic Surgery)

Initial hospital consultation for a 39-year-old female with nephrolithiasis requiring extensive opioid analgesics, whose vital signs are now elevated. She initially denied any drug use, but today gives history of multiple substance abuse, including opioids and prior treatment for a personality disorder. (Psychiatry)

Initial hospital consultation for a 70-year-old female without previous psychiatric history, who is now experiencing nocturnal confusion and visual hallucinations following hip replacement surgery. (Psychiatry)

99255 Initial inpatient consultation for 76-year-old female with massive, life-threatening gastrointestinal hemorrhage and chest pain. (Gastroenterology)

Initial inpatient consultation for a 75-year-old female, admitted to intensive care with acute respiratory distress syndrome, who is hypersensitive, has a moderate metabolic acidosis and a rising serum creatinine. (Nephrology)

Initial hospital consultation for patient with a history of complicated low back pain and neck problems with previous multiple failed back surgeries. (Orthopaedic Surgery/Neurosurgery)

Initial hospital consultation for a 66-year-old female, two days post-abdominal aneurysm repair, with oliguria and hypertension of one day duration. (Nephrology/Internal Medicine)

Initial hospital consultation for a patient with shotgun wound to face with massive facial trauma and airway obstruction. (Oral & Maxillofacial Surgery)

Initial hospital consultation for patient with severe pancreatitis complicated by respiratory insufficiency, acute renal failure and abscess formation. (General Surgery/Colon & Rectal Surgery)

Initial hospital consultation for 35-year-old multiple-trauma male patient with complex pelvic fractures, to evaluate and formulate management plan. (Orthopaedic Surgery)

Initial inpatient consultation for adolescent patient with fractured femur and pelvis who pulled out IVs and disconnected traction in attempt to elope from hospital. (Psychiatry)

Initial hospital consultation for 16-year-old primigravida at 32 weeks gestation requested by a family practitioner for evaluation of severe hypertension, thrombocytopenia and headache. (Obstetrics & Gynecology)

Initial hospital consultation for a 58-year-old insulin-dependent diabetic with multiple antibiotic allergies, now with multiple fascial plane abscesses and airway obstruction. (Oral & Maxillofacial Surgery)

Initial inpatient consultation for 55-year-old male with known cirrhosis and ascites; now with jaundice, encephalopathy and massive hematemesis. (Gastroenterology)

Initial hospital consultation for 25-year-old male, seen in emergency room with severe, closed head injury. (Neurosurgery)

Initial hospital consultation for 2-day-old male with single ventricle physiology and subaortic obstruction. Family counseling following evaluation for multiple, staged surgical procedures. (Thoracic Surgery)

Initial hospital consultation for 45-year-old male admitted with subarachnoid hemorrhage and intracranial aneurysm on angiogram. (Neurosurgery)

Initial inpatient consultation for myxedematous patient who is hypoventilating and obtunded. (Endocrinology)

Initial hospital consultation for a 45-year-old patient with widely metastatic lung carcinoma, intractable back pain, and a history that includes substance dependence, NSAID allergy, and two prior laminectomies with fusion for low back pain. (Pain Medicine)

Initial hospital consultation for evaluation of treatment options in a 50-year-old patient with cirrhosis, known peptic ulcer disease, hypotension, encephalopathy, and massive acute upper gastrointestinal bleeding which cannot be localized by endoscopy. (Interventional Radiology)

Follow-up Inpatient Consultations

Established Patient

99261 Follow-up consultation for a 78-year-old female nursing home resident for evaluation of medical management of pruritus ani. (Colon & Rectal Surgery/Geriatrics/General Surgery)

Follow-up hospital consultation on first post-op day for a 64-year-old male who has undergone uneventful CABG. (Anesthesiology)

Follow-up inpatient consultation for 67-year-old female admitted several days ago for bleeding ulcer; now stable. (Gastroenterology)

Follow-up hospital consultation for a 35-year-old female with history of mitral valve prolapse. (Cardiology)

Follow-up inpatient consultation to complete initial consultation for dental pain after review of radiographs. (Oral & Maxillofacial Surgery)

Follow-up inpatient consultation for evaluation of response to therapy for moniliasis. (Oral & Maxillofacial Surgery)

Follow-up inpatient consultation for a 22-year-old female with recurrent aphthous ulcers. (Oral & Maxillofacial Surgery)

Follow-up hospital consultation for 37-year-old female to complete review of previously unavailable studies. (Therapeutic Radiology & Oncology)

Follow-up consultation for highly functional 75-year-old female with urinary incontinence to review preliminary results of diagnostic evaluation. (Geriatrics)

Follow-up inpatient consultation for a 1-week-old premature female infant with patent ductus arteriosus. The murmur has disappeared. (Cardiology)

Follow-up hospital consultation to review the results of an audiogram. (Otolaryngology, Head & Neck Surgery)

99262 Follow-up inpatient consultation for a 6-year-old female child, established patient, with endocarditis and changing heart murmur. (Cardiology)

Follow-up inpatient consultation on a 2-year-old male, one day postoperative ventricular septal defect closure with signs of tachycardia. (Cardiology)

Follow-up inpatient consultation for a 63-year-old man, established patient, with moderately severe pulmonary insufficiency, 10 days postoperative coronary artery bypass for unstable angina. Patient has developed severe dyspnea, fever and a new exudative right pleural effusion. (Cardiology)

Follow-up inpatient consultation for a 67-year-old woman with lung cancer and syndrome of inappropriate secretion of antidiuretic hormone (SIADH) who has had a seizure following intravenous saline. (Endocrinology)

Follow-up inpatient consultation for a 22-year-old female, established patient, with steroid-dependent systemic lupus erythematosus, arthritis, and glomerulonephritis. Patient is reevaluated for loss of consciousness and chest pain. (Rheumatology)

Follow-up inpatient consultation for a 75-year-old diabetic with fever, chills, a gangrenous heel ulcer, rhonchi, and dyspnea who appears lethargic and tachypneic. (Endocrinology)

Follow-up inpatient consultation for a 30-year-old established patient, with intractable neck and low back pain, who is excessively sedated after institution of methadone therapy. (Pain Medicine)

Follow-up inpatient consultation for a 65-year-old man with a history of hypertension and MI who is five days post uncomplicated GI procedure with an unremarkable postoperative recovery. He has just been resuscitated from a cardiopulmonary arrest. (Cardiology)

99263 Follow-up hospital consultation of an AIDS patient admitted with a sore throat who now has enlarging neck mass. (Otolaryngology, Head & Neck Surgery)

Follow-up hospital consultation of a pansinusitis patient with sudden onset of proptosis. (Otolaryngology, Head & Neck Surgery)

Follow-up inpatient consultation for a 53-year-old man with known angina who develops crescendo angina post cholecystectomy. (Cardiology)

Critical Care Services

99291 First hour of critical care of a 65-year-old man with septic shock following relief of ureteral obstruction caused by a stone.

First hour of critical care of a 15-year-old with acute respiratory failure from asthma.

First hour of critical care of a 45-year-old who sustained a liver laceration, cerebral hematoma, flailed chest and pulmonary contusion after being struck by an automobile.

First hour of critical care of a 65-year-old woman who, following a hysterectomy, suffered a cardiac arrest associated with a pulmonary embolus.

First hour of critical care of a 6-month-old child with hypovolemic shock secondary to diarrhea and dehydration.

First hour of critical care of a 3-year-old child with respiratory failure secondary to pneumocystis carinii pneumonia.

Prolonged Services

Prolonged Physician Service With Direct (Face-to-Face) Patient Contact

Office or Other Outpatient

99354/ Twenty-year-old female with history of asthma presents
99355 with acute bronchospasm and moderate respiratory distress. Initial evaluation shows respiratory rate 30, labored breathing and wheezing heard in all lung fields. Office treatment is initiated which includes intermittent bronchial dilation and subcutaneous epinephrine. Requires intermittent physician face-to-face time with patient over a period of 2-3 hours. (Family Medicine/ Internal Medicine)

Inpatient

99356 34-year-old primigravida presents to hospital in early labor. Admission history and physical reveals severe preeclampsia. Physician supervises management of preeclampsia, IV magnesium initiation and maintenance, labor augmentation with pitocin, and close maternal-fetal monitoring. Physician face-to-face involvement includes 40 minutes of continuous bedside care until the patient is stable, then is intermittent over several hours until the delivery. (Family Medicine/Internal Medicine/Obstetrics & Gynecology)

Prolonged Physician Service Without Direct Patient (Face-to-Face) Contact

99358/ A 65-year-old new patient with multiple problems, is
99359 seen and evaluated. After the visit, the physician requires extensive time to talk with the patient's daughter, to review complex, detailed medical records transferred from previous physicians and to complete a comprehensive treatment plan. This plan also requires the physician to personally initiate and coordinate the care plan with a local home health agency and a dietician. (Family Medicine/Internal Medicine)

Physician Standby Services

99360 A 24-year-old patient is admitted to OB unit attempting VBAC. Fetal monitoring shows increasing fetal distress.

Patient's blood pressure is rising and labor progressing slowly. A primary care physician is requested by the OB/GYN to standby in the unit for possible cesarean delivery and neonatal resuscitation. (Family Medicine/Internal Medicine)

Care Plan Oversight Services

99375 First month of care plan oversight for terminal care of a 58-year-old woman with advanced intraabdominal ovarian cancer. Care plan includes home oxygen, diuretics IV for edema and ascites control and pain control management involving IV morphine infusion when progressive ileus occurred. Physician phone contacts with nurse, family and MSW. Discussion with MSW concerning plans to withdraw supportive measures per patient wishes. Documentation includes review and modification of care plan and certifications from nursing, MSW, pharmacy and DME. (Family Medicine/Internal Medicine)

Index

Instructions for the Use of the CPT Index

Main Terms

The index is organized by main terms. Each main term can stand alone, or be followed by up to 3 modifying terms. There are 4 primary classes of main entries:

1. Procedure or service.
For example: Endoscopy; Anastomosis; Splint

2. Organ or other anatomic site.
For example: Tibia; Colon; Salivary Gland

3. Condition.
For example: Abscess; Entropion; Tetralogy of Fallot

4. Synonyms, Eponyms and Abbreviations.
For example: EEG; Bricker Operation; Clagett Procedure

Modifying Terms

A main term may be followed by a series of up to 3 indented terms that modify the main term. When modifying terms appear, one should review the list, as these subterms do have an effect on the selection of the appropriate code for the procedure.

Code Ranges

Whenever more than one code applies to a given index entry, a code range is listed. If two sequential codes or several non-sequential codes apply, they will be separated by a comma. For example:

Debridement
  Mastoid Cavity. 69220, 69222

If more than two sequential codes apply, they will be separated by a hyphen. For example:

Antibody
  Antitrypsin, Alpha-1 86064-86067

Cross References

Cross references provide instructions to the user. There are 2 types of cross references.

1. "See"—This directs the user to refer to the term listed after the word "See." This type of reference is used primarily for synonyms, eponyms and abbreviations.

2. "See Also"—This directs the user to look under another main term if the procedure is not listed under the first main index entry.

Other Conventions

As a space saving convention, certain words infer some meaning. This convention is primarily used when a procedure or service is listed as a sub-term. For example:

Knee
  Incision (of)

In this example, the word in parentheses (of) does not appear in the index, but it is inferred. As another example:

Pancreas
  Anesthesia (for procedures on)

In this example, as there is no such entity as pancreas anesthesia, the words in parentheses are inferred. That is, anesthesia for procedures on the pancreas.

The alphabetic index is NOT a substitute for the main text of CPT. Even if only one code appears, the user must refer to the main text to ensure that the code selection is accurate.

A

Patch
    Application Tests 95044
Photo Patch 95052
Photosensitivity 95056
Provocative Testing 95078
Skin Tests
    Allergen Extract 95004
    Biologicals 95010
    Drugs 95010
    End Point Titration. 95027
    Venoms. 95010

Allograft
with Lung Transplant 32850
Skin. 15350
Spine Surgery
    Morselized 20930
    Structural 20931

Alloplastic Dressing
Burns. 16040–16042

Allotransportation
Renal. 50360–50365
    Removal 50370

Almen Test
See Blood, Feces

Alpha-2 Antiplasmin 85410

Alpha-1 Antitrypsin. . . . 82103–82104

Alpha-Fetoprotein 82105
Amniotic Fluid 82106

Alphatocopherol. 84446

Altemeier Procedure
See Rectum, Prolapse, Excision

Aluminum
Blood 82108

Alveolar Cleft
Ungrafted Bilateral. 21147
Ungrafted Unilateral. 21146

Alveolar Nerve
Avulsion 64738
Incision 64738
Transection. 64738

Alveolar Ridge
Fracture
    Closed Treatment. 21440
    Open Treatment 21445

Alveolectomy. 41830

Alveoli
Fracture
    Closed Treatment. 21421
    Open Treatment 21422–21423

Alveoloplasty. 41874

Alveolus
Excision 41830

Amikacin
Assay 80150

Amino Acid 82131
Blood or Urine 82128–82130

Aminolevulinic Acid (ALA)
Blood or Urine 82135

Amitriptyline
Assay 80152

Ammonia
Blood 82140
Urine. 82140

Amniocentesis. 59000
See also Chromosome Analysis
Anesthesia 00842
Induced Abortion 59850
    with Dilation and Curettage 59851
    with Dilation and Evacuation. . . . 59851
    with Hysterectomy. 59852

Amnion
Amniocentesis 59000

Amniotic Fluid
Alpha-Fetoprotein. 82106
Scan 82143
Testing 83661

Amobarbital 82205–82210

AMP
See Adenosine Monophosphate (AMP)

Amphetamine
Blood or Urine 82145

Amputation
See also Radical Resection; Replantation
Ankle 27888
Arm, Lower 24900–24920,
                        25900, 25905, 25915
    Cineplasty 24940
    with Implant 24931–24935
    Revision. 24925–24930,
                        25907, 25909
Arm, Upper 24900–24920
    with Implant 24931–24935
    Revision. 24925–24930
    and Shoulder 23900–23921
Cervix
    Total 57530
Ear
    Partial. 69110
    Total 69120
Femur
    Anesthesia 01232
Finger 26910, 26951–26952
Foot. 28800, 28805
Hand
    at Metacarpal. 25927
    Revision 25924, 25929, 25931
    at Wrist 25920, 25922
Interpelviabdominal
    Anesthesia 01140
Interthoracoscapular 23900
    Anesthesia 01636
Leg, Lower 27598, 27880–27882
    Revision 27884, 27886

Leg, Upper 27590–27592
    at Hip 27290, 27295
    Revision 27594, 27596
Metatarsal 28810
Penis
    Anesthesia 00932–00936
    Partial. 54120
    Radical 54130, 54135
    Total 54125
Thumb. 26910, 26951–26952
Toe 28810, 28820, 28825
Tuft of Distal Phalanx 11752

Amylase
Blood 82150
Urine. 82150

ANA
See Antinuclear Antibodies (ANA)

Anabolic Steroid
See Androstenedione

Analgesia
See also Anesthesia
Cesarean Section 00857
Epidural
    Drug Administration. 01996
    Labor. 00857, 00955
Subarachnoid Drug Administration . . . 01996
Vaginal Delivery 00955

Anal Sphincter
Dilation. 45905
Incision 46080

Analysis
Computer Data. 99090
Electroencephalogram
    Digital. 95957
Electronic
    Cardioverter-Defibrillator . 93737–93738
    Drug Infusion Pump 62367–62368
    Pulse Generator 63690–63691

Anastomosis
Arteriovenous Fistula
    Direct 36821
    with Graft 36825, 36830, 36832
Artery
    to Aorta 33606
    to Artery
        Cranial. 61711
Bile Duct
    to Bile Duct 47800
    to Intestines 47760, 47780
Bile Duct to Gastrointestinal 47785
Broncho-Bronchial 32486
Caval to Mesenteric. 37160
Epididymis
    to Vas Deferens
        Bilateral. 54901
        Unilateral. 54900
Excision
    Trachea 31775, 31780
Fallopian Tube 58750
Gallbladder to Intestines. . . . 47720–47721,
                                    47740

Anderson Tibial Lengthening
See Tibia, Osteoplasty, Lengthening

Androstanediol Glucuronide

Androstenedione

Androsterone

Anesthesia
See also Analgesia

Aneurysm Repair

Angiography

See also Aortography

Angioplasty

Carpometacarpal Joint 26070, 26100
Elbow 24000
   Capsular Release 24006
   with Joint Exploration 24101
   with Synovectomy 24101
   with Synovial Biopsy 24100
Finger Joint 26075, 26105, 26110
Glenohumeral Joint 23040
Hip 27030, 27033, 27052, 27054
Interphalangeal Joint 26080, 26110
   Toe 28024, 28054
Intertarsal Joint 28020, 28050
Knee 27310, 27330–27335, 27403
Metacarpophalangeal Joint . . 26075, 26105
Metatarsophalangeal Joint 28022
Sacroiliac Joint 27050
Shoulder Joint
   Exploration and/or Removal of Loose
   or Foreign Body 23107
Sternoclavicular Joint 23044
with Synovectomy
   Glenohumeral Joint 23105
   Sternoclavicular Joint 23106
Tarsometatarsal Joint 28020,
                    28050, 28052
Temporomandibular Joint 21010
Wrist 25040, 25100–25101,
                     25105, 25107

Artificial Eye
See Prosthesis

Artificial Insemination 58976
See also In Vitro Fertilization
Intra-Cervical 58321
Intra-Uterine 58322
Sperm Washing 58323

Arytenoid
Excision
   Endoscopic 31560–31561

Arytenoid Cartilage
Excision 31400
Repair 31400

Arytenoidectomy 31400, 31560

Arytenoidopexy 31400

Ascorbic Acid
Blood 82180

Aspartate Aminotransferase 80002–80019

Aspergillus
Antibody 86606

Aspiration
See also Puncture Aspiration
Bladder 51000–51010
Bone Marrow 85095
Brain Lesion
   Stereotactic 61750–61751
Bronchi
   Endoscopy 31645–31646
Bronchus
   Nasotracheal 31720

Catheter
   Nasotracheal 31720
   Tracheobronchial 31725
Cyst
   Bone 20615
   Kidney 50390
   Pelvis 50390
   Spinal Cord 62268
   Thyroid 60001
Duodenal 89100–89105
Laryngoscopy
   Direct 31515
Lens Material 66840
Liver 47015
Lung 32420
Nucleus of Disk
   Lumbar 62287
Orbital Contents 67415
Pelvis
   Endoscopy 56306
Pericardium 33010–33011
Pleural Cavity 32000–32002
Puncture
   Cyst
      Breast 19000–19001
Spinal Cord
   Stereotaxis 63615
Syrinx
   Spinal Cord 62268
Thyroid 60001
Trachea
   Nasotracheal 31720
   Puncture 31612
Tunica Vaginalis
   Hydrocele 55000
Vitreous 67015

Astragalectomy 28130

Ataxia Telangiectasia
Chromosome Analysis 88248

Atherectomy
See also X-Ray, Artery, Atherectomy
Open
   Aorta 35481
   Brachiocephalic 35484
   Femoral 35483
   Iliac 35482
   Popliteal 35483
   Renal 35480
   Tibioperoneal 35485
   Visceral 35480
Percutaneous
   Aorta 35491
   Brachiocephalic 35494
   Coronary 92995–92996
   Femoral 35493
   Iliac 35492
   Popliteal 35493
   Renal 35490
   Tibioperoneal 35495
   Visceral 35490
X-Ray
   Peripheral Artery 75992–75993
   Renal Artery 75994
   Visceral Artery 75995–75996

Atomic Absorption Spectroscopy 82190

Atresia, Congenital
Auditory Canal, External
   Reconstruction 69320

Atria
Reconstruction 33253

Atrial Electrogram
Esophageal Recording 93615–93616

Atticotomy 69631, 69635

Audiologic Function Tests
See also Hearing Evaluation
Acoustic Reflex 92568
Acoustic Reflex Decay 92569
Audiometry
   Bekesy 92560, 92561
   Comprehensive 92557
   Conditioning Play 92582
   Groups 92559
   Pure Tone 92552, 92553
   Select Picture 92583
   Speech 92555–92556
   Visual Reinforcement 92579
Central Auditory Function 92589
Electrocochleography 92584
Evoked Otoacoustic Emission 92587,
                         92588
Filtered Speech 92571
Lombard Test 92573
Loudness Balance 92562
Screening 92551
Sensorineural Acuity 92575
Short Increment Sensitivity Index 92564
Staggered Spondaic Word Test 92572
Stenger Test 92565, 92577
Synthetic Sentence Test 92576
Tone Decay 92563

Audiometry
Bekesy 92560, 92561
Brainstem Evoked Response 92585
Comprehensive 92557
Conditioning Play 92582
Groups 92559
Pure Tone 92552, 92553
Select Picture 92583
Speech 92555–92556
Tympanometry 92567

Auditory Canal
Decompression 61591
External
   Abscess
      Incision and Drainage 69020
   Biopsy 69105
   Lesion
      Excision 69140, 69145,
                  69150, 69155
   Reconstruction
      for Congenital Atresia 69320
      for Stenosis 69310

B

Bicuspid Valve
See Mitral Valve

Bifid Digit
Repair........................26585

Bifrontal Craniotomy 61557

Bile Acids..................82239
Blood 82240

Bile Duct
See also Gallbladder
Anastomosis
    Cyst 47716
    with Intestines 47760,
               47780, 47785
Biopsy
    Endoscopy 47553
Catheterization.................75982
Change Catheter Tube 75984
Cyst
    Excision 47715
    Repair....................47716
Destruction
    Calculi (Stone) 43265
Dilation
    Endoscopy...... 43271, 47555–47556
Drainage
    Transhepatic................75980
Endoscopy
    Biopsy....................47553
    Destruction
        Calculi (Stone) 43265
        Tumor 43271
    Dilation....... 43271, 47555–47556
    Exploration 47552
    Intraoperative...............47550
    Removal
        Calculi (Stone)....... 43264, 47554
        Foreign Body.............43269
        Stent 43269
    Specimen Collection 43260
    Sphincterotomy 43262
    Sphincter Pressure............43263
    Tube Placement 43267–43268
Exploration
    Atresia 47700
    Endoscopy 47552
Incision
    Sphincter 43262, 47460
Incision and Drainage...... 47420, 47425
Insertion
    Catheter............ 47510, 47525,
               47530, 75982
    Stent................ 47511, 47801
Nuclear Medicine
    Imaging...................78223
Reconstruction
    Anastomosis................47800
Removal
    Calculi (Stone)........ 43264, 47420,
           47425, 47554, 47630
    Foreign Body 43269
    Stent....................43269
Repair........................47701
    Cyst 47716

Gastrointestinal Tract...........47785
    with Intestines 47760, 47780
Tube Placement
    Nasobiliary.................43267
    Stent.....................43268
Tumor
    Destruction.................43271
    Excision 47711–47712
Unlisted Services and Procedures....47999
X-Ray
    with Contrast 74300–74320
        Guide Catheter 74328, 74330
        Guide Stone Removal........ 74327
        Guide Dilation 74360

Bilirubin
Blood...................82250–82251
Feces 82252

Billroth I or II
See Gastrectomy, Partial

Binet-Simon Test 96100

Binet Test....................96100

Binocular Microscopy 92504

Biofeedback
Anorectal 90911
Blood Flow 90906
Blood Pressure.................90904
Brainwaves....................90908
EEG (Electroencephalogram) 90908
Electromyogram 90900
Electro-oculogram..............90910
EMG (with Anorectal)............90911
Eyelids 90910
Nerve Conduction...............90902
Unlisted Services and Procedures....90915

Biometry
Eye 76516–76519

Biopsy
See also Brush Biopsy; Needle Biopsy
Abdomen 49000
Adrenal Gland............60540–60545
Anal
    Endoscopy 46606
Ankle............ 27613–27614, 27620
Anorectal
    Anesthesia 00902
Arm, Lower.............. 25065–25066
Arm, Upper.............. 24065–24066
Artery
    Temporal..................37609
with Arthrotomy
    Acromioclavicular Joint 23101
    Glenohumeral Joint 23100
    Sternoclavicular Joint 23101
Auditory Canal, External 69105
Back/Flank 21920–21925
Bile Duct
    Endoscopy 47553
Bladder.......................52204
    Cystourethroscopy 52224, 52250
Blood Vessel
    Transcatheter 75970

Bone 20220–20245
Bone Marrow 85102
Brain.........................61140
    Stereotactic 61750–61751
Brainstem 61575–61576
Breast 19100–19101
    Stereotactic 76095
Bronchi
    Catheterization...............31717
    Endoscopic 31625–31629
Brush
    Bronchi....................31717
    with Cystourethroscopy .. 52204, 52338
    Renal Pelvis.................52007
    Ureter.....................52007
Carpometacarpal Joint
    Synovium 26100
Cervix 57500, 57520
Chorionic Villus 59015
Clavicle
    Anesthesia 00454
Colon............... 44025, 44100
    Endoscopy 44389, 45380
    Multiple 44322
Colon-Sigmoid
    Endoscopy 45305, 45331
Conjunctiva....................68100
Cornea 65410
Duodenum 44010
Ear
    Anesthesia 00120
    External 69100
Elbow 24065–24066, 24101
Endometrium 56351, 58100
Epididymis 54820
Esophagus
    Endoscopy 43202
Eyelid 67810
Eye Muscle....................67350
Gallbladder
    Endoscopy 43261
Gastrointestinal, Upper
    Endoscopy 43239
Genital System
    Anesthesia 00900
Hand Joint
    Synovium 26100
Heart.........................93505
Hip 27040–27041
    Joint......................27052
Hypopharynx...................42802
Ileum
    Endoscopy 44382
Integumentary System,
    Anesthesia 00100
Interphalangeal Joint
    Finger Synovium 26110
    Toe Synovium...............28054
Intertarsal Joint
    Synovial 28050
Intestines, Small.......... 44020, 44100
    Endoscopy 44361, 44377
Intraoral Procedures
    Anesthesia 00170
Kidney........................50205

Birthing Room

Bischof Procedure
See Laminectomy, Surgical

Bladder

Blalock-Hanlon

Blalock-Taussig Procedure
See Shunt, Great Vessel

Blastomyces

Bleeding
See Hemorrhage

Bleeding Time 85002

Bleeding Tube
Passage and Placement 91100

Blepharoplasty 15820–15823
See also Canthoplasty
Anesthesia 00103
Ectropion
    Excision Tarsal Wedge 67916
    Extensive 67917
Entropion 67923–67924
    Excision Tarsal Wedge 67923
    Extensive 67924

Blepharoptosis
Repair 67901–67909
    Frontalis Muscle Technique 67901
    with Fascial Sling 67902
    Superior Rectus Technique with Fascial
    Sling 67906
    Tarso Levator Resection/Advancement
    External Approach 67904
    Internal Approach 67903

Blepharospasm
Chemodenervation 64612

Blepharotomy 67700

Blom-Singer Prosthesis 31611

Blood
Bleeding Time 85002
Collection, for Autotransfusion
    Intraoperative 86891
    Preoperative 86890
Feces 82270
Gastric Contents 82273
Harvesting of Stem Cells 38231
Nuclear Medicine
    Flow Imaging 78445
    Plasma Iron 78160
    Red Cell 78140
    Survival 78130–78135
Osmolality 83930
Other Source 82273
Plasma
    Exchange 36520
Platelet
    Aggregation 85576
    Automated Count 85595
    Count 85585
    Manual Count 85590
Stem Cell Transplantation . . . 38240–38241
Transfusion 36430, 36440
    Exchange 36455
        Newborn 36450
    Fetal 36460
Unlisted Services and Procedures 85999
Urine 83491
Viscosity 85810

Blood Banking
Frozen Blood Preparation 86930–86932
Frozen Plasma Preparation 86927

Physician Services 86077–86079

Blood Cell
Exchange 36520
Sedimentation Rate
    Automated 85652
    Manual 85651
Stem 38231

Blood Cell Count 85014
Differential WBC Count 85007, 85009
Hemoglobin 85018
Hemogram
    Added Indices 85029–85030
    Automated 85021–85027
    Manual 85031
Manual Blood Smear 85008
Microhematocrit 85013
Other 85014
Red Blood Cells 85041
Reticulocyte 85044–85045
T-Cells 86359, 86360
White Blood Cells 85048

Blood Clot
Clot Lysis Time 85175
Clot Retraction 85170
Clotting Factor 85250–85293
Clotting Factor Test 85210–85244
Clotting Inhibitors . . . 85300–85302, 85305
Coagulation Time 85345–85348

Blood Flow Check, Graft 15860

Blood Gases
CO_2 82803
HCO_2 82803
O_2 Saturation 82805–82810
pCO_2 82803
pH 82800–82803
pO_2 82803

Blood Pool Imaging
Cardiac 78472–78473, 78481–78483

Blood Pressure
Monitoring 93784–93790
Venous 93770

Blood Products
Irradiation 86945
Pooling 86965
Splitting 86985

Blood Sample
Fetal 59030

Blood Smear 85060

Blood Syndrome
Chromosome Analysis 88245–88248

Blood Tests
Iron, Chelatable 78172
Nuclear Medicine
    Iron Absorption 78162
    Plasma Volume 78110–78111
    Platelet Survival 78190–78191
    Red Cell Iron 78170
    Red Cell Volume 78120–78121

Whole Blood Volume 78122
Panels
    Arthritis Panel 80072
    General Health Panel 80050
    Hepatic Function 80058
    Hepatitis 80059
    Lipid Panel 80061
    Obstetric Panel 80055
    Torch Antibody Panel 80090
Volume Determination 78122

Blood Typing
ABO Only 86900
Antigen Screen 86903–86904
Crossmatch 86920, 86921–86922
Other RBC Antigens 86905
Paternity Testing 86910
Rh (D) 86901
Rh Phenotype 86906

Blood Urea Nitrogen . . . 84520–84525

Blood Vessels
See also Artery; Vein
Abdomen
    Anesthesia 00770, 00880–00884
Chest
    Anesthesia 00560–00562
Excision
    Arteriovenous
    Malformation 63250–63252
Exploration
    Abdomen 35840
    Chest 35820
    Extremity 35860
    Neck 35800
Great
    Suture 33320, 33321
Kidney
    Repair 50100
Repair
    See also Aneurysm Repair; Fistula,
    Repair
    Abdomen 35221, 35251, 35281
    Aneurysm 61705, 61708
    Arteriovenous
    Malformation 61680–61692,
      61705, 61708, 63250–63252
    Chest 35211, 35216, 35241,
        35246, 35271, 35276
    Finger 35207
    Graft Defect 35870
    Hand 35207
    Lower Extremity 35226,
        35256, 35286
    Neck 35201, 35231, 35261
    Upper Extremity 35206,
        35236, 35266
Shunt Creation
    Direct 36821
    with Graft 36825, 36830
    Thomas Shunt 36835
Shunt Revision
    with Graft 36832

Bloom Syndrome
Chromosome Analysis 88245

Repair
Abdomen 35907
Extremity 35903
Neck 35901
Thorax 35905
Revascularization
Extremity 35903
Neck 35901
Thorax 35905
Secondary Repair 35870
Splenic Artery 35536, 35636
Subclavian Artery 35506–35507,
35511, 35515–35516,
35526, 35606–35616,
35626, 35638, 35645
Thrombectomy 35875–35876
Tibial Artery 35566, 35571,
35623, 35666, 35671
Vertebral Artery 35508, 35515,
35637–35638, 35642, 35645

Bypass In-Situ
Femoral Artery 35582–35583, 35585
Peroneal Artery 35585, 35587
Popliteal Artery 35582–35583, 35587
Tibial Artery 35585, 35587

C

CABG
See Coronary Artery Bypass Graft (CABG)

Cadmium
Urine 82300

Calcaneus
Craterization 28120
Cyst
Excision 28100, 28102–28103
Diaphysectomy 28120
Excision 28118–28120
Fracture
with Manipulation 28405–28406
without Manipulation 28400
Open Treatment 28415, 28420
Repair
Osteotomy 28300
Saucerization 28120
Tumor
Excision 27647, 28100,
28102–28103
X-Ray 73650

Calcareous Deposits
Subdeltoid
Removal 23000

Calcifediol
Blood or Urine 82306

Calciferol
Blood or Urine 82307

Calcitonin
Blood or Urine 82308
Stimulation Panel 80410

Calcium
Blood
Infusion Test 82331
Deposits
See Calcareous Deposits; Removal,
Calculi (Stone)
Ionized 82330
Total 82310
Urine 82335–82340

Calcium-Pentagastrin Stimulation .
80410

Calculus
Analysis 82355–82370
Removal
Bladder 51050, 52310–52315,
52317–52330
Kidney 50060–50081,
50130, 50561, 50580
Ureter . 50610–50630, 50961, 50980,
52320–52330, 52336
Urethra 52310–52315

Caldwell-Luc Procedure
See also Sinus, Maxillary; Sinusotomy;
Sternum, Fracture
Orbital Floor Blowout Fracture 21385
Sinusotomy 31030–31032

Caliper
Application/Removal 20660

Callander Knee Disarticulation
See Disarticulation, Knee

Caloric Vestibular Test 92533,
92543

Calycoplasty 50405

Camey Enterocystoplasty 50825

Campbell Procedure 27422

Campylobacter
Antibody 86625

Canaloplasty 69631, 69635

Candida
Antibody 86628
Skin Test 86485

Cannulation 36821
Arterial 36620, 36625
Sinus
Maxillary 31000
Sphenoid 31002
Thoracic Duct 38794

Cannulization
See also Catheterization
Arteriovenous 36145, 36810, 36815
Declotting 36860–36861
ECMO 36822
Vas Deferens 55200
Vein to Vein 36800

Canthoplasty 67950
See also Blepharoplasty; Capsulodesis
Lateral 21282
Medial 21280

Canthorrhaphy 67880, 67882

Canthotomy 67715

Canthus
Reconstruction 67950

Capsule
See also Capsulodesis
Elbow
Arthrotomy 24006
Foot 28264
Interphalangeal Joint
Excision 26525
Incision 26525
Knee 27435
Metacarpophalangeal Joint
Excision 26520
Incision 26520
Shoulder 23020
Wrist
Excision 25320

Capsulodesis
Metacarpophalangeal Joint . . 26516–26518

Capsulorrhaphy
Anterior 23450–23462
Multi-Directional Instability 23466
Posterior 23465
Wrist 25320

Capsulotomy
Breast
Periprosthetic 19370–19371
Foot 28260–28262
Metacarpophalangeal Joint 26520
Toe 28270, 28272
Wrist 25085

Captopril 80416

Carbamazepine
Assay 80156

Carbon Dioxide
Blood or Urine 82374

Carbon Monoxide
Blood 82375–82376

Carbon Tetrachloride 84600

Carboxyhemoglobin . . . 82375–82376

Carbuncle
Incision and Drainage 10060–10061

Carcinoembryonic Antigen . . . 82378

Cardiac Catheterization
Anesthesia 01920
Balloon Catheter 93536
for Biopsy 93505
for Dilation Study 93561–93562
Imaging 93555–93556
Injection 93539–93540

Fracture
  Closed Treatment with
    Manipulation 21355
    Open Treatment 21360–21365
  Muscle Graft. 15841–15845
  Muscle Transfer 15845
  Reconstruction 21270
  Rhytidectomy 15828
  Skin Graft
    Delay of Flap 15620
    Full Thickness. 15240–15241
    Pedicle Flap 15574
  Tissue Transfer, Adjacent . . . 14040–14041

Chemical Cauterization
Granulation Tissue 17250

Chemical Exfoliation. 17360

Chemical Peel 15788–15793

Chemiluminescent Assay 82397

Chemistry Tests
Clinical
  Automated
    Blood or Urine 80002–80019
  Unlisted Services and
    Procedures 84999

Chemocauterization
Corneal Epithelium 65435
  with Chelating Agent 65436

Chemodenervation
Cervical Spinal Muscle 64613
Extraocular Muscle 67345
Facial Muscle 64612

Chemonucleolysis 62292
Anesthesia 00634

Chemosurgery
Moh's Technique 17304–17310

Chemotaxis Assay 86155

Chemotherapy
Arterial Catheterization 36640
Bladder Instillation. 51720
CNS 96450
Intra-Arterial 96420–96425
Intralesional 96405–96406
Intramuscular 96400
Intravenous 96408–96414
Peritoneal Cavity 96445
Pleural Cavity 96440–96445
Pump Services
  Implantable 96530
  Portable 96520
Subcutaneous 96400, 96542
Supply of Agent 96545
Unlisted Services and Procedures 96549

Chest
See also Mediastinum; Thorax
Anesthesia 00400–00410,
                         00470–00474,
          00520–00530, 00540–00548

Artery
  Ligation. 37616
CAT Scan 71250–71270
Exploration
  Blood Vessel 35820
Magnetic Resonance Imaging (MRI) . 71550
Repair
  Blood Vessel . . . 35211, 35216, 35241,
                   35246, 35271, 35276
Ultrasound 76604
Wound Exploration
  Penetrating. 20100
X-Ray. 71010–71038, 71090
  with Fluoroscopy 71023, 71034,
                      71038, 71090
  Guide Biopsy 71036, 71038
  Insertion Pacemaker 71090
  Stereo. 71015

Chest Cavity
Bypass Graft. 35905
Endoscopy
  Exploration 32601–32606
  Therapeutic. 32654–32665

Chest Wall
Anesthesia 00400–00474
Manipulation 94667–94668
Reconstruction 49905
  Trauma 32820
Repair 32905
  Closure 32810
  Fistula. 32906
Tumor
  Excision 19260–19272
Unlisted Services and Procedures. . . . 32999

Chevron Procedure 28296

Chicken Pox (Varicella)
Immunization 90716

Childbirth
Cesarean Section
  Analgesia 00857
  Anesthesia 00850
Vaginal Delivery
  Analgesia 00955
  Anesthesia 00946

Child Procedure
See Excision, Pancreas, Partial

Chin
Repair
  Augmentation. 21120
  Osteotomy 21121–21123
Rhytidectomy 15828
Skin Graft
  Delay of Flap 15620
  Full Thickness. 15240–15241
  Pedicle Flap 15574
Tissue Transfer, Adjacent . . . 14040–14041

Chlamydia
Antibody 86631–86632
Culture 87110

Chloramphenicol 82415

Chloride
Blood 82435
Other Source 82438
Spinal Fluid 82438
Urine. 82436

Chlorinated Hydrocarbons . . . 82441

Chlorpromazine. 84022

Choanal Atresia
Repair 30540–30545

Cholangiography
  with Bile Duct Exploration. 47700
    with Cholecystectomy . . . 47605, 47620
Injection 47500, 47505
Intraoperative 74300, 74301
Percutaneous 74320
  with Peritoneoscopy. 56362–56363
Postoperative 74305

Cholangiopancreatography . . . 43260
See also Bile Duct; Pancreatic Duct
  with Biopsy 43261
  with Surgery 43262–43265,
                 43267, 43269

Cholecystectomy 47600–47620
Any Method 56340
  with Cholangiography 56341
  with Exploration Common Duct. . 56342
  with Peritoneoscopy 56362

Cholecystenterostomy 56324

Cholecystography 74290–74291

Cholecystostomy 47480

Cholecystotomy 47480, 48001
Percutaneous 47490

Choledochoscopy 47550

Choledochostomy 47420, 47425

Choledochotomy 47420, 47425

Cholera Vaccine 90725

Cholesterol
Measurement 83721
Serum. 82465
Testing 83718–83719

Cholinesterase
Blood. 82480–82482

Chondroitin Sulfate. 82485

Chopart Procedure
See Amputation, Foot

Chorionic Gonadotropin. 80414,
                   84702–84703
Stimulation. 80415

Chorionic Villus
Biopsy. 59015

Choroid Plexus
Excision 61544

Christmas Factor 85250

X-Ray 72220

Cochlear Device
Insertion 69930

Codeine
Alkaloid Screening 82101

Codeine Screen 82486

Coffey Operation
See Uterus, Repair, Suspension

Cognitive Function Tests 96115

Cognitive Skills Development .
97770

Cold Agglutinin 86156–86157

Cold Pack Treatment 97010

Colectomy
Partial 44140
   with Anastomosis 44140
   with Coloproctostomy . . . 44145–44146
   with Colostomy . . 44141, 44143–44144
   with Ileostomy 44144
   with Transcanal Approach 44147
Total
   with Anastomosis 44152
   with Ileal Reservoir 44153
   with Ileostomy 44150–44151
   with Ileum Removal 44160
   with Proctectomy 44155–44156

Collagen Injection 11950–11954

Collar Bone
See Clavicle

Collateral Ligament
Ankle
   Repair 27695–27696
Interphalangeal Joint 26545
Knee Joint
   Repair 27407
Knee Repair 27405
Metacarpophalangeal Joint . . 26540–26542
Repair
   Ankle 27698

Collection and Processing
Autologous Blood
   Harvesting of Stem Cells 38231
   Intraoperative 86891
   Preoperative 86890
Specimen
   Venous Blood 36415
Washings
   Esophagus 91000
   Stomach 91055

Colles Fracture 25600, 25605,
25611, 25620

Collis Procedure
See Gastroplasty with Esophagogastric
Fundoplasty

Colon
See also Colon-Sigmoid

Biopsy 44025, 44100, 44322
   Endoscopic 44389, 45380
Colotomy 44320, 44322
   Revision 44340, 44345–44346
Destruction
   Lesion 44393, 45383
   Tumor 44393, 45383
Endoscopy
   Biopsy 44389, 45380
   via Colotomy 45355
   Destruction
      Lesion 44393
      Tumor 44393, 45383
   Exploration 44388, 45378
   Hemorrhage 44391, 45382
   Removal
      Foreign Body 44390, 45379
      Polyp 44392, 45384–45385
      Tumor 45384–45385
   Specimen Collection 45380
   via Stoma 44388–44394
Excision
   Partial . . 44140–44141, 44143–44147
   Total 44150–44160
Exploration 44025
   Endoscopy 44388, 45378
Hemorrhage
   Endoscopic Control 44391, 45382
Hernia 44050
Incision
   Creation
      Stoma 44320, 44322
   Exploration 44025
   Revision
      Stoma 44340, 44345–44346
Lesion
   Destruction 45383
   Excision 44110–44111
Lysis
   Adhesions 44005
Obstruction 44025, 44050
Reconstruction
   Bladder from 50810
Removal
   Foreign Body 44025, 44390, 45379
   Polyp 44392
Repair
   Diverticula 44605
   Fistula 44650, 44660–44661
   Hernia 44050
   Malrotation 44055
   Obstruction 44050
   Ulcer 44605
   Volvulus 44050
   Wound 44605
Stoma Closure 44620, 44625
Suture
   Diverticula 44605
   Fistula 44650, 44660–44661
   Plication 44680
   Stoma 44620, 44625
   Ulcer 44605
   Wound 44605
Tumor
   Destruction 45383

Unlisted Services and Procedures 44799
X-Ray with Contrast
   Barium Enema 74270–74280

Colonna Procedure
See Acetabulum, Reconstruction

Colonoscopy
Biopsy 45380
Collection Specimen 45380
   via Colotomy 45355
Destruction
   Lesion 45383
   Tumor 45383
Hemorrhage Control 45382
Removal
   Foreign Body 45379
   Polyp 45384–45385
   Tumor 45384–45385
via Stoma 44388–44390
   Biopsy 44389
   Destruction
      of Lesion 44393
      of Tumor 44393
   Exploration 44388, 45378
   Hemorrhage 44391
   Removal
      Foreign Body 44390
      Polyp 44392, 44394
      Tumor 44392, 44394

Colon-Sigmoid
See also Colon
Biopsy
   Endoscopy 45331
Endoscopy
   Ablation
      Polyp 45339
      Tumor 45339
   Biopsy 45331
   Exploration 45330
   Hemorrhage 45334
   Removal
      Foreign Body 45332
      Polyp 45333, 45338
      Tumor 45333, 45338
      Volvulus 45337
Exploration
   Endoscopy 45330
Hemorrhage
   Endoscopy 45334
Removal
   Foreign Body 45332
Repair
   Volvulus
      Endoscopy 45337

Colorrhaphy 44604

Color Vision Examination 92283

Colostomy 45563
Abdominal
   Establishment 50810
Perineal
   Establishment 50810

Colotomy 44025, 44320, 44322
Revision 44340, 44345–44346

Colpectomy
Anesthesia ... 00942
with Hysterectomy ... 58275
    with Repair of Enterocele ... 58280
Partial ... 57108
Total ... 57110

Colpocentesis ... 57020

Colpocleisis ... 57120

Colpoperineorrhaphy ... 57210

Colpopexy ... 57280

Colporrhaphy
Anesthesia ... 00942
Anterior ... 57240, 57289
Anteroposterior ... 57260
    with Enterocele Repair ... 57265
Nonobstetrical ... 57200
Posterior ... 57250

Colposcopy
Biopsy ... 57454
Exploration ... 57452
Loop Electrode Excision ... 57460

Colpotomy
Anesthesia ... 00942
Drainage
    Abscess ... 57010
Exploration ... 57000

Colpo-Urethrocystopexy ... 58152, 58267
Marshall-Marchetti-Krantz
Procedure ... 58152, 58267
Pereyra Procedure ... 58267

Combined Vaccine ... 90710–90711

Comedones
Removal ... 10040

Commissurotomy
Right Ventricle ... 33476, 33478

Community/Work Reintegration
Training ... 97537

Compatibility Test
Blood ... 86920

Complement ... 86162
Antigen ... 86160
Fixation Test ... 86171
Functional Activity ... 86161

Complete Blood Count (CBC) ... 85022–85025
See also Blood Cell Count
Manual ... 85031

Composite Graft ... 15760–15770

Computer Data Analysis ... 99090

Computerized Axial Tomography (CAT)
See CAT Scan

Concentration of Specimen ... 87015

Concentration Test for Renal Function
Water Load Test

Concentric Procedure ... 28296

Concha Bullosa Resection
with Nasal/Sinus Endoscopy ... 31240

Condyle
Humerus
    Fracture ... 24576–24577, 24579, 24582
Phalanges
    Toe
        Excision ... 28126

Condylectomy ... 21050
with Skull Base Surgery ... 61596–61597
Temporomandibular Joint ... 21050

Condyloma
Destruction ... 54050, 54065

Conference
Medical
    with Interdisciplinary
    Team ... 98910–98912, 99361–99362
    with Patient ... 98900–98902
Telephone
    Brief ... 98920
    Complex ... 98922
    Intermediate ... 98921

Confirmation
Drug ... 80102

Confirmatory Consultations
New or Established Patient ... 99271–99275

Congenital Kidney Abnormality
Nephrolithotomy ... 50070
Pyeloplasty ... 50405
Pyelotomy ... 50135

Conization
Cervix ... 57520–57522

Conjoint Psychotherapy ... 90847

Conjunctiva
Biopsy ... 68100
Cyst
    Incision and Drainage ... 68020
Fistulize for Drainage
    with Tube ... 68750
    without Tube ... 68745
Insertion Stent ... 68750
Lesion
    Destruction ... 68135
    Excision ... 68110–68130
Reconstruction ... 68320–68335
    with Flap
        Bridge or Partial ... 68360
        Total ... 68362
    Symblepharon
        with Graft ... 68335
        without Graft ... 68335
Repair
    Symblepharon
        Division ... 68340

    with Graft ... 68335
    without Graft ... 68330
Wound
    Direct Closure ... 65270
    Mobilization and
    Rearrangement ... 65272–65273
Unlisted Services and Procedures ... 68399

Conjunctivoplasty ... 68320–68330

Conjunctivorhinostomy
    with Tube ... 68750
    without Tube ... 68745

Conjunctivo-Tarso-Muller Resection ... 67908

Construction
Neobladder ... 51596
Vagina
    with Graft ... 57291
    without Graft ... 57292

Consultation
See also Second Opinion; Third Opinion
Confirmatory ... 99271–99275
    New or Established
    Patient ... 99271–99275
Follow-up Inpatient
    Established Patient ... 99261–99263
Initial Inpatient ... 99251–99255
    New or Established
    Patient ... 99251–99255
Office and/or Other
Outpatient ... 99241–99245
    New or Established
    Patient ... 99241–99245
Psychiatric, with Family ... 90887
Radiation Therapy
    Radiation Physics ... 77336, 77370
Surgical Pathology ... 80500–80502, 88321–88325
    Intraoperation ... 88329–88332
X-Ray ... 76140

Contact Lens Services
Fittings and Prescription ... 92070, 92310–92313
Modification ... 92325
Prescription ... 92314–92317
Replacement ... 92326
Supply ... 92391, 92396

Continuous Epidural Analgesia ... 00857, 00955

Continuous Negative Pressure Breathing (CNPB) ... 94662
See also Continuous Positive Airway Pressure (CPAP);
    Intermittent Positive Pressure
    Breathing (IPPB)

Continuous Positive Airway Pressure (CPAP) ... 94660
See also Continuous Negative Pressure Breathing (CNPB);
    Intermittent Positive Pressure
    Breathing (IPPB)

Contouring
Silicone Injections 11950–11954

Contraception
Cervical Cap
    Fitting 57170
Diaphragm
    Fitting 57170
Intrauterine Device (IUD)
    Insertion 58300
    Removal 58301

Contraceptive Capsules, Implantable
Insertion 11975
Removal 11976
    with Reinsertion 11977

Contracture
Palm
    Release 26121, 26123, 26125

Contrast Bath Therapy 97034

Contrast Material
Instillation
    Bronchography 31708
    Laryngography 31708

Coombs Test 86880

Copper 82525

Coprobilinogen
Feces 84577

Coproporphyrin 84120

Coracoacromial Ligament Release 23415

Coracoid Process Transfer 23462

Cordectomy 31300

Cordocentesis 59012

Cordotomy 63194–63199

Coreoplasty 66762

Cornea
Biopsy 65410
Curettage 65435–65436
    with Chelating Agent 65436
Epithelium
    Excision 65435–65436
        with Chelating Agent 65436
Lesion
    Destruction 65450
    Excision 65400
        without Graft 65420
Prosthesis 65770
Pterygium
    Excision 65420
Puncture 65600
Relaxing Incisions 65772–65775
Repair
    Astigmatism 65772–65775
    with Glue 65286
    Wedge Resection 65775

Wound
    Nonperforating 65275
    Perforating 65280, 65285–65286
Reshape
    Epikeratoplasty 65765
    Keratomileusis 65760
    Keratoprosthesis 65767
Scraping
    Smear 65430
Tattoo 65600
Transplantation
    Anesthesia 00144
    for Aphakia 65750
    Autograft or Homograft
        Lamellar 65710
    Penetrating . . . 65730, 65750, 65755

Coronary Arteriography
Anesthesia 01920

Coronary Artery
Insertion
    Stent 92980–92981
Ligation 33502
Repair 33500–33502, 33506

Coronary Artery Bypass Graft (CABG) 33503–33505,
             33510–33516, 33518–33519,
             33521–33523, 33533–33536
Arterial 33531–33534
Arterial-Venous 33517–33523
Reoperation 33530
Venous 33510–33516

Coroner's Exam 88045

Coronoidectomy 21070
Temporomandibular Joint 21070

Corpora Cavernosa
Corpus Spongiosum Shunt 54430
Glans Penis Fistulization 54435
Injection 54235
Irrigation
    Priapism 54220
Saphenous Vein Shunt 54420
X-Ray with Contrast 74445

Corpora Cavernosography 74445

Corpus Callosum
Transection 61541

Corpus Uteri 58120

Cortical Mapping
by Electric Stimulation 95961

Corticosteroids
Blood 83491
Urine 83491

Corticosterone
Blood or Urine 82528

Corticotropic Releasing Hormone (CRH) 80412

Cortisol 80400–80406,
        80418–80420, 80436, 82530

Stimulation 80412
Total 82533

Costotransversectomy 21610

Cotte Operation
See Repair, Uterus, Suspension

Counseling
Group 99411–99412
Individual 99401–99404
Medical
    with Interdisciplinary
        Team 98910–98912
    with Patient 98900–98902
Telephone
    Brief 98920
    Complex 98922
    Intermediate 98921

Counterimmuno-electrophoresis 86185

Coventry Tibial Wedge Osteotomy
See Osteotomy, Tibia

Cowper's Gland
Excision 53250

Coxiella Burnetii
Antibody 86638

Coxsackie
Antibody 86658

CPAP
See Continuous Positive Airway Pressure (CPAP)

C-Peptide 80432, 84681

CPK
Blood 82550–82552

CPR (Cardiopulmonary Resuscitation) 92950

Cranial Bone
Reconstruction 21181–21182
Tumor
    Excision 61563–61564

Cranial Halo 20661

Cranial Nerve
See also Specific Nerve
Avulsion 64155, 64732, 64734,
               64736, 64738, 64740,
               64742, 64744, 64746,
          64752, 64755, 64760, 64771
Decompression 61458, 64716
Implantation
    Electrode 64553, 64573
Incision 64155, 64732–64746,
             64752, 64760, 65771
Injection
    Anesthetic 64400, 64402,
              64405, 64408, 64412
    Neurolytic 64600, 64605, 64610
Insertion
    Electrode 64553, 64573
Neuroplasty 64716

Other 87102
Skin 87101
Lymphocyte
Chromosome Analysis 88230
Mycobacteria 87116–87118
Pathogen
by Kit 87082–87085
Skin
Chromosome Analysis 88233
Tissue
Toxin/Antitoxin 87230
Virus 87252–87253
Tubercle Bacilli 87116–87117
Typing 87140–87158
Unlisted Services and
Procedures 87163, 87999

Curettage 58120
See also Dilation and Curettage
Cervix
Endocervical 57454, 57505
Cornea 65435–65436
Chelating Agent 65436
Hydatidiform Mole 59870
Postpartum 59160

Curettement
Skin Lesion
Benign Hyperkeratotic . . . 11050–11052

Custodial Care
See Nursing Facility Services

Cyanide
Blood 82600
Tissue 82600

Cyanocobalamin 82607–82608

Cyclic AMP 82030

Cyclic GMP 83008

Cyclodialysis
Destruction
Ciliary Body 66740

Cyclophotocoagulation
Destruction
Ciliary Body 66710

Cyclosporine
Assay 80158

Cyst
Abdomen
Destruction/Excision 49200–49201
Ankle
Capsule 27630
Tendon Sheath 27630
Aspiration
CAT Scan Guide 76365
Bartholin's Gland
Excision 56740
Repair 56440
Bile Duct 47715, 47716
Bladder
Excision 51500
Bone
Drainage 20615

Injection 20615
Brain
Drainage 61150–61151, 61156
Excision 61516, 61524
Branchial Cleft
Excision 42810, 42815
Breast
Incision and Drainage 19020
Puncture Aspiration 19000–19001
Calcaneus 28100, 28102–28103
Carpal 25130, 25135–25136
Choledochal 47715–47716
Ciliary Body
Destruction 66770
Conjunctiva 68020
Dermoid
Nose
Excision 30124–30125
Excision
Clavicle 23140
with Allograft 23146
with Autograft 23145
Humerus
with Allograft 23156
with Autograft 23155
Mediastinum 32662
Olecranon Process
with Allograft 24126
with Autograft 24125
Pericardial 32661
Pilonidal 11770–11772
Radius
with Allograft 24126
with Autograft 24125
Scapula 23140
with Allograft 23146
with Autograft 23145
Ulna
with Allograft 24126
with Autograft 24125
Facial Bones
Excision 21030
Femur 27065–27067
Fibula 27635, 27637–27638
Gums
Incision and Drainage 41800
Hip 27065–27067
Humerus
Excision 24110
with Allograft 24116
Anesthesia 01758
with Autograft 24115
Ileum 27065–27067
Incision and Drainage 10060–10061
Pilonidal 10080–10081
Puncture Aspiration 10160
Iris
Destruction 66770
Kidney
Aspiration 50390
Excision 50280–50290
Injection 50390
X-Ray 74470
Knee
Excision 27345

Leg, Lower
Capsule 27630
Tendon Sheath 27630
Liver 47010
Drainage 47010
Repair 47300
Lung
Incision and Drainage 32200
Removal 32140
Lymph Node
Axillary/Cervical
Excision 38550–38555
Mandible
Excision 21040–21041
Mediastinal
Excision 39200
Metacarpal 26200, 26205
Metatarsal 28104, 28106–28107
Mouth 41005–41009, 41015–41018
Incision and Drainage 40800–40801
Mullerian Duct
Excision 55680
Nose
Excision 30124–30125
Ovarian
Excision 58925
Incision and Drainage 58800–58805
Pancreas 48500
Anastomosis 48520, 48540
Excision 48120
Pelvis
Aspiration 50390
Injection 50390
Pericardial
Excision 33050
Phalanges
Finger 26210, 26215
Toe 28108
Pilonidal
Excision 11770–11772
Pubis 27065–27067
Radius 25120, 25125–25126
Removal 10040, 27355–27358
Retroperitoneal
Destruction/Excision 49200–49201
Salivary Gland
Creation
Fistula 42325–42326
Drainage 42409
Excision 42408
Seminal Vesicle
Excision 55680
Spinal Cord
Aspiration 62268
Incision and Drainage 63172–63173
Sublingual Gland
Drainage 42409
Excision 42408
Talus 28100, 28102–28103
Tarsal 28104, 28106–28107
Thyroglossal Duct
Excision 60280–60281
Incision and Drainage 60000
Thyroid Gland
Aspiration 60001

Ureter 52338
Urethra 53265
Uvula 42160
Vagina
   Extensive 57065
   Simple 57061
Vascular 17106–17108
Vulva
   Extensive 56515
   Simple 56501
Molluscum Contagiosum 17110
Muscle Endplate
   Cervical Spine 64613
   Extraocular 67345
   Facial 64612
Nerve 64600–64680
   Laryngeal, Recurrent 31595
Polyp
   Aural 69540
   Nose 30110–30115
   Urethra 53260
Sinus
   Frontal 31080–31085
Skene's Gland 53270
Skin Tags . . . 11200–11201, 17200–17201
Tonsil
   Lingual 42870
Tumor
   Abdomen 49200–49201
   Bile Duct 43272
   Chemosurgery 17304–17310
   Colon 45383
   Intestines
      Large 44393
      Small 44369
   Pancreatic Duct 43272
   Rectum 45190, 45320,
               46937–46938
   Retroperitoneal 49200–49201
   Urethra 53220
Turbinate Mucosa 30801–30802
Unlisted Services and Procedures 17999
Ureter
   Endoscopic 50957, 50976
Urethra 52214–52224
   Prolapse 53275
Warts
   Flat 17110

Developmental Testing
Brain Function 96110–96111

Development Evaluation 99178

Device Handling 99002

DEXA
See Dual Energy X-Ray
Absorptiometry (DEXA)

Dexamethasone
Suppression Test 80420

DHEA
See Dehydroepiandrosterone

DHT
See Dihydrotestosterone

Dialysis
Arteriovenous Shunt 36145
End Stage Renal Disease . . . 90918–90925
Hemodialysis 90935, 90937
Hemoperfusion 90997
Patient Training
   Completed Course 90989
   Per Session 90993
Peritoneal 90945–90947
Unlisted Services and Procedures 90999

Diaphragm
Anesthesia 00540
   Hernia Repair 00756
Repair
   Anesthesia 00756
   for Eventration 39545
   Hernia 39502–39541
   Laceration 39501
Unlisted Procedures 39599
Vagina
   Fitting 57170

Diaphysectomy
Calcaneus 28120
Clavicle 23180
Femoral 27360
Fibula 27360
Humerus 24140
Metacarpal 26230
Metatarsal 28122
Olecranon Process 24147
Phalanges
   Finger 26235–26236
   Toe 28124
Radius 24145
Scapula 23182
Talus 28120
Tarsal 28122
Tibia 27360, 27640–27641
Ulna 25150–25151

Diathermy 97024
Destruction
   Ciliary Body 66700
Lesion
   Retina 67208, 67227
Retinal Detachment
   Prophylaxis 67141
   Repair 67101

Dibucaine Number 82638

Dichloroethane 84600

Dichloromethane 84600

Diethylether 84600

Differential Count
See White Blood Cell Count

Digits
See also Finger; Toe
Pinch Graft 15050
Replantation 20816–20822
Skin Graft
   Split 15120–15121

Digoxin
Assay 80162
Blood or Urine 82643

Dihydrocodeinone 82646

Dihydrocodeinone Screen . . . 82486

Dihydromorphinone 82486, 82649

Dihydrotestosterone 82651

Dihydroxyvitamin D 82652

Dilation 58120
See also Dilation and Curettage
Anal
   Endoscopy 46604
   Sphincter 45905
Bile Duct
   Endoscopy 43271, 47555–47556
   Stricture 74363
Bladder
   Cystourethroscopy 52260–52265
Bronchi
   Endoscopy 31630
Cervix
   Canal 57800
Curettage 57820
Esophagus 43450, 43453,
              43456, 43458
   Endoscopy 43220–43249
   Surgical 43510
Kidney 50395
Lacrimal Punctum 68800
Larynx
   Endoscopy 31528–31529
Pancreatic Duct
   Endoscopy 43271
Rectum
   Endoscopy 45303
   Sphincter 45910
Salivary Duct 42650, 42660
Stenosis 52281
Trachea
   Endoscopy 31630–31631
Ureter 50395, 52335
   Endoscopic 50553, 50572,
              50953, 50972
Urethra 52260–52265
   General 53665
   Suppository and/or
   Instillation 53660–53661
Urethral
   Stricture 52281, 53600–53621
Vagina 57400

Dilation and Curettage 59840
See also Curettage; Dilation
with Amniotic Injections 59851
Cervical Stump 57820
Corpus Uteri 58120
Hysteroscopy 56350
Postpartum 59160
with Vaginal Suppositories 59856

Dilation and Evacuation 59841
with Amniotic Injections 59851

Lower Extremity 93925–93926
Penile 93980–93981
Upper Extremity 93930–93931
Visceral 93975–93979
Hemodialysis Access 93990
Venous Studies
Extremity 93970–93971
Penile 93980–93981

Dupuy-Dutemp Operation
See Reconstruction, Eyelid

Dupuytren's Contracture 26040, 26045

Dwyer Procedure
See Osteotomy, Calcaneus

D-Xyclose Absorption Test . . . 84620

Dynamometry
with Ophthalmoscopy 92260

E

Ear
Anesthesia 00120–00126
Collection of Blood 36415
Drum
See Tympanic Membrane
External
Abscess
Incision and Drainage
Complicated 69005
Simple 69000
Biopsy 69100
Excision
Partial 69110
Total 69120
Hematoma
Incision and Drainage . 69000, 69005
Reconstruction 69300
Unlisted Services and
Procedures 69399
Inner
CAT Scan 70480, 70481, 70482
Excision
Labyrinth 69905, 69910
Exploration
Endolymphatic Sac 69805–69806
Incision 69820
Labyrinth 69801–69802
Semicircular Canal 69840
Insertion
Cochlear Device 69930
Semicircular Canal 69820
Unlisted Services and
Procedures 69949
Middle
Catheterization 69405
CAT Scan 70480, 70481, 70482
Exploration 69440

Inflation
with Catheterization 69400
without Catheterization 69401
Insertion
Baffle 69410
Catheter 69405
Lesion
Excision 69540
Reconstruction
Tympanoplasty with Antrotomy or
Mastoidectomy 69635–69637
Tympanoplasty with
Mastoidectomy 69641–69646
Tympanoplasty without
Mastoidectomy 69631–69633
Removal
Ventilating Tube 69424
Repair
Oval Window 69666
Round Window 69667
Revision
Stapes 69662
Tumor
Excision 69550, 69552, 69554
Unlisted Services and
Procedures 69799
Outer
CAT Scan 70480–70482
Skin Graft
Delay of Flap 15630
Full Thickness 15260–15261
Pedicle Flap 15576
Split 15120–15121
Tissue Transfer, Adjacent . . . 14060–14061

Ear, Nose, and Throat
See also Otorhinolaryngology, Diagnostic
Audiologic Function Tests
Acoustic Reflex 92568
Acoustic Reflex Decay . . . 92561, 92569
Audiometry
Bekesy 92560–92561
Comprehensive 92557
Conditioning Play 92582
Evoked Response 92585
Groups 92559
Pure Tone 92552, 92553
Select Picture 92583
Speech 92555–92556
Brainstem Evoked Response 92585
Central Auditory Function 92589
Ear Protector Evaluation 92596
Electrocochleography 92584
Filtered Speech 92571
Hearing Aid Evaluation . . 92590–92595
Lombard Test 92573
Loudness Balance 92562
Screening Test 92551
Sensorineural Acuity 92575
Short Increment Sensitivity
Index (SISI) 92564
Staggered Spondaic Word Test . . . 92572
Stenger Test 92565, 92577
Synthetic Sentence Test 92576
Tone Decay 92563

Tympanometry 92567
Binocular Microscopy 92504
Facial Nerve Function Study 92516
Hearing Evaluation 92506
Language Evaluation 92506
Laryngeal Function Study 92520
Nasal Function Study 92512
Nasopharyngoscopy 92511
Speech Evaluation 92506
Vestibular Function Tests
Additional Electrodes 92547
Caloric Tests 92533, 92543
Nystagmus
Optokinetic 92534, 92544
Positional 92532, 92542
Spontaneous 92531, 92541
Torsion Swing Test 92546
Tracking Tests 92545

Ear Cartilage
Graft
to Face 21235

Ear Lobes
Pierce 69090

Ear Protector Attenuation 92596

Ebstein Anomaly Repair 33468

ECG
See Electrocardiogram

Echinococcosis 86171, 86280

Echocardiography
Cardiac 93307–93314,
93320–93321, 93350
Doppler 93307–93314, 93320–93321
Fetal Heart 76825–76828
M Mode and Real Time 93307–93314,
93350
Transesophageal 93313–93314

Echoencephalography 76506

Echography
Abdomen 76700–76705
Arm 76880
Breast 76645
Cardiac 93307–93314,
93320–93321, 93350
Guidance 76932
Chest 76604
Extracranial Arteries 93880–93882
Eyes 76511–76529
Follow-up 76970
Head 76536
Intracranial Arteries 93886–93888
Intraoperative 76986
Kidney
Transplant 76778
Leg 76880
Neck 76536
Pelvis 76856–76857
Placement Therapy Fields . . . 76950–76960
Pregnant Uterus 76805–76816
Prostate 76872
Radiologic 76932

Electrophysiology Procedure 93600–93640, 93650, 93660

Electroretinography 92275

Electrosurgery
Trichiasis
    Correction................... 67825

Elliot Operation
See Excision, Lesion, Sclera

Eloesser Procedure
See Thoracostomy, Empyema

Eloesser Thoracoplasty
See Thoracoplasty

Embolectomy
Anesthesia .. 01274, 01502, 01772, 01842
Aortoiliac Artery.................. 34151
Axillary Artery 34101
Brachial Artery................... 34101
Carotid Artery.................... 34001
Celiac Artery 34151
Femoral......................... 34201
Iliac........................... 34201
Innominate Artery... 34001, 34051, 34101
Mesentery Artery.................. 34151
Peroneal Artery 34203
Popliteal Artery 34203
Radial Artery 34111
Renal Artery 34151
Subclavian Artery... 34001, 34051, 34101
Tibial Artery..................... 34203
Ulnar Artery 34111

Embryo Transfer
In Vitro Fertilization 58974, 58976
    Intrafallopian Transfer 58976
    Intrauterine Transfer 58974

Emergency Department Services 99281–99285, 99288
See also Critical Care; Emergency Department Services
Anesthesia 99140
    in Office 99058
Physician Direction of Advanced Life Support....................... 99288

Emesis Induction 99175

EMG
See Electromyography, Needle

Emission Computerized Tomography 78607, 78652

Emmet Operation
See Perineum, Repair; Vagina, Repair

Empyema
Closure
    Chest Wall 32810
Thoracostomy 32020, 32035–32036

Empyemectomy 32540

Encephalitis
Antibody 86651–86654

Encephalocele
Repair....................... 62120
    Craniotomy................. 62121

Endarterectomy
Pulmonary 33916

Endocrine System
Unlisted Services and Procedures 60699, 78099

Endolymphatic Sac
Exploration
    with Shunt 69806
    without Shunt 69805

Endometrial Ablation
via Hysteroscopy 56356

Endometrioma
Abdomen
    Destruction/Excision 49200–49201
Retroperitoneal
    Destruction/Excision 49200–49201

Endometrium
Biopsy................... 56351, 58100

Endorectal Pull-Through
See Proctectomy, Total

Endoscopy
See also Arthroscopy; Thoracoscopy
Anal
    Biopsy..................... 46606
    Dilation.................... 46604
    Exploration................. 46600
    Hemorrhage 46614
    Removal
        Foreign Body.............. 46608
        Polyp 46610, 46612
        Tumor............. 46610, 46612
Bile Duct
    Biopsy..................... 47553
    Destruction
        Calculi (Stone) 43265
        Tumor 43272
    Dilation....... 43271, 47555–47556
    Exploration................. 47552
    Intraoperative............... 47550
    Percutaneous 47552–47555
    Removal
        Calculi (Stone)....... 43264, 47554
        Foreign Body.............. 43269
        Stent 43269
    Specimen Collection 43260
    Sphincterotomy 43262
    Sphincter Pressure............ 43263
    Tube Placement 43267, 43268
Bladder 52000, 52010
    Biopsy................. 52007, 52204
    Catheterization.............. 52005
    Resection 52340
Bronchi
    Aspiration............ 31645–31646
    Biopsy............... 31625–31629

Destruction
    Lesion 31640
    Tumor 31641
    Dilation............... 31630–31631
    Exploration................. 31622
    Injection................... 31656
    Lesion
        Destruction 31640, 31656
    Needle Biopsy 31629
    Placement
        Stent 31631
    Stenosis 31641
    Tumor
        Destruction 31641
Chest Cavity
    Exploration 32601–32606
    Therapeutic........... 32654–32665
Colon
    Biopsy.............. 44389, 45380
    via Colotomy 45355
    Destruction
        Lesion 44393, 45383
        Tumor............. 44393, 45383
    Exploration 45378
    Hemorrhage 44391, 45382
    Removal
        Foreign Body......... 44390, 45379
        Polyp 44392, 45384–45385
        Tumor....... 44392, 45384–45385
    Specimen Collection 45380
    via Stoma 44388–44393
Colon-Sigmoid
    Ablation
        Polyp 45339
        Tumor 45339
    Biopsy..................... 45331
    Exploration................. 45330
    Hemorrhage 45334
    Removal
        Foreign Body.............. 45332
        Polyp 45333, 45338
        Tumor............. 45333, 45338
    Specimen Collection 45331
    Volvulus 45337
Esophagus
    Biopsy..................... 43202
    Dilation.............. 43220, 43226
    Exploration................. 43200
    Hemorrhage 43227
    Injection................... 43204
    Insertion Stent................ 43219
    Removal
        Foreign Body.............. 43215
        Polyp 43216, 43217, 43228
        Tumor............. 43216, 43228
    Vein Ligation 43205
Gastrointestinal
    Upper
        Anesthesia 00740
        Biopsy.................... 43239
        Catheterization 43241
        Destruction of Lesion 43258
        Dilation 43245, 43248, 43249
        Exploration.......... 43234–43235
        Hemorrhage............... 43255

Abscess
Incision and Drainage 54700
Anastomosis
to Vas Deferens
Bilateral.................... 54901
Unilateral.................. 54900
Epididymography 74440
Excision
Bilateral 54861
Unilateral 54860
Exploration
Biopsy....................... 54820
Hematoma
Incision and Drainage 54700
Lesion
Excision
Local 54830
Spermatocele 54840
Needle Biopsy 54800
Spermatocele
Excision 54840
Unlisted Services and Procedures.... 55899
X-Ray with Contrast.............. 74440

Epididymograms............. 55300

Epididymography 74440

Epididymovasostomy
Bilateral 54901
Unilateral 54900

Epidural
Analgesia
Continuous 00857, 00955
Drug Administration............ 01996
Electrode
Insertion...................... 61531
Removal 61535
Injection......... 62275, 62278–62279,
62281–62282, 62289, 62298

Epigastric
Hernia Repair.................... 49572

Epiglottidectomy 31420

Epiglottis
Excision 31420

Epikeratoplasty.............. 65767

Epinephrine
See also Catecholamines
Blood.................... 82383–82384
Urine......................... 82384

Epiphyseal Arrest
Femur.................. 27185, 27475,
27479, 27485, 27742
Fibula........... 27477, 27479, 27485,
27732, 27734, 27740, 27742
Radius................ 25450, 25455
Tibia........... 27477, 27479, 27485,
27730, 27734, 27740, 27742
Ulna.................. 25450, 25455

Epiphyseal Separation
Radius.................. 25600, 25620

Epiphysiodesis
See Epiphyseal Arrest

Epiploectomy................. 49255

Episiotomy 59300

Epispadias
Penis
Reconstruction................ 54385
Repair........................ 54380
with Exstrophy of Bladder....... 54390
with Incontinence............. 54385

**Epistaxis with Nasal/Sinus
Endoscopy**................... 31238

Epstein-Barr Virus
Antibody 86663–86665

ERCP
See Cholangiopancreatography

**Ergonovine Provocation
Test**....................... 93024

Erythropoietin 82668

Escharotomy
Burns 16035

**Esophageal Acid Infusion
Test**....................... 91030
See also Esophagus, Acid Perfusion Test

Esophageal Varices
Ligation................. 43205, 43400
Transection/Repair............... 43401

Esophagectomy
Partial 43116–43118,
43121–43124
Total.................... 43107–43108,
43112–43113, 43124

Esophagogastric Tests
Manometry.................... 91020

Esophagogastrostomy........ 43320

Esophagojejunostomy . 43340–43341

Esophagomyotomy.......... 32665,
43330–43331

Esophagoscopy
Anesthesia 00520

Esophagostomy........ 43350–43352

Esophagotomy........ 43020, 43045

Esophagus
Acid Perfusion Test 91030
Acid Reflux Tests 91032–91033
Anesthesia 00320, 00500
Biopsy
Endoscopy 43202
Cineradiography 74230
Dilation 43450, 43453, 43456, 43458
Endoscopic 43220, 43226,
43248–43249
Surgical 43510

Endoscopy
Biopsy........................ 43202
Dilation.............. 43220, 43226
Exploration 43200
Hemorrhage 43227
Injection...................... 43204
Insertion Stent................ 43219
Removal
Foreign Body............... 43215
Polyp 43216–43217, 43228
Tumor................. 43216, 43228
Vein Ligation 43205
Excision
Diverticula 43130, 43135
Partial 43116–43118,
43121–43124
Total............... 43107–43108,
43112–43113, 43124
Exploration
Endoscopy 43200
Hemorrhage
Endoscopic Control 43227
Incision 43020, 43045
Muscle 43030
Injection
Sclerosing Agent 43204
Insertion
Stent....................... 43219
Tamponade................. 43460
Tube 43510
Intubation with Specimen Collection .. 91000
Lesion
Excision 43100–43101
Ligation...................... 43405
Motility Study...... 78258, 91010–91012
Nuclear Medicine
Imaging...................... 78258
Reflux Study................. 78262
Reconstruction 43300, 43310
Creation
Stoma 43350–43352
Esophagostomy 43350
Fistula............ 43305, 43312
Gastrointestinal 43360–43361
Removal
Foreign Bodies 43020, 43045,
43215, 74235
Lesion..................... 43216
Polyp......... 43216–43217, 43228
Repair..................... 43300, 43310
Esophagogastric
Fundoplasty 43324–43325
Esophagogastrostomy 43320
Esophagojejunostomy ... 43340–43341
Fistula... 43305, 43312, 43420, 43425
Muscle 43330–43331
Varices 43401
Wound 43410, 43415
Suture....................... 43405
Wound 43410, 43415
Unlisted Services and Procedures.... 43499
Vein
Ligation............... 43205, 43400
Video 74230
X-Ray 74220

Established Patient
Confirmatory Consultations . . 99271–99275
Domiciliary or
Rest Home Visit 99331–99333
Emergency Department
Services 88288, 99281–99285
Home Services 99351–99353
Initial Inpatient
Consultations 99251–99255
Office and/or Other Outpatient
Consultations 99241–99245
Office Visit 99211–99215
Outpatient Visit 99211–99215

Establishment
Colostomy
   Abdominal 50810
   Perineal 50810

Estlander Procedure 40525
See also Excision, Lip

Estradiol 82670
Response 80415

Estriol
Blood or Urine 82677

Estrogen
Blood or Urine 82671–82672
Receptor 84233

Estrone
Blood or Urine 82679

Ethanol
Blood 82055
Breath 82075
Urine 82055

Ethchlorvynol
Blood 82690
Urine 82690

Ethmoid, Sinus
See Sinus, Ethmoid

Ethmoidectomy 31200–31205
Endoscopic 31254
with Nasal/Sinus
Endoscopy 31254–31255
Skull Base Surgery 61580–61581

Ethosuximide 80168
Assay 80168

Ethyl Alcohol
See Ethanol

Ethylene Glycol 82693

Etiocholanolone 82696

Euglobulin Lysis 85360

Eustachian Tube
Catheterization 69405
Inflation
   with Catheterization 69400
   without Catheterization 69401
   Myringotomy 69420
     Anesthesia 69421

Insertion
   Catheter 69405

Evacuation
Hydatidiform Mole 59870

Evaluation and Management
Basic Life and/or Disability Evaluation
Services 99450
Care Plan Oversight
Services 99375–99376
Case Management 99361–99362,
                  99371–99373
Consultation 99241–99245,
   99251–99255, 99261–99263,
                  99271–99275
Critical Care 99291–99292
Domiciliary 99321–99323,
                  99331–99333
Emergency Department 99281–99285,
                      99288
Home 99341–99343, 99351–99353
Hospital 99221–99223, 99231–99233
   Discharge 99238–99239
Hospital Discharge 99239
Insurance Exam 99450, 99455–99456
Neonatal Critical Care 99295–99297
Newborn Care 99431–99433
Nursing Facility 99301–99303,
                  99311–99313
Observation Care 99217–99220
Office and Other
Outpatient 99201–99205,
                  99211–99215
Physician Standby Services 99360
Preventive Services 99381–99387,
                  99391–99397,
   99401–99404, 99411–99412
Prolonged Services 99356–99357
Psychiatric Residential Treatment Facility
Care 99301–99303, 99311–99313
Rest Home 99321–99323,
                  99331–99333
Unlisted Services and Procedures 99499

Evisceration
Ocular Contents
   with Implant 65093
   without Implant 65091

Evocative/Suppression
Test 80400–80408, 80412–80440
Stimulation Panel 80410

Evoked Potential
Auditory Brainstem 92585

Ewart Procedure
See Palate, Reconstruction, Lengthening

Exchange
Arterial Catheter 37209, 75900
Intraocular Lens 66986

Excision
See also Debridement; Destruction
Abscess
   Brain 61514, 61522
   Olecranon Process 24138

Radius 24136
Ulna 24138
Acromion
   Shoulder 23130
Adenoids . . . 42830–42831, 42835–42836
Adenoma
   Thyroid Gland 60200
Adrenal Gland 60540
   with Excision Retroperitoneal
   Tumor 60545
Alveolus 41830
Anal Crypt 46210–46211
Anal Fissure 46200
Anal Tab 46220, 46230
Aorta
   Coarctation 33840, 33845,
                 33851–33853
Appendix 44950, 44955, 44960
Arteriovenous Malformation
   Spinal 63250–63252
Arytenoid Cartilage 31400
   Endoscopic 31560–31561
Atrial Septum 33735–33739
Bartholin's Gland 56740
Bladder
   Diverticulum 51525
   Neck 51520
   Partial 51550–51565
   Total . . . 51570, 51580, 51590–51597
     with Nodes 51575, 51585
   Transurethral 52640
   Tumor 51530
Bone Abscess
   Facial 21026
   Mandible 21025
Brain
   Hemisphere 61542–61543
   Other Lobe 61539
   Temporal Lobe 61538
Breast
   Biopsy 19100–19101
   Chest Wall Tumor 19260–19272
   Cyst 19120
   Lactiferous Duct Fistula 19112
   Lesion 19120–19126
   Mastectomy 19140–19240
   Nipple Exploration 19110
Bulbourethral Gland 53250
Bullae
   Lung 32141
Burns 16040–16042
Bursa
   Elbow 24105
   Excision 27060
   Femur 27062
   Ischial 27060
   Knee 27340
   Wrist 25115–25116
Bypass Graft 35901, 35903,
                  35905, 35907
Calcaneus 28118–28120
Calculi (Stone)
   Parotid Gland 42330, 43340
   Salivary Gland . . . 42330, 42335, 42340
   Sublingual Gland 42330

Ankle 27610, 27620
Arm, Lower 25248
Artery
    Carotid 35701
    Femoral 35721
    Popliteal 35741
    Unlisted Services and
    Procedures 35761
Bile Duct
    Atresia 47700
    Endoscopy 47552–47553
Blood Vessel
    Abdomen 35840
    Chest 35820
    Extremity 35860
    Neck 35800
Brain
    via Burr Hole 61250, 61253
    Infratentorial 61305
    Supratentorial 61304
Breast 19020
Bronchi
    Endoscopy 31622
Bronchoscopy 31622
Cauda Equina 63005, 63011, 63017
Colon
    Endoscopic 44388, 45378
Colon-Sigmoid
    Endoscopic 45330
Duodenum 44010
Ear, Inner
    Endolymphatic Sac
      with Shunt 69806
      without Shunt 69805
Ear, Middle 69440
Elbow 24000, 24101
Epididymis 54820
Esophagus
    Endoscopy 43200
Finger Joint 26075, 26080
Gallbladder 47480
Gastrointestinal Tract, Upper
    Endoscopy 43234–43235
Hand Joint 26070
Heart 33310, 33315
Hepatic Duct 47400
Hip 27033
Interphalangeal Joint
    Toe 28024
Intertarsal Joint 28020
Intestines, Small
    Endoscopy 44360
    Enterotomy 44020
Kidney 50010, 50045, 50120, 50135
Knee 27310, 27331
Lacrimal Duct 68820
    with Anesthesia 68825
    Canaliculi 68840
    with Insertion Tube or Stent 68830
Laryngoscopy 31575
Larynx 31320
    Endoscopy 31505,
              31520–31526, 31576
Liver
    Wound 47361–47362

Mediastinum 39000–39010
Metatarsophalangeal Joint 28022
Nasolacrimal Duct 68820
    with Anesthesia 68825
    with Insertion Tube or Stent 68830
Neck
    Lymph Nodes 38542
Nipple 19110
Nose
    Endoscopy 31231–31235
Orbit 61332–61334
    without Bone Flap 67400
    with/without Biopsy 67450
Parathyroid Gland 60500–60505
Pelvis 56300
Peritoneum
    Endoscopic 56360
Prostate 55860
    with Nodes 55862, 55865
Rectum
    Endoscopic 45300
    Injury 45562–45563
Retroperitoneal Area 49010
Scrotum 55110
Shoulder Joint 23040–23044, 23107
Sinus
    Frontal 31070–31075
    Maxillary 31020–31030
Skull 61105
Spinal Cord 63001, 63003, 63005,
       63011, 63015–63017, 63040, 63042
Stomach 43500
Tarsometatarsal Joint 28020
Testis 54560
    Undescended 54550
Ureter 50600, 50650–50660
Vagina 57000
    Endocervical 57452
Wrist 25101, 25248
    Joint 25040

Expression
Lesion
    Conjunctiva 68040

External Cephalic Version 59412

External Fixation
Adjustment/Revision 20693
Application 20690–20692
Mandibular Fracture
    Open Treatment 21454
    Percutaneous Treatment 21452
Removal 20694

Extracorporeal Circulation 33960–33961

Extracorporeal Membrane Oxygenation
Cannulization 36822

Extraction
Lens
    Extracapsular 66940
    Intracapsular 66920
      for Dislocated Lens 66930

Extraperitoneal Procedures
Anesthesia 00860

Extremity
Lower
    Repair
      Blood Vessel 35206
Upper
    Repair
      Blood Vessel 35206

Extremity Testing
Physical Therapy 97750
Vascular Diagnostics 93924

Eye
See also Ciliary Body; Cornea; Iris; Lens;
Retina; Sclera; Vitreous
Anesthesia 00140–00148
Biometry 76516–76519
Drainage
    Anterior Chamber
      with Diagnostic Aspiration of
      Aqueous 65800
      with Removal of Blood 65815
      with Removal of Vitreous and/or
      Discission of Anterior
      Hyaloid Membrane 65810
      with Therapeutic Release of
      Aqueous 65805
Goniotomy 65820
Incision
    Adhesions
      Anterior Synechiae 65860, 65870
      Corneaovitreal Adhesions 65880
      Goniosynechiae 65865
      Posterior Synechiae 65875
      Anterior Chamber 65820
      Trabeculae 65850
Injection
    Air 66020
    Medication 66030
Insertion
    Implantation
      Foreign Material for
      Reinforcement 65155
      Muscles Attached 65140
      Muscles not Attached 65135
      Reinsertion 65150
      Scleral Shell 65130
Lesion
    Excision 65900
Nerve
    Destruction 67345
Paracentesis
    Anterior Chamber
      with Diagnostic Aspiration of
      Aqueous 65800
      Removal of Blood 65815
      Removal or Vitreous and/or Discission
      Anterior Hyaloid
      Membrane 65810
      with Therapeutic Release of
      Aqueous 65805
Radial Keratotomy 65771

Vaginal Approach 57320
X-Ray 76080

Fistulectomy
See also Hemorrhoids
Anal 46060, 46270,
46275, 46280, 46285

Fistulization
Esophagus 43350–43352
Intestines 44300–44346
Penis 54435
Pharynx 42955
Salivary Cyst
Sublingual 42325–42326
Tracheopharyngeal 31755

Fistulotomy
Anal 46270, 46280

Fitting
Cervical Cap 57170
Contact Lens 92070, 92310–92313
Diaphragm 57170
Low Vision Aid 92354–92355
Ocular Prosthesis 92330
Spectacle Prosthesis 92352–92353
Spectacles 92340–92342

Fitzgerald Factor 85293

Fixation (Device)
See also Application; Bone, Fixation; Spinal
Instrumentation
Pelvic
Insertion 22848
Sacrospinous Ligament
Vaginal Prolapse 57282
Shoulder 23700
Spinal
Insertion 22841–22844
Prosthetic 22851
Reinsertion 22849

Flank
See Back/Flank

Flap
See also Skin Graft and Flap
Free
Breast Reconstruction 19364
Microvascular Transfer 15755
Grafts 15580–15650
Latissimus Dorsi
Breast Reconstruction 19361
Transverse Rectus Abdominis Myocutaneous
Breast Reconstruction . . . 19367–19369

Fletcher Factor 85292

Flow Cytometry 88180–88182

Flow-Volume Loop
Pulmonary 94375

Fluid Collection
Incision and Drainage 10140

Fluorescein
Intravenous Injection
Blood Flow Check, Graft 15860

Fluorescent Antibody . 83255–83256

Fluoride
Blood 82735
Urine 82735

Fluoroscopy
Bile Duct
Guide Catheter 74328, 74330
Guide Stone Removal 74327
Chest 71023, 71034, 71038
Drain Abscess 75989
GI Tract
Guide Intubation 74340
Hourly 76000–76001
Introduction
GI Tube 74340
Larynx 70370
Needle Biopsy 76003
Pancreatic Duct
Guide Catheter 74329, 74330
Pharynx 70370
Ureter
Guide Catheter 74480
X-Ray with Contrast
Guide Catheter 74475

Flurazepam
Blood or Urine 82742

Flush Aortogram 75722–75724

Flu Shots 90724, 90737

Foam Stability Test 83662

Foley Y-Pyeloplasty . . . 50400–50405

Folic Acid 82747
Blood 82746

Follicle Stimulating Hormone
(FSH) 80418, 80426, 83001

Follow-up Services
Inpatient Consultations 99261–99263
Post-Op 99024

Fontan Procedure
See Repair, Heart, Anomaly; Repair,
Tricuspid Valve

Food Allergy Test 95075

Foot
See also Metatarsal; Tarsal
Amputation 28800, 28805
Anesthesia 01460–01522
Bursa
Incision and Drainage 28001
Capsulotomy 28260–28262, 28264
Cast 29450
Fasciectomy 28060, 28062
Fasciotomy 28008
Incision 28002–28003, 28005
Joint
See also Talotarsal Joint; Tarsometatarsal
Joint
Magnetic Resonance Imaging
(MRI) 73721

Lesion
Excision 28080, 28090
Magnetic Resonance Imaging (MRI) . . 73720
Nerve
Excision 28030
Incision 28035
Neuroma
Excision 28080
Reconstruction
Cleft Foot 28360
Removal
Foreign Body 28190, 28192–28193
Repair
Muscle 28250
Tendon 28200, 28202, 28208,
28210, 28220, 28222,
28225–28226, 28230, 28234, 28238
Replantation 20838
Sesamoid
Excision 28315
Skin Graft
Delay of Flap 15620
Full Thickness 15240–15241
Pedicle Flap 15574
Split 15100–15101
Splint 29590
Strapping 29590
Suture
Tendon 28208, 28210
Tendon Sheath
Excision 28086, 28088
Tenotomy 28230, 28234
Tissue Transfer, Adjacent . . . 14040–14041
Tumor
Excision 28043, 28045–28046
Unlisted Services and Procedures 28899
X-Ray 73620–73630

Forehead
Reconstruction 21172–21175,
21182–21184
Midface 21159–21160
Reduction 21137–21139
Rhytidectomy 15824, 15826
Skin Graft
Delay of Flap 15620
Full Thickness 15240–15241
Pedicle Flap 15574
Tissue Transfer, Adjacent . . . 14040–14041

Forensic Exam 88040
Cytopathology 88125
Phosphatase, Acid 84061

Fowler-Stephens Orchiopexy
See Orchiopexy

Fowler-Stephens
Procedure 54650

Fox Operation
See Entropion, Repair

Fracture
Acetabulum
Closed Treatment 27220, 27222
with Manipulation 27220, 27222
without Manipulation 27220

Phalanges
Articular 26740, 26742, 26746
Closed Treatment 26740, 26742,
26750, 26755, 28510
Distal. . . 26750, 26755–26756, 26765
Finger/Thumb
Closed Treatment 26720, 26725
with Manipulation. 26725, 26727
Percutaneous Fixation. 26727
Shaft 26720, 26725, 26727
Great Toe 28490
Closed Treatment 28495
without Manipulation . 28495–28496
Open Treatment 28505
Percutaneous Fixation. 28496
with Manipulation 26742, 26755
without Manipulation. . . . 26740, 26750
Open Treatment . 26735, 26746, 26765
Percutaneous Fixation 26756
Shaft. 26735
Toe
Closed Treatment 28515
without Manipulation . 28510, 28515
Open Treatment 28515
Radius
Closed Treatment 25500, 25505,
25520, 25560,
25565, 25600, 25605
Distal. . . 25600, 25605, 25611, 25620
Head/Neck
Closed Treatment 24650–24655
Open Treatment. 24665–24666
with Manipulation 25565, 25605
without Manipulation. . . . 25560, 25600
Open Treatment 25515,
25525–25526,
25574, 25575, 25620
Percutaneous Fixation 25611
Shaft 25500, 25505,
25515, 25520, 25525–25526, 25574
with Ulna 25560, 25565, 25575
Rib
Closed Treatment. 21800
External Fixation 21810
Open Treatment 21805
Scaphoid. 25622, 25624, 25628
with Dislocation. 25680, 25685
Scapula
Closed Treatment
with Manipulation. 23575
without Manipulation. 23570
Open Treatment 23585
Sesamoid
Closed Treatment. 28530
Foot 28530
Open Treatment 28531
Skull 62000–62010
Closed Treatment. 21300
Talus
Closed Treatment 28430, 28435
without Manipulation. 28430,
28435–28436
Open Treatment 28445
Tarsal
without Manipulation. . . . 28455–28456

Open Treatment 28465
Percutaneous Fixation 28456
Thumb
with Dislocation 26645,
26650, 26665
Tibia
Arthroscopic Treatment . . 29855–29856
Closed Treatment 27530, 27532,
27538, 27750, 27752, 27760,
27808, 27810, 27824–27825
Distal 27824–27828
Intercondylar. 27538, 27540
Malformation 27810
Malleolus. 27760, 27762,
27766, 27808, 27814
with Manipulation 27752,
27810, 27824
without Manipulation. . . 27530, 27750,
27760, 27808, 27824
Open Treatment. 27535–27536,
27540, 27758–27759,
27814, 27826–27828
Percutaneous Fixation 27756
Plateau 27530, 27532,
27535–27536, 29855–29856
Shaft 27750, 27752,
27756, 27758–27759
Trachea
Endoscopy 31630
Ulna
Closed Treatment 25530, 25535,
25560, 25565, 25645
with Dislocation
Closed Treatment 24620
with Manipulation 25535, 25565
without Manipulation. . . . 25530, 25560
Olecranon
Closed Treatment 24670–24675
Open Treatment 24685
Open Treatment 25545,
25574–25575
with Radius 25560, 25565, 25575
Shaft 25530, 25535,
25545, 25574
Styloid Process 25650
Vertebra
Additional Segment
Open Treatment 22328
Cervical
Open Treatment 22326
Closed Treatment. 22305
without Manipulation. 22310
with Manipulation, Casting and/or
Bracing 22315
Lumbar
Open Treatment 22325
Thoracic
Open Treatment 22327
Wrist
with Dislocation. 25680, 25685
Zygomatic Arch
with Manipulation 21355
Open Treatment 21356–21365

Fragile-X
Chromosome Analysis 88250

Fragility
Red Blood Cell
Mechanical. 85547
Osmotic 85555–85557

Francisella 86000
Antibody. 86668

Franconi Anemia
Chromosome Analysis 88248

Fredet-Ramstedt Procedure . . 43520
See also Incision, Pyloric Sphincter

Frenectomy 40819, 41115

Frenotomy 40806, 41010

Frenulectomy 40819

Frenum
See also Lip
Lip
Incision. 40806

Frenumectomy 40819

Frickman Operation
See Proctopexy

Frontal Craniotomy 61556

Frontal Sinus
See Sinus, Frontal

Frost Suture 67875
See also Eyelid, Closure by Suture

**Frozen Blood
Preparation** 86930–86932

Fructose 84375
Semen. 82757

FSF 85290–85291

FT-4 84439

Fulguration 50957
See also Destruction
Bladder. 51020
Cystourethroscopy with 52214
Lesion. 52224
Tumor 52234–52240
Ureterocele. 52300

Full Thickness Graft . . . 15200–15261

Fundoplasty 43324–43325
Esophagogastric
with Gastroplasty. 43326

Fungus
Antibody. 86671
Culture
Blood 87103
Identification 87106
Other 87102
Skin 87101
Tissue Exam. 87220

Furuncle
Incision and Drainage. 10060–10061

Repositioning 43761

Gastrotomy 43500–43501, 43510

Gel Diffusion 86331

Genioplasty 21120
Osteotomy 21121–21123

Genitalia
Female
   Anesthesia 00940–00952
Male
   Anesthesia 00920–00938
Skin Graft
   Delay of Flap 15620
   Full Thickness 15240–15241
   Pedicle Flap 15574
   Split 15120–15121
Tissue Transfer, Adjacent . . . 14040–14041

Gentamicin 80170
Assay 80170

Giardia Lamblia
Antibody 86674

Gibbons Stent 52332

GIFT 89250
See also In Vitro Fertilization

Giles Approach
Fracture
   Zygomatic Arch 21356

Gill Operation 63012
See also Laminectomy, Lumbar

Gingiva
See Gums

Gingivectomy 41820

Gingivoplasty 41872

Girdlestone Laminectomy
See Arthrodesis; Laminectomy

Girdlestone Procedure
See Acetabulum, Reconstruction

Glabellar Frown Lines
Rhytidectomy 15826

Gland
See Specific Gland

Glaucoma
Fistulization of Sclera 66150
Provocative Test 92140

Glenn Procedure 33766–33767
See also Shunt, Great Vessel, Vena Cava to
Pulmonary

Glenohumeral Joint
Arthrotomy 23040
   with Biopsy 23100
   with Synovectomy 23105
Exploration 23107
Removal
   Foreign or Loose Body 23107

Glenoid Fossa
Reconstruction 21255

Globulin
Antihuman 86880–86886
Blood 82942
Sex Hormone Binding 84270

Glucagon 82943
Tolerance Panel 80422, 80424
Tolerance Test 82946

Glucose . . 80422–80424, 80430–80435
Blood Test 82947–82950, 82962
Joint Fluid 82947
Spinal Fluid 82947
Tolerance Test 82951–82952
   With Tolbutamide 82953

Glucose-6-Phosphate
Dehydrogenase 82955–82960

Glucosidase 82963

Glucuronide Androstanediol . 82154

Glue
Cornea Wound 65286
Sclera Wound 65286

Glutamate Dehydrogenase
Blood 82965

Glutamine 82975

Glutamyltransferase, Gamma .
                          82977

Glutathione 82978

Glutathione Reductase 82979

Glutethimide 82980

Glycated Protein 82985

Glycohemoglobin 83036

Goeckerman Treatment 96910
See also Photochemotherapy

Gold
Assay 80172
Blood 82995

Goldwaite Procedure 27422
See also Reconstruction, Patella, Instability

Gol-Vernet Operation
See Pyelotomy, Exploration

Gonadotropin
Chorionic 84702–84703
FSH 83001
ICSH 83002
LH 83002

Gonadotropin Panel 80426

Gonioscopy 92020

Goniotomy 65820

**Goodenough Harris Drawing
Test** 96100
See also Psychiatric Diagnosis

Graft
Anal 46753
Aorta 33860–33861, 33863,
              33870, 33875, 33877
Artery
   Coronary 33503–33505
Bone
   See also Bone Graft
   Harvesting 20900–20902
   Microvascular
   Anastomosis 20955–20962
   Osteocutaneous Flap with Microvascular
   Anastomosis 20969–20973
Bypass
   See Bypass Graft
Cartilage
   See also Cartilage Graft
   Harvesting 20910–20912
Cornea Transplant
   Lamellar 65710
   Penetrating 65730
   in Aphakia 65750
   in Pseudophakia 65755
Dura
   Spinal Cord 63710
Facial Nerve Paralysis 15840–15845
Fascia
   Cheek 15840
Fascia Lata
   Harvesting 20920–20922
Gum Mucosa 41870
Muscle
   Cheek 15841–15845
Nail Bed
   Reconstruction 11762
Nerve 64885–64907
Oral Mucosa 40818
Skin
   See also Skin Graft and Flap
   Blood Flow Check, Graft 15860
Tendon
   Finger 26392
   Hand 26392
   Harvesting 20924
Tissue
   Harvesting 20926
Vein
   Cross-Over 34520

Graft, Bypass
See Bypass Graft

Granulation Tissue
Cauterization, Chemical 17250

Greater Tuberosity Fracture
with Shoulder Dislocation
   Closed Treatment 23665
   Open Treatment 23670

Great Toe
Free Osteocutaneous Flap with Microvascular
Anastomosis 20973

Great Vessels
Anesthesia 00560–00562
Shunt

Aorta to Pulmonary Artery 33755, 33762
Central 33764
Subclavian to Pulmonary Artery . . 33750
Vena Cava to Pulmonary
Artery 33766–33767
Unlisted Services and Procedures 33999

Gritti Operation
See Amputation, Leg, Upper

Groin Area
Repair
Hernia 49550–49557

Group Health Education 99078

Growth Hormone 83003
Human 80428–80430, 86277

GSP
See Guanosine Monophosphate

Guaiac Test
See Blood, Feces

Guanosine Monophosphate . . 83008

Guard Stain 88313

Gums
Abscess
Incision and Drainage 41800
Alveolus
Excision 41830
Cyst
Incision and Drainage 41800
Excision
Gingiva 41820
Operculum 41821
Graft
Mucosa 41870
Hematoma
Incision and Drainage 41800
Lesion
Destruction 41850
Excision 41822–41828
Mucosa
Excision 41828
Reconstruction
Alveolus 41874
Gingiva 41872
Removal
Foreign Body 41805
Tumor
Excision 41825–41827
Unlisted Services and Procedures 41899

Gunning-Lieben Test
See Acetone, Blood or Urine

Guthrie Test 84030
See also Phenylalanine

H

HAA
See Hepatitis Antigen, B

HAAb
See Hepatitis Antibody, A

Hageman Factor 85280
See also Clotting Factor

Hair
Electrolysis 17380
Transplant
Punch Graft 15775–15776
Strip Graft 15220

HAI Test
See Hemagglutination Inhibition Test

Halo
Body Cast 29000
Cranial 20661
Femur 20663
Pelvis 20662
Removal 20665

Halsted Mastectomy
See Mastectomy, Radical

Halsted Repair
See Hernia, Repair, Inguinal

Hammertoe Repair 28285–28286

Hamster Penetration Test 89329
See also Sperm Analysis

Ham Test
See Hemolysins

Hand
See also Carpometacarpal Joint; Intercarpal Joint
Amputation
at Metacarpal 25927
Revision 25924, 25929, 25931
at Wrist 25920, 25922
Anesthesia 01800–01860
Arthrodesis
Carpometacarpal Joint . . 26843–26844
Intercarpal Joint 25820, 25825
Bone
Incision and Drainage 26034
Cast 29085
Decompression 26035, 26037
Excision
Excess Skin 15837
Fracture
Metacarpal 26600
Insertion
Tendon Graft 26392
Magnetic Resonance Imaging
(MRI) 73220, 73221
Reconstruction
Tendon Pulley . . . 26500, 26502, 26504

Removal
Implantation 26320
Tube 26392
Tube/Rod 26416
Repair
Blood Vessel 35207
Cleft Hand 26580
Muscle 26591, 26593
Scar Contracture 26597
Tendon 26350, 26352,
26356–26358, 26370,
26372–26373, 26410,
26412, 26415, 26416, 26426,
26428, 26433, 26434, 26437,
26440, 26442, 26445, 26449,
26450, 26460, 26476–26479,
26480, 26483, 26485, 26489
Replantation 20808
Skin Graft
Delay of Flap 15620
Full Thickness 15240–15241
Pedicle Flap 15574
Split 15100–15101
Strapping 29280
Tendon
Excision 26390, 26415
Tenotomy 26450, 26460
Tissue Transfer, Adjacent . . . 14040–14041
Tumor
Excision 26115–26117
Unlisted Services and Procedures 26989
X-Ray 73120–73130

Handling
Device 99002
Radioelement 77790
Specimen 99000–99001

Haptoglobin 83010–83012

Harrington Rod
Anesthesia 00670
Insertion 22840
Removal 22850

Hartmann Procedure 44143
See also Colectomy, Partial, with Colostomy

Harvesting
Bone Graft 20900–20902
Bone Marrow 38230
Cartilage Graft 20910–20912
Eggs
In Vitro Fertilization 58970
Fascia Lata Graft 20920–20922
Kidney 50300–50320
Liver 47133, 47134
Stem Cell 38231
Tendon Graft 20924
Tissue Grafts 20926

Hauser Procedure 27420
See also Reconstruction, Patella, Instability

Haygroves Procedure
See Reconstruction, Acetabulum

HBcAb
See Hepatitis Antibody, B

HBcAg
See Hepatitis Antigen, B

HBeAb
See Hepatitis Antibody, Be

HBeAg
See Hepatitis Antigen, Be

HBsAb
See Hepatitis Antibody, B

HBsAg
See Hepatitis Antigen, B

HBs AIg.....................86293

HDL
See Lipoprotein

Head
Anesthesia 00100–00222
CAT Scan.........70450, 70460, 70470
Excision..................21015–21070
Fracture and/or Dislocation . 21300–21497
Incision.......................21010
Introduction or Removal.....21076–21116
Lipectomy, Suction Assisted 15846
Nerve
   Graft 64885–64886
Other Procedures 21299, 21499
Repair/Revision and/or
Reconstruction 21120–21296
Ultrasound Exam 76506, 76536
X-Ray 70350

Headbrace
Application/Removal 20661

Heaf Test
See TB Test

Health Risk Assessment Instrument...................99420

Hearing Aid
Bone Conduction
   Implantation..................69710
   Removal 69711
   Repair.......................69711
   Replacement 69710
Checking.................92592–92593

Hearing Aid Services
Electroacoustic Test 92594–92595
Examination 92590–92591

Hearing Evaluation.... 92506, 92510
See also Otorhinolaryngology; Specific
Audiologic Tests

Hearing Tests
See Audiologic Function Tests; Hearing
Evaluation

Hearing Therapy 92507–92508,
                   92510

Heart
Anesthesia 00560–00580
Angiography
   Injection 93542–93543

Aortic Valve
   Repair.......................33414
   Replacement 33405–33406,
                  33411–33413
Arrhythmogenic Focus
   Catheter Ablation.......93650–93652
   Destruction...........33251, 33261
Balloon Catheterization 93536
Biopsy........................93505
Blood Vessel
   Repair........33320, 33321, 33322
Cardiac Output
   Measurements 93561–93562
Cardiac Rehabilitation 93797–93798
Cardioassist 92970–92971
Cardiopulmonary Bypass
   with Lung Transplant 32852, 32854
Catheterization 93501, 93510–93529
   Flow-directed 93503
Closure
   Septal Defect................33615
   Valve 33600, 33602
Commissurotomy 33476, 33478
Defibrillator
   Insertion 33245–33246
Destruction
   Arrhythmogenic Focus 33250
Electrical Recording
   Atria 93602
   Bundle of His 93600
   Comprehensive........93619–93622
Electroconversion 92960
Electrophysiologic Follow-up Study... 93624
Evaluation of Device 93640
Excision 33460
   Donor 33930, 33940
   Tricuspid Valve........33460, 33465
Fibrillation
   Atrial 33253
Implantation
   Ventricular Assist
     Device...............33975–33976
Incision
   Atrial 33253
   Exploration 33310, 33315
Injection
   Radiologic............93542–93543
Insertion
   Balloon Device................33973
   Defibrillator...........33212, 33246
   Electrode 33210–33211,
           33214, 33216–33217
   Pacemaker...........33200–33208,
             33212–33213
   Catheter 33210
   Pulse Generator 33214
Intraoperative Pacing and Mapping...93631
Ligation
   Fistula.......................37607
Magnetic Resonance Imaging (MRI)...75552
Myocardium
   Imaging, Nuclear 78466–78469
   Perfusion Study 78460–78465
Nuclear Medicine
   Blood Flow Study.............78414

Blood Pool Imaging..... 78472–78473,
              78481–78483
Myocardial Imaging 78466–78469
Myocardial Perfusion 78460–78465
Shunt Test 78428
Unlisted Services and
   Procedures 78499
Open Chest Massage..............32160
Pacemaker
   Conversion 33214
   Insertion 33200–33201,
      33206–33208, 33212–33213
   Removal.............33232–33238,
         33241, 33243–33244
   Repair.......................33242
   Replacement ... 33206, 33208, 33210,
       33240–33241, 33247, 33249
   Revision.....................33223
Pacing
   Arrhythmia Induction 93618
   Atria.......................93610
   Transcutaneous
     Temporary 92953
   Ventricular 93612
Positron Emission Tomography (PET) . 78459
Radiologic.....................76932
Reconstruction
   Atrial Septum.........33735–33739
   Vena Cava 34502
Recording
   Left Ventricle 93607
   Right Ventricle...............93603
   Tachycardia Sites..............93609
Removal
   Balloon Device................33974
   Ventricular Assist
     Device...............33977–33978
Repair
   Anomaly 33615, 33617
   Aortic Sinus 33702, 33710, 33720
   Atrial Septum...33253, 33641, 33647
   Atrioventricular Canal..........33660,
            33665, 33670
   Atrioventricular Valve....33660, 33665
   Cor Triatriatum................33732
   Infundibular 33476, 33478
   Mitral Valve.........33420, 33422,
           33425–33430
   Myocardium..................33542
   Outflow Tract 33478
   Postinfarction.........33542, 33545
   Septal Defect 33608, 33610,
        33660, 33813–33814
   Sinus of Valsalva 33702,
           33710, 33720
   Sinus Venosus 33645
   Tetralogy of Fallot 33692, 33694,
         33697, 33924
   Tricuspid Valve.........33460–33468
   Ventricle 33611–33612, 33619
   Ventricular Septum 33545, 33647,
       33681–33688, 33692, 33694
   Ventricular Tunnel 33722
   Wound 33300–33305

Hydroxyindoleacetic Acid 83497
Urine............................83497

Hydroxypregnenolone 84143

Hydroxyprogesterone .80402–80406,
83498–83499
See also Progesterone

Hydroxyproline 83500–83505

Hygroma
Cystic
   Axillary/Cervical
    Excision............38550–38555

Hymen
Excision 56700
Incision........................56720

Hymenal Ring
Revision 56700

Hymenectomy 56700

Hymenotomy 56720

Hyoid Bone
Fracture
   Closed Treatment
    with Manipulation...........21494
    without Manipulation........21493
   Open Treatment 21495

**Hyperbaric Oxygen
Pressurization** 99183
See also Pulmonology, Therapeutic, Pressure
Ventilation

**Hypercycloidal
X-Ray**.................76101–76102

**Hyperthermia
Treatment**............77600–77620

Hypoglossal Nerve
Anastomosis
   to Facial Nerve...............64868

Hypopharynx
Biopsy.........................42802

Hypophysectomy 61546, 61548

Hypospadias
Repair...................54300, 54352
   Complications........54340–54348
   First Stage 54304
    Meatal Advancement 54322
    Perineal....................54336
    Proximal Penile or Penoscrotal .54332
   Urethroplasty
    Local Skin Flaps 54324
    Local Skin Flaps and Mobilization of
    Urethra 54326
    Local Skin Flaps, Skin Graft Patch
    and/or Island Flap 54328
   Urethroplasty for Second
   Stage 54308, 54312
    Free Skin Graft 54316
   Urethroplasty for Third Stage 54318

Hypothermia..........99185–99186

Hysterectomy
Abdominal
   Radical 58210
   Supracervical 58180
   Total 58150, 58200
    with Colpo-Urethrocystopexy ...58152
   Resection of Ovarian
    Malignancy..................58951
Cesarean
   Anesthesia 00855
   after Cesarean Section 59525
   with Closure of Vesicouterine
    Fistula.....................51925
Induced Abortion
   with Amniotic Injections 59852
   with Vaginal Suppositories 59857
Radical
   Anesthesia 00846
Removal
   Lesion......................59100
Vaginal 56308, 58260
   Anesthesia 00944
   with Colpectomy 58275–58280
   with Colpo-Urethrocystopexy.....58267
   Laparoscopic 56308
   Radical 58285
   Removal Tubes/Ovaries........58262
    Repair of Enterocele 58263

Hysteroplasty 58540

Hysterorrhaphy 58520, 59350

Hysterosalpingography 74740
Anesthesia 01900
Catheterization.................58345
Injection Procedure 58340

Hysteroscopy
Diagnostic 56350
with Endometrial Ablation.........56356
with Lysis of Adhesions...........56352
Removal
   Impacted Foreign Body 56355
   Leiomyomata 56354
Resection
   of Intrauterine Septum.........56353
Surgical with Biopsy 56351

I

ICU Care...............99160–99162

Ideal Conduit
Visualization....................50690

IDH
See Isocitric Dehydrogenase, Blood

IgE..................86003–86005

Ileostomy....................44310

Continent (Kock Procedure)........44316
Revision 44312, 44314

Iliac Crest
Free Osteocutaneous Flap with Microvascular
Anastomosis....................20970

Iliohypogastric Nerve
Injection
   Anesthetic 64425

Ilioinguinal Nerve
Injection
   Anesthetic 64425

Ilium
Craterization 27070–27171
Cyst
   Excision 27065–27067
Excision..............27070–27171
Fracture
   Open Treatment 27215, 27218
Saucerization 27070–27171
Tumor
   Excision 27065–27067

Ilizarov Procedure
See also Application, Bone Fixation Device
Monticelli Type.................20692

Imaging
See Vascular Studies

Imbrication
Diaphragm 39545

Imipramine
Assay 80174

Immune Complex Assay.....86332

**Immune Serum Globulin
Immunization**................90741

Immunization
See also Allergen Immunotherapy
Active
   Acellular Pertussis.............90721
   BCG 90728
   Cholera.....................90725
   Diphtheria.............90719, 90721
   Diphtheria, Tetanus 90702
   Diphtheria, Tetanus, and Pertussis (DTP)
   and Injectable Poliomyelitis Vaccine
  90711
   Diphtheria, Tetanus, Pertussis ...90701
   Diphtheria, Tetanus, Pertussis,
   Hemophilus Influenza B........90720
   Diphtheria, Tetanus Toxoids,
   Acellular....................90700
   Hemophilus Influenza B........90721
   Hepatitis A..................90730
   Hepatitis B 90744–90747
   Influenza....................90724
   Influenza B 90737
   Measles 90705
   Measles, Mumps, Rubella.......90707
   Measles, Mumps, Rubella,
   Varicella 90710
   Measles and Rubella..........90708

Kidney 50010, 50045,
50120, 50130–50135
Knee
Capsule...................... 27435
Exploration................... 27310
Fasciotomy................... 27305
Removal of Foreign Body....... 27310
Lacrimal Punctum................ 68440
Larynx................... 31300–31320
Leg, Lower
Fasciotomy........... 27600–27602
Leg, Upper
Fasciotomy................. 27305
Tenotomy........... 27306–27307,
27390–27392
Lip
Frenum..................... 40806
Lung
Biopsy............... 32095–32100
Decortication
Partial.................. 32225
Total................... 32220
Lymphatic Channels............ 38308
Medullary Tract 61470
Mesencephalic Tract 61480
Metacarpophalangeal Joint
Capsule.................... 26520
Mitral Valve 33420, 33422
Nerve 64155–64772
Foot 28035
Root 63185, 63190
Vagus 43640–43641
Palm
Fasciotomy........... 26040, 26045
Pancreas
Sphincter 43262
Penis
Prepuce 54001
Newborn 54000
Pericardium.............. 33030–33031
with Clot Removal........... 33020
with Foreign Body Removal..... 33020
with Tube.................. 33015
Pharynx
Stoma..................... 42955
Pleura....................... 32320
Biopsy............. 32095–32100
Pleural Cavity
Empyema 32035–32036
Pneumothorax 32020
Prostate
Exposure
Bilateral Pelvic
Lymphadenectomy 55865
Insertion Radioactive Substance .
55860
Lymph Node Biopsy 55862
Transurethral 52450
Pterygomaxillary Fossa 31040
Pulmonary Valve.... 33470, 33472, 33474
Pyloric Sphincter 43520
Retina
Encircling Material............ 67115

Sclera
Fistulization
Iridencleisis or Idirotasis 66165
Sclerectomy with Punch or Scissors with
Iridectomy 66160
Thermocauterization with
Iridectomy 66155
Trabeculectomy ab Externo in Absence
Previous Surgery 66170
Trephination with Iridectomy..... 66150
Semicircular Canal
Fenestration 69820
Revision 69840
Seminal Vesicle 55600
Complicated 55605
Shoulder
Bone...................... 23035
Capsular Contracture Release 23020
Removal
Calcareous Deposits.......... 23000
Sinus
Frontal............... 31070–31087
Maxillary............. 31020–31032
Endoscopic 31256
Multiple 31090
Sphenoid
Sinusotomy 31050–31051
Skin................... 10040–10180
Skull
Suture............... 61550–61553
Spinal Cord................... 63200
Tract 63170, 63194–63199
Stomach
Creation
Stoma 43830–43832
Exploration................. 43500
Pyloric Sphincter 43520
Synovectomy 26140
Temporomandibular Joint.... 21015–21070
Tendon
Arm, Upper.................. 24310
Thigh
Fasciotomy.................. 27025
Thorax
Empyema 32035–32036
Pneumothorax 32020
Tibia 27607
Toe
Capsule............. 28270, 28272
Tendon 28232, 28234
Tenotomy 28010–28011
Tongue
Frenum 41010
Trachea
Emergency 31603–31605
with Flaps................. 31610
Planned.............. 31600–31601
Tympanic Membrane 69420
with Anesthesia.............. 69421
Ureterocele................... 51535
Urethra 53000–53010
Meatus 53020–53025
Uterus
Remove Lesion.............. 59100

Vagina
Exploration................... 57000
Vas Deferens 55200
for X-Ray 55300
Vitreous Strands
Laser Surgery................ 67031
Pars Plana Approach 67030
Wrist............ 25100–25101, 25105
Capsule.................... 25085
Decompression........ 25020, 25023
Tendon Sheath............... 25000

Incision and Drainage
See also Drainage; Incision
Abdomen
Fluid 49080–49081
Pancreatitis 48000
Abscess
Abdomen 49020, 49040
Anal 46045, 46050
Ankle 27603
Appendix 44900
Arm, Lower 25028
Arm, Upper........... 23930–23931
Auditory Canal, External 69020
Bartholin's Gland.............. 56420
Bladder..................... 51080
Brain............... 61320–61321
Breast..................... 19020
Ear, External
Complicated 69005
Simple................... 69000
Elbow 23930
Epididymis 54700
Eyelid 67700
Finger 26010–26011
Gums 41800
Hip 26990
Kidney 50020
Knee 27301
Leg, Lower 27603
Leg, Upper 27301
Liver 47010
Lung 32200
Lymph Node 38300–38305
Mouth 40800–40801,
41005–41009, 41015–41018
Nasal Septum................. 30020
Neck 21501–21502
Nose 30000–30020
Ovary
Abdominal Approach......... 58822
Vaginal Approach 58820
Palate 42000
Paraurethral Gland............. 53060
Parotid Gland 42300, 42305
Pelvis 26990, 45000
Perineum 56405
Peritoneum................. 49020
Prostate 55720, 55725
Rectum 45005, 45020,
46040, 46050, 46060
Retroperitoneal 49060
Salivary Gland........ 42300, 42305,
42310, 42320
Scrotum 54700, 55100

Vocal Cords
Therapeutic..... 31513, 31570–31571
Wrist
Radiologic 25246

Inkblot Test.................. 96100
See also Psychiatric Diagnosis

Innominate
Tumor
Excision 27077

Insemination
Artificial 58321–58322

Insertion
See also Implantation; Intubation;
Transplantation
Baffle
Ear, Middle 69410
Balloon
Intra-Aortic.................. 33973
Breast
Implants 19340–19342
Cannula
Arteriovenous.......... 36810, 36815
ECMO..................... 36822
Thoracic Duct............... 38794
Vein to Vein 36800
Cardioverter/Defibrillator
Anesthesia.................. 00534
Catheter
Abdomen 49420–49421
Abdominal Artery....... 36245–36248
Bile Duct............ 47510, 47525,
47530, 75982
Bladder.................... 51045
Brachiocephalic Artery... 36215–36218
Brain................. 61210, 61770
Bronchi............. 31710, 31717
Ear, Middle 69405
Eustachian Tube.............. 69405
Flow Directed................ 93503
Gastrointestinal, Upper 43241
Jejunum 44015
Kidney 50392
Lower Extremity Artery . 36245–36248
Nasotracheal 31720
Pelvic Artery.......... 36245–36248
Portal Vein 36481
Prostate 55859
Pulmonary Artery....... 36013–36015
Right Heart.................. 36013
Skull...................... 61107
Spinal Cord.......... 62350–62351
Suprapubic.................. 51010
Thoracic Artery........ 36215–36218
Trachea.................... 31700
Tracheobronchial 31725
Ureter via Kidney............. 50393
Urethra 53670–53675
Vein.............. 36489, 36491
Vena Cava 36010
Venous............. 36011–36012,
36400–36425, 36488,
36489, 36491, 36500, 36510
Cervical Dilation................ 59200

Cochlear Device.................. 69930
Contraceptive Capsules 11975, 11977
Defibrillator
Heart......... 33212, 33245–33246
Electrode
Brain 61531, 61533,
61760, 61850–61875
Heart 33210–33211,
33214, 33216–33217
Nerve 64553–64580
Sphenoidal 95830
Spinal Cord............ 63650–63655
Endotracheal Tube 31500
Filiform
Urethra 53640
Gastrostomy Tube 43750
Graft
Aorta............... 33330, 33335
Heart Vessel.......... 33330, 33335
Guide
Kidney Pelvis 50395
Guide Wire
Endoscopy 43248
Esophagoscopy......... 43226, 43248
Infusion Pump
Intraarterial 36260
Intravenous................. 36530
Spinal Cord............ 62361–62362
Intracatheter/Needle
Aorta............... 36160, 36200
Arteriovenous Shunt 36145
Intraarterial 36100–36101,
36120, 36140
Intravenous................. 36000
Kidney 50392
Intraocular Lens 66983
not Associated with Concurrent Cataract
Removal 66985
Manual or Mechanical
Technique.................. 66984
Intrauterine Device (IUD).......... 58300
IVC Filter 75940
Jejunostomy Tube
Endoscopy 44372
Keel
Laryngoplasty............... 31580
Laminaria 59200
Nasobiliary Tube
Endoscopy 43267
Nasopancreatic Tube
Endoscopy 43267
Needle
Bone 36680
Intraosseous................ 36680
Prostate 55859
Needle Wire
Trachea................... 31730
Neurostimulator
Pulse Generator 64590
Receiver 64590
Nose
Septal Prosthesis............. 30220
Obturator
Larynx.................... 31527

Ocular Implant
with/without Conjunctival Graft . 65150
with Foreign Material 65155
Muscles Attached 65140
Muscles not Attached 65135
in Scleral Shell.............. 65130
Orbital Transplant.................. 67550
Oviduct
Chromotubation 58350
Hydrotubation............... 58350
Pacemaker
Anesthesia.................. 00530
Fluoroscopy/Radiography 71090
Heart 33200–33208, 33210,
33212–33213, 33240, 33247, 33249
Packing
Vagina.................... 57180
Penile Prosthesis
Anesthesia.................. 00938
Pessary
Vagina.................... 57160
Pin
Skeletal Traction 20650
Prostate
Radioactive Substance 55860
Prosthesis
Nasal Septal................. 30220
Palate.................... 42281
Penis
Inflatable 54401, 54405
Noninflatable............... 54400
Speech 31611
Testis 54660
Pulse Generator
Brain.................... 61885
Heart............. 33212, 33214
Spinal Cord................. 63685
Radioactive Material
Bladder................... 51020
Cystourethroscopy 52250
Kidney........... 50559, 50578
Urethral Endoscopic..... 50959, 50978
Receiver
Brain.................... 61885
Spinal Cord................. 63685
Reservoir
Brain............. 61210, 61215
Spinal Cord................. 62360
Shunt 36835
Abdomen
Vein..................... 49425
Venous................... 49426
Spinal Instrumentation
Anterior...........22845–22847
Internal Spinal Fixation 22841
Pelvic Fixation 22848
Posterior Nonsegmental
Harrington Rod Technique 22840
Posterior Segmental.....22842–22844
Prosthetic Device.............22851
Stent
Bile Duct....... 43268, 47511, 47801
Bladder..................51045
Conjunctiva 68750
Esophagus 43219

In Vitro Fertilization
See also Artificial Insemination
Culture Oocyte 89250
Fertilize Oocyte 89250
Retrieve Oocyte 58970
Transfer Embryo 58974, 58976
Transfer Gamete 58976

Iodide Test
See Nuclear Medicine, Thyroid, Uptake

Iodine Test
See Starch Granules, Feces

Iontophoresis 97033

IP
See Allergen Immunotherapy

Ipecac Administration 99175

IPPB
See Intermittent Positive Pressure Breathing

Iridectomy
Anesthesia 00147
with Corneoscleral or Corneal
Section 66600
by Laser Surgery 66761
Peripheral for Glaucoma 66625
with Sclerectomy with Punch or
Scissors 66160
with Thermocauterization 66155
with Transfixion as for
Iris Bombe 66605
with Trephination 66150

Iridencleisis 66165

Iridodialysis 66680

Iridoplasty 66762

Iridotasis 66165

Iridotomy
with Cyclectomy 66505
Excision
with Corneoscleral or Corneal
Section 66600
with Cyclectomy 66605
Optical 66635
Peripheral 66625
Incision
Stab 66500
with Transfixion as for
Iris Bombe 66505
by Laser Surgery 66761
Optical 66635
Peripheral 66625
Sector 66630
by Stab Incision 66500

Iris
Anesthesia 00147
Cyst
Destruction 66770
Excision
Iridectomy
with Corneoscleral or Corneal
Section 66600

with Cyclectomy 66605
Optical 66635
Peripheral 66625
Sector 66630
Incision
Iridotomy
Stab 66500
with Transfixion as for
Iris Bombe 66505
Lesion
Destruction 66770
Repair
with Ciliary Body 66680
Suture 66682
Revision
Laser Surgery 66761
Photocoagulation 66762
Suture
with Ciliary Body 66682

Iron 83540
Absorption 78162
Chelatable
Total Body Iron 78172
Turnover 78160
Utilization 78170

Iron Binding Capacity 83550

Iron Hematoxylin Stain 88312

Iron Stain 85535

Irradiation
Blood Products 86945

Irrigation
Bladder 51700
Caloric Vestibular Test 92533, 92543
Catheter
Brain 62194, 62225
Corpora Cavernosa
Priapism 54220
Penis
Priapism 54220
Shunt
Spinal Cord 63744
Sinus
Maxillary 31000
Sphenoid 31002
Vagina 57150

Irving Sterilization
See Ligation, Fallopian Tube, Oviduct

Ischial
Tumor
Excision 27060, 27078, 27079

Ischiectomy 15941

Ischium
Pressure Ulcer 15940–15946

ISG Immunization 90741
See also Immunization, Passive, Immune
Serum Globulin

Island Pedicle Flaps 15740

Islet Cell
Antibody 86341

Isocitric Dehydrogenase
Blood 83570

Isopropyl Alcohol 84600

Isthmusectomy
Thyroid Gland 60210–60225

IUD
See Intrauterine Device

IV
See Intravenous

IVC Filter
Placement 75940

IVF
See In Vitro Fertilization

IV Infusion Therapy
See Injection, Chemotherapy

Ivy Bleeding Time 85002

J

Jaboulay Operation
See Gastroduodenostomy

Jannetta Procedure
See Decompression, Cranial Nerve

Jatene Procedure
See Repair, Great Arteries

Jatene Type 33778–33781

Jaw Joint
See Mandible; Maxilla; Temporomandibular
Joint (TMJ)

Jaws
Muscle Reduction 21295–21296
X-Ray
for Orthodontics 70355

Jejunostomy
Catheterization 44015
Insertion
Catheter 44015
Non-Tube 44310
with Pancreatic Drain 48001

Johannsen Procedure 53400
See also Urethroplasty

Joint
See also Specific Joint
Arthrocentesis 20600–20610
Drainage 20600–20610
Injection 20600–20610
Mobilization 97265
Nuclear Medicine
Imaging 78300, 78315

Jones and Cantarow Test
See Urea Nitrogen, Clearance

Jones Procedure 28760
See also Arthrodesis, Interphalangeal Joint,
Great Toe

Joplin Procedure 28292–28294
See also Repair, Hallux Valgus

K

Kader Operation
See Incision, Stomach, Creation, Stoma

Kala Azar Smear 87207

Kasai Procedure 47701
See also Portoenterostomy

Keel
Insertion/Removal
    Laryngoplasty 31580

Keen Operation
See Laminectomy

Kelikian Procedure 28280
See also Toes, Repair, Webbed

Keller Procedure 28292
See also Toes, Repair, Bunion

Kelly Urethral Plication 57220

Keratectomy
Partial
    for Lesion 65400

Keratomileusis 65760

Keratophakia 65765

Keratoplasty
Lamellar 65710
Penetrating 65730
    in Aphakia 65750
    in Pseudophakia 65755

Keratoprosthesis 65770

Keratotomy
Radial 65771

Ketogenic Steroids 83582

Ketone Body
Acetone 82009–82010

Ketosteroids 83586–83593

Kidner Procedure 28238

Kidney
Abscess
    Incision and Drainage 50020
Anesthesia 00862, 00868,
                00872–00873
Biopsy 50205

Catheterization
    Endoscopic 50572
Cyst
    Aspiration 50390
    Excision 50280–50290
    Injection 50390
    X-Ray 74470
Destruction
    Calculus 50590
    Endoscopic 50557, 50576
Dilation 50395
Endoscopy
    Biopsy 50555, 50574
    Catheterization 50553, 50572
    Destruction 50557, 50576
    Dilation
        Ureter 50553
    via Incision 50570–50580
    Radioactive Substance 50578
    Radiotracer 50559
    Removal
        Calculus 50561, 50580
        Foreign Body 50561, 50580
    via Stoma 50551–50561
Excision
    Donor 50300–50320
    Partial 50240
    Recipient 50340
    Transplantation 50370
    with Ureters 50220–50236
Exploration 50010, 50045,
                50120, 50135
Function Study 78725–78726
Incision 50010, 50045,
            50120, 50130, 50135
Incision and Drainage 50040, 50125
Injection
    Radiologic 50394
Insertion
    Catheter 50392, 50393
    Guide 50395
    Intracatheter 50392
    Stent 50393
    Tube 50398
Lithotripsy 50590
Manometry
    Pressure 50396
Needle Biopsy 50200
Nuclear Medicine
    Blood Flow 78715
    Function Study 78725–78726
    Imaging 78700–78707, 78710
    Transplant Evaluation 78727
    Unlisted Services and
      Procedures 78799
Removal
    Calculus 50060–50081, 50130
    Foreign Body 50561, 50580
Renal Pelvis 50405
Repair
    Blood Vessels 50100
    Fistula 50520–50526
    Horseshoe Kidney 50540
    Renal Pelvis 50400–50405
    Wound 50500

Solitary 50405
Suture
    Fistula 50520–50526
    Horseshoe Kidney 50540
Transplantation 00862, 00868, 01990
    See also Transplantation, Renal
    Anesthesia 00868
    Donor Nephrectomy 50300–50320
    Implantation of Graft 50360
    Recipient Nephrectomy .. 50340, 50365
    Reimplantation Kidney 50380
    Removal Transplant Renal
      Autograft 50370
Ultrasound 76770–76778
X-Ray with Contrast
    Arthrography 73580
    Guide Catheter 74475

Kidney Stone
See Calculus, Removal, Kidney

Killian Operation
See Sinusotomy, Frontal

Kineplasty
See Cineplasty

Kinetic Therapy 97530

Kininogen 85293

Kleihauer-Betke Test 85460
See also Hemoglobin, Fetal

Knee
See also Femur; Fibula; Patella; Tibia
Abscess 27301
Anesthesia 01300–01444
Arthrocentesis 20610
Arthrodesis 27580
Arthroplasty 27440–27443,
                 27445, 27446
    Revision 27486, 27487
Arthroscopy
    Diagnostic 29870–29871
    Surgical 29874–29877,
               29879–29889
Arthrotomy 27310, 27330–27331,
    27332–27333, 27334–27335, 27403
Biopsy 27323–27324, 27330–27331
    Synovium 27330
Bone
    Drainage 27303
Bursa 27301
    Excision 27340
Cyst
    Excision 27345
Disarticulation 27598
Dislocation 27550, 27552,
             27554, 27560, 27562
    Open Treatment 27556–27558
Drainage 27310
Excision 27350
    Cartilage 27332–27333
    Synovial Lung 27334–27335
Exploration 27310, 27331
Fasciotomy 27305, 27496–27499
Fracture 27520, 27524

Arthroscopic Treatment . . 29850–29851
Fusion 27580
Hematoma 27301
Incision
    Capsule 27435
Injection
    X-Ray 27370
Magnetic Resonance Imaging (MRI) . 73721
Manipulation 27570
Meniscectomy 27332–27333
Reconstruction 27437–27438
    with Implantation 27445
    Ligament 27427–27429
Removal
    Foreign Body 27310, 27331, 27370
    Loose Body 27331
    Prosthesis 27488
Repair
    Instability 27420, 27422, 27424
    Ligament 27405, 27407
    Meniscus 27403
    Tendon 27380–27381
Replacement 27447
Retinacular
    Release 27425
Strapping 29530
Suture
    Tendon 27380–27381
Tumor
    Excision 27327–27329, 27365
Unlisted Services and Procedures 27599
X-Ray 73560–73564
    with Contrast 73580
    Standing 73559

Knock-Knee Repair 27455, 27457

Kocher Operation
See Shoulder, Dislocation, Closed Treatment

Kocher Pylorectomy
See Gastrectomy, Partial

Kock Pouch 44316
Formation 50825

Kock Procedure 44316

KOH
See Tissue, Examination for Fungi

Kraske Procedure 45116
See also Proctectomy, Partial

Krause Operation
See Gasserian Ganglion, Sensory Root,
Decompression

Kroenlein Procedure 67420
See also Orbitotomy

Krukenberg Procedure 25915

Kuhlmann Test 96100
See also Psychiatric Diagnosis

**Kuhnt-Szymanowski
Procedure** 67917
See also Ectropion, Repair

K-Wire Fixation
Tongue 41500

L

Labial Adhesions
Lysis 56441

Labyrinthectomy 69905
with Mastoidectomy 69910
with Skull Base Surgery 61596

Labyrinthotomy
with/without Cryosurgery 69801
with Mastoidectomy 69802

Laceration Repair
See Specific Site

Lacrimal Duct
Canaliculi
    Repair 68700
Exploration 68820
    with Anesthesia 68825
    Canaliculi 68840
    Stent 68830
Insertion
    Stent 68830
Removal
    Dacryolith 68530
    Foreign Body 68530
X-Ray with Contrast 70170

Lacrimal Gland
Biopsy 68510
Close Fistula 68770
Excision
    Partial 68505
    Total 68500
Fistulization 68720
Incision and Drainage 68400
Injection
    X-Ray 68850
Nuclear Medicine
    Tear Flow 78660
Removal
    Dacryolith 68530
    Foreign Body 68530
Repair
    Fistula 68770
Tumor
    Excision
        without Closure 68540
        with Osteotomy 68550

Lacrimal Punctum
Closure
    by Plug 68761
    by Thermocauterization, Litigation
    or Laser Surgery 68760
Dilation 68800
Incision 68440
Repair 68705

Lacrimal Sac
Biopsy 68525
Excision 68520
Incision and Drainage 68420

Lacrimal System
Unlisted Services and Procedures 68899

Lacryoaptography
Nuclear 78660

**Lactase Deficiency Breath
Test** 91065

Lactic Acid 83605

**Lactic
Dehydrogenase** 83615–83625

Lactiferous Duct
Excision 19112
Exploration 19110

Lactogen, Human Placental . . . 83632

Lactose
Urine 83633–83634

Ladd Procedure 44055

Lambrinudi Operation
See Arthrodesis, Foot Joint

Laminaria
Insertion 59200

Laminectomy 62351, 63001,
    63005, 63011, 63015–63042,
    63180–63200, 63265–63655
Anesthesia 00604
with Facetectomy 63045–63048
Lumbar 63012
Surgical 63170, 63172

Language Evaluation 92506

Language Therapy 92507–92508

LAP
See Leucine Aminopeptidase

Laparoscopy
Anesthesia 00790, 00840
Appendectomy 56315
Aspiration 56306
Biopsy 56305, 56311
    Peritoneal Surface 56305
Cholecystectomy 56340–56342
Destruction
    Lesion 56303
Diagnostic 56300
Ectopic Pregnancy 59150
    with Salpingectomy and/or
    Oophorectomy 59151
Fimbrioplasty 56344
Hernia Repair
    Initial 56316
    Recurrent 56317
In Vitro Fertilization 58976
    Retrieve Oocyte 58970
    Transfer Embryo 58974
    Transfer Gamete 58976

Pressure Ulcer 15950–15958
Skin Graft
    Delay of Flap 15610
    Full Thickness 15220–15221
    Muscle, Myocutaneous, or
    Fasciocutaneous Flaps 15738
    Pedicle Flap 15572
    Split 15100–15101
Tissue Transfer, Adjacent . . . 14020–14021
Upper
    See also Femur
    Abscess 27301
    Amputation 27590–27592
      at Hip 27290, 27295
      Revision 27594, 27596
    Anesthesia 01200–01274
    Artery
      Ligation 37618
    Biopsy 27323–27324
    Bursa 27301
    Bypass Graft 35903
    Cast 29345, 29355, 29365, 29450
    Cast Brace 29358
    CAT Scan 73700–73702
    Exploration
      Blood Vessel 35860
    Fasciotomy 27305,
      27496–27499, 27892–27894
    Hematoma 27301
    Magnetic Resonance Imaging
    (MRI) 73720
    Neurectomy 27315, 27320
    Removal
      Cast 29705
      Foreign Body 27370
    Repair
      Blood Vessel . . 35226, 35256, 35286
      Muscle 27385–27386,
        27400, 27430
      Tendon 27393–27395,
        27396–27397, 27400
    Splint 29505
    Strapping 29580
    Suture
      Muscle 27385–27386
    Tenotomy 27306–27307,
      27390–27392
    Tumor
      Excision 27327–27329
    Ultrasound 76880
    Unlisted Services and
    Procedures 27599
    Unna Boot 29580
    X-Ray 73592
Wound Exploration
    Penetrating 20103

Legionella
Antibody 86713

Leiomyomata
Removal 56309, 56354

Leishmania
Antibody 86717

Lens
Anesthesia 00142
Extracapsular 66940
Intracapsular 66920
    Dislocated 66930
Intraocular
    Exchange 66986
    Reposition 66825
Prosthesis
    Insertion 66983
    not Associated with Concurrent
    Cataract Removal 66985
    Manual or Mechanical
    Technique 66984
Removal
    Lens Material
      Aspiration Technique 66840
      Extracapsular 66940
      Intracapsular 66920, 66930
      Pars Plana Approach 66852
      Phacofragmentation Technique . 66850

Lens Material
Aspiration Technique 66840
Pars Plana Approach 66852
Phacofragmentation Technique 66850

Leptospira
Antibody 86720

Leriche Operation
See Sympathectomy, Thoracolumbar

Lesion
See also Tumor
Anal
    Destruction 46900, 46910,
      46916–46917, 46924
    Excision 45108, 46922
Ankle
    Tendon Sheath 27630
Arm, Lower
    Excision 25110
Auditory Canal, External
    Excision
      Exostosis 69140
      Radical with Neck Dissection . . 69155
      Radical without Neck
      Dissection 69150
      Soft Tissue 69145
Brain
    Excision 61534, 61536,
      61600–61608, 61615–61616
    Radiation Treatment 77432
Brainstem
    Excision 61575–61576
Breast
    Excision 19120
Carotid Body
    Excision 60600–60605
Chemotherapy 96405–96406
Ciliary Body
    Destruction 66770
Colon
    Destruction 44393, 45383
    Excision 44110–44111

Conjunctiva
    Destruction 68135
    Excision 68110–68130
    Expression 68040
Cornea
    Destruction 65450
    Excision 65400
    of Pterygium 65420
Destruction
    Bladder 51030
    Ureter 52338
Ear, Middle
    Excision 69540
Epididymis
    Excision 54830, 54840
Esophagus
    Ablation 43228
    Excision 43100–43101
    Removal 43216
Excision 59100
    Bladder 52224
    Urethra 52224, 53265
Eye
    Excision 65900
Eyelid
    Destruction 67850
    Excision
      under Anesthesia 67808
      without Closure 67840
      Multiple, Different Lids 67805
      Multiple, Same Lid 67801
      Single 67800
Facial
    Destruction 17000–17010
Femur
    Excision 27062
Finger
    Tendon Sheath 26160
Foot
    Excision 28080, 28090
Gums
    Destruction 41850
    Excision 41822–41823,
      41825–41828
Hand
    Tendon Sheath 26160
Intestines, Small
    Destruction 44369
    Excision 44110–44111
Iris
    Destruction 66770
Leg, Lower
    Tendon Sheath 27630
Lymph Node
    Incision and Drainage 38300–38305
Mesentery
    Excision 44820
Mouth
    Destruction 40820
    Excision 40810, 40812,
      40814, 40816, 41116
    Vestibule
      Destruction 40820
      Repair 40830

Nasopharynx
  Excision 42880
Nerve
  Excision 64774–64792
Nose
  Intranasal
    External Approach........... 30118
    Internal Approach 30117
Orbit
  Excision 61333, 67412
Palate
  Destruction................. 42145
  Excision.................... 42104,
        42106–42107, 42120
Pancreas
  Excision 48120
Pelvis
  Destruction................. 56303
Penis
  Destruction
    Any Method 54065
    Cryosurgery............... 54056
    Electrodesiccation.......... 54055
    Laser Surgery 54057
    Simple.................... 54050
    Surgical Excision........... 54060
  Excision 54060
    Penile Plaque........ 54110–54112
Pharynx
  Destruction................. 42808
  Excision 42808
Rectum
  Excision 45108
Removal
  Larynx.............. 31512, 31578
  Resection 52338
Retina
  Destruction
    Extensive........... 67227–67228
    Localized 67208, 67210
  Radiation by Implantation of
    Source 67218
Sclera
  Excision 66130
Skin
  Abrasion 15786–15787
  Biopsy............... 11100–11101
  Destruction
    Malignant 17260–17286
  Excision
    Benign............. 11400–11471
    Malignant 11600–11646
  Injection 11900–11901
  Paring or Curettement
    Benign Hyperkeratotic . 11050–11052
  Removal 11200–11201
  Shaving............. 11300–11313
Skull
  Excision 61400, 61500,
     61600–61608, 61615–61616
Spermatic Cord
  Excision 55520
Spinal Cord
  Destruction.......... 62280–62282

Excision 63265–63268,
            63270–63273
Stomach
  Excision 43611
Testis
  Excision 54510
Toe
  Excision 28092
Tongue
  Excision....... 41110, 41112–41114
Uvula
  Destruction................. 42145
  Excision....... 42104, 42106–42107
Vagina
  Destruction.......... 57061, 57065
Vulva
  Destruction
    Extensive................. 56515
    Simple................... 56501
Wrist Tendon
  Excision 25110

Leucine Aminopeptidase ... 83670

Leukoagglutinins 86021

Leukocyte
See also White Blood Cell
Alkaline Phosphatase............. 85540
Antibody...................... 86021
Histamine Release Test 86343
Phagocytosis 86344
Transfusion................... 86950

**Leukocyte Histamine Release
Test**........................ 86343

Levator Muscle Rep
See Blepharoptosis, Repair

LeVeen Shunt
Insertion 49425
Patency Test................... 78291
Revision 49426

LH
See Luteinizing Hormone

LHR
See Leukocyte Histamine Release Test

Lidocaine
Assay 80176

Lid Suture
See Blepharoptosis, Repair

Life Support
Organ Donor................... 01990

Ligament
See also Specific Site
Dentate
  Incision............. 63180–63182
  Section............. 63180–63182
Injection 20250

Ligation
Artery
  Abdomen 37617
  Carotid 37600, 37605–37606

  Chest 37616
  Coronary.................. 33502
  Coronary Artery 33502
  Extremity 37618
  Fistula.................... 37607
  Neck..................... 37615
  Temporal.................. 37609
Fallopian Tube
  Oviduct 56301, 58600–58611
Gastroesophageal............... 43405
Hemorrhoids........... 46945–46946
Oviducts 59100
Salivary Duct 42665
Shunt
  Aorta
    Pulmonary............... 33924
  Peritoneal
    Venous.................. 49428
Thoracic duct 38380
  Abdominal Approach 38382
  Thoracic Approach........... 38381
Vas Deferens 55450
Vein
  Esophagus...... 43205, 43244, 43400
  Gastric 43244
  Iliac..................... 37660
  Jugular, Internal............ 37565
  Perforate.................. 37760
  Saphenous........... 37700, 37720,
       37730, 37735, 37780
  Secondary 37785
  Vena Cava............ 37620, 37650

Ligature Strangulation
Skin Tags 11200–11201

Limited Neck Dissection
with Thyroidectomy 60252

Limulus Lysate............... 87175

Lingual Nerve
Avulsion 64740
Incision...................... 64740
Transection................... 64740

Linton Procedure 37760

Lip
Biopsy........................ 40490
Excision............ 40500–40530
  Frenum 40819
Incision
  Frenum 40806
Reconstruction 40525, 40527
Repair 40650, 40652, 40654
  Cleft Lip............ 40700–40702,
        40720, 40761
  Fistula.................... 42260
Unlisted Services and Procedures.... 40799

Lipase 83690

Lipectomy 15831
Suction Assisted.......... 15876–15879

Lipids
Feces.................. 82705–82710

Lipoprotein
Blood....................83715–83719
LDL...........................83721

Liposuction 15876–15879
See also Lipectomy

Lips
Repair
  Cleft
    Anesthesia 00102
  Cleft Palate
    Anesthesia 00172
Skin Graft
  Delay of Flap 15630
  Full Thickness.........15260–15261
  Pedicle Flap 15576
Tissue Transfer, Adjacent ...14060–14061

Lisfranc Operation
See Amputation, Foot

Listeria Monocytogenes
Antibody.......................86723

Lithium
Assay 80178

Litholapaxy 52317–52318

Lithotripsy
Anesthesia 00872–00873
Bile Duct Calculi (Stone)
  Endoscopy 43265
with Cystourethroscopy 52337
Kidney.........................50590
Pancreatic Duct Calculi (Stone)
  Endoscopy 43265

Liver
See also Hepatic Duct
Abscess
  Aspiration..................47015
  Incision and Drainage 47010
  Injection...................47015
Anesthesia...........00792, 00796
Aspiration.....................47015
Biopsy.......................47100
  Anesthesia..................00702
Cyst
  Aspiration..................47015
  Incision and Drainage 47010
Excision
  Extensive 47122
  Partial 47120, 47125,
              47130, 47134
  Total 47133
Injection......................47015
  Radiologic..................47505
  X-Ray.....................47500
Lobectomy 47125, 47130
  Partial.....................47120
Needle Biopsy 47000–47001
Nuclear Medicine
  Function Study...............78220
  Imaging...........78201–78216
Repair
  Abscess 47300

Cyst 47300
Wound............47350, 47360,
            47361–47362
Suture
  Wound............47350, 47360,
            47361–47362
Transplantation..........47135, 47136
  Anesthesia 00796, 01990
Trisegmentectomy 47122
Unlisted Services and Procedures....47399

Lobectomy
Brain..........................61539
Contralateral Subtotal
  Thyroid Gland.........60212, 60225
Liver......47120, 47122, 47125, 47130
Lung 32480–32482
  Sleeve.....................32486
Parotid Gland 42410, 42415
Segmental 32663
Sleeve........................32486
Temporal Lobe 61538
Thyroid Gland
  Partial..............60210, 60212
  Total 60220, 60225
Total 32663

Lobotomy
Frontal 61490

Localization of Nodule
Radiographic
  Breast..............76096–76097

Lombard Test 92573

Longmire Operation
See Anastomosis, Hepatic Duct to Intestine

Long Term Care Facility Visits
See Nursing Facility Services

Loose Body
Removal
  Elbow.....................24101

Lord Procedure
See Anal Sphincter, Dilation

Low Vision Aids
Fitting.................92354–92355
Supply........................92392

LRH
See Luteinizing Releasing Factor

LSD
See Lysergic Acid Diethylamide

L/S Ratio
Amniotic Fluid 83661

Lumbar
See also Spine
Aspiration, Disk
  Percutaneous 62287

Lumbar Plexus
Decompression.................64714
Neuroplasty 64714
Release.......................64714
Repair/Suture..................64862

Lumen Dilation 74360

Lunate
Arthroplasty
  with Implant.................25444
Dislocation 25690, 25695

Lung
Abscess
  Incision and Drainage 32200
Anesthesia 00522, 00540–00548
  Transplant...................00580
Angiography
  Injection...................93541
Aspiration......................32420
Biopsy.............32095–32100
Bullae
  Excision 32141
Cyst
  Incision and Drainage 32200
  Removal....................32140
Decortication......32320, 32651–32652
  Partial.....................32225
  Total......................32220
Empyema
  Excision 32540
Excision..........32440–32445, 32488
  Bronchus Resection............32486
  Chest Resection.......32520–32525
  Donor.....................33930
  Lobe 32480–32482
  Segment....................32484
  Wedge Resection.......32500, 32657
Hemorrhage 32110
Injection
  Radiologic..................93541
Lysis
  Adhesions...................32124
Needle Biopsy 32405
Nuclear Medicine
  Imaging, Perfusion......78580–78585
  Imaging, Ventilation.....78586–78594
  Unlisted Services and
    Procedures 78599
Pneumocentesis..................32420
Pneumolysis.....................32940
Pneumothorax 32960
Puncture.......................32420
Removal
  Bronchoplasty 32501
  Completion Pneumonectomy.....32488
  Extrapleural 32445
  Single Lobe 32480
  Single Segment 32484
  Sleeve Lobectomy 32486
  Sleeve Pneumonectomy.........32442
  Total Pneumonectomy 32440
  Two Lobes 32480
  Wedge Resection.............32500
Repair
  Hernia.....................32800
Segmentectomy 32484
Tear
  Repair.....................32110
Thoracotomy 32095–32100, 32110
  Cardiac Massage.............32160

Bone Marrow Study 76400
Brain 70551–70553
Breast 76093–76094
Chest 71550
Elbow 73221
Face 70540
Finger Joint 73221
Foot Joints 73721
Hand 73220
Heart 75552
   Complete Study 75554
   Flow Mapping 75556
   Limited Study 75555
Knee 73721
Leg 73720
Neck 70540
Orbit 70540
Pelvis 72196
Radiology
   Diagnostic
     Unlisted Services and
     Procedures 76499
Spine
   Cervical 72141–72142, 72156
   Lumbar 72148–72149, 72158
   Thoracic 72146–72147, 72157
Temporomandibular Joint (TMJ) 70336
Toe 73721
Wrist 73221

Magnet Operation
See Eye, Removal, Foreign Body

Magnuson Procedure 23450
See also Capsulorrhaphy, Anterior

Magpi Operation 54322

Magpi Procedure
See Hypospadias, Repair

Malar Area
Bone Graft 21210
Fracture
   with Bone Graft 21366
   with Manipulation 21355

Malaria Antibody 86750

Malaria Smear 87207

Malate Dehydrogenase 83775

Malleolus
See Ankle; Fibula; Tibia

Mallet Finger Repair 26432

Maltose
Tolerance Test 82951–82952

Mammary Duct
X-Ray with Contrast 76086–76088

Mammary Ductogram 19030

Mammary Node
Dissection
   Anesthesia 00406

Mammography 76090–76091
Screening 76092

Mammoplasty
Anesthesia 00402
Augmentation 19324–19325
Reduction 19318

Mandible
See also Facial Bones; Maxilla;
Temporomandibular Joint (TMJ)
Abscess
   Excision 21025
Bone Graft 21215
Fracture
   Closed Treatment
     with Interdental Fixation 21453
     with Manipulation 21451
     without Manipulation 21450
   Open Treatment 21465, 21470
     with Interdental Fixation 21462
     without Interdental Fixation 21461
   Percutaneous Treatment 21452
Osteotomy 21198
Reconstruction
   with Implant 21248–21249
Removal
   Foreign Body 41806
Tumor
   Excision 21040–21045
X-Ray 70100–70110

Mandibular Body
Augmentation
   with Bone Graft 21127
   with Prothesis 21125

Mandibular Condyle
Fracture
   Open Treatment 21465, 21470
Reconstruction 21247

Mandibular Ramis
Reconstruction
   with Bone Graft 21194
   without Bone Graft 21193
   with Internal Rigid Fixation 21196
   without Internal Rigid Fixation . . . 21195

Mandibular Resection
Prosthesis 21081

Mandibular Staple Bone Plate
Reconstruction
   Mandible 21244

Manganese 83785

Manipulation
See also Manipulation, Dislocation and/or
Fracture
Dislocation and/or Fracture 25535
   Acetabulum 27222
   Acromioclavicular 23545
   Ankle 27810, 27818, 27860
   Carpometacarpal 26670,
                 26675–26676
   Chest Wall 94667–94668
   Clavicle 23505
   Elbow 24640
   Epicondyle 24565

   Femoral 27232, 27502,
                27510, 27517
   Pertrochanteric 27240
   Fibula 27781, 27788
   Finger 26725, 26727,
                26742, 26755
   Greater Tuberosity 23625
   Hand 26670, 26675–26676
   Heel 28405–28406
   Hip 27257
   Hip Socket 27222
   Humeral 23605, 24505,
                24535, 24577
   Hyoid 21494
   Intercarpal 25660
   Interphalangeal Joint 26770,
                26775–26776
   Larynx 31586
   Lunate 25690
   Malar Area 21355
   Mandibular 21451
   Metacarpal 26605, 26607
   Metacarpophalangeal 26700,
         26705–26706, 26742
   Metatarsal 28475–28476
   Nasal Bone 21315–21320
   Orbit 21401
   Phalangeal Shaft 26727
     Distal, Finger or Thumb 26755
     Phalanges, Finger/Thumb 26725
   Phalanges
     Finger 26742, 26755,
           26770, 26775–26776
     Finger/Thumb 26727
     Great Toe 28495–28496
     Toes 28515
   Radial 25565
   Radial Shaft 25505
   Radiocarpal 25660
   Radioulnar 25675
   Scapula 23575
   Shoulder 23650–23655
     with Greater Tuberosity 23665
     with Surgical or Anatomical
     Neck 23675
   Sternoclavicular 23525
   Talus 28435–28436
   Tarsal 28455–28456
   Thumb 26641, 26645,
             26650, 26659
   Tibial 27532, 27752
   Trans-Scaphoperilunar 25680
   Ulna 24675
   Ulnar 25535, 25565
   Vertebral 22315
   Wrist 25624, 25635, 25660,
         25675, 25680, 25690
Foreskin 54450
Globe 92018–92019
Hip 27275
Interphalangeal Joint, Proximal 26742
Knee 27570
Osteopathic 98925–98929
Physical Therapy 97260–97261

Transposition 64721

Mediastinoscopy 39400
Anesthesia 00528

Mediastinotomy
Cervical Approach 39000
Transthoracic Approach 39010

Mediastinum
See also Chest; Thorax
Anesthesia 00528, 00540
Cyst
    Excision 32662, 39200
Endoscopy
    Biopsy 39400
    Exploration 39400
Exploration 39000–39010
Incision and Drainage 39000–39010
Needle Biopsy 32405
Removal
    Foreign Body 39000–39010
Tumor
    Excision 32662, 39220
Unlisted Procedures 39488

**Medical Disability Evaluation
Services** 99455–99456

Medical History
Office and/or Other Outpatient
Services 99201–99205

Medical Testimony 99075

Medulla
Tractotomy 61470

Medullary Tract
Incision 61470
Section 61470

Meninges
Tumor
    Excision 61512, 61519

Meningioma
Excision 61512, 61519
Tumor
    Excision 61512, 61519

Meningocele Repair . . . 63700, 63702

**Meningococcal Polysaccharide
Vaccine** 90733

Meniscectomy 21060
Knee Joint 27332–27333
Temporomandibular Joint 21060

Meniscus
Knee
    Excision 27332–27333
    Repair 27403

Mental Nerve
Avulsion 64736
Incision 64736
Transection 64736

Meprobamate 83805

Mercury 83015, 83825

Merskey Test
See Fibrin Degradation Products

Mesencephalic Tract
Incision 61480
Section 61480

Mesencephalon
Tractotomy 61480

Mesentery
Lesion
    Excision 44820
Repair 44850
Suture 44850
Unlisted Services and Procedures 44899

Metabisulfite Test
See Red Blood Cell, Sickling

Metabolite 82520

Metacarpal
Craterization 26230
Cyst
    Excision 26200, 26205
Diaphysectomy 26230
Excision 26230, 26250, 26255
Fracture
    Closed Treatment 26605, 26607
    with Manipulation 26605, 26607
    without Manipulation 26600
    Open Treatment 26615
    Percutaneous Fixation 26608
Ostectomy 26250, 26255
Repair
    Lengthening 26568
    Osteotomy 26565
Saucerization 26230
Tumor
    Excision 26200, 26205

Metacarpophalangeal Joint
Arthrodesis 26850, 26852
Arthroplasty 26530–26531
Arthrotomy 26075
Biopsy
    Synovium 26105
Capsule
    Excision 26520
    Incision 26520
Capsulodesis 26516–26518
Dislocation 26700, 26705–26706
    Open Treatment 26715
Exploration 26075
Fracture 26740, 26742, 26746
Fusion 26516–26518, 26850, 26852
Removal of Foreign Body 26075
Repair
    Collateral Ligament 26540–26542
Synovectomy 26135

Metanephrine 83835

Metatarsal
See also Foot
Amputation 28810
Condyle
    Excision 28288

Craterization 28122
Cyst
    Excision 28104, 28106–28107
Diaphysectomy 28122
Excision 28110–28114, 28122, 28140
Fracture
    Closed Treatment
        without Manipulation 28470,
                                      28475–28476
        Open Treatment 28485
Free Osteocutaneous Flap with Microvascular
Anastomosis 20972
Repair 28322
    Lengthening 28306–28307
    Osteotomy 28306–28308, 28309
Saucerization 28122
Tumor
    Excision 28104,
                            28106–28107, 28173

Metatarsophalangeal Joint
Arthrotomy 28022
Dislocation 28630, 28635, 28645
    Percutaneous Fixation 28636
Exploration 28022
Great Toe
    Arthrodesis 28750
    Fusion 28750
Removal
    of Foreign Body 28022
    of Loose Body 28022
Synovial
    Excision 28072
Toe 28270

Methadone 83840

Methamphetamine
Blood or Urine 82145

Methanol 84600

Methemalbumin 83857

Methemoglobin 83045–83050

Methsuximide 83858

Metyrapone 80436

MIC
See Minimum Inhibitory Concentration

Microalbumin
Urine 82043–82044

Microbial Identification
with Nucleic Acid Probe 87178–87179

Microbiology
Unlisted Services and Procedures 87999

Microglobulin, Beta 2
Blood 82232
Urine 82232

Micrographic Surgery
Moh's Technique 17304–17310

Micro-Ophthalmia
Orbit Reconstruction 21256

Mucocele
Sinusotomy
    Frontal 31075

Mucopolysaccharides . 83864–83866

Mucormycosis
Antibody. 86732

Muller Procedure
See Sleep Study

**Multiple Sleep Latency Testing
(MSLT)** 95805

Multiple Valve Procedures
See Valvotomy; Valvuloplasty

Mumps
Antibody. 86735
Immunization 90704, 90707,
                    90709, 90710

Muramidase 85549

Murine Typhus 86000

Muscle
See also Specific Muscle
Biopsy. 20200–20206
Removal
    Foreign Body 20520–20525
Revision
    Arm, Upper. 24330, 24331
Transfer
    Arm, Upper. 24301, 24320
    Elbow 24301

Muscle Compartment Syndrome
Detection 20950

Muscle Division
Scalenus Anticus 21700–21705
Sternocleidomastoid. 21720–21725

Muscle Flaps 15732–15738

Muscle Grafts 15841–15842

Muscles
Repair
    Extraocular 65290

Muscle Testing
Dynamometry, Eye. 92260
Extraocular Multiple Muscles 92265
Manual 95831–95834

Muscle Transfer
Shoulder 23395–23397

Musculoskeletal System
Unlisted Services and
Procedures 20999, 21499

Musculotendinous (Rotator) Cuff
Repair 23410–23412

Mustard Procedure
See Repair, Great Arteries

Mustard Type 33774–33777

Mycobacteria
Culture 87116–87117
    Identification 87118

Mycoplasma
Antibody. 86738

Myelin Basic Protein
Cerebrospinal Fluid. 83873

Myelography
Anesthesia 01906–01910
Brain 70010
Spine
    Cervical 72240
    Lumbosacral 72265
    Thoracic 72255
    Total 72270

Myelomeningocele
Repair. 63704, 63706

Myelotomy 63170

Myocardial
Positron Emission Tomography (PET) . 78459

Myocardium
Repair
    Postinfarction. 33542

Myocutaneous Flaps. . . 15732–15738

Myofascial Release. 97250

Myoglobin 83874

Myomectomy. 58145
Anorectal 45108
Uterus. 58140

Myotomy
Esophagus 43030

Myringoplasty. 69620
See also Tympanoplasty

Myringotomy 69420–69421

N

Naffziger Operation
See Decompression, Orbit

Nagel Test
See Color Vision Examination

Nail Bed
Reconstruction. 11762
Repair. 11760

Nail Fold
Excision
    Wedge 11765

Nails
Avulsion 11730–11732
Biopsy. 11755

Debridement. 11700–11711
Evacuation
    Hematoma, Subungual. 11740
Excision. 11750–11752
    Cyst
        Pilonidal. 11770–11772
Removal. . . . 11730–11732, 11750–11752

Narcoanalysis 90835

Narcosynthesis
Diagnostic/Therapeutic 90835

Nasal Area
Bone Graft 21210

Nasal Bone
Fracture
    Closed Treatment 21310–21320
    Open Treatment 21325–21335
X-Ray 70160

Nasal Deformity
Repair 40700–40702, 40720, 40761

Nasal Function Study. 92512

Nasal Prosthesis 21087

Nasal Septum
Abscess
    Incision and Drainage 30020
Fracture
    Closed Treatment. 21337
    Open Treatment 21336
Hematoma
    Incision and Drainage 30020
Repair. 30680

Nasal Smear
Eosinophils. 89190

Nasal Turbinate
Fracture
    Therapeutic 30930

Nasoethmoid Complex
Fracture
    Open Treatment 21338–21339
    Percutaneous Treatment 21340
Reconstruction 21182–21184

Nasolacrimal Duct
Exploration 68820
    with Anesthesia. 68825
Insertion
    Stent. 68830
X-Ray
    with Contrast 70170

Nasomaxillary
Fracture
    Closed Treatment. 21345
    Open Treatment 21346–21348

Nasopharyngoscopy. 92511

Nasopharynx
See also Pharynx
Biopsy. 42804, 42806
Hemorrhage 42970–47072

Nodes
See Lymph Nodes

No Man's Land
Tendon Repair............26356–26358

Non-Invasive Vascular Imaging
See Duplex Scan; Vascular Studies

Non-Office Medical Services 99056

Non-Stress Test, Fetal.......59025

Noradrenalin
Blood..................82383–82384
Urine........................82384

Norepinephrine
See also Catecholamines
Blood..................82383–82384
Urine........................82384

Norwood Procedure
See Repair, Heart, Ventricle

Nose
Abscess
   Incision and Drainage....30000–30020
Anesthesia 00160–00164
Artery
   Incision..............30915–30920
Biopsy
   Intranasal...................30100
Dermoid Cyst
   Excision
     Complex 30125
     Simple....................30124
Displacement Therapy.............30210
Endoscopy
   Diagnostic............31231–31235
   Surgical.......31237–31294, 31254
Excision
   Rhinectomy...........30150–30160
Fracture
   Open Treatment 21338–21339
   Percutaneous Treatment 21340
Hematoma
   Incision and Drainage....30000–30020
Hemorrhage
   Cauterization 30901–30906
Insertion
   Septal Prosthesis..............30220
Intranasal
   Lesion
     External Approach............30118
     Internal Approach 30117
Lysis of Adhesions................30560
Polyp
   Excision
     Extensive...................30115
     Simple....................30110
Reconstruction
   Dermatoplasty 30620
   Primary.............30400–30420
   Secondary............30430–30462
   Septum.....................30520
Removal
   Foreign Body 30300

Anesthesia 30310
   Lateral Rhinotomy...........30320
Repair
   Adhesions...................30560
   Cleft Lip.............40700–40702,
               40720, 40761
   Fistula........30580–30600, 42260
   Rhinophyma 30120
   Septum 30540–30545, 30630
   Synechia....................30560
Skin
   Excision 30120
   Surgical Planing...............30120
Skin Graft
   Delay of Flap 15630
   Full Thickness..........15260–15261
   Pedicle Flap 15576
Submucous Resection Turbinate
   Excision 30130–30140
Tissue Transfer, Adjacent ...14060–14061
Turbinate
   Fracture 30930
   Injection....................30200
Turbinate Mucosa
   Cauterization 30801–30802
Unlisted Services and Procedures....30999

Nose Bleed
See Hemorrhage, Nasal

Notriptyline
Assay 80182

NTD
See Nitroblue Tetrazolium Dye Test

Nuclear Antigen
Antibody......................86235

Nuclear Imaging
See Nuclear Medicine

Nuclear Medicine.............78807
Abscess Localization 78805–78806
Adrenal Gland
   Imaging.....................78075
Automated Data..........78890–78891
Bile Duct
   Imaging.....................78223
Bladder
   Residual Study...............78730
Blood
   Flow Imaging 78445
   Iron
     Absorption..................78162
     Chelatable..................78172
     Plasma.....................78160
     Plasma Volume 78110–78111
     Platelet Survival 78190–78191
     Red Cells 78120–78121,
        78130–78135, 78140, 78170
     Unlisted Services and
     Procedures 78199
     Whole Blood Volume 78122
Bone
   Density Study..........78350–78351
   Imaging........78300–78315, 78320
   SPECT.....................78320

Unlisted Services and
   Procedures 78399
Bone Marrow
   Imaging..............78102–78104
Brain
   Blood Flow 78610–78615
   Cerebrospinal Fluid......78630–78650
   Imaging 78600–78607,
        78608–78609, 78610
Endocrine Glands
   Unlisted Services and
   Procedures 78099
Esophagus
   Imaging (Motility) 78258
   Reflux Study................78262
Gallbladder
   Imaging.....................78223
Gastric Mucosa
   Imaging.....................78261
Gastrointestinal
   Blood Loss Study.............78278
   Protein Loss Study............78282
   Shunt Testing................78291
   Unlisted Services and
   Procedures 78299
Genitourinary System
   Unlisted Services and
   Procedures 78799
Heart
   Blood Flow..................78414
   Blood Pool Imaging.....78472–78473,
             78481–78483
   Myocardial Imaging 78459,
             78466–78469
   Myocardial Perfusion ...78460–78465,
             78478–78480
   Shunt Test 78428
   Unlisted Services and
   Procedures 78499
Hepatic Duct
   Imaging.....................78223
Intestines
   Imaging.....................78290
Kidney
   Blood Flow..................78715
   Function Study 78725–78726
   Imaging.......78700–78707, 78710
   Transplant Evaluation...........78727
Lacrimal Gland
   Tear Flow 78660
Liver
   Function Study................78220
   Imaging.............78201–78216
Lung
   Imaging Perfusion.......78580–78585
   Imaging Ventilation 78586–78594
   Unlisted Services and
   Procedures 78599
Lymphatics 78195
   Unlisted Services and
   Procedures 78199
Lymph Nodes 78195
Musculoskeletal System
   Unlisted Services and
   Procedures 78399

O

Office Medical Services
After Hours 99050–99054
Emergency Care 99058
Normal Infant 90755
Normal Newborn 99432

Olecranon
See Elbow

Olecranon Bursa
Arthrocentesis 20605

Olecranon Process
Craterization 24147
Diaphysectomy 24147
Excision 24147
   Abscess 24138
Fracture
   Closed Treatment 24670–24675
   Open Treatment 24685
Osteomyelitis 24138, 24147
Saucerization 24147
Sequestrectomy 24138

Oligoclonal Immunoglobulin
Cerebrospinal Fluid 83916

Omentectomy . . . 49255, 58950–58952
Laparotomy 58960
Oophorectomy 58943
Resection Ovarian Malignancy 58950

Omentum
Excision 49255, 58950–58952
Flap 49905
Unlisted Services and Procedures 49999

Omphalectomy 49250

Omphalocele
Anesthesia 00754
Repair 49600, 49605–49606,
                    49610–49611

Omphalomesenteric Duct
Excision 44800

One Stage Prothrombin Time
See Prothrombin Time

Onychia
Drainage 10060–10061

Oocyte
Culture
   for In Vitro Fertilization 89250
Retrieval
   for In Vitro Fertilization 58970

Oophorectomy 56307,
         58262–58263, 58940, 58943
Ectopic Pregnancy
   Laparoscopic Treatment 59120
   Surgical Treatment 59120

Operculectomy 41821

Operculum
See Gums

Ophthalmic Mucous Membrane
Test 95060

Ophthalmology
See also Ophthalmology, Diagnostic
Unlisted Services and Procedures 92499

Ophthalmology, Diagnostic
Color Vision Exam 92283
Dark Adaptation 92284
Electromyography, Needle 92265
Electrooculography 92270
Electroretinography 92275
Eye Exam
   with Anesthesia 92018–92019
   Established Patient 92012–92014
   New Patient 92002–92004
Glaucoma Provocative Test 92140
Gonioscopy 92020
Ocular Photography
   External 92285
   Internal 92286–92287
Ophthalmoscopy 92225–92226
   with Angiography 92235
   with Angioscopy 92230
   with Dynamometry 92260
   with Fundus Photography 92250
Sensorimotor Exam 92060
Tonography 92120
   with Provocation 92130
Tonometry
   Serial 92100
Visual Field Exam 92081–92083

Ophthalmoscopy 92225–92226
Anesthesia 00148
with Dynamometry 92260
with Fundus Photography 92250

Opiates 83925

Optic Nerve
Decompression 67570
   with Nasal/Sinus Endoscopy 31294

Oral Lactose Tolerance Test
See Glucose, Tolerance Test

Oral Surgical Splint 21085

Orbit
See also Orbital Contents; Orbital Floor;
Periorbital Region
Biopsy 61332
   Exploration 67450
   Fine Needle Aspiration or Orbital
     Contents 67415
   Orbitotomy without Bone Flap . . . 67400
CAT Scan 70480, 70481, 70482
Decompression 61330
   Bone Removal 67414, 67445
Exploration 61332, 67400, 67450
Lesion
   Excision 61333
Fracture
   Closed Treatment
     with Manipulation 21401
     without Manipulation 21400
   Open Treatment 21406–21408
Incision and Drainage 67405, 67440

Injection
   Retrobulbar 67500–67505
   Tenon's Capsule 67515
Insertion
   Implant 67550
Lesion
   Excision 67412, 67420
Magnetic Resonance Imaging
(MRI) 70540
Removal
   of Bone, for
     Decompression 67414, 67445
   Exploration 61334
   Foreign Body 61334, 67413, 67430
   Implant 67560
Sella Turcica 70482
Unlisted Services and Procedures 67599
X-Ray 70190–70200

Orbital Contents
Aspiration 67415

Orbital Floor
See also Orbit; Periorbital Region
Fracture
   Blow Out 21385–21395

Orbital Hypertelorism
Osteotomy
   Periorbital 21260–21263

Orbital Implant
See also Ocular Implant
Insertion 67550
Removal 67560

Orbital Prosthesis 21077

Orbital Rim and Forehead
Reconstruction 21172–21175

Orbital Rims
Reconstruction 21182–21184

Orbital Transplant 67560

Orbital Walls
Reconstruction 21182–21184

Orbit Area
Reconstruction
   Secondary 21275

Orbitocraniofacial
Reconstruction 21275

Orbitotomy
with Bone Flap
   with Drainage 67440
   for Exploration 67450
   Lateral Approach 67420
   with Removal of Bone for
     Decompression 67445
   with Removal Foreign Body 67430
without Bone Flap
   with Drainage Only 67405
   for Exploration 67400
   with Removal Lesion 67412
with Removal of Bone for
   Decompression 67414
   with Removal Foreign Body 67413

Orbits
Skin Graft
   Split 15120–15121

Orbit Wall
Decompression
   with Nasal/Sinus
   Endoscopy 31292–31293

Orchiectomy
Anesthesia 00926–00928
Radical
   Abdominal Exploration 54535
   Inguinal Approach 54530
Simple 54520

Orchiopexy
Abdominal Approach 54650
Anesthesia 00930
Inguinal Approach 54640

Organ/Disease Panel
Arthritis Panel 80072
General Health Panel 80050
Hepatic Function Panel 80058
Hepatitis Panel 80059
Lipid Panel 80061
Obstetric Panel 80055
Thyroid Panel 80091–80092
Torch Antibody Panel 80090

Organ Donor
Life Support 01990

Organic Acids 83918

Oropharynx
Biopsy 42800

Orthodontic Cephalogram 70350

Orthopantogram 70355

Orthoptic Training 92065

Orthoroentgenogram 76040

Orthotics
Check-Out 97703
Training 97500–97501

Osmolality
Blood 83930
Urine 83935

Ossicles
Excision
   Stapes
     with Footplate Drill Out 69661
     without Foreign
     Material 69660–69661
Reconstruction
   Ossicular Chain
     Tympanoplasty with Antrotomy or
     Mastoidectomy 69636–69637
     Tympanoplasty with
     Mastoidectomy 69642, 69644, 69646
     Tympanoplasty without
     Mastoidectomy 69632–69633
Release
   Stapes 69650

Replacement
   with Prosthesis 69633, 69637

Ostectomy
Metacarpal 26250, 26255
Metatarsal 28288
Phalanges
   Finger 26260–26262
Pressure Ulcer
   Ischial 15941, 15945
   Sacral 15933, 15935, 15937
   Trochanteric 15951, 15953, 15958
Scapula 23190
Sternum 21620

Osteocalcin 83937

Osteocutaneous Flap
with Microvascular
Anastomosis 20969–20973

Osteoma
Sinusotomy
   Frontal 31075

Osteomyelitis 20000, 21510
Elbow
   Incision and Drainage 23935
Excision
   Clavicle 23180
   Facial 21026
   Humerus 23184
   Mandible 21025
   Scapula 23182
Humerus 24134
   Incision and Drainage 23935
Incision 23035
Olecranon Process 24138, 24147
Radius 24136, 24145
Sequestrectomy
   Clavicle 23170
   Humeral Head 23174
   Scapula 23172

Osteopathic Manipulation 98925–98929

Osteoplasty
Anesthesia 01484
Facial Bones
   Augmentation 21208
   Reduction 21209
Femur 27179
   Lengthening 27466, 27468
   Shortening 27465, 27468
Fibula
   Lengthening 27715
Humerus 24420
Metacarpal 26568
Phalanges, Finger 26568
Radius 25390–25393
Tibia
   Lengthening 27715
Ulna 25390–25393

Osteotomy
Anesthesia 01484, 01742
Calcaneus 28300

Chin 21121–21123
Clavicle 23480–23485
Femur 27140, 27151, 27156,
             27161, 27165, 27181,
             27448, 27450, 27454
Fibula 27707, 27709, 27712
with Graft
   Reconstruction
     Periorbital Region 21267–21268
Hip 27146–27147, 27151, 27156
   Femur 27151
Humerus 24400–24410
Mandible 21198
Maxilla 21206
Metacarpal 26565
Metatarsal 28306–28308, 28309
Orbit Reconstruction 21256
Pelvis 27158
Periorbital
   Orbital Hypertelorism 21260–21263
Phalanges
   Finger 26567
   Toe 28310, 28312
Radius 25350, 25355,
             25365, 25370, 25375
Skull Base 61582–61585, 61592
Talus 28302
Tarsal 28304–28305
Tibia 27455, 27457,
             27705, 27709, 27712
Ulna 25360, 25365, 25370, 25375
Vertebra
   Additional Segment
     Anterior Approach 22226
     Posterior/Posterolateral
     Approach 22216
   Cervical
     Anterior Approach 22220
     Posterior/Posterolateral
     Approach 22210
   Lumbar
     Anterior Approach 22224
     Posterior/Posterolateral
     Approach 22214
   Thoracic
     Anterior Approach 22222
     Posterior/Posterolateral
     Approach 22212

Otolaryngology
See Otorhinolaryngology, Diagnostic

Otolaryngology Examination . 92510

Otoplasty 69300

Otorhinolaryngology
Diagnostic
   Otolaryngology Exam 92502
Unlisted Services and Procedures 92599

Otoscopy
Anesthesia 00124

Ouchterlony Immunodiffusion 86331

Outpatient Visit
See Office and/or Other Outpatient Services

P

Removal
Calculi (Stone) 43264
Foreign Body 43269
Stent 43269
Sphincterotomy 43262
Sphincter Pressure 43263
Tube Placement 43267–43268
Incision
Sphincter 43262
Removal
Calculi (Stone) 43264
Foreign Body 43269
Stent 43269
Tube Placement
Nasopancreatic 43267
Stent 43268
Tumor
Destruction 43272
X-Ray with Contrast
Guide Catheter 74329–74330

Pancreaticojejunostomy 48180

Pancreatography 48400
Intraoperative 74300–74301
Postoperative 74305

Pancreatorrhaphy 48530

Pancreozymin-Secretin Test . 82938

Panniculectomy
Anesthesia 00802

Papillectomy 46220

Papilloma
Destruction 54050, 54065

Pap Smear 88150–88155

Paracentesis 49080
Eye
Anterior Chamber
with Diagnostic Aspiration of
Aqueous 65800
with Removal of Blood 65815
with Removal Vitreous and/or
Discission of Anterior Hyaloid
Membrane 65810
with Therapeutic Release of
Aqueous 65805

Paracervical Nerve
Injection
Anesthetic 64435

Paraffin Bath Therapy 97018

Parasites
Blood 87207
Smear 87177

Parathormone 83970

**Parathyroid
Autotransplantation** 60512

Parathyroidectomy 60500–60505

Parathyroid Gland
Autotransplant 60512

Excision 60500–60502
Exploration 60500–60505
Nuclear Medicine
Imaging 78070

Parathyroid Hormone 83970

Paraurethral Gland
Abscess
Incision and Drainage 53060

Paravertebral Nerve
Destruction 64622–64623
Injection
Anesthetic 64440–64443
Neurolytic 64622–64623

Parietal Cell Antibody . 83255–83256

Parietal Craniotomy 61556

Paring
Skin Lesion
Benign Hyperkeratotic . . . 11050–11052

Paronychia
Incision and Drainage 10060–10061

Parotid Duct
Diversion 42507–42510
Reconstruction 42507–42510

Parotid Gland
Abscess
Incision and Drainage 42300, 42305
Calculi (Stone)
Excision 42330, 42340
Excision
Partial 42410, 42415
Total 42420, 42425–42426
Tumor
Excision 42410, 42415,
42420, 42425–42426

Partial
Lung
Partial 32225

Partial Thromboplastin Time
See Thromboplastin, Partial, Time

**Particle
Agglutination** 86403, 86406

Parvovirus
Antibody 86747

Patch
Allergy Tests 95044

Patella
See also Knee
Anesthesia 01390–01392
Dislocation 27560, 27562
Excision 27350
Fracture 27520, 27524
Reconstruction 27437–27438
Repair
Instability 27420, 27422, 27424

**Patellar Tendon Bearing (PTB)
Cast** 29435

Paternity Testing 86910

Patey's Operation
See Mastectomy, Radical

Pathology
Clinical
Consultation 80500–80502
Surgical 88355
Consultation 88321–88325
Intraoperative 88329–88332
Decalcification Procedure 88311
Electron Microscopy 88348–88349
Histochemistry 88318–88319
Immunocytochemistry 88342
Immunofluorescent
Study 88346–88347
Morphometry
Nerve 88356
Skeletal Muscle 88355
Tumor 88358
Nerve Teasing 88362
Special Stain 88312–88314
Staining 88312–88314
Tissue Hybridization 88365
Unlisted Services and
Procedures 88399, 89399

Patient
Dialysis Training,
Completed Course 90989

Patterson's Test
See Blood Urea Nitrogen

Paul-Bunnell Test
See Antibody

PCP
See Phencyclidine

Peak Flow Rate 94160

Peans' Operation
See Amputation, Leg, Upper, at Hip

Pectus Carinatum
Reconstructive Repair 21740

Pectus Excavatum
Anesthesia 00474
Reconstructive Repair 21740

Pedicle Fixation
Insertion 22842–22844

Pedicle Flap
Formation 15570–15576
Island 15740
Neurovascular 15750
Transfer 15650

Peet Operation
See Nerve, Sympathetic, Excision

Pelvic Exam 57410

Pelvic Exenteration 51597
Anesthesia 00848

Pelvic Fixation
Insertion 22848

Perineorrhaphy
Repair
    Rectocele 57250

Perineum
Abscess
    Incision and Drainage 56405
Anesthesia 00900–00908
Removal
    Prosthesis. 53442
Repair. 56810
X-Ray with Contrast. 74775

Periorbital Region
Reconstruction
    Osteotomy with Graft. . . . 21267–21268

Periprosthetic Capsulotomy
Breast 19370–19371

Peritoneal Dialysis 90945–90947

Peritoneal Lavage 49080

Peritoneocentesis 49080–49081

Peritoneoscopy
Biopsy. 56361, 56363
Exploration 56360
Unlisted Services and Procedures. . . . 56399
with X-Ray 56362

Peritoneum
Abscess
    Incision and Drainage 49020
Chemotherapy Administration 96445
Endoscopy
    Biopsy. 56361, 56363
    Exploration 56360
    X-Ray 56362
Ligation
    Shunt 49428
Removal
    Cannula/Catheter. 49422
    Foreign Body 49085
    Shunt 49429
Unlisted Services and Procedures. . . . 49999
Venous Shunt 49427
X-Ray 74190

Pertussis Immunization 90701,
          90711, 90720–90721, 90742

Pessary
Insertion 57160

Pesticides
Chlorinated Hydrocarbons 82441

PET
See Positron Emission Tomography (PET)

Petrous Temporal
Excision
    Apex. 69530

Peyronie Disease
with Graft 54110–54112
Injection 54200
Surgical Exposure. 54205

pH
See also Blood; pH
Other Fluid 83986
Urine. 83986

Phacoemulsification
Removal
    Extracapsular Cataract. 66984
    Secondary Membranous
    Cataract 66850

Phagocytosis
White Blood Cells 86344

Phalanx
Craterization 26235–26236
Cyst
    Excision 26210, 26215
Diaphysectomy 26235–26236
Excision. 26235–26236
Fracture
    Articular 26740, 26742, 26746
    Distal . . . 26750, 26755–26756, 26765
    Open Treatment 26735, 26765
    Shaft. 26735
Saucerization 26235–26236
Thumb
    Fracture
      Shaft 26720, 26725, 26727
Tumor
    Excision 26210, 26215

Phalanx, Finger
Excision. 26260–26262
Fracture
    Shaft 26720, 26725, 26727
Incision and Drainage 26034
Ostectomy. 26260–26262
Repair
    Lengthening 26568
    Osteotomy 26567

Phalanx, Great Toe
See also Phalanx, Toes
Fracture. 28490
    without Manipulation. . . . 28495–28496
    Open Treatment 28505
without Manipulation 28490

Phalanx, Toes
Condyle
    Excision 28126
Craterization 28124
Cyst
    Excision 28108
Diaphysectomy. 28124
Excision. . . . 28124, 28150, 28153, 28160
Fracture
    without Manipulation. . . . 28510, 28515
    Open Treatment 28515
Repair
    Osteotomy 28310, 28312
Saucerization 28124
Tumor
    Excision 28108, 28175

Pharyngectomy
Partial. 42890

Pharyngo-
laryngectomy 31390–31395

Pharyngoplasty 42950

Pharyngostomy 42955

Pharynx
See also Nasopharynx; Throat
Anesthesia 00174–00176
Biopsy 42800, 42802, 42804, 42806
Cineradiography 70371, 74230
Creation
    Stoma. 42955
Excision 42145
    with Larynx. 31390
    Partial. 42890
    with Pharynx 31395
    Resection 42892, 42894
Hemorrhage 42960–42962
Lesion
    Destruction. 42808
    Excision 42808, 42880
Reconstruction 42950
Repair
    with Esophagus 42953
Unlisted Services and Procedures. . . . 42999
Video Study 70371, 74230
X-Ray 70370, 74210

Phencyclidine. 83992

Phenobarbital. 82205–82210
Assay 80184

Phenothiazine 84022

Phenylalanine 84030

Phenylalanine-Tyrosine
Ratio 84030

Phenylketones. 84035

Phenytoin
Assay 80185–80186

Pheochromocytoma 80424

Phleborrhaphy
Anesthesia 01782, 01852

Phlebotomy
Therapeutic. 99195–99199

Phonocardiogram
Evaluation . . 93201, 93204–93205, 93209
Intracardiac. 93210
Tracing 93202, 93208

Phosphatase
Alkaline. 84075, 84080
    Blood 84078
Forensic Examination. 84061

Phosphatase Acid 84060
Blood 84066

Phosphatidylglycerol 84081

Phosphogluconate-6
Dehydrogenase. 84085

Phosphohexose Isomerase . . . 84087

Retropubic..........55831, 55840, 55842, 55845	
Suprapubic.................55821	
Transurethral....52601, 52612–52630	
Exploration	
Exposure.................55860	
with Nodes..........55862, 55865	
Incision	
Exposure......55860, 55862, 55865	
Transurethral.............52450	
Insertion	
Radioactive Substance.........55860	
Needle Biopsy................55700	
Ultrasound...................76872	
Unlisted Services and Procedures....55899	
Urinary System.............53899	
Urethra	
Transurethral Balloon Dilation....52510	
Vaporization	
Laser....................52648	

Prostatectomy...............52601
Anesthesia...............00865, 00908
Perineal
    Partial......................55801
    Radical.......55810, 55812, 55815
Retropubic
    Partial......................55831
    Radical.......55840, 55842, 55845
Suprapubic
    Partial......................55821
Transurethral..............52612–52630

Prostate Specific Antigen..............84153, 86316

Prostatotomy.........55720, 55725

Prosthesis
Augmentation
    Mandibular Body..............21125
Auricular.......................21086
Breast
    Insertion.............19340–19342
    Removal.............19328–19330
    Supply....................19396
Check-Out......................97703
Cornea.........................65770
Facial.........................21088
Hernia
    Mesh......................49568
Hip
    Removal.............27090–27091
Lens
    Insertion.............66983–66985
    not Associated with Concurrent Cataract
    Removal....................66985
    Manual or Mechanical
    Technique..................66984
Mandibular Resection............21081
Nasal..........................21087
Nasal Septum
    Insertion..................30220
Obturator......................21076
    Definitive.................21080
    Interim...................21079

Ocular
    Fitting and Prescription.........92330
    Loan......................92358
    Prescription...............92335
    Supply....................92393
Orbital........................21077
Ossicle
    Total Orbit Partial.............69637
Ossicle Reconstruction
    Chain.....................69633
Palatal Augmentation.............21082
Palatal Lift...................21083
Palate.....................42280–42281
Penile
    Insertion............54400, 54405
    Removal............54402, 54407
    Repair....................54409
Perineum
    Removal...................53442
Skull Plate
    Removal...................62142
    Replacement...............62143
Spectacle
    Fitting.............92352–92353
    Repair....................92371
Speech Aid.....................21084
Spinal
    Insertion..................22851
Synthetic......................69633
Temporomandibular Joint
    Arthroplasty................21243
Testicular
    Insertion..................54660
Training...................97520–97521
Urethral Sphincter
    Removal...................53447
Wrist
    Removal.............25250–25251

Protein
Glycated.......................82985
Osteocalcin....................83937
Serum.....................84160–84165
Total..........................84155
Western Blot..............84181–84182

Protein Analysis, Tissue
Western Blot..............88370–88371

Protein C Actiator..........85337

Protein C Antigen...........85302

Protein C Assay............85303

Protein S
Assay..........................85306
Total..........................85305

Prothrombin...............85210

Prothrombin Time.....85610–85612

Prothrombokinase..........85230

Protoporphyrin.......84202–84203

Protozoa
Antibody.......................86753

Provocation Test
for Allergies...................95078
for Glaucoma...................92140

Provocation Tonography......92103

PSA
See Prostate Specific Antigen

Psoriasis Treatment
See Photochemotherapy

Psychiatric Diagnosis
Evaluation of Records, Reports,
    Tests......................90825
Interview and Evaluation....90801, 90820
Narcosynthesis.................90835
Psychological Testing............96100
Unlisted Services and Procedures....90899

Psychiatric Treatment
Consultation with Family..........90887
Drug Management...............90862
Electroconvulsive Therapy...90870–90871
Environmental Intervention........90882
Hypnotherapy...................90880
Narcosynthesis/Analysis..........90835
Psychoanalysis
    Medical...................90845
Psychotherapy
    Family...............90846–90849
    Group...............90853, 90857
    Individual......90841–90844, 90855
Report Preparation...............90889
Residential
    Facility Care..........99301–99303, 99311–99313
Unlisted Services and Procedures....90899

Psychoanalysis
Medical........................90845

Psychotherapy
Family...............90846–90849
Group................90853, 90857
Individual........90841–90844, 90855

PTA...........................85270

PTA (Factor XI)
See Clotting Factor

PTCA
See Percutaneous Transluminal Angioplasty

PTC Factor..................85250

Pterygium
Excision.......................65420

Pterygomaxillary Fossa
Incision.......................31040

Pubic Symphysis.............27282

Pubis
Craterization.............27070–27171
Cyst
    Excision..............27065–27067
Excision..................27070–27171
Saucerization.............27070–27171

Q

R

Septum. 30520
Orbital Rims 21182–21184
Orbital Walls. 21182–21184
Orbit Area
　　Secondary 21275
Orbitocraniofacial
　　Secondary Revision 21275
Oviduct
　　Fimbrioplasty 58760
Palate
　　Cleft Palate. 42200–42225
　　Lengthening 42226–42227
Parotid Duct
　　Diversion. 42507–42510
Patella. 27437–27438
　　Instability 27420, 27422, 27424
Penis
　　Angulation 54360
　　Chordee 54300, 54304
　　Complications. 54340–54348
　　Epispadias 54380–54390
　　Hypospadias. 54332, 54352
　　　One Stage Distal with
　　　Urethroplasty. 54328
　　　One Stage Perineal. 54336
Periorbital Region
　　Osteotomy with Graft. . . . 21267–21268
Pharynx. 42950
Pyloric Sphincter 43800
Radius 24365, 25390–25393, 25441
　　Arthroplasty
　　　with Implant 24366
Scaphoid. 25443
Shoulder Joint
　　with Implant 23470–23472
Skull 61555
　　Defect 62140–62141, 62145
Sternum 21740
Stomach
　　with Duodenum. 43810,
　　　　　　　　　　　　43850, 43855
　　Gastric Bypass. 43846
　　with Jejunum 43820, 43825,
　　　　　　　　　　　　43860, 43865
　　for Obesity 43846–43848
　　Roux-En-Y. 43846
Superior-Lateral Orbital Rim and
Forehead. 21172–21175
Supraorbital Rim and
Forehead. 21179–21180
Symblepharon. 68335
Temporomandibular Joint
　　Arthroplasty 21240–21243
Throat. 42950
Thumb
　　from Finger. 26550
　　Opponensplasty. 26296, 26490,
　　　　　　　　　26492, 26494, 26496
　　from Toe. 26552
Tibia
　　Lengthening 27715
　　Tubercle 27418
Toe
　　Angle Deformity. 28313
　　Extra. 28344

Hammertoe. 28285–28286
Macrodactyly 28340–28341
Supernumerary. 26587
Syndactyly 28345
Webbed Toe. 28345
Tongue
　　Frenum 41520
Trachea. 31750
　　Carina. 31766
　　Fistula. 31755
　　Graft Repair 31770
　　Intrathoracic. 31760
Trapezium 25445
Tympanic Membrane 69620
Ulna. 25390–25393, 25442
　　Radioulnar 25337
Ureter 50700
　　with Intestines 50840
Urethra. 53410–53440,
　　　　　　　53440, 53443–53445
　　Complications. 54340–54348
　　Hypospadias. 54308
　　　One Stage Distal with Meatal
　　　Advancement 54322
　　　One Stage Distal with
　　　Urethroplasty . 54324, 54326, 54328
　　　Urethroplasty for Second
　　　Stage. 54312, 54316
　　　Urethroplasty for Third Stage. . . 54318
　　Meatus 53450–53460
　　Suture to Bladder 51840, 51841
Uterus. 58540
Vena Cava. 34502
Wound Repair. 13100–13300
Wrist. 25330–25332
　　Capsulectomy. 25320
　　Capsulorrhaphy 25320
　　Realign 25335
Zygomatic Arch 21255

Rectal Sphincter
Dilation. 45910

Rectocele
Repair. 45560

Rectum
See also Anus
Abscess
　　Incision and Drainage . . . 45005, 45020,
　　　　　　　　　　　46040, 46060
Biopsy. 45100
Dilation
　　Endoscopy 45303
Endoscopy
　　Destruction
　　　Tumor 45320
　　Dilation. 45303
　　Exploration 45300
　　Hemorrhage 45317
　　Removal
　　　Foreign Body. 45307
　　　Polyp 45308–45309, 45315
　　　Tumor 45308–45309, 45315
　　Volvulus 45321

Excision
　　Partial 45111, 45113,
　　　　　　　　45114, 45116, 45123
　　Total 45110, 45112, 45120
　　with Colon 45121
Exploration
　　Endoscopic. 45300
Hemorrhage
　　Endoscopic. 45317
Injection
　　Sclerosing Solution 45520
Lesion
　　Excision 45108
Manometry. 91122
Prolapse
　　Excision 45130, 45135
Removal
　　Fecal Impaction 45915
　　Foreign Body 45307, 45915
Repair
　　Fistula 45800, 45805,
　　　　　　　　　　　45820, 45825
　　Injury. 45562–45563
　　Prolapse. 45505, 45520,
　　　　　　　　45540–45541, 45900
　　Rectocele. 45560
　　with Sigmoid Excision. 45550
　　Stenosis 45500
Stricture
　　Excision 45150
Suture
　　Fistula 45800, 45805,
　　　　　　　　　　　45820, 45825
　　Prolapse 45540–45541
Tumor
　　Destruction 45190, 45320,
　　　　　　　　　　　46937–46938
　　Excision 45160, 45170
Unlisted Services and Procedures. . . . 45999

Red Blood Cell (RBC)
Antibody. 86850–86870
　　Pretreatment. 86970–86972
Count 85041
Fragility. 85547, 85555–85557
　　Mechanical. 85547
　　Osmotic 85555–85557
Hematocrit 85014
Iron Utilization 78170
Sedimentation Rate
　　Automated 85652
　　Manual. 85651
Sequestration. 78140
Sickling. 85660
Survival Test. 78130–78135
Volume Determination 78120–78121

Reduction
Forehead. 21137–21139
Mammoplasty. 19318
Masseter Muscle/Bone 21295–21296
Osteoplasty
　　Facial Bones. 21209
Skull
　　Craniomegalic. 62115–62117

Talus
Osteotomy 28302
Tarsal 28320
Osteotomy 28304–28305
Testis
Injury 54670
Suspension 54620, 54640
Torsion 54600
Throat 42953
Wound 42900
Thumb
Muscle 26508
Tendon 26510
Tibia 27720, 27722,
27724–27725
Epiphysis 27477, 27479,
27485, 27730,
27734, 27740, 27742
Osteotomy 27455, 27457,
27705, 27709, 27712
Pseudoarthrosis 27727
Toes
Bifid Toe 26585
Bunion 28290, 28292–28294,
28296–28299
Macrodactylia 26590
Muscle 28240
Supernumerary 26587
Tendon 28240
Webbing 28280, 28345
Tongue 41250–41252
Fixation 41500
Laceration 41250–41252
Mechanical 41500
Suture 41510
Trachea
Fistula 31755, 31825
with Plastic Repair 31825
without Plastic Repair 31820
Stenosis 31780, 31781
Stoma 31613–31614, 31825
with Plastic Repair 31825
without Plastic Repair 31820
Scar 31830
Wound
Cervical 31800
Intrathoracic 31805
Tricuspid Valve 33460,
33463–33465, 33468
Truncus Arteriosus 33786, 33788
Tunica Vaginalis
Hydrocele 55060
Tympanic Membrane 69450, 69610
Ulna 25400, 25415
Epiphyseal 25450, 25455
with Graft 25405, 25420,
25425–25426
Osteotomy 25360, 25370, 25375
Umbilicus
Omphalocele 49600,
49605–49606, 49610–49611
Ureter
Anastomosis 50740–50825
Continent Diversion 50825
Deligation 50940

Fistula 50920–50930
Lysis Adhesions 50715–50725
Suture 50900, 50940
Urinary Undiversion 50830
Ureterocele 51535
Urethra
Artificial Sphincter 43449
Diverticulum 53240, 53400–53405
Fistula 45820, 45825,
53400–53405, 53520
Stoma 53520
Stricture 53400–53405
Urethrocele 57230
Wound 53502–53515
Urethral Sphincter 57220
Urinary Incontinence 53440,
53443–53445, 57284
Uterus
Fistula 51920–51925
Rupture 58520, 59350
Suspension 58400, 58410
Presacral Sympathectomy 58410
Vagina
Cystocele 57240, 57260
Enterocele 57265
Fistula 46715–46716, 51900
Rectovaginal . . 57300, 57305, 57307
Urethrovaginal 57310–57311
Vesicovaginal 57320, 57330
Hysterectomy 58267
Incontinence 57284, 57288
Pereyra Procedure 57289
Postpartum 59300
Prolapse 57282, 57284
Rectocele 57250, 57260
Suspension 57280, 57284
Wound 57200, 57210
Vas Deferens
Suture 55400
Vein
Angioplasty 35460, 35476, 75978
Femoral 34501
Graft 34520
Pulmonary 33730
Transposition 34510
Vulva
Postpartum 59300
Wound
Complex 13100–13300
Intermediate 12031–12057
Simple 12001–12021
Wound Dehiscence
Complex 13160
Simple 12020–12021
Wrist 25260, 25263,
25265, 25270,
25272, 25274, 25447
Bone 25440
Cartilage 25107
Removal
Implant 25449
Tendon 25280, 25290,
25295, 25300–25301,
25310, 25312, 25315–25316
Total Replacement 25446

Replacement
Ankle
Anesthesia 01486
Aortic Valve 33405–33406,
33411–33413
Cerebrospinal Fluid Shunt 62194,
62225, 62230
Contact Lens 92326
Elbow
Anesthesia 01760
Electrode
Heart 33211, 33217
Gastrostomy Tube 43760
Hearing Aid
Bone Conduction 69710
Heart
Pacemaker 33240
Hip 27130, 27132
Anesthesia 01214
Revision 27134, 27137–27138
Knee
Anesthesia 01402
Mitral Valve 33430
Nerve 64726
Ossicles
with Prosthesis 69633, 69637
Pacemaker 33206, 33208
Catheter 33210
Electrode 33210, 33216
Heart 33247, 33249
Prosthesis
Skull 62143
Pulmonary Valve 33475
Skull Plate 62143
Tissue Expanders 11970
Tricuspid Valve 33465
Ureter
with Intestines 50840
Wrist
Anesthesia 01832

Replantation
Arm, Upper 20802
Digits 20816–20822
Foot 20838
Forearm 20805
Hand 20808
Thumb 20824–20827

Report Preparation
Extended, Medical 99080
Psychiatric 90889

Repositioning
Electrode
Heart 33216, 33217
Gastrostomy Tube 43761
Intraocular Lens 66825
Tricuspid Valve 33468

Reptilase Test 85635

Resection
Bladder 52340
Bladder Diverticulum 52305
Humeral Head 23195

Rotavirus
Antibody........................86759

Round Window
Repair Fistula...................69667

Roux-En-Y............47741, 47785

Roux-En-Y Procedure........43621,
43633–43634, 43846,
47740, 47780, 48540

RPR..........................86592

Rubella
Antibody........................86762

Rubella HI Test
See Hemagglutination Inhibition Test

Rubella Immunization.90706–90710

Rubeola
Antibody........................86765

Russell Viper Venom
Time...................85612–85613

S

Saccomanno Technique......88108
See also Cytopathology, Fluids, Washings,
Brushings

Sacroiliac Joint
Anesthesia......................01160
Arthrodesis.....................27280
Arthrotomy......................27050
Biopsy..........................27050
Dislocation
    Open Treatment..............27218
Fusion..........................27280
X-Ray...................72200–72202

Sacrum
Pressure Ulcer..........15931–15937
Tumor
    Excision....................49215
X-Ray...........................72220

Sahli Test....................91055
See also Stomach, Intubation with Specimen
Prep

Salabrasion...........15810–15811

Salicylate
Assay...........................80196

Saline Load Test.............91060

Salivary Duct
Catheterization.................42660
Dilation.................42650, 42660
Ligation........................42665
Repair..................42500, 42505
    Fistula.....................42600

Salivary Glands
Abscess
    Incision and Drainage....42310, 42320
Anesthesia......................00100
Biopsy..........................42405
Calculi (Stone)
    Excision........42330, 42335, 42340
Cyst
    Creation
        Fistula.........42325–42326
    Drainage....................42409
    Excision....................42408
Injection
    X-Ray.......................42550
Needle Biopsy...................42400
Nuclear Medicine
    Function Study..............78232
    Imaging..............78230–78231
Parotid
    Abscess.............42300, 42305
Unlisted Services and Procedures....42699
X-Ray...................70380–70390
    with Contrast...............70390

Salmonella
Antibody........................86768

Salpingectomy..............56307,
58262–58263, 58700
Ectopic Pregnancy
    Laparoscopic Treatment.........59151
    Surgical Treatment.............59120
Oophorectomy....................58943

Salpingolysis................58740

Salpingoneostomy.....56343, 58770

Salpingo-Oophorectomy......58720
Resection Ovarian Malignancy......58950

Salpingostomy........56343, 58770
Laparoscopic....................56343

Sampling
See Biopsy

Sang-Park Procedure........33739
See also Septectomy, Atrial

Saucerization
Calcaneus.......................28120
Clavicle........................23180
Femoral.........................27360
Femur...................27070–27171
Fibula..........................27360
Hip.....................27070–27171
Humerus.........................24140
Ileum...................27070–27171
Metacarpal......................26230
Metatarsal......................28122
Olecranon Process...............24147
Phalanges
    Finger..............26235–26236
    Toe.....................28124
Pubis...................27070–27171
Radius..........................24145
Talus...........................28120
Tarsal..........................28122

Tibia............27360, 27640–27641
Ulna....................25150–25151

Saundby Test
See Blood, Feces

Scalenus Anticus
Division.................21700–21705

Scalp
Skin Graft
    Delay of Flap...............15610
    Full Thickness........15220–15221
    Pedicle Flap................15572
    Split.................15100–15101
Tissue Transfer, Adjacent...14020–14021
Tumor Resection
    Radical.....................21015

Scalp Blood Sampling........59030

Scanogram...................76040

Scaphoid
Arthroplasty
    with Implant................25443
Fracture..........25622, 25624, 25628
Repair..........................25440

Scapula
Anesthesia......................00450
Craterization...................23182
Cyst
    Excision....................23140
        with Allograft.........23146
        with Autograft.........23145
Diaphysectomy...................23182
Excision
    Partial.....................23182
Fracture
    Closed Treatment
        with Manipulation......23575
        without Manipulation...23570
    Open Treatment..............23585
Ostectomy.......................23190
Repair
    Scapulopexy.................23400
Saucerization...................23182
Tumor
    Excision....................23140
        with Allograft.........23146
        with Autograft.........23145
    Radical Resection..........23210
X-Ray...........................73010

Scapulopexy..................23400

Schauta Operation
See Hysterectomy, Vaginal, Radical

Schede Procedure.....32905–32906
See also Thoracoplasty

Scheie Procedure
See Iridectomy

Schilling Test...............78270
See also Vitamin, B12, Absorption Study

Schlicter Test...............87197
See also Bactericidal Titer, Serum

Serum
Antibody Identification
    Pretreatment 86975–86978

Serum Globulin
Immunization 90741

Sesamoid Bone
Excision 28315
Fracture 28530–28531

Sever Procedure
See Contracture, Palm, Release

Sex Change Operation
Female to Male 55980
Male to Female 55970

Sex Chromatin
Identification 88130, 88140

Sex Hormone Binding
Globulin 84270

SGOT 84450
See also Aspartate Aminotransferase

SGPT 84460
See also Alanine Aminotransferase

Shaving
Skin Lesion 11300–11313

SHBG
See Sex Hormone Binding Globulin

Shelf Procedure
See Osteotomy, Hip

Shigella
Antibody 86771

Shirodkar Operation
See Repair, Cervix, Cerclage

Shock Wave Lithotripsy 50590

Shoulder
See also Clavicle; Scapula
Abscess
    Drainage 23030
Amputation 23900–23921
Anesthesia 00450–00454,
                        01600–01682
Arthrocentesis 20610
Arthrodesis 23800
    with Autogenous Graft 23802
Arthrography
    Injection 23350
Arthroplasty
    with Implant 23470–23472
Arthroscopy
    Diagnostic 29815
    Surgical 29819–29823,
                       29825–29826
Arthrotomy
    with Biopsy 23100–23101
    with Synovectomy 23105–23106
Biopsy
    Deep 23066
    Soft Tissue 23065

Bone
    Incision 23035
Bursa
    Drainage 23031
Capsular Contracture Release 23020
Cast
    Figure Eight 29049
    Removal 29710
    Spica 29055
    Velpeau 29058
Dislocation
    Closed Treatment
      with Manipulation 23650–23655
    with Greater Tuberosity Fracture
      Closed Treatment 23665
      Open Treatment 23670
    Open Treatment 23660
    with Surgical or Anatomical Neck
    Fracture
      Closed Treatment with
      Manipulation 23675
      Open Treatment 23680
Excision
    Acromion 23130
    Torn Cartilage 23101
Exploration 23040–23044, 23107
Hematoma
    Drainage 23030
Incision and Drainage 23040–23044
Joint
    X-Ray 73050
Manipulation
    Application of Fixation
    Apparatus 23700
Prophylactic Treatment 23490–23491
Radical Resection 23077
Removal
    Calcareous Deposits 23000
    Cast 29710
    Foreign Body 23040–23044
      Complicated 23332
      Deep 23331
      Subcutaneous 23330
    Foreign or Loose Body 23107
Repair
    Capsule 23450–23466
    Ligament Release 23415
    Muscle Transfer 23395–23397
    Rotator Cuff 23420
    Tendon 23410–23412,
                   23430–23440
    Tenomyotomy 23405–23406
Strapping 29240
Tumor
    Excision 23075–23077
Unlisted Services and Procedures 23929
X-Ray 73020–73030
X-Ray with Contrast 73040

Shoulder Girdle
Anesthesia 00400–00474

Shunt
Aqueous
    to Extraocular Reservoir 66180
      Revision 66185

Brain
    Creation 62180–62223
    Removal 62256, 62258
    Replacement 62194, 62225,
                    62230, 62258
Creation
    Arteriovenous
      Direct 36821
      ECMO 36822
      with Graft 36825, 36830
      Thomas Shunt 36835
      Thomas Shunt 36835
    Great Vessel
      Aorta
        Pulmonary 33924
      Aortic Pulmonary Artery . 33755, 33762
      Central 33764
      Subclavian Pulmonary Artery 33750
      Vena Cava to Pulmonary
      Artery 33766–33767
    Intraatrial 33735–33739
    Nonvascular
      X-Ray 75809
    Peritoneal
      Venous
        Injection 49427
        Ligation 49428
        Removal 49429
        X-Ray 75809
    Revision
      Arteriovenous 36832
    Spinal Cord
      Creation 63740–63741
      Irrigation 63744
      Removal 63746
      Replacement 63744
    Spinal Fluid
      Anesthesia 00220
    Ureter to Colon 50815

Shuntogram 75809

Sialic Acid 84275

Sialodochoplasty 42500, 42505

Sialography 70390

Sickling
Electrophoresis 83020

Siderocytes 85535

Sigmoid Bladder
Cystectomy 51590

Sigmoidoscopy
Ablation
    Polyp 45339
    Tumor 45339
Biopsy 45331
Collection
    Specimen 45331
Exploration 45330
Hemorrhage Control 45334
Removal
    Foreign Body 45332
    Polyp 45333, 45338
    Tumor 45333, 45338

Manipulation
Anesthesia 22505
Myelography
Cervical 72240
Lumbosacral 72265
Thoracic 72255
Total 72270
Standing X-Ray 72069
Ultrasound 76880
Unlisted Services and Procedures 22899
X-Ray 72020, 72090
Cervical 72040–72052
with Contrast
Cervical 72240
Lumbosacral 72265
Thoracic 72255
Total 72270
Lumbosacral 72100–72120
Thoracic 72070–72074
Thoracolumbar 72080
Total 72010

Spine Chemotherapy
Administration 96450

Spirometry 94010–94070

Spleen
Excision 38100–38102
Injection
Radiologic 38200
Nuclear Medicine
Imaging 78185, 78215–78216
Repair 38115

Splenectomy 38115
Partial 38101
Total 38100, 38102

Splenoportography 75810
Injection Procedures 38115

Splenorrhaphy 38115

Splint
See also Cast; Strapping
Arm
Long 29105
Short 29125–29126
Finger 29130–29131
Foot 29590
Leg
Long 29505
Short 29515
Oral Surgical 21085

Split Grafts 15100–15121

Split Renal Function Test
See Cystourethroscopy, Catheterization,
Ureteral

Splitting
Blood Products 86985

Sprengel's Deformity 23400

Sputum Analysis 89350

Ssabanejew-Frank Operation
See Incision, Stomach, Creation, Stoma

Stable Factor 85230

Stallard Procedure
See Conjunctivorhinostomy

Stamey Procedure 51845
See also Repair, Bladder, Neck

Standby Services
Physician 99360

Stanford-Binet Test
See Psychiatric Diagnosis

Stapedectomy
with Footplate Drill Out 69661
without Foreign Material 69660
Revision 69662

Stapedotomy
with Footplate Drill Out 69661
without Foreign Material 69660
Revision 69662

Stapes
Excision
with Footplate Drill Out 69661
without Foreign Material 69660
Release 69650
Revision 69662

Staphyloma
Sclera
Repair
with Graft 66225
without Graft 66220

Starch Granules
Feces 89355

State Operation
See Proctectomy

Steindler Stripping 28250

Stellate Ganglion
Injection
Anesthetic 64510

Stem Cell
Harvesting 38231
Transplantation 38240–38241

Stenger Test 92565, 92577
See also Audiologic Function Tests, Stenger

Stenosis
Bronchi 31641
Reconstruction 31775
Excision
Trachea 31781
Laryngoplasty 31582
Reconstruction
Auditory Canal, External 69310
Repair
Trachea 31780

Stent
Indwelling
Insertion
Ureter 50605

Placement
Bronchoscopy 31631

Stereotactic Frame
Application/Removal 20660

Stereotaxis
Aspiration
Brain Lesion 61750
with Cat Scan 61751
Spinal Cord 63615
Biopsy
Aspiration
Brain Lesion 61750
Brain 61750
with Cat Scan 61751
Breast 76095
Spinal Cord 63615
Cat Scan
Aspiration 61751
Biopsy 61751
Computer Assisted
Brain Surgery 61795
Creation Lesion
Brain
Deep 61720, 61735
Percutaneous 61790
Gasserian Ganglion 61790
Spinal Cord 63600
Trigeminal Tract 61791
Excision Lesion
Spinal Cord 63615
Focus Beam
Radiosurgery 61793
Localization
Brain 61770
Radiation Therapy 77432
Stimulation
Spinal Cord 63610

Sternoclavicular Joint
Anesthesia 01620, 01630–01638
Arthrotomy 23044
with Biopsy 23101
with Synovectomy 23106
Dislocation
Closed Treatment
with Manipulation 23525
without Manipulation 23520
Open Treatment 23530–23532
with Fascial Graft 23532

Sternocleidomastoid
Division 21720–21725

Sternotomy
Closure 21750

Sternum
Debridement 21627
Excision 21620, 21630
Fracture
Closed Treatment 21820
Open Treatment 21825
Ostectomy 21620
Radical Resection 21630–21632
X-Ray 71120–71130

Submaxillary Gland
Abscess
    Incision and Drainage.... 42310, 42320

Submental Fat Pad
Excision
    Excess Skin 15838

Subperiosteal Implant
Reconstruction
    Mandible 21245–21246
    Maxilla 21245–21246

Sucrose Hemolysis Test
See Red Blood Cell (RBC), Fragility, Osmotic

Sugars 84375

Sugiura Procedure
See Esophagus, Repair, Varices

Sulfate
Urine......................... 84392

Superficial Musculoaponeurotic System (SMAS) Flap
Rhytidectomy 15829

Supernumerary Digit
Reconstruction 26587
Repair......................... 26587

Supply
Chemotherapeutic Agent 96545
Contact Lenses........... 92391, 92396
Educational Materials 99071
Low Vision Aids................. 92392
Materials 99070
Ocular Prosthesis................ 92393
Prosthesis
    Breast..................... 19396
Radionuclide................... 78990
Radionuclide Therapy 79900
Radiopharmaceutical
Therapy................. 78990, 79900
Spectacle Prosthesis 92395
Spectacles 92390

Suppression 80400

Suppression/Testing
See Evocative/Suppression Test

Suprahyoid 38700

Supraorbital Nerve
Avulsion 64732
Incision....................... 64732
Transection.................... 64732

Supraorbital Rim and Forehead
Reconstruction 21179–21180

Suprascapular Nerve
Injection
    Anesthetic 64418

Surgical Planing
Nose
    Skin 30120

Surgical Services
Post-Op Visit 99024

Suspension
Aorta........................ 33800

Suture
See also Repair
Abdomen 49900
Aorta................... 33320–33321
Bile Duct
    Wound 47900
Bladder
    Fistulization........... 44660–44661,
        45800, 45805, 51880, 51900
    Vesicouterine........ 51920–51925
    Vesicovaginal 51920
    Wound 51860–51865
Cervix 57720
Colon
    Diverticula 44604–44605
    Fistula........ 44650, 44660–44661
    Plication 44680
    Stoma.............. 44620, 44625
    Ulcer 44604–44605
    Wound 44604–44605
Esophagus
    Wound 43410, 43415
Eyelid 67880
    Closure of.................. 67875
    with Transposition of Tarsal
    Plate...................... 67882
    Wound
        Full Thickness 67935
        Partial Thickness 67930
Facial Nerve
    Intratemporal
        Lateral to Geniculate Ganglion . 69740
        Medial to Geniculate Ganglion . 69745
Foot
    Tendon 28210
Gastroesophageal................. 43405
Great Vessel 33320–33321
Hemorrhoids........... 46945–46946
Intestines
    Large
        Diverticula.................. 44604
        Ulcer 44604
        Wound.................... 44604
    Small
        Diverticula 44602–44603, 44605
        Fistula........... 44640, 44650,
            44660–44661
        Plication 44680
        Stoma 44620, 44625
        Ulcer........ 44602–44603, 44605
        Wound...... 44602–44603, 44605
Iris
    with Ciliary Body 66682
Kidney
    Fistula............... 50520–50526
    Horseshoe 50540
    Wound 50500
Leg, Upper
    Muscle 27385–27386
Liver
    Wound 47350, 47360, 47361
Mesentery 44850
Nerve 64831–64876

Pancreas....................... 48530
Rectum
    Fistula.............. 45800–45825
    Prolapse 45540–45541
Removal
    Anesthesia 15850–15851
Stomach
    Fistula.................... 43880
    Laceration............. 43501, 43502
    Stoma.................... 43870
    Ulcer 43501, 43840
    Wound 43840
Tendon
    Foot.......... 28200, 28202, 28208
    Knee 27380–27381
Testis
    Injury 54670
    Suspension............ 54620–54640
Thoracic Duct.................... 38380
    Abdominal Approach 38382
    Thoracic Approach............ 38381
Throat
    Wound 42900
Tongue
    to Lip 41510
Trachea
    Fistula.................... 31825
        with Plastic Repair........... 31825
        without Plastic Repair 31820
    Stoma..................... 31825
        with Plastic Repair........... 31825
        without Plastic Repair 31820
    Wound
        Cervical................... 31800
        Intrathoracic 31805
Ulcer.................... 44604–44605
Ureter 50900, 50940
    Fistula.............. 50920–50930
Urethra
    to Bladder............. 51840–51841
    Fistula........ 45820, 45825, 53520
    Stoma..................... 53520
    Wound 53502–53515
Uterus
    Fistula............... 51920–51925
    Rupture.............. 58520, 59350
    Suspension............ 58400–58410
Vagina
    Cystocele 57240, 57260
    Enterocele 57265
    Fistula.................... 51900
        Rectovaginal .. 57300, 57305, 57307
        Urethrovaginal........ 57310–57311
        Vesicovaginal......... 57320, 57330
    Rectocele 57250, 57260
    Suspension.................. 57280
    Wound 57200, 57210
Vas Deferens 55400
Vein
    Femoral.................... 37650
    Iliac...................... 37660
    Vena Cava 37620
Wound 44604–44605

Swallowing Evaluation 92525–92526

Telangiectasia
Chromosome Analysis 88248
Injection 36468

Telephone
Case Management Services . 99371–99373
Pacemaker Analysis 93733, 93736
Transmission of ECG 93012

Teletherapy
Dose Plan 77305–77321

Temperature Gradient Studies .
93740

Temporal, Petrous
Excision
    Apex 69530

Temporal Bone
Electromagnetic Bone Conduction Hearing Device
    Implantation/Replacement 69710
    Removal/Repair 69711
Excision 69535
Resection 69535
Tumor
    Removal 69970
Unlisted Services and Procedures 69979

Temporomandibular Joint (TMJ)
Arthrocentesis 20605
Arthrography 70328–70332
    Injection 21116
Arthroplasty 21240–21243
Arthroscopy 29800, 29804
Arthrotomy 21010
Condylectomy 21050
Coronoidectomy 21070
Dislocation
    Closed Treatment 21480–21485
    Open Treatment 21490
Magnetic Resonance Imaging (MRI) . 70336
Meniscectomy 21060
X-Ray with Contrast 70328–70332

Tenago Procedure 53443

Tendon
Arm, Upper
    Revision 24320
Finger
    Excision 26180
Graft
    Harvesting 20924
Insertion
    Biceps Tendon 24342
Lengthening
    Arm, Lower 25280
    Arm, Upper 24305
    Elbow 24305
    Finger 26476, 26478
    Hand 26476, 26478
    Leg, Upper 27393–27395
    Toe 28240
    Wrist 25280
Palm
    Excision 26170

Release
    Arm, Lower 25295
    Wrist 25295
Shortening
    Finger 26477, 26479
    Hand 26477, 26479
Transfer
    Arm, Lower 25310, 25312, 25316
    Arm, Upper 24301
    Elbow 24301
    Finger 26497, 26498
    Hand . . . 26480, 26483, 26485, 26489
    Leg, Lower 27690–27692
    Leg, Upper 27400
    Pelvis 27098
    Thumb 26490, 26492, 26510
    Wrist 25310, 25312, 25316

Tendon Sheath
Finger
    Incision 26055
    Incision and Drainage 26020
    Lesion 26160
Foot
    Excision 28086, 28088
Hand
    Lesion 26160
    Injection 20250
Palm
    Incision and Drainage 26020
Removal
    Foreign Body 20520
Wrist
    Excision 25115–25116
    Incision 25000

Tennis Elbow
Repair 24350–24356

Tenodesis
Anesthesia 01716
Biceps Tendon
    at Elbow 24340
    Shoulder 23430
Finger 26471, 26474
Wrist 25300–25301

Tenolysis
Ankle 27680–27681
Arm, Lower 25295
Finger 26440, 26442, 26445, 26449
Foot 28220, 28222, 28225–28226
Hand 26440, 26442, 26445, 26449
Leg, Lower 27680–27681
Wrist 25295

Tenomyotomy 23405–23406

Tenon's Capsule
Injection 67515

Tenoplasty
Anesthesia 01712

Tenotomy
Achilles Tendon 27605–27606
Anesthesia 01712
Ankle 27605–27606

Arm, Lower 25290
Arm, Upper 24310
Finger 26060, 26455, 26460
Foot 28230, 28234
Hand 26450, 26460
Hip
    Iliopsoas Tendon 27005
Hip/Adductor 27000–27001,
                    27003, 27006
Leg, Upper . 27306–27307, 27390–27392
Toe 28010–28011,
           28232, 28234, 28240
Wrist 25290

TENS
See Application, Neurostimulation

Tensilon Test 95857–95858

Tentorium Cerebelli
Section 61440

Terman Test 96100

Testimony, Medical 99075

Testing
Neuropsychological 96117

Testing, Neurophysiologic 95920

Testis
Abscess
    Incision and Drainage 54700
Anesthesia 00924–00930
Biopsy 54505
Excision
    Radical 54530, 54535
    Simple 54520
Hematoma
    Incision and Drainage 54700
Insertion
    Prosthesis 54660
Lesion
    Excision 54510
Needle Biopsy 54500
Nuclear Medicine
    Imaging 78760–78761
Repair
    Injury 54670
    Suspension 54620, 54640
    Torsion 54600
Suture
    Suspension 54620, 54640
Transplantation
    to Thigh 54680
Tumor
    Excision 54530, 54535
Undescended
    Anesthesia 00924
    Exploration 54550, 54560
Unlisted Services and Procedures 55899

Testosterone 84402
Response 80414
    Stimulation 80414–80415
Total 84403

Tetanus 86280
Antibody 86774

Replacement 11970
Grafts
Harvesting 20926
Hybridization In Situ 88365
Preparation
Drug Analysis. 80103
Soft
Abscess 20000–20005

Tissue Transfer
Adjacent
Arms. 14020–14021
Axillae. 14040–14041
Cheeks 14040–14041
Chin 14040–14041
Ears. 14060–14061
Eyelids 14060–14061, 67961
Face 14040–14061
Feet. 14040–14041
Finger 14350
Forehead. 14040–14041
Genitalia 14040–14041
Hand 14040–14041
Legs 14020–14021
Limbs 14020–14021
Lips 14060–14061
Mouth 14040–14041
Neck 14040–14041
Nose 14060–14061
Scalp. 14020–14021
Trunk. 14000–14001
Unusual/Complicated 14300
Facial Muscles 15845
Finger Flap 14350
Toe Flap 14350

Tissue Typing
HLA Antibodies 86812–86817
Lymphocyte Culture 86821–86822

TLC Screen 84375
See also Sugars

TMJ
See Temporomandibular Joint (TMJ)

Tobramycin 84810
Assay 80200

Tocolysis 59412
External Cephalic Version 59412

Tocopherol 84446

Toe Flap
Tissue Transfer. 14350

Toes
See also Interphalangeal Joint, Toe;
Metatarsophalangeal Joint
See also Phalanx
Amputation 28810, 28820, 28825
Arthrocentesis 20600
Capsulotomy. 28270, 28272
Dislocation
See Specific Joint
Lesion
Excision 28092
Magnetic Resonance Imaging (MRI). . 73721

Reconstruction
Angle Deformity. 28313
Extra Digit 26587
Extra Toes 28344
Hammer Toe 28285–28286
Macrodactyly 28340–28341
Syndactyly 28345
Webbed Toe 28345
Repair. 26590
Bifid Toe 26585
Bunion 28290, 28292–28294,
28296–28299
Extra Digit 26587
Muscle 28240
Tendon 28232, 28234, 28240
Webbed 28280, 28345
Reposition. 26557–26559
Strapping 29550
Tenotomy. 28010–28011,
28232, 28234
Unlisted Services and Procedures. . . . 28899
X-Ray 73660

Tolbutamide Tolerance Test. . . 82953

Tolerance Test
Glucagon. 82946
Glucose 82951–82952
With Tolbutamide. 82953
Heparin-Protamine 85530
Insulin 80434–80435
Maltose. 82951–82952
Tolbutamide 82953

Tomographic SPECT
Myocardial Imaging 78469

Tompkins Metroplasty
See Uterus, Reconstruction

Tongue
Abscess
Incision and Drainage. 41000,
41005–41006, 41015
Biopsy. 41100, 41105
Cyst
Incision and Drainage. 41000,
41005–41006, 41015, 60000
Excision
Complete 41140, 41145,
41150, 41153, 41155
Frenum 41115
with Mouth Resection . . . 41150, 41153
Partial 41120, 41130, 41135
with Radical Neck. 41135, 41145,
41153, 41155
Fixation. 41500
Hematoma
Incision and Drainage. 41000,
41005–41006, 41015
Incision
Frenum 41010
Lesion
Excision 41110, 41112–41114
Reconstruction
Frenum 41520

Repair
Laceration. 41250–41252
Suture. 41510
Suture. 41510
Unlisted Services and Procedures. . . . 41599

Tonography 92120
with Provocation 92130

Tonometry, Serial 92100

Tonsillectomy 42820–42821,
42825–42826

Tonsils
Abscess
Incision and Drainage 42700
Excision. 42825–42826
with Adenoids 42820–42821
Lingual 42870
Radical 42842, 42844–42845
Tab 42860
Lingual
Destruction. 42870
Unlisted Services and Procedures. . . . 42999

TORCH Antibody Panel 80090

Torek Procedure
See Orchiopexy

Torkildsen Procedure 62180
See also Ventriculocisternostomy

**TORP (Total Ossicular Replacement
Prosthesis)** 69633, 69637
See also Prosthesis

Torsion Swing Test 92546

Torus Mandibularis
Tumor Excision. 21031

Total Catecholamines
See Catecholamines, Urine

Touroff Operation
See Ligation, Artery, Neck

Toxicology Screen 80100–80103

Toxin Assay. 87230

Toxoplasma
Antibody 86777–86778

Trabeculectomy Ab Externo
in Absence of Previous Surgery. 66170
with Scarring Previous Surgery. 66172

Trabeculoplasty
by Laser Surgery 65855

Trabeculotomy Ab Externo
Eye 65850

Trachea
Anesthesia 00320, 00542
Aspiration. 31720
Catheter 31720–31725
Catheterization. 31700
Dilation. 31630–31631

Renal
  Allotransplantation............50360
    with Recipient Nephrectomy ...50365
    Autotransplantation............50380
    Donor Nephrectomy.....50300–50320
    Recipient Nephrectomy........50340
    Removal Transplanted Renal
    Allograft....................50370
  Stem Cells........38231, 38240–38241
Testis
  to Thigh....................54680

Transposition
Arteries
  Carotid..............35637, 35691,
                        35694–35695
  Subclavian.....35638, 35693–35695
  Vertebral.............35637–35638,
                        35691, 35693
Cranial Nerve...................64716
Eye Muscles.....................67320
Great Arteries
  Repair..33770–33771, 33774–33781
Nerve.....................64718–64721
Ovary..........................58825
Vein Valve......................34510

Trans-Scaphoperilunar
Fracture/Dislocation........25680, 25685

Transureteroureterostomy....50770

Transurethral Balloon Dilation
Prostatic Urethra.................52510

Transurethral Fulguration
Postoperative Bleeding............52606

Transurethral Procedure
See also Specific Procedure
Anesthesia...............00910–00918
Prostate
  Incision.....................52450

Trapezium
Arthroplasty
  with Implant..................25445

Travel, Unusual..............99082

Treacher-Collins Syndrome
Midface Reconstruction.....21150–21151

Trendelenburg Operation
See Pulmonary Artery, Embolism; Varicose
Vein, Removal, Secondary Varicosity; Vein,
Ligation, Saphenous

Trephine Procedure
Sinusotomy
  Frontal.....................31070

Treponema Pallidum
Antibody.......................86781

TRH
See Thyrotropin Releasing Hormone (TRH)

Trichiasis
Repair.........................67825
  Epilation, by Forceps.........67820

Epilation, by Other than Forceps .67825
Incision of Lid Margin.........67830
  with Free Mucous Membrane
  Graft......................67835

Trichinella
Antibody.......................86784

Trichrome Stain..............88312

Tricuspid Valve
Excision................33460, 33465
Repair.....33460, 33463–33465, 33468
Replacement....................33465
Repositioning..................33468

Trigeminal Nerve
Destruction........64600, 64605, 64610
Injection
  Anesthetic...................64400
  Neurolytic............64600–64610

Trigeminal Tract
Stereotactic
  Create Lesion................61791

Trigger Finger Repair.........26055

Trigger Point Injection.......20250

Triglycerides.................84478

Trigonocephaly...............21175

Triiodothyronine
Free...................84479, 84481
Resin Uptake...................84479
Reverse........................84482
Total..........................84480
True...........................84480

Trisegmentectomy............47122

Trocar Biopsy
Bone Marrow....................85102

Trochanter
Pressure Ulcer...........15950–15958

Truncus Arteriosus
Repair..................33786, 33788

Trunk
Lipectomy, Suction Assisted........15877
Skin Graft
  Delay of Flap................15600
  Full Thickness...............15200
  Muscle, Myocutaneous, or
  Fasciocutaneous Flaps.........15734
  Split.................15100–15101
Tissue Transfer, Adjacent...14000–14001

Trypanosomiasis.......86171, 86280

Trypsin
Duodenum......................84485
Feces..................84488–84490

TSH
See Thyroid Stimulating Hormone

TT-3
See Triiodothyronine, True

TT-4
See Thyroxine, True

Tubal Ligation................58600
  with Cesarean Section.........58611
Laparoscopic...................56301
Postpartum.....................58605

Tubal Pregnancy.............59121
  with Salpingectomy and/or
  Oophorectomy.................59120

Tube Change
Tracheotomy....................31502

Tubed Pedicle Flap
Formation...............15570–15576

Tube Placement
Gastrostomy Tube...............43750

Tubercle Bacilli
Culture.................87116–87117

Tuberculosis
Culture.................87116–87117
Skin Test...............86580–86585

Tuberculosis Vaccine (BCG) ..90728

Tudor 'Rabbit Ear'
See Urethra, Repair

Tuffier Vaginal Hysterectomy
See Hysterectomy, Vaginal

Tumor
See also Lesion
Abdomen
  Destruction/Excision....49200–49201
Abdominal Wall
  Excision.....................22900
Acetabulum
  Excision.....................27076
Ankle.........27615, 27618–27619
Arm, Lower..............25075–25077
Arm, Upper
  Excision..............24075–24077
Back/Flank
  Excision.....................21930
  Radical Resection............21935
Bile Duct
  Destruction..................43272
  Extrahepatic..........47711–47712
Bladder..........51530, 52234–52240
  Anesthesia...................00912
Brain..........................61510
  Excision......61518, 61520–61521,
                 61526, 61530, 61545
Breast
  Excision.....................19120
Bronchi
  Excision..............31640–31641
Calcaneus........28100, 28102–28103
  Excision.....................27647
Carpal.......25130, 25135–25136
Chest Wall
  Excision..............19260–19272
Clavicle.......................23140
  with Allograft...............23146

Tympanoplasty

See also Myringoplasty

with Antrotomy and Mastoidectomy	69635
with Ossicular Chain Reconstruction	69636
and Synthetic Prosthesis	69637
with Mastoidectomy	69641
with Intact or Reconstructed Wall	69643
and Ossicular Chain Reconstruction	69644
with Ossicular Chain Reconstruction	69642
without Mastoidectomy	69631
with Ossicular Chain Reconstruction	69632
and Synthetic Prosthesis	69633
Radical or Complete	69645
with Ossicular Chain Reconstruction	69646

Tympanostomy 69433, 69436

Tympanotomy
Anesthesia 00126

Typhoid Vaccine 90714

Tyrosine 84510

Tzank Smear 87207
See also Inclusion Bodies, Smear

U

Uchida Procedure
See Tubal Ligation

UFR
See Uroflowmetry

Ulcer
Pinch Graft	15050
Pressure	15920–15999
Stomach Excision	43610

Ulcer, Decubitus
See Pressure Ulcer (Decubitus)

Ulna
See also Arm, Lower; Elbow; Radius

Arthroplasty with Implant	25442
Craterization	25150–25151
Cyst Excision	25120, 25125–25126
Diaphysectomy	25150–25151
Excision Abscess	24138
Complete	25240
Partial	25145, 25150–25151, 25240

Fracture	25605
Closed Treatment	25530, 25535, 25650
with Dislocation Closed Treatment	24620
Open Treatment	24635
with Manipulation	25535
without Manipulation	25530
Open Treatment	24685, 25545, 25574
with Radius	25560, 25565, 25575
Shaft	25530, 25535, 25545, 25574
Styloid Process	25650
Incision and Drainage	25035
Osteoplasty	25390–25393
Prophylactic Treatment	25491–25492
Reconstruction Radioulnar	25337
Repair	25400, 25415
Epiphyseal Arrest	25450, 25455
with Graft	25405, 25420, 25425–25426
Osteotomy	25360, 25365, 25370, 25375
Saucerization	25150–25151
Sequestrectomy	25145
Tumor Excision	25120, 25125–25126, 25170

Ulnar Nerve
Decompression	64718
Neuroplasty	64718–64719
Reconstruction	64718–64719
Release	64718–64719
Repair/Suture Motor	64836
Transposition	64718–64719

Ultrasonic Procedure 52325

Ultrasound
See also Echocardiography; Echography

Abdomen	76700–76705
Arm	76880
Breast	76645
Chest	76604
Drainage	75989
Eye	76511–76513, 76529
Arteries	93875
Biometry	75616–75619
Fetus	76818
Follow-up	76970
Gastrointestinal	76975
Gastrointestinal, Upper	43259
Guidance Amniocentesis	76946
Arteriovenous Fistulae	76936
Aspiration	76938
Chorionic Villus Sampling	76945
Heart Biopsy	76932
Needle Biopsy	76942
Ova Retrieval	76948
Pericardiocentesis	76930
Pseudoaneurysm	76936
Radiation Prescription	76950–76960

Radioelement	76965
Thoracentesis	76934
Head	76506, 76536
Heart Fetal	76825–76828
Intraoperative	76986
Kidney	76778
Leg	76880
Neck	76536
Pelvis	76856–76857
for Physical Therapy	97035
Pregnant Uterus	76805–76816
Prostate	76872
Retroperitoneal	76770–76775
Scrotum	76870
Spine	76880
Unlisted Services and Procedures	76999
Vagina	76830

Ultraviolet A Therapy 96912

Ultraviolet B Therapy 96910

Ultraviolet Light Therapy
for Dermatology	96900
for Physical Medicine	97028

Umbilectomy 49250

Umbilicus
Excision	49250
Repair Hernia	49580–49587
Omphalocele	49600, 49605–49606, 49610–49611

Unlisted Services and Procedures .
	99499
Abdomen	22999, 49999
Allergy/Immunology	95199
Anal	46999
Anesthesia	01999
Ankle	27899
Arm	25999
Arm, Upper	24999
Arthroscopy	29909
Autopsy	88099
Bile Duct	47999
Brachytherapy	77799
Breast	19499
Bronchi	31899
Cardiac	33999
Cardiovascular Studies	93799
Cervix	58999
Chemistry Procedure	84999
Chemotherapy	96549
Chest	32999
Colon	44799
Conjunctiva Surgery	68399
Craniofacial	21299
Cytogenetic Study	88299
Cytopathology	88199
Dermatology	96999
Dialysis	90999
Diaphragm	39599
Ear External	69399
Inner	69949

Temperature Gradient. 93740
Thermogram
    Cephalic. 93760
    Peripheral. 93762
Unlisted Services and Procedures. . . . 93799
Venous Studies
    Extremity 93965–93971
    Venous Pressure. 93770
Visceral Studies 93975–93979

Vascular Surgery
Abdomen
    Anesthesia 00770, 00880–00884
Arm, Lower
    Anesthesia 01840–01852
Arm, Upper
    Anesthesia 01770–01782
Brain
    Anesthesia 00216
Central Venous Circulation
    Anesthesia 00532
Elbow
    Anesthesia 01770–01782
Hand
    Anesthesia 01840–01852
Heart
    Anesthesia 01921
Knee
    Anesthesia 01430–01444
Leg, Lower
    Anesthesia 01500–01522
Leg, Upper
    Anesthesia 01260–01274
Neck
    Anesthesia 00350–00352
Shoulder
    Anesthesia 01650–01670
Unlisted Services and Procedures. . . . 37799
Wrist
    Anesthesia 01840–01852

Vas Deferens
Anastomosis
    to Epididymis 54900–54901
Excision 55250
Incision. 55200
    for X-Ray 55300
Ligation. 55450
Repair
    Suture. 55400
Unlisted Services and Procedures. . . . 55899
Vasography. 74440
X-Ray with Contrast. 74440

Vasectomy. 55250
Contact Laser Vaporization with/without
Transurethral Resection
    of Prostate 52648
Non-Contact Laser Coagulation of
Prostate 52647
Transurethral Electrosurgical Resection of
Prostate. 52601, 52647–52648

Vasoactive Drugs
Injection 54231

Vasoactive Intestinal Peptide .
                                     84586

Vasography. 74440

Vasopneumatic Device Therapy .
                                     97016

Vasopressin 84588

Vasotomy 55200, 55250, 55300

Vasovasorrhaphy 55400

Vasovasostomy. 55400

VATS
See Thoracoscopy

VCG
See Vectorcardiogram

VDRL 86593

Vectorcardiogram
Evaluation. 93220, 93222
Tracing 93221

Vein
Adrenal
    Venography. 75840–75842
Anastomosis
    Caval to Mesenteric. 37160
    Portocaval 37140
    Reniportal. 37145
    Vein. 34530, 37180–37181
    to Vein. 37140, 37145, 37160
Angioplasty. 75978
    Transluminal. 35460
Arm
    Venography. 75820–75822
Axillary
    Thrombectomy 34490
Biopsy
    Transcatheter 75970
Cannulization
    to Artery. 36810–36815
    to Vein 36800
Catheterization
    Cutdown. 36490–36491
    Organ Blood 36500
    Percutaneous 36488–36489
    Umbilical 36510
Femoral
    Repair. 34501
Femoropopliteal
    Thrombectomy 34421, 34451
Hepatic Portal
    Splenoportography. 75810
    Venography. 75885–75887
Iliac
    Thrombectomy . . 34401, 34421, 34451
Injection
    Sclerosing Agent 36468–36471
Insertion
    IVC Filter 75940
Interrupt
    Femoral. 37650
    Iliac. 37660

Vena Cava 37620
Jugular
    Venography. 75860
Leg
    Venography. 75820–75822
Ligation
    Esophagus 43205
    Jugular 37565
    Perforation 37760
    Saphenous. 37700, 37720,
                    37730, 37735, 37780
    Secondary 37785
Liver
    Venography. 75889–75891
Neck
    Venography. 75860
Nuclear Medicine
    Thrombosis Imaging. 78455–78458
Orbit
    Venography. 75880
Placement
    IVC Filter 75940
Portal
    Catheterization. 36481
Pulmonary
    Repair. 33730
Removal
    Saphenous. 37720, 37730,
                     37735, 37780
    Secondary 37785
Renal
    Venography. 75831–75833
Repair
    Aneurysm. 36834
    Angioplasty 75978
    Graft. 34520
Sampling
    Venography. 75893
Sinus
    Venography. 75870
Skull
    Venography. 75870–75872
Spermatic
    Excision 55530
    Ligation. 56320
Splenic
    Splenoportography. 75810
Stripping
    Saphenous 37720, 37730, 37735
Subclavian
    Thrombectomy 34471, 34490
Unlisted Services and Procedures. . . . 37799
Valve Transposition 34510
Vena Cava
    Thrombectomy . . 34401, 34421, 34451
    Venography. 75825–75827

Velpeau Cast 29058

Vena Cava
Reconstruction. 34502
Resection with Reconstruction 37799

Vena Caval
Thrombectomy. 50230

with Focal Endolaser
Photocoagulation 67039
Pars Plana Approach 67036
Subtotal 67010

Vitreous
Aspiration 67015
Excision
    with Epiretinal Membrane
    Stripping 67038
    with Focal Endolaser
    Photocoagulation 67039
    Pars Planta Approach 67036
Incision
    Strands 67030–67031
Injection
    Fluid Substitute 67025
    Pharmacologic Agent 67028
Removal
    Anterior Approach 67005
    Subtotal 67010
Strands
    Discission 67030
    Severing 67031
Subtotal 67010

Vitreous Humor
Anesthesia 00145

VLDL
See Lipoprotein, Blood

Vocal Cords
Injection
    Endoscopy 31513
    Therapeutic 31570–31571

Voice Button 31611
See also Speech Prosthesis, Creation

Voiding Pressure Studies
Abdominal 51797
Bladder 51795

Volatiles 84600

Volhard's Test
See Water Load Test

Volkman Contracture . . 25315–25316

Von Kraske Proctectomy
See Proctectomy, Partial

VP
See Voiding Pressure Studies

Vulva
Abscess
    Incision and Drainage 56405
Anesthesia 00906
Excision
    Complete 56625, 56632–56634
    Partial 56620, 56632
    Radical 56630–56631, 56640
Lesion
    Destruction 56501, 56515
Perineum
    Biopsy 56605–56606

Incision and Drainage 56405
Radical
    Complete 56634, 56637, 56640
    Partial 56630–56632
Repair
    Obstetric 59300
Simple
    Complete 56625
    Partial 56620

Vulvectomy
Anesthesia 00906
Complete 56625, 56632–56634
Partial 56620, 56632
Radical 56630–56631, 56640
Complete
    with Bilateral Inguinofemoral
    Lymphadenectomy 56637
    with Inguinofemoral, Iliac, and Pelvic
    Lymphadenectomy 56640
    with Unilateral Inguinofemoral
    Lymphadenectomy 56634
Partial
    with Bilateral Inguinofemoral
    Lymphadenectomy 56632
    with Unilateral Inguinofemoral
    Lymphadenectomy 56631
Simple
    Complete 56625
    Partial 56620
Tricuspid Valve 33460, 33465

V-Y Plasty
See Skin, Adjacent Tissue Transfer

W

WADA Activation Test 95958

WAIS-R 96100
See also Psychiatric Diagnosis

Waldius Procedure 27445
See also Arthroplasty, Knee, Implantation

**Walsh Modified Radical
Prostatectomy**
See Prostatectomy

Warts
Flat
    Destruction 17110

Washing
Sperm 58323

Wasserman Test
See Syphilis Test

Wassmund Procedure
Osteotomy
    Maxilla 21206

Water Load Test 89365

Waterson Procedure
See Shunt, Great Vessel

Waterston Procedure 33755

Watson-Jones Procedure 27698
See also Repair, Ankle, Ligament

WBC
See White Blood Cell

Wedge Excision
Osteotomy 21122

Wedge Resection
Ovary 58920

Well-Baby Care 90757,
99391, 99432

Wertheim Operation
See Hysterectomy, Radical

Westergren Test
See Sedimentation Rate, Blood Cell

Western Blot
HIV 86689
Protein 84181–84182
Tissue Analysis 88370–88371

**Wheelchair Management/
Propulsion**
Training 97542

Wheeler Knife Procedure
See Discission, Cataract

Wheeler Procedure
See also Blepharoplasty, Entropion
Blepharoplasty 67924
Discission Secondary Membranous
Cataract 66820

Whipple Procedure 48150
See also Excision, Pancreas, Partial

Whirlpool Therapy 97022

White Blood Cell
Alkaline Phosphatase 85540
Antibody 86021
Count 85048
Histamine Release Test 86343
Phagocytosis 86344

White Blood Cell Count
with Alkaline Phosphatase 85540
Differential 85007, 85009

Whitemead Operation
See Hemorrhoidectomy, Complex

Whitman Astragalectomy
See Talus, Excision

Whitman Procedure 27120
See also Acetabulum, Reconstruction

Wick Catheter Technique 20950

Widal Serum Test
See Agglutinin, Febrile

X